Medical neurotoxicology

Medical neurotoxicology

Occupational and environmental causes of neurological dysfunction

Edited by

PETER G BLAIN BMedSci, MBBS, PhD, FiBiol, FFOM, FRCP (Lond), FRCP (Edin)

Professor of Environmental Medicine, University of
Newcastle upon Tyne, Department of Environmental and Occupational
Medicine, The Medical School, Newcastle upon Tyne, UK

JOHN B HARRIS BPharm, PhD, MRPharmS, FiBiol

Professor of Experimental Neurology, School of Neurosciences
and Psychiatry, The Medical School, Newcastle upon Tyne, UK

A member of the Hodder Headline Group
LONDON • SYDNEY • AUCKLAND
Co-published in the United States of America by
Oxford University Press Inc., New York

First published in Great Britain in 1999 by
Arnold, a member of the Hodder Headline Group,
338 Euston Road, London NW1 3BH

http://www.arnoldpublishers.com

Co-published in the United States of America by
Oxford University Press Inc.,
198 Madison Avenue, New York, NY 10016
Oxford is a registered trademark of Oxford University Press

British Library Cataloguing in Publication Data
A catalogue record for this book is available from the British Library

Library of Congress Cataloging-in-Publication Data
A catalog record for this book is available from the Library of Congress

ISBN 0 340 59665 1

1   2   3   4   5   6   7   8   9   10

Commissioning Editor: Georgina Bentliff
Project Editor: Catherine Barnes
Project Manager: Lesley Gray
Production Editor: Liz Gooster
Production Controller: Sarah Kett

Produced and typeset by Gray Publishing, Tunbridge Wells, Kent
Printed and bound in Great Britain by The Bath Press, Bath

Contents

Colour plates appear between pages 116 and 117

Contributors

Sandra L Allen BSc, PhD, CBiol, MIBiol
Neurotoxicologist/Study Reviewer, Zeneca Central Toxicology Laboratory, Macclesfield, Cheshire, UK

David Bates MA, MB, Bchir, FRCP
Consultant Neurologist and Senior Lecturer in Neurology, The Royal Victoria Infirmary and Associated Hospitals NHS Trust, Newcastle upon Tyne, UK

John P Birchall MD, FRCS
Professor of Otorhinolaryngology, Nottingham University Hospital, Nottingham, UK

Peter G Blain BMedSci, MBBS, PhD, FiBiol, FFOM, FRCP (Lond), FRCP (Edin)
Professor of Environmental Medicine, University of Newcastle upon Tyne, Department of Environmental and Occupational Medicine, The Medical School, Newcastle upon Tyne, UK

Walter G Bradley DM, FRCP
Professor and Chairman of Neurology, University of Miami School of Medicine, Jackson Memorial Hospital, and Miami VA Medical Center, Miami, Florida, USA

Niall EF Cartlidge MBBS, FRCP
Consultant Neurologist and Senior Lecturer in Neurology, University of Newcastle, Medical School, Framlington Place, Newcastle upon Tyne, UK

Andrew Eisen MD, FRCP(C)
Professor and Head, Division of Neurology, Vancouver Hospital and University of British Columbia, Vancouver, Canada

Christopher G Goetz MD
Rush University/Rush Presbyterian St Luke's Medical Center, Chicago, USA

A Goonetilleke MBBS, MRCP
Consultant Neurologist and Senior Lecturer in Neurology, Newcastle General Hospital, Newcastle upon Tyne, UK

John M Gray PhD
Chartered Clinical Psychologist, Consultant Clinical Neuropsychologist and Honorary Clinical Lecturer, School of Neurosciences and Psychiatry, University of Newcastle upon Tyne, UK

John B Harris BPharm, PhD, MRPharmS, FiBiol
Professor of Experimental Neurology, School of Neurosciences and Psychiatry, The Medical School, Newcastle upon Tyne, UK

John Harrison MBChB, BSc, MRCP, FFOM
Senior Lecturer in Occupational Medicine, University of Newcastle upon Tyne, The Medical School, Newcastle upon Tyne, UK

G Jean Harry PhD
Neurotoxicology Group Leader, Laboratory of Toxicology, National Institute of Environmental Health Sciences, Research Triangle Park, North Carolina, USA

JW Howe MB, DO, FRCS, FRCSEd, FRCOphth
Consultant Ophthalmologist, Royal Victoria Infirmary, Newcastle upon Tyne, UK

Don Gerard Rohan Jayamanne MBBS, FRCOpth
Specialist Registrar, Royal Victoria Infirmary, Newcastle upon Tyne, UK

Haruo Kobayashi PhD, DVM
Faculty of Agriculture, Iwate University, Morioka, Japan

Malcolm Lader OBE, DSc, PhD, MD, FRCPsych
Professor of Clinical Psychopharmacology, Institute of Psychiatry, Section of Clinical Psychopharmacology, Denmark Hill, London, UK

Masashi Nakajima MD
Director, Stroke Unit, Cerebrovascular Disorders Centre, Nanasawa Rehabilitation Hospital, Nanasawa, Atsugi, Japan

Peter K Newman MBChB, FRCP
Consultant Neurologist, Middlesbrough General Hospital, Middlesbrough, UK

Thomas P Nikolopoulos PhD, MD
Lecturer in Otorhinolaryngology, Nottingham University Hospital, Nottingham, UK

Sarah J O'Brien MBBS, MFPHM, DTM&H
Consultant Epidemiologist, PHLS Communicable Disease Surveillance Centre, London, UK, formerly Consultant Epidemiologist, Scottish Centre for Infection and Environmental Health, Glasgow, UK

John R Silver MBBS, FRCP (Edin & Lond)
Fellow of the Institute of Sports Medicine and Emeritus Consultant in Spinal Injuries, National Spinal Injuries Centre, Stoke Mandeville Hospital and formerly Consultant in Charge, Liverpool Regional Paraplegic Centre and Lecturer in Surgery, University of Liverpool, UK

Tadahiko Suzuki PhD, DVM
Faculty of Agriculture, Iwate University, Morioka, Japan

M Anthony Verity MD
Professor of Neuropathology, University of California, Center for the Health Sciences, Los Angeles, California, USA

Ashok Verma MD, DM
Assistant Professor of Neurology, University of Miami School of Medicine, Jackson Memorial Hospital, and Miami VA Medical Center, Miami, Florida, USA

Kurt R Washburn MD
Rush University/Rush Presbyterian St Luke's Medical Center, Chicago, USA

Faith M Williams MA, PhD
Reader in Biochemical Toxicology, Department of Environmental and Occupational Medicine, The Medical School, University of Newcastle upon Tyne, UK

Martin Zeidler BM, MRCP
Research Registrar, National Creutzfeld–Jakob Disease Surveillance Unit, Western General Hospital, Edinburgh, UK

Foreword

When one is honored by being invited to write a foreword for a major textbook, there is an inevitable temptation, after reading the work, to end up by penning a passage which might well resemble a critical review, with the consequential risk of giving offence to the authors and/or editors. If, as is the case with this volume, the editors and many of the contributors are erstwhile colleagues and friends, this is a risk which the writer may attempt to avoid by 'damning with faint praise', bearing in mind that foreword-writing, like blurb-writing, is a special art-form, as many publishers will no doubt acknowledge. However, in the case of this book, detailed, comprehensive, well-written and edited, no such risks or even qualms arise. We live in an age when concerns about the environmental damage associated with increasing fossil-fuel consumption and consequential global warming are increasing, as are, very properly, anxieties about the effects of many toxic agents on human health, whether biological, chemical, psychological or physical. Sometimes these agents are released into the environment, deliberately or accidentally; sometimes exposure is occupational.

This carefully designed volume of over 350 pages considers in depth those agents in all of these categories which are capable of affecting, and in many instances damaging, the structure and function of the central and peripheral nervous system, and of the neuromuscular apparatus in human subjects. The first, and longest, section of the book contains 11 excellent chapters on clinical neurotoxicology, the second (four chapters) reviews fully specific environmental hazards, and the third, in six chapters, covers investigations, whether neuropsychological, electrophysiological, neuropathological, neurochemical, or epidemiological, while the final chapter very properly deals with regulatory testing. While at first sight chapters on parasitic disease, prions and spinal injury seem to sit a little oddly in a work on toxicology, the approach and content of the relevant chapters more than justify their inclusion.

Logically planned, carefully executed, and attractively produced (despite its relative sparsity of illustrations) and printed in a readable format, this work will, in my view, be an invaluable work of reference, not just for neurologists and for doctors and scientists working in public, environmental, industrial and occupational health, but also for lawyers and for those associated with a variety of environmental agencies. It is welcome, timely, and, in my opinion, assured of success.

John Walton
(Walton of Detchant)
Oxford

Preface

Toxicology is that branch of science dealing with toxin agents that damage the structural or functional integrity of cells, tissues and organs. Neurotoxicology is the highly specialized branch of general toxicology that concerns itself with toxin-induced structural or functional damage to the nervous system. As a formal science it is relatively new, its roots residing in the pioneering work of clinical scientists such as J.B. Cavanagh and the late Pamela Le Quesne in Great Britain and P.S. Spencer in the United States of America.

The use of neurotoxins extracted from venomous and poisonous animals and from poisonous plants and algae is, however, an ancient art and it is clear from historical records that many societies had an excellent empirical understanding of the chemistry, biology and pharmacology of naturally occurring neurotoxins. Empirical knowledge, however, is not well suited to a proper understanding of why certain compounds are neurotoxic, how neurotoxic 'injury' is identified and how the toxic effects should be managed. Understanding neurotoxicology at this level requires a comprehensive understanding of many varied disciplines at a highly specialized level.

We felt that there was a need for a new approach to the presentation of neurotoxicology as a discipline: an approach that would emphasize the environmental and occupational causes of damage to the nervous system in humans; one that would explain to the younger clinician or scientists how to examine a patient and how to differentiate between organic and toxin-induced disease; one that would enable him/her to interpret epidemiological data; and one that would enable an understanding of the complexities of regulatory testing of new compounds.

We have attempted to meet this need by producing a multi-authored text that divides easily into three major sections. The first concerns the clinical expression of poisoning by neurotoxic agents, the second deals with specific environmental and occupational hazards, some of which are rarely dealt with in a book of this kind, and the third deals with the techniques used during the formal investigation of patients with neurological or psychiatric illness that may be environmental in origin.

We have not attempted to compete with the longer comprehensive texts of neurotoxicology, which we consider to be primarily of interest to the professional neurotoxicologist or neuropathologist, or with the numerous texts concerning animal toxins and venoms. Neither have we been able to address every neurotoxic agent. We hope we have provided a text that will be interesting, informative and stimulating. There is a growing need for more skilled clinical neurotoxicologists.

We have been greatly helped in this venture by the enthusiasm of our contributors from around the world. Georgina Bentliff and Catherine Barnes of Arnold were our Commissioning and Project Editors, and Lesley Gray and Annette Bruno of Gray Publishing were responsible for the project management and production of this text. We thank them all for their management of this project.

PART 1

Clinical neurotoxicology

Diagnosis of neurotoxic syndromes

DAVID BATES

INTRODUCTION

The nervous system is particularly susceptible to the effects of exogenous toxins because of its high metabolic rate. In addition, neurones, being postmitotic cells, do not divide. The tissues of the nervous system, therefore, have a relatively inadequate process of repair and regeneration. However, the central nervous system is protected by the 'blood–brain barrier' and the peripheral nervous system by the 'blood–nerve barrier,' although some tissues within the nervous system lie outside these barriers: the choroid plexus, neurohypophysis, area postrema, pineal gland, and locus caeruleus in the central nervous system; the dorsal root ganglia, autonomic ganglia, and neuromuscular junctions in the peripheral nervous system. Toxins which enter the nervous system at these points may spread to other areas by axonal transport and trans-synaptic transfer. In general those chemical compounds which are non-polar and more lipid soluble will have greater access to the nervous system (Norton, 1986; Berger and Schaumburg, 1996).

The link between a specific toxin and damage to an area of the nervous system may be difficult to determine because the ingested toxin may be a protoxin, rather than the primary neurotoxin, as with the exposure to MPTP (1-methyl-4-phenyl-1,2,3,6-tetrahydropyridine) which causes an extrapyramidal syndrome (Langston *et al.*, 1982). In addition, the susceptibility of any particular area of the central nervous system will depend upon its vascularity, its metabolic activities and requirements, and the local neurotransmitters and receptors. In general, neurones, with their high metabolic rate, are the most vulnerable cells followed by oligodendrocytes, astrocytes, microglia and the endothelial cells. The toxic effects of an individual chemical will vary depending upon the cellular or sub-cellular target: changes in membrane structure will impair excitability and impede impulse transmission; alterations in membrane proteins and channels may cause swelling of cells, damage to endothelium and edema; specific neurotransmitter toxins may block or hyperstimulate receptors or may alter the synthesis, storage, release, re-uptake and enzymatic inactivation of the natural neurotransmitter (Spencer and Schaumburg, 1984).

Neurotoxins may not damage the nervous system directly but rather will be a secondary effect following injury to vascular endothelium with a consequent effect upon neuronal function. The clinical effect of any agent will therefore depend upon the agent, the dose and possibly the length of exposure, the vulnerability of the target tissue, the organism's ability to metabolize, excrete or neutralize the agent, which may vary genetically with age or in the presence of other disease, and the ability of target tissues to repair. There is an enormous range of potential neurotoxins which vary greatly in their molecular complexity. At one extreme, neurotoxins can be elemental, such as mercury or lead, or simple compounds such as carbon monoxide but they may be as complex as the toxin of *Clostridium botulinum* which has a molecular weight of 150 000.

For the clinical neurologist there are several important steps in recognizing the possibility that a neurotoxin may be relevant to the symptoms of an individual patient (Figure 1.1). First, there should be recognition and proof, on clinical examination or investigation, that there is a disease process present which is not explained on the basis of a constitutional or natural condition, reasonable historical evidence of adequate exposure to the specific toxin, evidence that the neurotoxin is capable of generating the clinical syndrome (biological

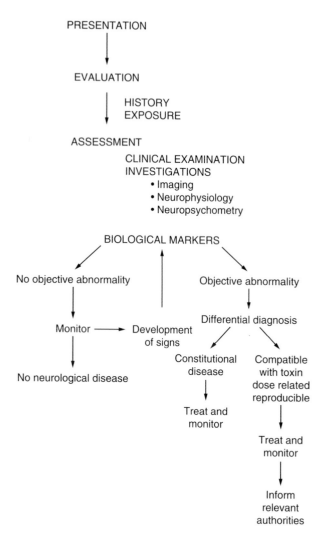

PRESENTATION

EVALUATION

HISTORY
EXPOSURE

ASSESSMENT

CLINICAL EXAMINATION
INVESTIGATIONS
• Imaging
• Neurophysiology
• Neuropsychometry

BIOLOGICAL MARKERS

No objective abnormality   Objective abnormality

Differential diagnosis

Monitor ⟶ Development
of signs

Constitutional   Compatible
disease   with toxin
dose related
reproducible

No neurological disease

Treat and
monitor

Treat and
monitor

Inform
relevant
authorities

Figure 1.1 *Management of patient with suspected neurotoxic disease.*

plausability), and exclusion through monitoring or follow-up of any other causative agent or diagnosis. In some instances, such as with the acute effects of agents such as ethanol, an association and relationship is abrupt and evident but in others, particularly where the neurological condition is similar to a degenerative process, it may be extremely difficult to identify a causal relationship between exposure and the subsequent development and progression of symptoms and signs. In general, it can be assumed that toxic neuronal loss will occur abruptly and at the time of exposure to the toxic agent, whereas neuronal loss, which is more progressive and degenerative, is likely to be age related or related to an underlying and constitutional illness (Baker and Smith, 1984). It must, however, be remembered that whilst in many syndromes, such as Parkinson's disease, it has been assumed that there is a progressive loss of cells with time there are increasing suggestions that an abrupt loss of dopaminergic cells may occur relatively acutely. There is a natural

progressive loss of neuronal function with age which may result in an earlier development of signs following the additional loss from neurotoxic damage when a threshold of deficit is crossed.

CLINICAL FEATURES OF TOXIC DISORDERS

Encephalopathy

Many neurotoxins affect cerebral function, giving rise to a syndrome of encephalopathy for which the underlying pathophysiological basis is not always known. Perhaps the most common mild encephalopathy is that caused by ethanol taken to reduce inhibition and induce a sense of relaxation. These social benefits occur at the cost of reduced judgement and slower reaction times. The intake of greater quantities of ethanol results in greater inebriation and ultimately in coma and acute ethanol toxicity which, by causing cerebral edema, can be fatal. Chronic consumption of ethanol can result in physical addiction. Methanol is more toxic than ethanol and frequently present in 'social alcohol' made to circumvent legislation surrounding the production of ethanol. Methanol can cause a severe encephalopathy with a metabolic acidosis as well as its principal toxic effect on the optic nerves (Anderson *et al.*, 1989).

Hallucinogens obtained from mushrooms were frequently used in ancient civilizations to induce social encephalopathy and the use of 'magic mushrooms' in the twentieth century, or the taking of agents such as lysergic acid diethylamide (LSD) create similar deliberate encephalopathies which may result in dysarthria, ataxia and seizures, and can be fatal due to gross cerebral edema.

Organic solvents, widely used in industry and recently in the recreational drug context, can cause encephalopathy in addition to other more peripheral effects on the nervous system. Toluene is probably a major chemical in this respect and euphoria may occur, followed by headache, nausea, dizziness and incoordination. Habituation has been reported (Knox and Nelson, 1966). Chronic exposure to other volatile organic compounds such as methyl chloride has been identified as the cause of seizures, nausea, and intellectual or cognitive change. The ingestion of domoic acid from algae-infected shell fish has been associated with loss of short-term memory and seizures (Nunn and O'Brien, 1991).

The simple elemental chemicals, mercury, thallium, and aluminum have all been implicated in the development of encephalopathy, seizures, and dementia. There have been suggestions that chronic bismuth injection, and the use of gold in the treatment of rheumatoid arthritis may also result in an encephalopathy.

The clinical problems relating to the causal association of neurotoxins and encephalopathies are most important for those occasions when the severity of dysfunction or the neurological sequelæ persist beyond the immediate exposure period. Most of the acute effects of exposure to a toxin result from the direct toxicological effect of the chemical but some agents may have a more prolonged effect and their toxicity can continue and increase even when they are removed from the environment. When residual structural brain damage occurs in relation to acute exposure, as can be seen with carbon monoxide poisoning, the prolonged effect of the encephalopathy can be understood, but in the absence of such evidence of structural damage there is inevitable concern about the validity of symptoms such as mood disorders, problems with cognition and memory, and frank dementia.

Depressive symptoms are not uncommon in patients who have been exposed to possible neurotoxins (Baker, 1989). They are often associated with psychomotor slowing and reduced psychomotor accuracy. There may be associated cognitive dysfunction and the problems may result in deterioration in job performance and in activities of daily living (Baker and White, 1985). The recognition of such disability demands careful medical evaluation, including a formal assessment of psychological and psychiatric symptomatology. The evolution of the syndrome may be insidious and the symptoms will always be difficult to distinguish from other mild neurobehavorial conditions. In general, the symptoms should resolve when exposure to the offending agent, or agents, is ceased and although it may be difficult to identify a specific chemical etiology and completely to exclude constitutional psychological or psychiatric illness, a close and reversible relationship between the development of symptoms and exposure to an agent should be reasonably persuasive.

There is some suggestion that conditioned responses may underlie the development of symptoms following exposure to odors in the 'multiple chemical sensitivity syndrome.'

There is a continuum between the mild encephalopathy which may present with mood disorders during the period of exposure and the chronic toxic encephalopathy associated with some degree of memory and psychomotor function impairment which can be confirmed on formal psychometry. Such patients may show neurobehavioral abnormalities affecting visuospacial ability and abstract concept formation. The diagnosis of a chronic toxic encephalopathy requires a careful clinical assessment: first, to establish that there is evidence for abnormality on sophisticated neuropsychological testing and preferably supported with objective evidence of neurophysiological abnormality on electroencephalogram; second, to provide good evidence of a relationship with exposure to a potentially hazardous toxin; and, third, to exclude any other underlying causes. Although mild toxic encephalopathy may not be fully reversible when exposure to the chemical is ended, it seems reasonable to suggest that there should not be further deterioration after removal from exposure and that if there is a continuation and worsening of an encephalopathy this militates in favor of an underlying constitutional diagnosis.

The important question of whether a toxic encephalopathy can become chronic and progress to, or presage, the development of dementia is not fully explained. There is increasing evidence suggesting that most forms of 'degenerative' dementia have a multifactorial cause involving genetic, biological, and chemical factors. It is recognized that chronic exposures to heavy metals, manganese, and aluminum may be associated with damage to the central nervous system, including impaired mental capacity and these problems can be irreversible. A question which arises is whether exposure to neurotoxic agents may themselves result in presenile dementia and whether lower chronic levels of exposure may contribute to neuronal depletion which, when coupled with other neuronal insults or aging, over time may culminate in a form of dementia. The diagnostic dilemma between the effects of solvents versus degenerative dementias, such as Alzheimer's disease, can sometimes be resolved by a neurological investigation when imaging studies, neurophysiology or biochemical studies reveal a focal lesion or a recognizable syndrome. However, in those cases where the neurological examination is normal, scanning shows only mild atrophy and an electroencephalogram (EEG) shows no more than mild slowing, conditions which may be seen in both Alzheimer's disease or with chronic exposure to solvents. This means that problems in differentiation may arise. It is suggested that neuropsychological testing may be useful in this situation in helping to differentiate between the two conditions since studies with patients exposed to chronic solvent use indicate relative sparing of language functions in the psychometric subtests, unlike Alzheimer's disease where language ability is usually affected (Baker et al., 1990). It should, however, be recognized that psychometric testing is, to some extent, a subjective assessment and there will remain problems in the true differentiation of Alzheimer's disease from a possible neurotoxin-related dementia, unless and until a specific biological marker is established for the former or histopathological features are identified on biopsy.

Cerebellar syndromes

Progressive cerebellar ataxia is seen classically in methyl mercury poisoning, now often termed 'Minamata disease,' in which there is atrophy of cerebellar folia with loss of the granule cell layer (Tokuomi et al., 1982). Similar syndromes have been reported in chronic exposure to toluene, although, as so often is the case with organic solvents, there must remain some doubt as to whether the neuropathological agent is toluene itself or some contaminant or impurity. Ataxia is commonly seen as part of the syndrome of chronic ethanol abuse where some question still exists as to whether the ataxia is due to the toxic effect of ethanol or related to an associated dietary insufficiency. Ataxia may be seen in patients treated with agents such as 5-fluorouracil and in those who have been treated to toxic levels with lithium and with phenytoin.

The important differentiation from inflammatory diseases like multiple sclerosis is unlikely to create problems but differentiation from hereditary and degenerative ataxias may be difficult.

Extrapyramidal syndromes

PARKINSON'S DISEASE

Manganese toxicity has been documented to cause a clinical syndrome resembling Parkinson's disease, although whether its toxicity results from its role in electron transfer and therefore as part of the development of free radicals remains uncertain. Perhaps the most classic example of an extrapyramidal syndrome due to neurotoxins, and certainly the one which has been subjected to most experimental work, is the development of a Parkinson's disease-like syndrome following exposure to MPTP, a contaminant of a so-called 'designer drug.' Its importance lies in the fact that MPTP is the precursor of the toxin MPP+ and is metabolized, probably in the glial tissues, before exerting its toxic effect in the neurone. It also highlights the possible existence of a neurotoxic effect causing damage to cells within the central nervous system which became manifest some years later due to a natural and progressive decline in neurone population with increasing age (Langston et al., 1982).

Acute carbon monoxide poisoning can result in a delayed extrapyramidal syndrome which begins two to three weeks after recovery from the initial exposure. The extrapyramidal disturbance can be progressive and is associated with symmetrical necrosis of the globus pallidus and demyelination of the sub-cortical white matter. Abnormalities may be shown on a computerized tomography (CT) head scan and on magnetic resonance imaging (MRI) scanning. Similar changes have occasionally been demonstrated with methanol poisoning.

PROGRESSIVE SUPRANUCLEAR PALSY

This syndrome described by Steele et al. (1964) is usually degenerative. However, there have been reports of patients exposed to organic solvents developing such a syndrome with the classical appearance of the eyes,

the loss of voluntary but not reflex conjugate gaze, and features of rigidity and bradykinesia with a tendency to fall backwards. There are also suggestions that one of the phenotypic forms of the Guamian Parkinson dementia complex, which resembles supranuclear palsy, may possibly be related to a constituent or contaminant of the cycad which is a dietary staple on the island. The relationship between potential neurotoxins in the cycad and the development of the disease is not proven but might theoretically involve prolonged exposure (McCrank and Rabheru, 1989).

TREMOR

Tremulousness, most commonly action tremor, is seen with several forms of chemical intoxication. It may be seen with heavy metal poisoning, particularly with mercury, and also with the use of some organic solvents. Differentiation from hyperthyroidism, hypercapnia and extrapyramidal disease is important.

Cranial nerves and brain stem

VISUAL PATHWAY

Methanol is probably the most widely recognized cause of acute visual loss. It seems probable that the injury to the optic nerves occurs due to the formation of formic acid and formates that are metabolites of methanol which can therefore be regarded as a protoxin. Organic mercury poisoning, as in 'Minamata disease,' tends to cause concentric constriction of the visual fields and the presence of optic atrophy, although damage may not be confined only to the optic nerves since there is histological evidence of injury to the calcarine cortex.

A dietary cause of peripheral visual field loss is seen in African populations exposed to Cassava root – the toxic material may be a cyanogenetic glycoside – and a similar toxicity seen in Caribbean populations appears to affect central vision rather than peripheral (Osuntokun and Osuntokun, 1971). The use of clioquinol as an oral intestinal amoebicide has been associated with the development of the subacute myelo-optico neuropathy which usually causes asymmetrical visual loss with impairment of color vision and an evident optic neuropathy. The variability in the frequency of the syndrome in differing populations using clioquinol raises questions as to its causative role in this condition but also highlights the possibility of genetic differences in presentation of toxic syndromes. Carbon disulfide, which is used in the rayon and film industries, may cause optic neuropathy and can result in enlargement of the blind spot. Patients may have central scotomata, red/green color blindness and occasionally manifest nystagmus implying a central brain stem disturbance as well as the optic nerve abnormality. Differentiation from inflammatory, structural and inherited optic neuropathy is necessary.

TRIGEMINAL NERVE

Trichloroethylene can cause a unique neurotoxic syndrome affecting predominantly the cranial nerves and principally the trigeminal nerve (Feldman *et al.*, 1970). It is used as an industrial solvent and degreasing agent and tends to cause a centripetal, or 'onion skin,' pattern of sensory loss on the face. This may spread to involve the entire distribution of the trigeminal nerve, and may be associated with weakness of the muscles of mastication. Recovery usually follows removal from exposure and, although electrophysiological studies have suggested a demyelinating change in the nerve, pathological studies have shown both axonal and demyelination of the nerve, pathologies which may occasionally also affect the optic and facial nerves. Differentiation of brain stem lesions and inflammatory vasculitis is relevant. There is some clinical evidence that trichlorethylene may be associated with the development of extrapyramidal syndromes such as multiple system atrophy.

AUDITORY NERVE

Several pharmacological agents, particular the aminoglycoside antibiotics (Prosen and Stebbins, 1980) are recognized to cause damage to the auditory nerve and which may also rarely be seen with the diuretics, ethacrynic acid, and frusemide. Salicylate toxicity can occur with massive doses which may occasionally result in hearing loss, as may the use of quinine.

SPINAL CORD

Neurolathyrism, which is most commonly seen in East Africa and Asia, is thought to be related to the amino acid beta-*N*-oxalylamino-L-alanine (BOAA) found in the chickling pea (*Lathyrus sativa*) (Allen *et al.*, 1990). It causes damage to the pyramidal tracts and usually manifests as a spastic paraparesis. There are occasional changes seen in the anterior horn cells and suggestions have been made that it may relate to some of the variants of motor neurone disease seen in the Pacific basin. Differentiation from structural or inflammatory paraparesis and demyelination or human T-cell lymphocytotrophic virus (HTLV) 1 infection is necessary.

The toxin tetanospasmin, produced by *Clostridium tetani*, enters the nervous system at the neuromuscular junction but its effects are mediated at the spinal cord level where it acts to cause specific blockade of the release of the inhibitory transmitter glycine, probably by an effect on membrane-binding proteins. The resulting dysinhibition of the spinal motor neurones results in spasms and trismus, which are the clinical manifestations of the illness. It is also possible that the venom of the black widow spider, which also affects the neuromuscular junction, may spread by axonal transport to the central nervous system and affect the spinal cord.

The use of bismuth, by intramuscular injection, can cause thrombosis and vasoconstriction and has been associated with an ischemic myelopathy.

Peripheral nervous system

CENTRAL PERIPHERAL AXONOPATHY

The fact that many toxins can affect both central and peripheral axons and that dorsal root ganglion cells have a prolonged central axon process has led to the recognition that a combination of central and peripheral effects of toxins may be seen. The dorsal columns are most commonly affected in the central aspect of a mixed axonopathy, but spinocerebellar and corticospinal tracts may also be involved, presumably by axonal transport of the toxin and transsynaptic spread. The neuropathy of clioquinol in subacute myelo-optic neuropathy (SMON) is predominantly in the proximal axon and the appearance is that of a posterior column syndrome with deafferentation and sensory ataxia, often associated with dysaesthesiae and either a flaccid or a spastic paraparesis (Tsubaki *et al.*, 1971). Sphincter control may be affected and optic neuropathy is common.

Another central and peripheral axonopathy is hexacarbon-induced neurotoxicity, which is seen in industrial exposure and in relation to 'glue sniffing,' in which the toxic compounds are believed to be *n*-hexane and methyl *n*-butyl ketone (Cianchetii *et al.*, 1976). They may act as protoxins producing the common metabolite 2,5-hexanedione but cause a predominantly dorsal root ganglioneuropathy, although there may be some peripheral demyelinating component in addition.

Acrylamide, which is used in industry, has been associated with a similar dorsal root ganglioneuropathy in relation to cutaneous absorption. There is some suggestion that organophosphorus compounds, including triorthocresyl phosphate, whilst having their major effect as inhibitors of anticholinesterase at the neuromuscular junction, may also cause a delayed central and peripheral axonopathy by a mechanism which does not seem to depend upon the inhibition of acetyl cholinesterase.

The tropical ataxic neuropathy which may be seen in African populations in relation to the use of a bitter cassava root, may be due to chronic cyanide toxicity and arsenic neurotoxicity, which commonly presents as a subacute neuropathy with sensory symptoms and pain but with preserved deep tendon reflexes. It is also likely to be a central peripheral axonopathy. The peripheral effects of thallium neurotoxicity are similar and can be confused clinically with the Guillain–Barré syndrome, although whether the mechanism is in relation to a depletion of flavoprotein or direct toxicity at the mitochondrial level is unknown.

PERIPHERAL NEUROPATHY

Peripheral neuropathies are reported with the heavy metals lead, in which segmental demyelination is believed to be the cause of the neuropathy, and gold, used in the treatment of rheumatoid arthritis in which a combination of segmental demyelination and axonal degeneration has been reported. There is also some suggestion that hexacarbon-induced neurotoxicity may cause demyelination as well as axonal changes in the peripheral nervous system.

An unusual manifestation of neurotoxicity occurs with the industrial catalyst dimethylamino-proprionitrile (DMAPN) which causes a neuropathy in the bladder resulting in urinary retention and hesitancy resembling an autonomic neuropathy.

The pathological effects of diphtheria toxin are delayed by some 5–40 days from the acute pharyngitis and results in demyelination due to progressive disruption of protein synthesis within the Schwann cell. Demyelination is also the main cause of peripheral neuropathy with Buckthorn toxin and in hexachlorophene poisoning, where there is vesiculation of the myelin sheath, splitting of lamellae, and consequent slowing of conduction and development of a neuropathy. Some neurotoxins, like perhexiline, can cause intracellular inclusion bodies within the Schwann cells mimicking storage diseases.

AUTONOMIC NEUROPATHY

Thallium is reported to cause autonomic disturbances resulting in sphincter problems, paralytic ileus, and postural hypotension. The agent muscarine, which is found in some mushrooms, affects the acetyl choline receptors at parasympathetic cholinergic nerve terminals and can cause an autonomic syndrome of perspiration, salivation, lacrimation, myosis with blurring of vision, vomiting, diarrhea, and hypotension. The organophosphates used in industry as plasticizers and flame retardants, in warfare as nerve gases, and in agriculture as insecticides and sheep dips cause inhibition of acetylcholinesterase with resulting overactivity of the cholinergic components of the autonomic nervous system. Acute toxicity will cause an identical syndrome.

NEUROMUSCULAR JUNCTION

The neuromuscular junction is one of those areas of the nervous system not protected by a 'blood–nerve barrier.' It is therefore particularly vulnerable to neurotoxins and many such toxins are part of naturally occurring agents in animal, plant, and unicellular species. The toxins may act at the presynaptic, synaptic or postsynaptic level, and can have an effect directly on the muscle membrane. Natural toxins have been identified which affect sodium channels by causing blockade, such as saxitoxin and tetrodotoxin, prolonged opening of the channels, such as siguatoxin, or prevention of closure of the channels, such as batrachotoxin. They may also cause increased permeability of the channel, such as tityus toxin. Alternatively they may affect the calcium channels by causing blockade, most classically with botulinum toxin, and they may affect acetylcholine release either by causing blockade, as with tic venom or beta-bungarotoxin, or by excessive release with alpha-laterotoxin. Acetylcholine receptor blockade is seen with the natural toxins alpha-bungarotoxin and curare (Mitchell, 1994).

Acetyl cholinesterase inhibition is most commonly seen with organophosphate compounds and with carbamates which are industrial chemicals developed as insecticides and, in the case of the former, nerve gases. Acute intoxication will cause autonomic effects together with the inhibition of conduction across the myoneural junctions and interference with central nervous system synaptic transmission (Feldman, 1988). Most toxins which affect neuromuscular junction function may be associated with autonomic disturbance, many cause initial symptoms of peripheral tingling and paraesthesiae followed by myalgia, then paralysis which most importantly involves the respiratory muscles and bulbar muscles. All are life threatening and require respiratory support whilst the differential diagnosis from myasthenia gravis, Lambert Eaton myasthenic syndrome, or an ascending demyelinating radiculopathy of Guillain–Barré type is established. Neurophysiology will help to identify the site of the abnormality and measurement of peripheral red blood cell acetylcholinesterase concentrations may be of value in acute anticholinesterase intoxication.

Both the organophosphates, which inhibit acetyl cholinesterase, and the carbamates, another group of pesticides which cause carbamylation and consequent inhibition of anticholinesterase, can cause an acute syndrome of overstimulation of neuromuscular junctions and other synaptic connections. Although the inhibition with organophosphates is more complete and more persistent, both can be associated in the human with an acute toxic syndrome of fatigue, malaise, and autonomic disturbances. Organophosphates have also been associated with a syndrome of delayed neurotoxicity developing one to four weeks after exposure to the compounds in which there is progressive weakness beginning in the lower extremities, spreading to the upper extremities and associated with minimal sensory change and depression of deep tendon reflexes. The syndrome can persist for months and shows slow recovery. This is sometimes called the 'intermediate syndrome' in which the change at the neuromuscular junction has been shown to be non-depolarizing and there may be some muscle fiber necrosis. Single fiber electromyography (SF EMG) studies have demonstrated abnormalities in 'jitter' in such patients. In patients exposed to very low concentrations of the organophosphates consistent with the development of a sub-clinical non-depolarizing neuromuscular block, changes are reversible over months returning to normal within two years and are not associated with any clinical neuromuscular symptoms or signs (Baker and Sedgwick, 1996).

MUSCLE SYNDROMES

Several natural toxins including sea snake venom and cobra venom are reported to cause acute rhabdomyolosis in addition to disturbance of function at the neuromuscular junction (Senanayake and Roman, 1992).

Paralytic syndromes of muscle related to changes in potassium within the intracellar and extracellular compartments are seen in poisoning with barium and poisoning with cotton plants which contain a phenolic compound, gossypol, associated with loss of potassium from the intracellular space and through the kidney. The abuse of liquorice, either medicinally or from habituation, can also be associated with renal potassium loss and can result in a flaccid paralysis which resembles clinically the hypocalaemic periodic paralysis which is genetically determined.

MANAGEMENT

History

When the possibility of a neurotoxin as the cause of a neurological syndrome in an individual patient occurs, it is essential that an adequate history is established. This must explore the possibility of symptoms beginning before the time of exposure, the relationship of the development of symptoms to the time of exposure, and the length and quantity of the exposure to the putative toxin. It is appropriate that a combination of the skills of the clinical neurologist to determine the relevance, timing, and significance of individual clinical symptoms together with that of an occupational physician to establish and evaluate the significance of exposure be combined in the individual assessment. It is important that patients be interviewed not only in respect of their known exposure to substances with neurotoxic potential but also their employment in certain trades which are linked with the liability to such exposure (Baker *et al.*, 1990).

In those instances where there has been an acute illness in association with a specific, identified exposure to a toxin there should be little problem in relating the two phenomena. Greater problems arise when symptoms have developed either following a latency from the exposure or if they have developed during the time of exposure and have then continued and progressed when the offending agent has been eliminated or avoided. If it can be established that the syndrome is progressing after the time of exposure it is important that information be obtained either from precedent or from experimental evidence that the toxin implicated can cause such a delay in the development of the symptoms. There are certain agents, such as carbon monoxide, in which it is clearly recognized that the extrapyramidal syndrome may develop after a delay and may progress despite the removal of the agent. There are others, such as organophosphorous compounds, where there continues to be great debate about the possibility of long-term effects following single or repeated exposure to the compounds which are now avoided.

Examination

Following the obtaining of a careful history, clinical examination should establish the degree of dysfunction. In those situations in which neurological signs are identified, it becomes important to try to identify which of the syndromes are due to the putative toxin and which might represent part of an intercurrent or unrelated constitutional process. These neurological signs can include clear evidence of optic neuropathy, evident cranial nerve dysfunction, objective changes in reflexes, tone, power or sensory dysfunction, the development of primitive reflexes or objective, and measurable changes in informal psychometry. It is recognized that although Koch's postulates cannot exist fully for toxic exposure certain clinical syndromes are recognized to occur with some toxins. The occurrence of a novel neurological syndrome should indicate the need for exhaustive exclusion of other explanations.

When there are no objective neurological signs, and even in the presence of those signs, their validity can be increased by investigations.

Investigations

HEMATOLOGICAL AND BIOCHEMICAL INVESTIGATIONS

When the patient is seen close to the time of exposure it may be possible to obtain tissue samples from blood or urine which demonstrate that there has been exposure to the relevant toxin and that the exposure was of sufficient severity to give rise to a clinical syndrome. It is obligatory in those cases in which there is an acute illness in relation to exposure that some attempt be made to assess the level of putative toxin within the blood. However, problems will undoubtedly occur in those cases where there is a delay between exposure and the development of clinical symptoms, or where the relationship is only tenuous. There may occasionally be paraclinical features in the hematological and biochemical tests indicating red blood cell changes as in the case of lead poisoning, liver function test abnormalities as in the case of some organic solvent problems, and direct measurement of the offending chemical may be possible.

NEURO-IMAGING

The advent of CT scanning and more recently of MRI scanning has made enormous changes to the ability of the clinical neurologist, with the assistance of radiological colleagues, to identify structural pathologies and the underlying cause of many previously puzzling neurological syndromes. The finding of significant structural changes, those seen with some examples of carbon monoxide poisoning and in relation to hypoxia or ischemia which may be induced by toxins, should always raise the possibility of an alternative diagnosis as the cause of the syndrome under investigation. However, the absence of abnormality on scanning or the finding of non-specific changes such as atrophy does not necessarily exclude an underlying neurotoxic cause.

NEUROPHYSIOLOGY

For those syndromes which are predominantly subjective and related to changes in mood, cognition, fatigue, or purely sensory symptoms, neurophysiology is of great value in demonstrating whether there is underlying pathology. An abnormal EEG demonstrating an underlying encephalopathic process does not necessarily indicate the nature of the pathology. However, the finding of an entirely normal EEG in someone presenting with significant abnormalities of mood, cognition, or memory would militate against the likelihood of an organic, and therefore neurotoxic, cause for those symptoms. Similarly, the finding of neurophysiological abnormalities on tests of central conduction, such as visual evoked potentials, brain stem auditory evoked potentials, somato sensory evoked potentials, and motor evoked potentials or, in the peripheral nervous system, examination including neuromuscular junction testing, does not of itself demonstrate the nature of the underlying pathology. However, the absence of any significant abnormality on those tests militates against any organic cause for the patient's symptoms. It should be further recognized that many of the tests currently used in neurophysiology have a subjective basis to their assessment and their

evaluation requires an experienced neurophysiologist working in a laboratory in which there are good internal and external quality control measures. This means that changes which are identified will be known to be reproducible and to be significant.

NEUROPSYCHOMETRY

The use of formal neuropsychometry to assess standards of cognition, memory, alertness, and mood are important in identifying where there is a significant abnormality which may be explained on the basis of neurotoxic changes. Once again there is the requirement for an experienced neuropsychologist to undertake and evaluate the investigation. There should be the recognition on the part of all of those involved that neuropsychiatric tests are not absolute but must be interpreted within the clinical context of the individual patient. A lack of abnormality in the tests militates strongly against any organic underlying disease including toxicity; the presence of an abnormality is not necessarily indicative of an organic problem and may occur in the absence of overt underlying pathology.

BIOLOGICAL MARKERS

It is probable that in the future diagnostic biological markers will be developed to allow the detection of biochemical signals in peripheral tissues which can be easily and ethically obtained and which will provide surrogate indicators of equivalent parameters in the central nervous system (Manzo et al., 1996). Measurement of neurotransmission and second messenger systems in peripheral blood cells, such as cholinergic muscarinic receptors and calcium signaling in peripheral blood lymphocytes, myelin basic protein in cerebrospinal fluid, and the presence of polyamines in the blood, are potential surrogate indicators based on animal studies of neurotoxic elements, organic compounds, drugs of abuse, and potentially epileptogenic compounds. The measurement of serum prolactin, type B monoamine oxidase and dopamine beta hydroxylase may help identify potential problems arising within the basal ganglia. It is also to be expected that neurochemical markers may be used in animal studies as a complement to conventional laboratory tests to improve both sensitivity and specificity. Such a research approach could be expected to establish which markers will offer the greater promise.

BIOPSY

The final recognition of a relationship between a clinical syndrome and a neurotoxin will depend upon examination of pathology. In some instances, particularly in those situations involving the peripheral nerve or muscle part of the investigation, this may involve biopsy of nerve, muscle or neuromuscular junction with an assessment of the tissues, histopathologically and metabolically. There are characteristic changes in some of the peripheral neuropathies such as that related to *n*-hexane which enable a diagnosis to be suggested strongly from the histological evidence. There are few circumstances in which brain biopsy can be indicated but the importance of prolonged follow-up and final autopsy information is of great importance in establishing ultimately a relationship between the putative toxin and the clinical syndrome.

CONFIRMATION OF DISEASE

When the required investigations are complete it should be possible for the clinician to determine the probability of an association between the putative neurotoxin and the clinical syndrome by the patient. Where such a relationship is believed to be established it is obligatory that relevant authorities be informed of the source and nature of exposure to the toxin and, in those cases where the exposure has been accidental, environmental or industrial, appropriate warnings may be given and legalization undertaken.

In those situations where chronic disability persists following exposure to the toxin it will be the responsibility of the clinician to maintain observation of the patient. The clinician will need to try to gain more information about the natural history of the underlying condition and, if necessary, to consider further investigation and the possible revision of the diagnosis should the progress of the condition make it unlikely that the putative neurotoxin was responsible for the neurological condition.

REFERENCES

Allen, C.N., Ross, S.M. and Spencer, P.S. 1990: In *New Advances in Toxicology and Epidemiology*, Rose, F.C. and Norris, F.H. (eds), pp 41–8. London: Smith Gordon.

Anderson, T.J., Shuaib, A. and Becker, W.J. 1989: Methanol poisoning: factors associated with neurological complications. *Canadian Journal of Neurological Sciences*, **16**, 432–5.

Baker, D.J. and Sedgwick, E.M. 1996: Single fiber electromyographic changes in man after organophosphate exposure. *Human and Experimental Toxicology*, **15**, 369–75.

Baker, E.L. 1989: Neurological and behavioral disorders. In *Occupational Health: Recognizing and Preventing Work-related Disease*, Levy, B. and Wegman, D. (eds). Boston, MA: Brown.

Baker, E.L., Feldman, R.G. and French, J.G. 1990: Environmentally related disorders of the nervous systems. *Medical Clinics of North America*, **74**, 325–45.

Baker, E.L. and Smith, T.J. 1984: Evaluation of exposure to organic solvents. In *Recent Advances in Occupational Health*, Harrington, J.M. (ed.). London: Churchill Livingstone.

Baker, E.L. and White, R.F. 1985: The use of neuropsychological testing in the evaluation of neurotoxic effects of organic solvents. In *Chronic Effects of Organic Solvents on the Central Nervous System and Diagnosis Criteria*. Report on joint WHO/NORDIC Council of Ministers Working Group, pp 224–41. Copenhagen: World Health Organization.

Berger, A.R. and Schaumburg, H.H. 1996: Effects of occupational and environmental agents on the nervous system. In *Neurology in Clinical Practice*, Bradley, W.G., Daroff, R.B., Fenichel, G.M. and Marsden, C.D. (eds). Boston, MA: Butterworth-Heinemann.

Cianchetii, C.G., Abbritti, G., Perticoni, A. *et al.* 1976: Toxic polyneuropathy of shoe industry workers. *Journal of Neurology, Neurosurgery and Psychiatry*, **39**, 1151–61.

Feldman, R.G. 1988: Effects of toxins and physical agents on the nervous system. In *Neurology in Clinical Practice*, Bradley, W.G., Daroff, R.B. and Fenichel, G.M. (eds). London: Butterworth.

Feldman, R.G., Mayer, R.M. and Taub, A. 1970: Evidence for peripheral neurotoxic effect of trichloroethylene. *Neurology*, **20**, 599–606.

Knox, J.W. and Nelson, J.B. 1966: Permanent encephalopathy from toluene inhalation. *New England Journal of Medicine*, **273**, 1494–6.

Langston, J.W., Ballard, P., Tetrud, J.W. and Irwin, L. 1982: Chronic parkinsonism in humans due to a product of meperidine analog synethesis. *Science*, **219**, 979–80.

Manzo, L., Artigas, F., Martinez, E. *et al.* 1996: Biochemical markers of neurotoxicity. A review of mechanistic studies and applications. *Human and Experimental Toxicology*, **15**, S20–S35.

McCrank, E. and Rabheru, K. 1989: Four cases of progressive supranuclear palsy in patients exposed to organic solvents. *Canadian Journal of Psychiatry*, **34**, 934–6.

Mitchell, J.L. 1994: Clinical neurotoxicology. In *Handbook of Clinical Neurology. Intoxications of the Nervous System*, deWolff, F.A. (ed.), Vol. 20. New York: Elsevier Science.

Norton, S. 1986: Toxic responses of the central nervous system. In Casarett and Doull's *Toxicology*, Klassen, C.D., Amdur, D.O. and Doull, J. (eds), 3rd edn. London: Churchill Livingstone.

Nunn, P.B. and O'Brien, P. 1991: In *New Evidence in MND/ALS Research*, Rose, F.C. (ed.), pp 229–36. London: Smith Gordon.

Osuntokun, B.O. and Osuntokun, O. 1971: Tropical amblyopia in Nigerians. *American Journal of Ophthalmology*, **72**, 708–16.

Prosen, C.A. and Stebbins, W.C. 1980: Ototoxicity. In *Experimental and Clinical Neurotoxicology*, Spencer, P.S. and Schaumburg, H.H. (eds). Baltimore, MD: Williams & Wilkins.

Senanayake, N.G. and Roman, G.C. 1992: Disorders of neuromuscular transmission due to natural environmental toxins. *Journal of the Neurological Sciences*, **107**, 1–13.

Spencer, P.S. and Schaumburg, H.H. 1984: An expanded classification of neurotoxic responses based on cellular targets of chemical agents. *Acta Neurologica Scandinavica*, **70**, 9–19.

Steele, J.C., Richardson, J.C. and Olszewski, J. 1964: Progressive supranuclear palsy. *Archives of Neurology*, **10**, 333–59.

Tokuomi, H., Echino, M., Imanura, S. *et al.* 1982: Minamata disease. *Neurology*, **32**, 1369–72.

Tsubaki, T., Honmay, Y. and Sushi, M. 1971: Neurological syndrome associated with clioquinol. *Lancet*, **i**, 696–8.

2

Developmental neurotoxicology

G JEAN HARRY

INTRODUCTION

Neurotoxicity has been defined as a structural change or a functionally adverse response of the nervous system to a chemical, biological, or physical agent. Due to the complexity of the nervous system and its activities to maintain the balance of all of the various organ systems of the body, characterization of toxicity encompasses multiple levels of organization and interactions. Such characterization includes structural, biochemical, physiological, and behavioral levels of effects. Complex cognitive functions such as speech, emotion, learning, memory, neuromuscular coordination, and autonomic control of organ functioning depend upon the normal integrative capacity of the nervous system. Interactions with the external environment are dependent upon the correct anatomical structure and cellular interactions at various levels of functioning. In order to accomplish these multiple tasks, the nervous system must develop a coordinated interactive communication system between functional sites. Temporal and spatial organization of nervous system development is a precise and complex process with the basic framework laid down in a stepwise fashion in which each step is dependent upon the proper completion of the previous one. Thus, a relatively minor disturbance resulting in a perturbation of developmental interactions between selective cells for a limited time period may result in a major deleterious outcome. In the developing animal, the pattern of toxic damage may differ from that seen following exposure of the mature nervous system. Major differences in sensitivity to insult are related to changing cell structure, the degree of development of the blood–brain barrier, the degree of myelination of tracts, the degree of arborization of dendritic and axonal processes, and the extent of development of the cerebral vascular bed and capillary endothelium.

During gestation, chemicals may affect maternal tissues and have indirect effects upon the fetus or they may have a direct effect on the embryonic cells; each can result in a specific pattern of abnormality. Teratogenic effects of drugs and chemicals have traditionally been noted as anatomic malformations. These effects are dose and time related and the susceptibility of the fetus is the greatest during the first few months of gestation. While congenital anatomic malformations do occur, it is crucial that concern also be given to events that include adverse effects that can be subtle, unexpected, delayed, and affect the neurobiological functioning of the offspring. In a rapidly developing tissue, chemicals may cause both an injury to an already developed structure, as well as a derangement of later development. Given the redundancy of the nervous system and the dynamic nature of its formation, a chemical can disrupt an ongoing process or stage of development resulting in subtle alterations rather than tissue destruction and gross morphological alterations. Often, this is a matter of exposure level and can be seen, for example, with many of the metals, such as inorganic lead producing myelin edema at high doses and subtle alterations in synaptic number and placement at lower exposure levels. While an insult occurring at the time of a developmental event may result in a given malformation, it may also result in an alteration in the developmental program thus affecting any events that are subsequent to the insult. Due to this feature of developmental insults, developmental event and developmental program, the concept of termination period was formulated. The termination period is the time in the development of an organ after which a specific malformation cannot occur by any teratogenic mechanisms. However, it has become clear over the years that drugs and chemicals can exert their effects upon the fetus at times during pregnancy other than during the first few months. This chapter will present information concerning the basic formation of the nervous system with emphasis placed on aspects of the system that may account for its increased susceptibility to environmental-induced perturbations.

BASIS OF NERVOUS SYSTEM DEVELOPMENT

The development of the nervous system starts in the embryo and for humans is not complete until approximately the time of puberty. Nervous system organogenesis occurs during the period from implantation through mid-gestation with synaptogenesis and myelination predominant during late gestation and the early neonatal period. The complex architecture of the brain requires that different cell types develop in a precise spatial relationship to one another. The embryo must not only establish a coordinate system for itself but must also ensure that the appropriate cell types are correctly generated (for review see Purves and Lichtman, 1985; Jacobson, 1991; Volpe, 1995). In the development of the human brain, the first two major processes of neural embryogenesis are the formation of the neural tube and the prosencephalon (Volpe, 1995). Primary neurulation refers to the formation of the neural tube and results in the formation of the brain and spinal cord. This occurs during weeks three to four of gestation. During this time the notochord and chordal mesoderm induce neural plate formation. The neural plate then invaginates and closes dorsally to form the neural tube. The neural plate is committed to develop into neural tissue and local areas of the plate along its anterior–posterior axis are predestined to develop into specific brain regions. Neural plate cells migrate toward the midline and acquire different cell shapes. Differential changes in cell morphology result in the edges of the neural plate folding in to form the neural groove and adhere to each other to form the neural tube. The folding of the neural plate involves a coordinated functioning of the cytoskeletal filaments, microtubules, and microfilaments. In addition, this process involves the interaction of various surface

glycoproteins, extracellular matrix proteins, and cell adhesion molecules to insure cell–cell recognition and adhesive interactions between the lips of the neural folds (Karfunkel, 1974; Hay, 1981; Morriss-Kay and Crutch, 1982; Copp and Bernfield, 1988a,b; Nagele et al., 1989; van Straaten et al., 1989; Jacobson, 1991).

The caudal neural tube forms the lower sacral and coccygeal segments by canalization and retrogressive differentiation. The process begins at approximately 28 days of gestation and continues until approximately seven weeks. This is followed by retrogressive differentiation until some time after birth resulting in a regression of the caudal cell mass. The pseudostratified epithelial cells continue to proliferate and increasing fluid pressure within the central canal leads to 'ballooning' of the rostral end of the tube to form the three brain vesicles that define the major divisions of the brain. The first fusion process of the neural tube occurs at approximately 22 days of gestation forming the lower medulla. This fusion continues with the anterior end of the neural tube closing at approximately 24 days and the posterior end at approximately 26 days at the lumbosacral level of the spinal cord. The skull and vertebrae form due to an interaction between the neural tube and the surrounding mesoderm. Disturbances of the inductive events involved in primary neurulation result in errors of neural tube closure. This is accompanied by alterations in the axial skeleton and the meningovascular and dermal coverings (Volpe, 1977). Cells on the margins of the plate migrate into the region between the surface ectoderm and the dorsal aspect of the neural tube and become the cells of the neural crest. The principal cell types in the central nervous system (CNS): the neurons and macroglia (astrocytes and oligodendrocytes), arise from a pseudostratified epithelium of ectodermal sheet origins. Cells emerge from the neural crest and migrate to specific sites giving rise to the dorsal root ganglia, sensory ganglia of the cranial nerves, autonomic ganglia, Schwann cells, and cells of the pia and arachnoid. The characteristic migration patterns of the neural crest cells are determined by the local environment with cell adhesion and extracellular matrix molecules having a regulatory effect on cell motility and morphology.

The cerebral hemispheres develop from the region of the rostral dorsal part of the neural tube; the telencephalic pallium. The continued proliferation of the clonogenic neuroepithelial germinal cells cause the outward bulging of the pallial walls to form the cerebral vesicles. This primary radial organization is distorted by differentiation, growth of neurons and glial cells, and nerve fibers. Neurogenesis begins during fetal development with temporal differences in cell production maintained with the first-generated neurons reaching their final position earlier than subsequent generations of neurons (for review see Purves and Lichtman, 1985;

Jacobson, 1991). The laminar features of the cortex are generated over time by differential movement of groups of neurons born at different times (Hicks and D'Amato, 1968; Smart and Smart, 1982; Luskin and Shatz, 1985; Bayer and Altman, 1991). By 20–24 weeks of gestation, the cerebral cortex in the human has its full complement of neurons and connection between hemispheres is established (Rakic and Yakovlev, 1968). Given that different populations of neurons in each structure are produced at different stages of development, the timing of any given environmental stimuli can have very different effects on the final formation of each brain region.

The subplate neurons elaborate a dendritic arbor with spines, receive synaptic inputs from ascending afferents from thalamus and distant cortical sites, and extend axonal collaterals to overlying cerebral cortex and to other cortical and subcortical sites. The subplate neuron layer in frontal human cortex reaches a peak number between approximately 23 and 24 weeks of gestation. Programmed cell death of this layer appears to begin late in the third trimester, and approximately 90% of the subplate neurons disappear after approximately the sixth month of postnatal life. A slightly different and later temporal pattern exists for somatosensory and visual cortices. Given the temporal association between the significant time of development for the subplate neurons or axonal collaterals and the time of occurrence of a variety of periventricular hemorrhagic and ischemic lesions, any such lesions could alter the final pattern of neuronal organization (Volpe, 1995).

NEURONAL MIGRATION

Neuronal migration is the highly ordered process whereby millions of nerve cells move from their sites of origin in the ventricular and subventricular zones to their final central nervous system loci. The migration of neuronal precursors plays a role in establishing the identity of some neurons and defining their functional properties and connections (Sidman and Rakic, 1973). Cell translocation is achieved by a combination of the extension of the cell process, its attachment to the substratum, and the subsequent pulling of the cell by contractile proteins associated with an intracellular network of microfilaments.

In the cerebrum, migration occurs in certain areas as early as the second month and can continue until shortly after the fifth month. Radial migration of cells from their origin is responsible for the formation of the cortex and the deep nuclear structures. The radial glial cell processes serve as directional controls to guide neurons from the zone of neuronal generation to the zones for final settlement (Sidman and Rakic, 1973;

O'Rourke et al., 1992). In studies of monkey cortex, Rakic showed that the first migrating cells occupy the deepest positions and they later take up more superficial positions (Rakic 1975a, b; 1988a, b; 1990). In addition, tangential migration has been described in cells that originate in the germinal zones like the olfactory regions and migrate over the surface of the cortex coming to termination at more inward sites (Brun, 1965; Gadisseau et al., 1992).

In the cerebellum, the external granular layer forms by tangential migration followed by a stage of radial migration inward. The location of Purkinje cells, the dentate nucleus and other outer nuclei are due to radial migration along the Bergmann glia. In the formation of the cerebral cortex, cells move along radial glial cells parallel to the pial surface by lateral migration. (Luskin et al., 1988; Walsh and Cepko, 1990; 1993; Austin and Cepko, 1990). While radial glial cells serve as guides for migration of neurons, extracellular matrix molecules may play a crucial role in signaling arriving migrating neurons of the next stage of development. Such molecules associated with radial glial fibers include laminin and fibronectin (Liesi, 1990; Sheppard et al., 1991) and those with neurons, cerebroglycan (Stipp et al., 1994), and astrotactin (Fishell and Hatten, 1991). Subtle alterations in the signaling process induced by chemical exposure could have detrimental effects on the final neural network. For example, development neurotoxicants such as cadmium can produce alterations in the cellular organization of the cerebellum. Whether this is due to an alteration in neuronal migration via neuron or glial signaling needs further examination.

In the human, disorders of neuronal migration result in overt alterations in neurological function evident very early in life. The most dominant early manifestation is seizures and with the use of magnetic resonance imaging (MRI) scanning, various stages of this disorder have been identified. One hallmark of altered neuronal migration in the cerebrum is an aberration of gyral development. The most rapid period of development of the major gyri occurs between 26 and 28 weeks of gestation with elaboration continuing until shortly after birth (Chi et al., 1977). In lissencephaly, no gyri develop due to a failure of all cortical layers to receive a full complement of neurons (Norman, 1967; Aicardi, 1991; Barth, 1992; Evrard et al., 1992). Based on the anatomical features of the lesions and associated temporal exposure to teratogenic agents, the onset of this abnormality is no later than the third and fourth months of gestation (Choi et al., 1978; Aicardi, 1991). Seizures develop in the first 6 to 12 months and are characterized by infantile spasms or akinetic–myoclonic seizures with a grossly disordered electroencephalogram (EEG) – Lennox–Gastaut syndrome. With MRI there is evidence of dilation of the trigone and occipital horns, due to absence of the corpus callosum and calcarine sulci. Dilation in temporal horns of the lateral ventricles occurs due to a failure of inversion of the hippocampus (Barkovich *et al.*, 1991).

CELL ADHESION MOLECULES

Interactions between cells in direct contact and between cells and components of the intercellular matrix are mediated by cell surface adhesion molecules and cell surface recognition molecules. Additional interactions are by means of diffusible molecules such as, growth factors and trophic agents or by agents that require transport over long distances. Migration is also influenced by adhesion properties of the cells with a direct interaction between a cell and the extracellular matrix. These adhesion molecules are cell adhesion molecules (CAMs), intracellular adhesion molecules (I-CAMs), integrins and cadherins. CAMs are a family of high molecular weight cell surface glycoproteins that possesses morphoregulatory properties during neural development. The members of this family include: neural CAM (*N*-CAM), neuronal-glial GAM (Ng-GAM – NILE or L1), tenascin (TAG-1), and adhesion molecule of glia (AMOG/beta 2 isoform of the membrane Na, K-ATPase pump). *N*-CAM is detected widespread early in embryogenesis and throughout the development of the nervous system in both glia and neuronal cells (Rutishauser *et al.*, 1988). As such, it may contribute to processes such as glial guidance of axonal processes, neurite fasciculation, axon–target cell interactions, and cell positioning relationships (Rutishauser *et al.*, 1988). *N*-cadherin (A-CAM) is a member of a family of non-Ig glycoproteins that are important in cell–cell interaction functioning in a calcium-dependent manner (Grunwald *et al.*, 1980; Hatta and Takeichi, 1986; Crittenden *et al.*, 1988; Lagunowich and Grunwald, 1991). The ectoderm shows an early expression of *N*-cadherin and may serve to induce the development of the neural plate (Detrick *et al.*, 1990) and mediate closure of the neural tube. During development, *N*-cadherin plays a role in the guidance of growth cones during neurite extension (Hatta and Takeichi, 1986; Matsunaga *et al.*, 1988a, b). Altered expression of *N*-cadherin during specific times of development results in a disruption of the normal pattern of nervous system development (Duband *et al.*, 1987; Fujimori and Takeichi, 1993). *N*-cadherin has been demonstrated to be altered by exposure to inorganic lead (Lagunowich *et al.*, 1994). L1 is involved in heterotypic binding between neuronal and neuroglial cells and may be involved in fragile-X syndrome. TAG-1 is a large extracellular matrix glycoprotein implicated in cell proliferation and neural cell attachment and possibly plays a role in neurite outgrowth and cell migration.

Adhesion molecules on the cell or on the extracellular matrix mediate neurite–neurite and neurite–glial interactions and influence neurite outgrowth. In addition, a significant role has been identified for *N*-type calcium channels and glutamate receptors of the *N*-methyl-D-aspartate (NMDA) type (Komuro and Rakic, 1992; 1993; Rossi and Slater, 1993). The selective blockage of *N*-type calcium channels which are involved in the release of neurotransmitters can inhibit neuronal migration.

NEURITE OUTGROWTH

The function of the mature nervous system depends on the actions of distinct neuronal circuits which function correctly because all are connected appropriately to each other. The diversity of connections formed by a single nerve cell is one of the key features that distinguishes neurons from cells in other tissues of the body. As neuronal migration ceases, lamination occurs to insure the proper alignment, orientation, and layering of cortical neurons (Marin-Padilla, 1992). This is followed by the elaboration of dendritic and axonal ramification. Elongation of neurites occurs exclusively at their growth cones, the actively growing tip of neurites which responds to environmental cues and guides the axon to a final terminal connection. As the dendrite or axon elongate, the cell body and proximal segments of the axon or dendrite are attached and stationary, the growth cone moves through the environment and, as such, is the site of most of the interactions of the developing neuron with its environment. Alterations in the signaling mechanisms associated with growth cone motility could significantly alter the interconnections of the nervous system. In each region, the axons grow out in a characteristic and consistent direction with the final network controlled by both stimulatory and inhibitory substances (Kapfhammer and Schwab, 1992). Growth of the axon can be modulated by matrix proteoglycans (Reichardt and Tomaselli, 1991), heparin proteoglycans (Unsicker *et al.*, 1993), and chondroitin sulfate (Snow *et al.*, 1991) each of which could serve as a target site for chemical neurotoxicity. It has also been postulated that there exist specific signals to stop axon movement and initiate synapse formation (Raper and Grunewald, 1990).

After the neurons have migrated to their final positions, there is often a long delay before full differentiation of the dendrites occurs. Dendritic spines are the main postsynaptic sites on most neurons and because inhibitory and excitatory inputs are often spatially segregated on different regions of the dendrites (for review see Kandel *et al.*, 1991), each type of neuron has a distinct size and pattern of dendritic branching. Extrinsic factors that can influence the final dendritic pattern include: passive guidance by oriented structures, local conditions, active modification of extra-cellular matrix by the growth cone, growth factors, inhibition by the target site, and modification in response to nerve activity. In the human brain, dendritic growth is maximal from the late fetal periods to about one year of age and it continues at a slower pace for several years (Schade and Groenigen, 1961). In the human, dendritic development occurs earlier in the thalamus and the brain stem than in the cerebral cortical regions (Takashima et al., 1990; Mojsilovic and Zecevic, 1991). The formation of spines can be modulated by such things as sensorimotor deprivation or increased functional activity producing an increase in spines in the cerebral cortex. In ventilator-dependent premature infants a decreased number of dendritic spines, abnormally thin dendrites, and long, thin dendritic spines in the medulla oblongata can occur (Takashima and Mito, 1985). The abnormalities in Down's syndrome are alterations in cortical lamination, reduced dendritic branching and diminished dendritic spines and synapses (Marin-Padilla, 1972; Purpura, 1975; Petit et al., 1984; Wisniewski, 1990). Neurons of layers II and IV which utilize gamma-aminobutyric acid (GABA) as a neurotransmitter are deficient in number resulting in a decreased inhibitory activity in the cerebral cortex. The sequence of excessive initial branching followed by deficits is similar to certain animal models of impaired dendritic development. Fragile-X syndrome is the most common form of inherited mental retardation and is a disorder of males (Goldson and Hagerman, 1992; Tarleton and Saul, 1993). The neuropathology is limited to abnormal dendritic spine morphology of neocortical neurons. Limited data in infantile autism suggest that cortical organizational events relating to neuronal differentiation and dendritic branching are impaired (Bauman and Kemper, 1985).

SYNAPTOGENESIS

The onset of synaptogenesis occurs according to a specific timetable during the same period as dendritic outgrowth and proceeds very rapidly. The temporal sequence of the formation of synaptic connections between different neurons is correlated with the times of neuronal origin and differentiation. Synaptogenesis follows a pattern of occurring earlier in the deeper layers of the cerebral cortex and cerebellum (Jones, 1983). From prenatal period to young adulthood there is an increase in the number of synapses in many regions of the central nervous system (Aghajanian and Bloom, 1967; Brand and Rakic, 1984; Petit et al., 1984). In the frontal cortex, the maximal synaptic density is reached at two years followed by a gradual synapse

elimination of approximately 40% (Huttenlocher et al., 1982; Huttenlocher and de Courten, 1987).

Nervous system organization and dendritic differentiation are critically dependent upon the establishment of afferent input and synaptic activity (Marin-Padilla, 1970; Goodman and Shatz, 1993; Schlaggar et al., 1993). Through the manipulation of functional activity, environmental stimuli can have significant effects upon the progress and final pattern (Harris, 1981; Wiesel, 1982). Any chemical or pharmaceutical agent that alters neurotransmitter levels or functioning can result in significant alterations in the developing nervous system. Endogenous factors which have been demonstrated to influence neuronal differentiation include a variety of growth factors, neuropeptides, hormones, and cytokines (Patterson and Nawa, 1993). Alterations in such endogenous factors can be associated with chemical-induced neurotoxicity.

GLIAL CELLS AND MYELINATION

The progenitor cells of glia are cells of the ventricular/subventricular zones and radial glia. The radial glial cells proliferate and differentiate into astrocytes and may contribute to the formation of the oligodendroglia. Unlike neurons, glia may proliferate at the site of origin, and locally both during and after migration. In the process of development, astrocytes migrate from the deep cortical layers to the superficial cortical region and are essential for normal development of neurons of the upper cortical layer (Gressens et al., 1992). In addition to their role in neuronal migration, glia cells are responsible for maintaining the extracellular ionic balance for neurons and modulate neuronal function in reaction to metabolic and structural insults (for review see Hettenmann and Ransom, 1995). A critical role for astrocytes in the protection of neurons from excitotoxic injury from such things as seizures, ischemia, hypoglycemia, or neurotoxic agents is the uptake and conversion of glutamate to glutamine by the astrocyte-specific enzyme, glutamine synthetase. In the case of heavy metal exposure, the astrocyte has been known to sequester such things as lead from the neuronal environment possibly as a protective mechanism. In addition, experimental animal data suggests that the active sequestration of glutamate by astrocytes can be an early event preceeding the onset of neurodegeneration. CNS-specific organizational events set the framework for the neural network and the process of myelination (for review see Martenson, 1992; Hettenmann and Ransom, 1995). In the human brain, these occur in a peak time period from approximately the fifth month of gestation to several years after birth and may continue for many more years. The time period of myelination in the human is very long. It is initiated in the second trimester of pregnancy and continues into adult life (Gilles *et al.*, 1983). In general, the process of myelination in the CNS occurs in a descending order of spinal cord, brain stem, cerebellum, and cerebrum (Raine, 1984). For each fiber tract, a specific spatiotemporal pattern of myelination exists. Thus, the degree of myelination differs in different fiber tracts at any given stage of development. For example, in the optic nerve, myelination progresses along a retinal-to-chiasmal gradient while the spinal cord progresses along a rostral to caudal gradient. The process begins with a rapid proliferation of glia and differentiation of a subpopulation into oligodendroglia. These cells then align themselves along the axon and following various signaling processes between the two cell types, oligodendroglia and the neuronal axon, the initiation of myelination occurs (Kinney *et al.*, 1988). The myelin membrane, the oligodendroglia plasmolemma, then continues to wrap in an organized fashion around the axon forming the myelin sheath. (Bunge, 1968). The presence of this myelin sheath allows for salutatory conduction along the axon, insuring rapid transmission of signals from the periphery to the nerve body and the initiation of the correct sensory or motor response. In the peripheral nervous system, the Schwann cells initially surround bundles of axons but as the Schwann cells proliferate they become associated with fewer axons, eventually establishing a one-to-one relationship with a single axon with each Schwann cell forming an internodal segment of a single axon (Webster, H. deF., 1975). In the central nervous system, the oligodendroglia myelinates one internodal segment of many axons. During the rapid deposition of myelin a large portion of the brain's metabolic activity and protein and lipid synthesis are involved. Thus, any metabolic insult during this 'vulnerable period' could result in decreased myelin formation. If a disruption occurs during the proliferation of myelinating cells there exists an irreversible deficit of myelin-forming cells and hypomyelination. This appears to often be the case following exposure to high levels of inorganic lead, triethyltin, or hexachlorophene (see following sections). At high doses, the basic alteration is massive cerebral edema and in newborns of various species, brains became swollen with evidence of petechial hemorrhages.

CELL DEATH

Morphogenic cell death is an important natural aspect of development occurring in most regions of the CNS (Cowan *et al.*, 1984) and it plays a critical role in determining the final pattern of the neural network. It occurs during cavitation, fusion, folding, and bending of the neural plate and neural tube. A large number of cells die during reduction in the thickness of the dorsal part of the neural tube. Cell death is highly dependent upon the extracellular environment, cell–cell interactions and on nutritional, hormonal, and trophic influences. Dying neurons can autophagosize or undergo apoptosis (Clarke and Hornung, 1989). Any alteration or failure of this process could have major deleterious effects on normal brain development and subsequent functioning.

Factors which seem to play a major role in determining this process are associated with the competition between neurons for a limited supply of trophic factors and target sites. The selective loss of neurons serves two major functions during development. First, it insures the proper number of interconnecting populations of neurons and second, it insures that any aberrant or incorrect connection is eliminated (Catsicas *et al.*, 1987; Oppenheim, 1991; Allsopp, 1993; Janner and Burke, 1993). Although neurons originate, migrate, and differentiate in the absence of their normal targets, such an absence of synaptic connections will result in a neuron's death. Multiple connections provide multiple sources of trophic factors and allow the cell to adjust for the loss of one synaptic target site by the retraction or elimination of the axon or of the collaterals.

In addition to the generation of an abundant number of neurons to maximize the occurrence of correct connections and network formation, the nervous system initially forms an abundance of neuronal processes and synapses. This second stage of neural organization refinement is characterized by the removal of terminal axonal branches and their synapses. While many of the factors involved in neuronal death are thought to play a role in synapse elimination, activation of the NMDA receptor has been demonstrated to play an important part (Rabacchi *et al.*, 1992). It is likely that these regressive events can be modified and various neurons and synapses retained if required. This process of 'plasticity' in the developing brain gradually decreases as the developing brain completes its process of organization (Purves and Lichtman, 1980; Kolb and Whishaw, 1989; Oppenheim, 1991; Oppenheim *et al.*, 1992). In addition, if the brain is still in the mode to carry out organizational events, an injury may stimulate the system to generate new projections and synapses. In support of this theory is the observation of the development of ipsilateral corticospinal tract projections following neonatal motor cortex ablation (Barth and Stanfield, 1990; Ono *et al.*, 1990, 1991). In children, it has been demonstrated that hemiparesis caused by cerebral anoxia at birth can be modified by motor neuron input from the spared ipsilateral motor cortex (Lewine *et al.*, 1994).

Development of the brain proceeds by a complex and regulated process. During this time, major features include the establishment and differentiation of the subplate neurons, proper alignment, orientation, and layering of cortical neurons, dendritic elaboration and axonal ramifications, synaptic contact formation, cell death and selective elimination of neuronal processes and synapses, and the proliferation and differentiation of glia. Perturbations at any stage of this process can manifest as a spectrum of effects including retardation, gross malformations, and dramatic or very subtle alterations in the motor, sensory, or cognitive functioning of the organism. Manifestation of neurotoxicity following developmental exposure can depend on the time at which exposure occurs including, not only the external exposure incident, but also the distribution and kinetics of the chemical in the nervous system. Many chemicals can have a relatively long half-life in the brain especially with regard to the active stages of development. The remainder of the chapter will present examples of known neurotoxic effects of pharmacological and environmental chemicals for consideration in any future evaluation of possible neurotoxicity during development. Both human clinical observations and limited examples of experimental animal data will be presented to demonstrate possible biological processes as chemical target sites.

ENVIRONMENTAL-INDUCED ALTERATIONS IN THE DEVELOPING NERVOUS SYSTEM: HUMAN CLINICAL OBSERVATIONS AND ANIMAL EXPERIMENTAL DATA

Chemical exposure during development

The developing human can be adversely affected by body burdens of environmental chemicals that do not affect the adult (Fein et al., 1984). The toxic effects seen in the developing human can be more varied, more severe, and more debilitating than those seen in the adult (Hara, 1985; Hsu et al., 1985; Rogan et al., 1988; Driscoll et al., 1990). In the human infant, several studies have provided evidence supporting the concept of a critical period from birth to about two years of age during which the nervous system is most vulnerable to malnutrition and not responsive to nutritional therapy. In addition, the developing nervous system can be much more susceptible to damage due to the immaturity of the blood–brain barrier (BBB). This immature barrier can allow passage of chemicals into the brain that may not gain access in the adult. For example, paraquat, exposure in two week old rats resulted in a higher brain concentration as compared to exposure of three month old animals (Corasaniti et al., 1991). The BBB of the developing animal has been reported to be 'less tight' with regard to cadmium than that of the mature animal (Arvidson, 1986). The pattern of susceptibility of neurons, petechial hemorrhages, and endothelial vacuolation following postnatal

exposure to cadmium is thought to parallel the maturation of capillaries in the brain parenchyma (Valois and Webster, 1987). The vulnerability of the developing nervous system to various factors is determined by the developmental stage of the cellular activities targeted by a specific insult. No one vulnerable period can be identified, it will vary depending on the agent and the timetable of developmental events in different species (for review see Davis and Dobbing, 1974). These toxic effects can alter the quality of life and productivity over an entire lifespan (Spyker, 1975).

Children can have exposure to chemicals by direct contact or indirectly through the parents. This exposure can occur during gestation, lactation and even from the clothing and body surfaces of parents exposed in an occupational setting. The fetus can be exposed to both nutrients and xenobiotics via the maternal circulation. The main route of exposure is trans-placental. The placenta is metabolically active toward xenobiotics and the nature of the compounds reaching the fetal circulation may depend on multiple placental biotransformation reactions. Chemical exposure in utero can be manifested as altered newborn growth and functional development. It needs to be noted that exposure to a chemical during pregnancy may not necessarily result in any observable alteration within a short time period after birth but may instead take years before the toxicity becomes overt. One classic example of this was the use of diethylstilbestrol during pregnancy to prevent miscarriage. It was found that female fetuses exposed to diethylstilbestrol are at an increased risk for adenocarcinoma of the vagina. This type of malignancy is not discovered until after puberty (Herbst et al., 1971). Additional clinical findings indicate that male offspring were not spared from the effects of the drug with abnormalities of the reproductive system.

It is well established that drugs are excreted into the breast milk and are bioavailable to the infant. In much the same fashion, environmental chemicals can be transferred to the nursing infant. Exposure during lactation has also been known to result in persistent toxicity. While breastfeeding offers many positive features to the newborn, it also can serve as a source of infant exposure to drugs and chemicals. Often the amount of drug present in maternal milk is only a small fraction of the adult intake (Riordan and Riordan, 1984). Environmental exposure via breastfeeding may be chronic and consequently more toxic, unlike therapeutic agents that can be voluntarily terminated (Wilson et al., 1980; Wilson, 1983). The amount of drug that is available for transfer to milk is dependent on certain maternal factors such as dosage, frequency, and route of administration and all other pharmacokinetic principles of absorption, distribution, metabolism, and excretion (Riordan and Riordan, 1984; Nation and Hotham, 1987). In addition to the pharmacokinetic factors of the mother, the flow and pH of blood to the breast, the composition and pH of milk, and the rate of milk production and resorption of the drug from milk into the maternal circulation are factors that affect the amount of drug delivery to the child. General factors that may influence breast milk concentrations include maternal age, parity, maternal body weight, and fat content of the breast milk (Sim and McNeil, 1992). Human milk is a suspension of fat and protein in a carbohydrate–mineral solution. Milk proteins are fully synthesized from substrate delivered from the maternal circulation with the major proteins identified as casein and lactalbumin. Drug excretion into milk may be accomplished by binding to the proteins, lipids, or onto the surface of the milk fat globule.

The physiochemical features of the compound are the most important factors influencing drug excretion into the breast milk (Giacola and Catz, 1979). Such things as degree of ionization, molecular weight, lipid solubility, and protein binding capacity will affect the ability of the chemical to traverse the mammary gland epithelium. The mechanisms that determine the concentration of a drug in breast milk are similar to those existing elsewhere within the organism. Drugs traverse membranes primarily by passive diffusion and the concentration achieved is dependent upon the concentration gradient and on the intrinsic lipid solubility of the drug and its degree of ionization, as well as binding to protein and other cellular constituents. In general, drugs and chemicals bind more readily to plasma proteins than to milk proteins thus, the dosage to the infant is dependent upon the degree of plasma protein binding of the drug.

For drugs that bind to milk proteins, accumulation and delayed responsiveness must be considered. For example, exposure via breast milk to the fungicide, hexachlorobenzene, resulted in manifestations of hexachlorobenzene-induced porphyria cutanea tarda including hyperpigmentation and severe scarring of the face and hands continuing for 25 years (Gocmen et al., 1989). The human maternal ingestion of hexachlorobenzene via treated wheat in Turkey resulted in chemical accumulation of the fungicide in breast milk and infants showing symptoms of a disease called pembe yara and the condition porphyria cutanea tarda. In rats, maternal transfer of hexachlorobenzene has been demonstrated. Tissue concentrations in rat fetuses reflect maternal blood concentrations whereas the tissue concentrations in neonates can be elevated up to 10-fold due to the storage of hexachlorobenzene in maternal adipose tissue and the rapid transfer to the suckling neonates via the milk (Goldey and Taylor, 1992). The evaluation of potential risk of toxicity on the child must consider all exposure routes both during pregnancy and after birth.

Undernutrition

General factors like undernutrition can have maximal effects on processes that are most active during what has been called the 'brain growth spurt' (Dobbing and Sands, 1979). Thus, the target site for chemical injury depends on the developmental process ongoing at the time of exposure. For example, myelination occurs mainly postnatally in both human and rat and continues for the same time relative to lifespan. This extended process of myelination appears to be extremely sensitive to undernutritional factors over a broad time frame of development. While the effects of malnutrition on the cerebral cortex of the rat are correlated with the times of development of different neurons, layer V pyramidal cells are affected most in the early postnatal age; layer III pyramidal cells at early and later postnatal ages; and interneurons during the late postnatal age.

The most striking effects of developmental undernutrition are the reduction in number of dendritic spines and number of synapses per neuron (Warren and Bedi, 1982; Bedi et al., 1980). In rats, malnutrition during the first two to three weeks after birth results in a 30% deficit in the synapse-to-neuron ratio in the cerebral cortex which is augmented by rearing in isolation (Warren and Bedi, 1982). In the mouse, severe neonatal malnutrition can result in the loss of neurons and axon terminals (Cragg, 1972). The reduced myelination in the corpus callosum is associated with a reduction in number of oligodendrocytes. There is a reduction in total myelin proteins and gangliosides. In the peripheral nervous system, the Schwann cell ultrastructure is abnormal and the number of myelin lamellae is reduced.

Alterations in thyroid hormone

The thyroid gland produces two hormones, L-thyroxine (T4) and L-triiodothyronine (T3). Thyroxine is the main circulating form but it is converted to T3 which is the active hormone. T3 receptors are expressed on neurons in the mammalian brain during the fetal period while neuron production is active. The receptors continue to be expressed on both neurons and glia throughout the postnatal period. Thyroid hormone stimulates neural development in several ways: increasing cell proliferation, synthesis of microtubule-associated proteins (MAPs) and tubulin, increasing microtubule assembly, inducing axonal and dendritic outgrowth, synaptogenesis, and myelination.

T3 receptors are detectable in the rat brain on gestational day 20 (Schwartz and Oppenheimer, 1978) and the density reaches a maximum at birth in the cerebellum and at postnatal day nine (PND9) in the cerebrum and falls to adult levels by PND30. In humans, the neuron production in the cerebral cortex continues until 25 weeks of gestation and the T3 receptors are detected as early as 10 weeks gestation and increase substantially for the next 6 weeks (Bernal and Pekonen, 1984). In the adult mammalian nervous system, there is a high level of expression of the T3 receptor in the hippocampus, amygdala, and cerebral neocortex (Ruel et al., 1985). T4 has a general action of increasing metabolic rate and enhancing tubulin synthesis thus promoting neurite outgrowth. There are several reports of reduced axonal and dendritic growth in hypothyroid rats and of the converse in hyperthyroid rats. In hypothyroid rats, there is a reduction in length of parallel fibers and diminished branching of Purkinje cell dendrites (Nicholson and Altman, 1972). Thyroid hormone treatment of neonatal rats increases the size of cell body and dendrites of pyramidal cells in area CA3 of the hippocampus (Gould et al., 1990).

Neonatal thyroidectomy of rats decreases myelination, reduces neuronal volume with no change in number, and decreases dendritic branching and number of axodendritic synapses in the cerebral cortex (Balaza et al., 1971) resulting in a decrease in brain growth after day 14. In the cerebellum of hypothroid rats there is a reduction in the number of synapses in the molecular layer (Nicholson and Altman, 1972). However, the cerebellar axodendritic synapses appear normal and the effect is on dendritic growth. The rate of migration of granule cells in the cerebellum and outgrowth of parallel fibers is slowed resulting in a decrease in length of fibers and possible inability to make adequate connections with Purkinje cell dendritic spines. This would lead to subsequent granule cell death. This retardation of neuronal migration may be associated with the concurrent retardation of differentiation of cerebellar astrocytes (Clos et al., 1982). This would include effects on the Bergmann glial cells which are necessary for granule cell migration. Postnatal treatment of rats with T4 produces a decrease in brain weight, body weight, acceleration in the histogenesis and morphogenesis of the cerebellar cortex (Nicholson and Altman, 1972), increase in the number of dendritic spines in layer IV of the visual cortex (Schapiro et al., 1973) and an increase in S100 astrocyte protein in the cerebellum (Clos et al., 1982). The decrease in brain weight has been found to be due to a 30–40% reduction in the number of brain cells formed after birth.

Thyroid hormone receptors are present in neurons of the hippocampal formation so this brain region is very sensitive to alterations in the levels of thyroid hormones during development. Hyperthyroidism in newborn rats results in overgrowth of the hippocampal granule cell axons, the mossy fibers, which synapse on the hippocampal pyramidal cell dendrites (Lauder and Mugnaini, 1980). In hypothyroidism, the mossy fibers appear normal while the volume of the hippocampus is decreased as the result of less granule cells. The primary effect of hypothyroidism of the developing cerebellum is the stunting of dendritic development, reduced outgrowth of parallel fibers leading to a failure in synaptogenesis, death of some granule cells, basket cells, and stellate cells. Similar effects are seen in the development of the cerebrum with retardation of differentiation and growth resulting in a reduction of dendritic growth and synaptogenesis.

Ionization

The effects of acute exposure to ionizing radiation on the brain and in the induction of cancer vary with the age at exposure. The developing brain is susceptible to severe mental retardation primarily from the eighth to the 15th week of gestation and to small head size from the fourth to 15th week (Plummer, 1952; Miller, 1956; Miller and Mulvihill, 1976). In these studies and on follow-up examinations, severe mental retardation was defined as the inability to perform simple calculations, to converse, and to care for oneself. The small head size was determined as a circumference of two or more standard deviations below normal mean size. The severe mental retardation was suggested to be due to impairment in the proliferation and migration of neurons from near the cerebral ventricles to the cortex (Otake and Schull, 1984). The small brain size in the absence of severe mental retardation was attributed to the death of glial cells. IQ test scores and school performance suggest a dose–response relationship with gestational age of exposure (Otake et al., 1988; Schull and Otake, 1986). From these studies and animal experimental data, it has been speculated that the outcome of exposure to ionizing radiation in humans of mental retardation and small head size lasts for 8 and 14 weeks, respectively. In contrast, susceptibility of other organs to teratogenesis induced by ionization is more time limited, for example, from the 20th to the 32nd day of gestation.

Hexachlorophene (HCP)

2,2′-Methylenebis (3,4,6-trichlorophenol) is an antimicrobial agent that has been previously used in soaps and detergents and was used in the bathing of newborn babies to prevent bacterial infections. Intoxication with hexachlorophene has resulted from either dermal application or ingestion of liquid detergents containing high concentrations. Dermal application has produced intoxication in patients with extensive epidermal damage due to burns or ichthyosis (Korloff and Winsten, 1967; Lockhart, 1972; Mullick, 1973). Dermal application of hexachlorophene as an antibacterial agent produces no adverse effects in the normal adult. However, the topical application to children resulted in severe neurological damage (Alder et al., 1974; Tyrala et al., 1977). In some infants, application of 3–6% HCP to normal skin in the diaper area resulted in excoriation which facilitated the absorption of HCP leading to fatal intoxication. Another source of exposure was the previous use of HCP-containing solutions to bathe infants (Curley et al., 1971; Abbott et al., 1972; Kopelman, 1973). While neuropathological changes in the white matter of the brain can be seen in adults with epidermal damage, the brains of low birth-weight premature infants are highly susceptible to the effects of HCP. In premature infants weighing less than 1400 g, bathing with HCP produced vacuolization of myelin in the brain stem (Powell et al., 1973; Shuman et al., 1975). Dermal hexachlorophene exposure produces edema of the myelin sheath in young rats. This is evident once a site for fluid accumulation, the interperiod line of the myelin wrapping, has developed and offers a hydrophobic reservoir for the compound (Nieminen et al., 1973).

Triethyltin (TET)

Another chemical which alters myelination in a manner similar to hexachlorophene is the organo-tin compound, triethyltin. When older animals (postnatal day 8) were exposed, both the hemorrhagic and necrotic changes occurred. However, damage was seen in the myelinated fibers of the brain stem and cerebellum. The morphological alteration in myelin dissipates over time but biochemical evidence suggests that the amount of myelin produced is decreased and myelin protein deficits persist until adulthood (Toews et al., 1983). Exposure of PND5 rat pups induced an anterior–posterior atrophy of the brain with cortical thinning and degenerative neuronal changes, infiltration of microglia, and increased cellular density in the cortex (Reuhl and Cranmer, 1984; Veronesi and Bondy, 1986).

Lead

One of the classic examples of differential susceptibility of the developing organism to the effects of an environmental chemical is that of inorganic lead exposure. By comparison to adults, children are more vulnerable to lead in terms of external exposure sources, internal levels of lead, timing of exposures during development, and exposure level at which an adverse effect occurs. Lead readily crosses the placenta so that the developing fetus may be at a high risk of exposure to toxic lead levels without any adverse effects being seen in the mother. Several studies have found significant correlation between maternal and neonatal/

umbilical cord blood lead levels. The coefficients are generally in the area of about 0.60 to 0.70 and neonatal concentrations usually averaging about 70–80% of maternal blood lead levels (Ong et al., 1985; Korpela et al., 1986; Schramel et al., 1988; Sikorski et al., 1988; Truska et al., 1989). In a long-term follow-up study, Needleman et al. (1990) found that lead-exposed children continued to show a significant inverse relationship between previous dentine lead concentrations and school performance. The follow-up data also revealed several neuropsychological deficits of poor eye–hand coordination, longer reaction times, and slower finger tapping rates.

While exposure occurs in utero it also occurs much earlier due to the fact that lead is stored in body compartments such as bone. This body burden of lead from previous exposure can be mobilized during pregnancy and transferred from the mother to the fetus (Manton, 1985; Silbergeld et al., 1988; Mahaffey, 1991). In utero, the fetus accumulates lead from about the 12th week of gestation (Baltrop, 1969) thus sufficient stores of lead in the bone and other tissues at birth provide an internal exposure to the neonate in the absence of any current exogenous exposure.

After birth and until about six months of age, exposure is dominated by dietary sources of lead via the mother's milk or formula although each is relatively low (Rye et al., 1983; Rabinowitz et al., 1985; Sternowsky and Wessolowski, 1985; Dabeka and McKenzie, 1987). However, use of lead-contaminated tap water in preparing infant formula can result in elevated exposure levels (Lacey et al., 1985; Shannon and Graef, 1989). Children can also be exposed to relatively high levels of lead via inhalation. While many of the exposure routes are similar for adults and children the internal levels of lead with exposure to a given concentration of lead in the external environment tend to be higher for children. Factors such as higher metabolic rate, turnover in blood lead, blood volume, affinity of fetal/neonatal hemoglobin for lead, and nutritional factors contribute to the greater uptake of lead in children (for review see US Environmental Protection Agency, 1986). Lead is absorbed in inverse relationship to the availability of iron, calcium, phosphorus, zinc, and copper in the diet (Mahaffey, 1980; 1990) and enhanced with diets rich in lipids (Barltrop and Khoo, 1975). Milk components and vitamin D levels can modulate lead absorption (Nzelibe et al., 1986; US Environmental Protection Agency, 1986; Fullmer, 1991).

The central nervous system has been identified as a target site for lead's adverse effects in the developing organism. Lead induces encephalopathy in children at high exposure levels and can be life threatening. The importance of calcium–lead interactions in lead neurotoxicity have been identified (Bressler and Goldstein, 1991) and its interference in the developmental sequence of events in the early structuring of the brain as directed by regulatory proteins (Markovac and Goldstein, 1988; Regan et al., 1989)

Experimental animal studies have allowed for the examination of various specific target sites and processes of development that may be susceptible to lead toxicity. Subtle neuronal changes following developmental exposure to lead include reduction in hippocampal axonal and dendritic arborization (Petit et al., 1983) and synaptic elaboration (Petit and LeBoutillier, 1979). Similar reductions have been reported for cortical ontogenesis (Krigman and Hogan, 1974) and synaptic elaboration (McCauley et al., 1982; Bull et al., 1983). Developmental alterations are not limited to the neuronal population. The astroglial cell population has been shown to be altered following lead exposure. Krigman and Hogan (1974) reported an increase in the number of astroglia in the cortex while others report both structural and functional changes of astroglia in response to lead exposure (Dave et al., 1993; Legare et al., 1993; Buchheim et al., 1994). Recently, it has been reported that early developmental exposure to lead acetate results in a disruption of the normal developmental profile of expression for both GAP-43 mRNA, a protein associated with the axonal growth cone (Schmitt et al., 1996) and the astrocyte-specific GFAP mRNA (glial fibrillary acidic protein; Harry et al., 1996). Postnatal lead exposure has been reported to cause abnormalities in the development of cerebellar Purkinje neuron dendrites which may be related to differences in the development of synaptic contacts with these neurons. During development, the accumulation of brain myelin is decreased resulting in a decrement of myelin in the adult nervous system (Toews et al., 1983).

Polyhalogenated biphenyls (PHBs)

The PHBs are found in all environments and populations throughout the world (Safe, 1984; Fries, 1985). Once in the environment they persist for decades in the soil and water (Safe, 1984; Fries et al., 1986). The PHBs are stored primarily in adipose tissue and bioaccumulate in mammals due to long half-lives of approximately 12 years. The half-lives in children have not been determined. The process of bioconcentration greatly adds to the exposure of the human. Due to transplacental passage, the newborn has serum PHB levels similar to the mother's serum level when expressed on a serum lipid basis (Masuda et al., 1978).

The PHBs are preferentially stored and excreted in the breast milk lipids. In the United States breast samples contain levels of PHB higher than the regulation levels in cow's milk intended for human consumption (for review see Rogan, 1996). Four-year-old children who are breastfed for at least 12 months have 17 times the PHB serum levels of children not breastfed. The continuation of breastfeeding for 12 months results in levels four times higher than in children who breastfeed for only six months (Jacobson et al., 1990a). Multigenerational PHB exposure is an important concern in humans. This is the result of a combination of the long half-lives of PHBs, their bioaccummulation, and bioconcentration, and their transfer through the placenta and breast milk. Compounds like polychlorinated biphenyls (PCBs) and dicophane (DDT), which are absorbable and resistant to metabolism or excretions and have become widespread environmental contaminants, can appear with high prevalence in the milk of the mother. Human milk is usually 1–4% fat and is in equilibrium with the other fat stores of the body, and highly lipid soluble chemicals like PCBs, DDT, and dieldrin have been shown to appear in the fat of a high percentage of human milk samples (Rogan, 1996). The amounts are generally in the milligram per kilogram of fat range, or in parts per billion of whole milk. While no disease has been associated with exposure at these levels, our knowledge and ability to detect subtle alterations limits our ability to discount this route of exposure as safe for the infant. In fact, high concentrations of other organochlorine insecticides including DDT, dieldrin, lindane, and chlordane have been found in breast milk. A metabolite of DDT, 1,1-dichloro-2,2-bis(4-chlorophenyl)ethylene (DDE), has been demonstrated to produce hyporeflexia in human infants (Rogan et al., 1986).

The toxic effects of PHBs in the human are dependent upon the congener-specific mixture of PHBs. The toxicity may be due to one PHB or the combination and interaction of several PHBs. The PHBs have been linked to toxicities of almost all organ systems (Masuda and Yoshimura, 1984). The most severe adverse effects seen in the human are the developmental toxicities. Intrauterine growth retardation has been reported in the Yu-cheng and Yusho populations (Yamaguchi et al., 1971; Rogan et al., 1988) and the PCB Michigan fish-eater population (Fein et al., 1984). Head circumference reduction at birth was noted in both populations and in the Michigan population the head circumference was at control size by four years of age (Jacobson et al., 1990b). The ingestion of polychlorinated biphenyl-contaminated rice oil during pregnancy and lactation resulted in low birth-weight infants, growth retardation, abnormal skin pigmentation, and bone and tooth defects (Yamaguchi et al., 1971). The levels of polychlorinated biphenyls in human milk were found to be associated with hypotonicity and hyporeflexia in the nursing infants (Rogan et al., 1986).

Neurobehavioral deficits have been the most common functional birth defect in the offspring exposed to various PHBs in utero (Tilson et al., 1990). Functional neurological deficits have been identified in the Michigan cohort (Jacobson *et al.*, 1984; 1985; 1990a; 1990b) the Yu-cheng cohort (Rogan *et al.*, 1988) and Yusho (Yamaguchi *et al.*, 1971, Yamashita and Hayashi, 1985). While neurobehavioral deficits of polybrominated biphenyls (PBB) have been noted, only one study demonstrated a dose–response relationship between PBB serum levels and subtle neurodevelopmental dysfunction (Weil *et al.*, 1981). In the North Carolina study, only pregnant females were evaluated (Rogan *et al.*, 1986). The newborns with the highest PCB breast milk levels (>3.5 ppm) had decreased scores on neurological tests and decreased motor tone and reflexes. What is interesting is that the PCB body burdens of even the highest group were well within the range of the general population. In the Michigan cohort, the newborns and children had similar altered neurological function with no effects in the mothers (Jacobson *et al.*, 1984, 1985, 1990a, b). The Yusho children exposed to PCBs and polychlorinated dibenzofurans (PCDFs) only through breast milk had decreased neurological function (Harada, 1976).

Mercury

Mercury can be categorized into inorganic and organic forms, and the toxicity can depend upon the form. In the inorganic form there is elemental mercury and its inorganic salts. Elemental mercury exists as a liquid and can readily vaporize to an odorless, colorless vapor which is heavier than air. Elemental mercury is poorly absorbed across skin, mucous membranes, and gastrointestinal epithelium and the major route of human exposure is via inhalation. Mercurous salts are also poorly absorbed following ingestion or dermal application but there have been reports of toxicity from calomel teething powders. For any form of mercury, exposure during childhood targets the nervous system producing irreversible neurologic abnormalities.

The organic form of mercury that produces major problems in the developing organism is methyl mercury (MeHg) which induces neuropathological and neurobehavioral effects that exhibit striking comparability across a number of species. During gestation, methyl mercury passes through the placenta resulting in fetal concentrations equal or exceeding the maternal concentrations (Snyder, 1971; Bakir *et al.*, 1973; Null *et al.*, 1973; Rustam and Hamdi, 1974). Some evidence suggests that mercury accumulates on the fetal side of the placenta resulting in higher concentrations in the fetus (Clarkson *et al.*, 1972; Viny *et al.*, 1990) and an accumulation in the brain (Choi, 1989). Congenital MeHg poisoning is also called fetal Minamata disease from the massive outbreak of methyl mercury poisoning in Minamata Bay and Niigata, Japan during the 1950s. Ingestion of mercury-contaminated fish from Minamata Bay resulted in contamination of the

mother's milk and severe neurological disorders in the human infant (Matsumoto *et al.*, 1965). Humans exposed to methyl mercury during development exhibit sensory deficits, mental deficiency, cerebral palsy, seizures, and spasticity at high exposure levels. At slightly lower doses (3–11 ppm) the effects are characterized by mental deficiency, reflex and muscle tone abnormalities, and delayed motor development. At even lower doses (0.1–3 ppm) a delay in psychomotor development was seen. The brains of a young child or infant with Minamata disease showed widespread neuronal damage with associated gliosis and cytoarchitectural abnormalities such as ectopic cell masses and disorganization of the cortical layers (Eto and Takeuchi, 1978). The cases of Minamata disease have similar disturbances in neuronal migration, defective lamination of the cerebral cortex, changes in the pattern of the cerebral gyri, and either gliosis or neuroglial heterotopias. It has been proposed that organomercurials induce their effects by inhibiting neuronal migration. Once neuronal migration has been disrupted, normal development cannot occur and the neurotoxic effects are not reversible. In addition to a disorganization in neurons, methyl mercury induces a reduction in brain size, ventricular dilation, disorganized cortical layering, ectopic cells, and necrosis resulting in altered behavioral functioning (Burbacher *et al.*, 1990).

The massive epidemic of methyl mercury poisoning in Iraq during 1971–1972 resulted in thousands of people poisoned and hundreds of deaths (Bakir *et al.*, 1973; Clarkson *et al.*, 1976). Symptoms of poisoning occurred a month or more after people started eating bread made from contaminated grain (Rustam and Hamdi, 1974; Clarkson *et al.*, 1976). Mothers were exposed for several months during pregnancy and 84 pairs of mothers and infants were evaluated (Marsh *et al.*, 1981). In general, the threshold for minimal abnormal neurologic signs was between 68 and 180 ppm methyl mercury in maternal hair. Severe neurologic impairment was seen in children when maternal peak hair mercury values were above 165 ppm and were the most severe with highest exposures during the second trimester of pregnancy (Marsh, 1987). The effects of paresthesis and anxiety were dose related and transient in the mothers while the infants suffered permanent, devastating, psychomotor retardation. Symptoms of poisoning included seizures and motor, speech, and mental retardation. Additional symptoms were manifest with higher peak maternal hair concentrations. The major neuropathological findings included disturbances of neuronal migration and laminar cortical organization in the cerebrum and cerebellum, and were reported in the infants born to mothers who had ingested methyl mercury-contaminated bread during pregnancy (Choi *et al.*, 1978). While this has been difficult to confirm in an experimental model, a transient inhibition of neuronal migration has been reported in exposed rodent pups. However, by weaning, the cytoarchitecture of the brain appears normal (Inouye et al., 1985; for review see Tilson and Sparber, 1987). Since it has been difficult to confirm permanent neuronal misplacement research efforts have been directed toward processes known to be intricately involved in neuronal migration. Interest has focused on components of the cytoskeleton, in particular the microtubular system. Microtubules are cytoplasmic organelles involved in mitosis, cell movement, process formation, and axonal transport. A loss of microtubules could interfere with neuronal migration in several ways including the disruption of microtubule-dependent cell–cell communication required for oriented neuronal movement. A delay in neuronal mitosis could result in neurons migrating asynchronously with other parts of the brain. In postmigratory neurons, exposure to MeHg could result in disassembled microtubules in neurites altering dendritic aborization, synaptic organization or cell activities.

Neural–immune interactions

Another newly identified link between the periphery and the nervous system is the presence of resident immune competent cells in the brain. A major initiator of the cytokine cascade is tumor necrosis factor (TNF). Cells in the brain make tumor necrosis factor in response to endotoxin or physical injury and thus may play a role in the host-resistance response of the brain. TNF has been found in the cerebrospinal fluid (CSF) of newborns with Gram-negative bacterial meningitis (McCracken et al., 1989) and in the blood of preterm infants with necrotizing enterocolitis (Caplan et al., 1990). In these conditions, TNF alpha may cause damage to the brain by hypotension/ischemia. Ischemic foci may be due to intravascular coagulation of macrocapillaries (Tracey et al., 1987), endothelial cell activation (Cavender et al., 1989) and increased expression of adhesion molecules (Parsons et al., 1989; Wellicome et al., 1990; Robaye et al., 1991). The production of platelet activating factor (PAF) by TNF alpha may result in cytotoxicity (Camussi et al., 1987; Kornecki and Ehrlich, 1988), membrane destruction (Sawyer and Andersen, 1989), vasoconstriction (Armstead et al., 1988) and increase the permeability of the blood–brain barrier (Kumar et al., 1988). TNF has dramatic effects on the various glial cells of the brain. It increases proliferation of astrocytes and initiates the destruction of the myelinating cells of the brain, the oligodendrocytes (Robbins et al., 1987; Selmaj et al., 1988) and is found in brain tissue in childhood subacute sclerosing panencephalitis (Hofman et al., 1991). Whether circulating levels of TNF in the maternal blood can cross the placental barrier and influence the developing fetus is still to be determined.

Lesions of the white matter in human newborn infants with Gram-negative sepsis (Gilles and Kassirer, 1976; Gilles et al., 1977) and the increased risk of periventricular leukomalacia in the newborn associated with maternal infection (Bejar et al., 1988, 1992) suggest that this is a entirely new area of examination that will need to be addressed. In addition, the multitude of chemicals that have been shown to increase cytokine levels in the body and the effect of stress on these factors identify a set of environmental factors that could contribute as some of the indirect effects of neurotoxicant exposure during development.

SUMMARY

In many cases, the underlying mechanisms responsible for neurotoxicity have yet to be determined. However, when a substance alters the sensory or motor functions, disrupts the processes of learning and memory, or produces detrimental behavioral effects, it is characterized as neurotoxic. The vulnerability of the developing nervous system to toxic substances is due to a number of characteristics inherent in the biological system, and minor changes in the structure and function of the nervous system can lead to profound consequences for neurological, behavioral, and related body functions. In the perinatal period, insults that frequently occur are premature birth, hypoxia-ischemia, acidosis, intracranial hemorrhage, posthemorrhagic hydrocephalus, infection, undernutrition, administration of various drugs and hormones, sensory deprivation or stimulation. Many of the insults known to damage the developing brain interfere with one or more of the developmental processes of the brain: neuronal proliferation and migration, formation of the blood–brain barrier, synaptogenesis, myelination, and development of the cerebral circulation and programmed cell death.

In a rapidly developing tissue, chemicals may cause both injury to an already developed structure as well as derangement of later development. Toxic agents with antimitotic action, such as X-rays and methyl mercury, have distinctly different effects on structure depending on which neurons are forming at the time of exposure. Vulnerability to agents that interfere with cell production decreases rapidly over the early postnatal period. Other toxic substances, such as lead, seem to have their greatest effects during even later stages of brain development perhaps by altering the process of synaptic pruning. It is also possible that a destructive event during early development may result in a less active cellular response to tissue destruction resulting in a less detectable morphological alteration. It is crucial that attention be given to events that include adverse effects that can be subtle, unexpected, delayed, and affect the psychological functioning of the offspring.

Studies designed to compare sensitivity to toxic agents during development with that of the adult must consider the above factors along with those that more directly influence sensitivity, for example, metabolic capability, growth and repair processes, functional maturity, or genetic differences in susceptibility.

REFERENCES

Abbott, L.M., Buckfield, P.M., Ferry, D.G., Malcolm, D.S. and McQueen, E.G. 1972: Blood levels of hexachlorophene in neonates. *Australian Pediatric Journal*, **8**, 246.

Aghajanian, G.K. and Bloom, F.E. 1967: The formation of developing junctions in developing rat brain. A quantitative electron microscopic study. *Brain Research*, **6**, 716–26.

Aicardi, J. 1991: The agyria-pachygyria complex: a spectrum of cortical malformations. *Brain Development*, **13**, 1–8.

Alder, V.G. and Gillespies, W.T. 1974: Proceedings: absorption of hexachlorophane from newborn infants' skin. *Journal of Clinical Pathology*, **27**, 931.

Allsopp, T. 1993: Life and death in the nervous system. *Trends in Neurosciences*, **16**, 1–4.

Armstead, W.M., Pourcyrous, M., Mirro, R., Leffler, C.W. and Busija, D.W. 1988: Platelet activating factor: a potent constrictor of cerebral arterioles in newborn pigs. *Circulation Research*, **62**, 1–7.

Arvidson, B. 1986: Autoradiographic localization of cadmium in the rat brain. *Neurotoxicology*, **7**, 89–99.

Austin, C.P. and Cepko, C.L. 1990: Cellular migration patterns in the developing mouse cerebral cortex. *Development*, **110**, 713–32.

Bakir, F., Damluji, S.F., Amin-Zaki, L. *et al.* 1973: Methyl mercury poisoning in Iraq. *Science*, **181**, 230–41.

Balaza, R., Kovacs, S., Cocks, W.A., Johnson, A.L. and Eayrs, J.T. 1971: Effect of thyroid hormone on the biochemical maturation of rat brain: postnatal cell formation. *Brain Research*, **25**, 555–70.

Baltrop, D. 1969: Transfer of lead to the human foetus. In *Mineral Metabolism in Pediatrics*, Baltrop, D. and Burland, W.L. (eds), pp 135–51. Philadelphia, PA: F.A. Davis Co.

Baltrop, D. and Khoo, H.E. 1975: Nutritional determinants of lead absorption. In *Trace Substances in Environmental Health – IX*, Hemphill, D.D. (ed.). Columbia, MO: University of Missouri.

Barkovich, A.J., Koch, T.K. and Carrol, C.L. 1991: The spectrum of lissencephaly: report of 10 patients analyzed by magnetic resonance imaging. *Annuals of Neurology*, **30**, 139–40.

Barth, P.G. 1992: Schizencephaly and nonlissencephalic cortical dysplasias. *American Journal of Neuroradiology*, **13**, 104–6.

Barth, T.M. and Stanfield, B.B. 1990: The recovery of forelimb-placing behavior in rats with neonatal unilateral cortical damage involves the remaining hemisphere. *Journal Neuroscience*, **10**, 3449–59.

Bauman, M. and Kemper, T.L. 1985: Histoanatomic observations of the brain in early infantile autism. *Neurology*, **35**, 866–74.

Bayer, S. and Altman, J. 1991: *Neocortical Development*. New York: Raven Press.

Bedi, K.A., Hall, R., Davies, C.A. and Dobbing, J. 1980: A steriological analysis of the cerebellar granule and Purkinje cells of 30-day-old and adult rats undernourished during early postnatal life. *Journal of Comparative Neurology*, **193**, 863–70.

Bejar, R., Wolzniak, P., Allard, M. *et al.* 1988: Antenatal origin of neurologic damage in newborn infants. I: Preterm infants. *American Journal of Obstetrics and Gynecology*, **159**, 357–63.

Bejar, R.F., Vaucher, T.E., Benirschke, K. and Berry, C.C. 1992: Postnatal white matter necrosis in preterm infants. *Journal of Perinatology*, **12**, 3–6.

Bernal, J. and Pekonen, F. 1984: Ontogenesis of the nuclear 3,5,3′-tri odothyromine receptor in the human fetal brain. *Endocrinology*, **114**, 677–9.

Brand, S. and Rakic, P. 1984: Cytodifferentiation and synaptogenesis in the neostriatum of fetal and neonatal rhesus monkeys. *Anatomical Embryology*, **196**, 21–34.

Bressler, J.P. and Goldstein, G.W. 1991: Mechanism of lead neurotoxicity. *Biochemical Pharmacology*, **41**, 479–84.

Brun, A. 1965: The subpial granular layer of the foetal cerebral cortex in man. *Acta Pathology Microbiology Scandanavia*, **179**, 3–98.

Buchheim, K., Noack, S., Stoltenburg, G., Lilienthal, H. and Winneke, G. 1994: Developmental delay of astrocytes in hippocampus of rhesus monkeys reflects the effect of pre- and postnatal chronic low-level lead exposure. *Neurotoxicology*, **15**, 665–9.

Bull, R., McCauley, P., Taylor, D. and Croften, K. 1983: The effects of lead on the developing central nervous system of the rat. *Neurotoxicology*, **4**, 1–18.

Bunge, R.P. 1968: Glial cells and the central myelin sheath. *Physiology Review*, **48**, 197–251.

Burbacher, T.M., Rodier, P.M. and Weiss, B. 1990: Methyl mercury developmental neurotoxicity: a comparison of effects in humans and animals. *Neurotoxicology and Teratology*, **12**, 191–202.

Camussi, G., Bussolino, F., Salvidio, G. and Baglinoni, C. 1987: Tumor necrosis factor/cachectin stimulates peritoneal macrophages, polymorphonuclear neurophils, and vascular endothelial cells to synthesize and release platelet activating factor. *Journal of Experimental Medicine*, **166**, 1390–404.

Caplan, M.S., Sun, X.M., Hsueh, W. and Hagerman, J.R. 1990: Role of platelet activating factor and tumor necrosis factor-alpha in neonatal necrotizing enterocolitis. *Journal of Pediatrics*, **116**, 960–4.

Catsicas, S., Thanos, S. and Clarke, P.G. 1987: Major role for neuronal death during brain development: refinement of topographical connections. *Proceedings of National Academy of Science of the United States of America*, **84**, 8165–8.

Cavender, D.E., Edelbaum, D. and Ziff, M. 1989: Endothelial cell activation induced by tumor necrosis factor and lymphotoxin. *American Journal of Pathology*, **134**, 551–60.

Chi, J.F., Dooling, E.C. and Gilles, F.H. 1977: Gyral development of the human brain. *Annuals of Neurology*, **1**, 86–93.

Choi, B.H. 1989: The effects of methyl mercury on the developing brain. *Progress in Neurobiology*, **32**, 447–70.

Choi, B.H., Lapham, L.W., Amin-Zaki, L. and Saleem, T. 1978: Abnormal neuronal migration deranged cerebral cortical organization, and diffuse white matter astrocytosis of human fetal brain: a major effect of methyl mercury poisoning *in utero*. *Journal of Neuropathology and Experimental Neurology*, **37**, 719–33.

Clarke, P.G.H. and Hornung, J.P. 1989: Changes in the nuclei of dying neurons as studied with thymidine autoradiography. *Journal of Comparative Neurology*, **283**, 438–49.

Clarkson, T.W., Amin-Zaki, L. and Al-Tikriti, S.K. 1976: An outbreak of methyl mercury poisoning due to consumption of contaminated grain. *Federation Proceedings*, **35**, 2395–9.

Clarkson, T.W., Magos, L. and Greenwood, M.R. 1972: The transport of elemental mercury into fetal tissues. *Biology of Neonate*, **21**, 239–44.

Clos, J., Legrand, C., Legrand, J. *et al.* 1982: Effects of thyroid state and undernutrition on S100 protein and astroglia development in rat cerebellum. *Developmental Neuroscience*, **5**, 285–92

Copp, A.J. and Bernfield, M. 1988a: Glycosaminoglycans vary in accumulation along the neuraxis during spinal neurulation in the mouse embryo. *Developmental Biology*, **130**, 573–82.

Copp, A.J. and Bernfield, M. 1988b: Accumulation of basement membrane-associated hyaluronate is reduced in the posterior neuropore region of mutant (curly tail) mouse embryos developing spinal neural tube defects. *Developmental Biology*, **130**, 583–90.

Corasaniti, M.T., Defilippo, R., Rodino, P., Nappi, G. and Nistico, G. 1991: Evidence that paraquat is able to cross the blood–brain barrier to a different extent in rats of various ages. *Functional Neurology*, **6**, 385–91.

Cowan, W.M., Fawcett, J.W., O'Leary, D.M. and Stanfield, B.B. 1984: Regressive events in neurogenesis. *Science*, **225**, 1258–65.

Cragg, G.G. 1972: The development of cortical synapses during starvation in the rat. *Brain*, **95**, 143–50.

Crittenden, S.L., Rutishauser, U. and Lilien, J. 1988: Identification of two structural types of calcium-dependent adhesion molecules in the chicken embryo. *Proceedings of the National Academy of Science of the United States of America*, **85**, 3464–8.

Curley, A., Hawk, R.E., Kimbrough, R.D., Nathenson, G. and Finberg, L. 1971: Dermal absorption of hexachlorophene in infants. *Lancet*, **2**, 296.

Dabeka, R.W. and McKenzie, A.D. 1987: Lead, cadmium, and fluoride levels in market milk and infant formulas in Canada. *Journal Association Official Analytical Chemist*, **70**, 754–7.

Dave, V., Vitarella, D., Aschner, J.L., Fletcher, P., Kimelberg, H.K. and Aschner, M. 1993: Lead increases inositol 1,4,5–triphosphate levels but does not interfere with calcium transients in primary astrocytes. *Brain Research*, **618**, 9–18.

Davis, J.A. and Dobbing, J. (eds) 1974: *Scientific Foundations of Pediatrics*. Philadelphia, PA: W.B. Saunders.

Detrick, R.J., Dickey, D. and Kintner, C. 1990: The effects of *n*-cadherin misexpression on morphogenesis in Xenopus embryos. *Neuron*, **4**, 493.

Dobbing, J. and Sands, J. 1979: Comparative aspects of the brain growth spurt. *Early Human Development*, **3**, 79–83.

Driscoll, C.D., Streissguth, A.P. and Riley, E.P. 1990: Prenatal alcohol exposure: comparability of effects in humans and animal models. *Neurotoxicology and Teratology*, **12**, 231–7.

Duband, J.L., Dufour, S., Hatta, K., Takeichi, M., Edelman, G.M. and Thiery, J.P. 1987: Adhesion molecules during somitogenesis in the avian embryo. *Journal of Cell Biology*, **104**, 1361–74.

Eto, K. and Takeuchi, T. 1978: A pathological study of prolonged cases of Minamata disease. With particular reference to 83 autopsy cases. *Acta Pathology Japan*, **28**, 565–84.

Evrard, P., Miladi, N. and Bonnier, C. 1992: Normal and abnormal development of the brain. In *Handbook of Neuropsychology*, Vol. 6: *Child Neuropsychology*, Rapin, I. and Segalowitz, S.J. (eds). Amsterdam: Elsevier Science.

Fein, G.G., Jacobson, J.L., Jacobson, S.W., Schwartz, P.M. and Dowler, J.K. 1984: Prenatal exposure to polychlorinated biphenyls: effects on birth size and gestational age. *Journal of Pediatrics*, **105**, 315–20.

Fishell, G. and Hatten, M.E. 1991: Astrotactin provides a receptor system for CNS neuronal migration. *Development*, **113**, 755–65.

Fishell, G., Mason, C.A. and Hatten, M.E. 1993: Dispersion of neural progenitors within the germinal zones of the forebrain. *Nature*, **362**, 636–8.

Fries, G.F. 1985: The PBB episode in Michigan: an overall appraisal. *CRC Critical Reviews in Toxicology*, **16**, 105–56.

Fries, D.S., de Vries, J., Hazelhoff, B. and Horn, A.S. 1986: Synthesis and toxicity toward nigrostriatal dopamine neurons of 1-methyl-4-phenyl-1,2,3,6-tetrahydropyridine (MPTP) analogues. *Journal of Medicinal Chemistry*, **29**, 424–7.

Fujimori, T. and Takeichi, M. 1993: Disruption of epithelial cell–cell adhesion by exogenous expression of a mutated nonfunctional N-cadherin. *Molecular Biology of the Cell*, **4**, 37–47.

Fullmer, C.S. 1991: Intestinal calcium and lead absorption: effects of dietary lead and calcium. *Environmental Research*, **54**, 159–69.

Gadisseux, J.-F., Goffinet, A.M., Lyson, G., Evrard, P. 1992: The human transient subpial granular layer: an optical, immunohistochemical, and ultrastructural analysis. *Journal of Comparative Neurology*, **32**, 94–114.

Giacola, G.P. and Catz, C.S. 1979: Drugs and pollutants in breast milk. *Clinical Perinatology*, **6**, 181–96.

Gilles, F.H. and Kassirer, M. 1976: Hydrocephalus. *Human Pathology*, **7**, 123–6.

Gilles, F.H., Averill, D.R. Jr and Kerr, C.S. 1977: Neonatal endotoxin encephalopathy. *Annuals of Neurology*, **2**, 49–56.

Gilles, F.H., Leviton, A. and Dooling, E.C. 1983: *The Developing Human Brain: Growth and Epidemiologic Neuropathology*. Boston, MA: John Wright.

Gocmen, A., Peters, H.A., Cripps, D.J., Bryan, G.T. and Morris, C.R. 1989: Hexachlorobenzene episode in Turkey. *Biomedical Environmental Science*, **2**, 36–43.

Goldey, E.S. and Taylor, D.H. 1992: Developmental neurotoxicity following premating maternal exposure to hexachlorobenzene in rats. *Neurotoxicology and Teratology*, **14**, 15–21.

Goldson, E. and Hagerman, R.J. 1992: The fragile-X syndrome. *Developmental Medicine Child Neurology*, **33**, 191–200.

Goodman, C.S. and Shatz, C.J. 1993: Developmental mechanisms that generate precise patterns of neuronal connectivity. *Cell*, **72**, 77–98.

Gould, E., Westlind-Danielsson, A., Frankfurt, M. and McEwen, B.S. 1990: Sex differences and thyroid hormone sensitivity of hippocampal pyramidal cells. *Journal of Neurosciences*, **9**, 996–1003.

Gressens, P., Richelme, C., Kadhim, H.J., Gadisseux, J.F. and Evrard, P. 1992: The germinative zone produces the most cortical astrocytes after neuronal migration in the developing mammalian brain. *Biology of the Neonate*, **61**, 1–24.

Grunwald, G.B., Geller, R.L. and Lilien, J. 1980: Enzymatic dissection of embryonic cell adhesive mechanisms. *Journal of Cell Biology*, **85**, 766–76.

Hara, I. 1985: Health status and PCBs in blood of workers exposed to PCBs and of their children. *Environmental Health Perspectives*, **59**, 85–90.

Harada, M. 1976: Intrauterine poisoning: clinical and epidemiological studies of the problem. *Bull Institution Constitutional Medicine (Kumamotoa University)*, **25**, 1–60.

Harris, W.A. 1981: Neural activity and development. *Annual Review of Physiology*, **43**, 689–710.

Harry, G.J., Schmitt, T.J., Gong, Z., Brown, H., Zawia, N. and Evans, H.L. 1996: Lead-induced alterations of glial fibrillary acidic protein (GFAP) in the developing rat brain. *Toxicology and Applied Pharmacology*, **139**, 84–93.

Hatta, K. and Takeichi, M. 1986: Expression of N-cadherin adhesion molecules associated with early morphogenetic events in chick development. *Nature*, **320**, 447–9.

Hay, E.D. 1981: Extracellular matrix. *Journal of Cell Biology*, **91**, S205–223.

Herbst, AL., Ulfelder, H. and Poskanzer, D.C. 1971: Adenocarcinoma of the vagina: association of maternal stilbestrol therapy with tumor appearance in young women. *New England Journal of Medicine*, **284**, 878–81.

Hettenmann, H. and Ransom, B.R. 1995: *Neuroglia*. New York: Oxford University Press.

Hicks, S.P. and D'Amato, C.J. 1968: Cell migrations to the isocortex in the rat. *Anatomical Record*, **160**, 619–34.

Hofman, F.M., Hinton, D.R., Baemayr, J., Weil, M. and Merrill, J.E. 1991: Lynphokines and immunoregulatory molecules in subacute sclerosing panencephalitis. *Clinical Immunology and Immunopathology*, **58**, 331–42.

Hsu, S.T., Ma, C.I., Hsu, S.K. *et al.* 1985: Discovery and epidemiology of PCB poisoning in Taiwan: a four-year follow-up. *Environmental Health Perspectives*, **59**, 5–10.

Huttenlocher, P.R. and de Courten, C. 1987: The development of synapses in striate cortex of man. *Human Neurobiology*, **6**, 1–9.

Huttenlocher, R.P., de Courten, C., Garey, L.J. and van der Loos, H. 1982: Synaptogenesis in human visual cortex – evidence for synapse elimination during normal development. *Neuroscience Letters*, **33**, 247–52.

Inouye, M., Murao, K. and Kajiwara, Y. 1985: Behavioral and neuropathological effects of prenatal methyl mercury exposure in mice. *Neurobehavioral Toxicology and Teratology*, **7**, 227–32.

Jacobson, J.L., Jacobson, S.W., Fein, G.G., Schwartz, P.M. and Dowler, J.K. 1984: Prenatal exposure to an environmental toxin: a test of the multiple effects model. *Developmental Psychology*, **20**, 523–32.

Jacobson, J.L., Jacobson, S.W. and Humphrey, H.E.B. 1990a: Effects of *in utero* exposure to polychlorinated biphenyls and related contaminants on cognitive functioning in young children. *Journal of Pediatrics*, **11**, 38–45.

Jacobson, J.L., Jacobson, S.W. and Humphrey, H.E.B. 1990b: Effects of exposure to PCBs and related compounds on growth and activity in children. *Neurotoxicology and Teratology*, **12**, 319–26.

Jacobson, M. 1991: *Developmental Neurobiology*. New York: Plenum Press.

Jacobson, S.W., Fein, G.G., Jacobson, J.L., Schwartz, P.M. and Dowler, J.K. 1985: The effect of intrauterine PCB exposure on visual recognition memory. *Child Development*, **56**, 853–60.

Janner, E. and Burke, R.E. 1993: Naturally occurring cell death during postnatal development of the substantia nigra pars compacta of rat. In *Molecular and Cellular Neurosciences*, Conn, P.M. (ed.). San Diego, CA: Academic Press.

Jones, D.G. 1983: Development, maturation and aging of synapses. In *Advances in Cellular Neurobiology*, Federoff, S. and Hertz, L., (eds), Vol. 4, pp 163–222. New York: Academic Press.

Kandel, E.R., Schwartz, J.H., Jessel, T.M. 1991: *Principles of Neural Science*, 3rd edn. New York: Elsevier.

Kapfhammer, J.P. and Schwab, M.E. 1992: Modulators of neuronal migration and neurite growth. *Current Opinions in Cell Biology*, **4**, 863–8.

Karfunkel, P. 1974: The mechanisms of neural tube formation. *International Review of Biology*, **38**, 245–71.

Kinney, H.C., Brody, B.A., Kloman, A.E., Gilles, F.H. 1988: Sequence of central nervous system myelination in human infancy. II. Patterns of myelination in autopsied infants. *Journal Neuropathology Experimental Neurology*, **47**, 217–34.

Kolb, B. and Whishaw, I.Q. 1989: Plasticity in the neocortex: mechanisms underlying recovery from early brain damage. *Progress in Neurobiology*, **32**, 235–76.

Komuro, H. and Rakic, P. 1992: Selective role of N-type calcium channels in neuronal migration. *Science*, **257**, 806–9.

Komuro, H. and Rakic, P. 1993: Modulation of neuronal migration by NMDA receptors. *Science*, **260**, 95–7.

Kopelman, A.E. 1973: Cutaneous absorption of hexachlorophene in low birth-weight infants. *Journal of Pediatrics*, **82**, 972–5.

Korlof, B. and Winsten, J. 1967: The complications of pHisoHex. *Scandinavian Journal of Plastic and Reconstructive Surgery*, **1**, 78.

Kornecki, R. and Ehrlich, Y.H. 1988: Neuroregulatory and neuropathological actions of the etherphospholipid platelet-activating factor. *Science*, **240**, 1792–4.

Korpela, H., Loueniva, R., Yrjanheikki, E. and Kauppila, A. 1986: Lead and cadmium concentrations in maternal and umbilical cord blood, amniotic fluid, placenta, and amniotic membranes. *American Journal of Obstetrics and Gynecology*, **155**, 1086–9.

Krigman, M.R. and Hogan, E.L. 1974: Effect of lead intoxication on the postnatal growth of the rat nervous system. *Environmental Health Perspectives*, May, 187–99.

Kumar, R., Harvey, A.K., Kester, M., Hanahan, D. and Olson, M.S. 1988: Production and effects of platelet-activating factor in the rat brain. *Biochimica et Biophysica Acta*, **963**, 375–83.

Lacey, R.F., Moore, M.R. and Richards, W.N. 1985: Lead in water, infant diet and blood: the Glasgow duplicate diet study. *Science Total Environment*, **4**, 235.

Lagunowich, L.A. and Grunwald, G.B. 1991: Tissue and age-specificity of post-translational modifications of N-cadherin during chick embryo development. *Differentiation*, **47**, 19–27.

Lagunowich, L.A., Stein, A.P. and Reuhl, K.R. 1994: N-cadherin in normal and abnormal brain development. *Neurotoxicology*, **15**, 123–32.

Lauder, J.M. and Mugnaini, E. 1980: Infrapyramidal mossy fibers in the hyperthyroid hippocampus: a light and electron microscopic study in the rat. *Developmental Neuroscience*, **3**, 248–65.

Legare M.E., Castiglioni A.J. Jr, Rowles, T.K., Calvin, J.A., Snyder-Armstead, C. and Tiffany-Castiglioni, E. 1993: Morphological alterations of neurons and astrocytes in guinea pigs exposed to low levels of inorganic lead. *Neurotoxicology*, **14**, 77–80.

Lewine, J.D., Astur, R.S., Davis, L.E., Knight, J.E., Maclin, E.L. and Orrison, W.W., Jr 1994: Cortical organization in adulthood is modified by neonatal infarct – a case study. *Radiology*, **190**, 93–6.

Liesi, P. 1990: Extracellular matrix and neuronal movement. *Experientia*, **46**, 900–7.

Lockhart, J.D. 1972: How toxic is hexachlorophene? *Pediatrics*, **50**, 229–35.

Luskin, M.B., Pearlman, A.L. and Sanes, J.R. 1988: Cell lineage in the cerebral cortex of the mouse studied *in vivo* and *in vitro* with a recomginant retrovirus. *Neuron*, **1**, 635–47.

Luskin, M.B. and Shatz, C.J. 1985: Neurogenesis of the cat's visual cortex. *Journal of Comparative Neurology*, **242**, 611–32.

Mahaffey, K.R. 1980: Nutrient lead interactions. In *Lead Toxicity*, Singhal, P.L. and Thomas, J.A. (eds), pp 425–59. Baltimore, MD: Urban and Schwarzenberg, Inc.

Mahaffey, K.R. 1990: Environmental lead toxicity: nutrition as a component of intervention. *Environmental Health Perspectives*, **89**, 75–8.

Mahaffey, K.R. 1991: Biokinetics of lead during pregnancy. *Fundamental and Applied Toxicology*, **16**, 15–16.

Manton, W.I. 1985: Total contribution of airborne lead to blood lead. *British Journal of Industrial Medicine*, **42**, 168–72.

Marin-Padilla, M. 1970: Prenatal and early postnatal ontogenesis of the human motor cortex: a Golgi study. I. The sequential development of the cortical layers. *Brain Research*, **23**, 167–83.

Marin-Padilla, M. 1972: Structural abnormalities of the cerebral cortex in human chromosomal aberrations: a Golgi study. *Brain Research*, **44**, 625–9.

Marin-Padilla, M. 1992: Ontogenesis of the pyramidal cell of the mammalian neocortex and developmental cytoarchitectonics: a unifying theory. *Journal Comparative Neurology*, **321**, 233–40.

Markovac, J. and Goldstein, G.W. 1988: Lead activates protein kinase C in immature rat brain microvessels. *Toxicology and Applied Pharmacology*, **95**, 14–23.

Marsh, D.O. 1987: Dose–response relationship in humans: methyl mercury epidemics in Japan and Iraq. In *The Toxicity of Methyl Mercury*, Eccles, C.U. and Annau, Z. (eds), pp 24–44. Baltimore, MD: Johns Hopkins.

Marsh, D.O., Myers, G.J., Clarkson, T.W. *et al.* 1981: Dose–response relationship for human fetal exposure to methylmercury. *Clinical Toxicology*, **18**, 1311–18.

Martenson, R.E. 1992: *Myelin: Biology and Chemistry*. Boca Raton, FL: CRC Press.

Masuda, Y., Kagawa, R., Kuroki, H. *et al.* 1978: Transfer of polychlorinated biphenyls from mothers and fetuses and infants. *Food and Cosmetic Toxicology*, **16**, 543–6.

Masuda, Y. and Yoshimura, H. 1984: Polychlorinated biphenyls and dibenzofurans in patients with yusho and their toxicological significance: a review. *American Journal of Industrial Medicine*, **5**, 31–44.

Matsumoto, H., Koya, G. and Takeuchi, T. 1965: Fetal Minamata disease. A neuropathological study of two cases of intrauterine intoxication by a methyl mercury compound. *Journal of Neuropathology and Experimental Neurology*, **24**, 563–74.

Matsunaga, M., Hatta, K., Nagafuchi, A. and Takeichi, M. 1988a: Guidance of optic nerve fibers by N-cadherin adhesion molecules. *Nature*, **334**, 62–4.

Matsunaga, M., Hatta, K. and Takeichi, M. 1988b: Role of N-cadherin cell adhesion molecules in the histogenesis of neural retina. *Neuron*, **1**, 289–95.

McCauley, P., Bull, R., Tonti, P., Lutkenhoff, S., Meister, M. and Doerger Stober, J. 1982: The effect of prenatal and postnatal lead exposure on neonatal synaptogenesis in the rat cerebral cortex. *Journal of Toxicology and Environmental Health*, **10**, 639–51.

McCracken, G.H. Jr, Mustafa, M.M., Ramilo, O., Olsen, K.D. and Risser, R.C. 1989: Cerebrospinal fluid interleukin 1-beta and tumor necrosis factor concentrations and outcome from neonatal Gram-negative enteric bacillary meningitis. *Pediatric Infectious Disease Journal*, **8**, 155–9.

Miller, R.W. 1956: Delayed effects occurring within the first decade after exposure of young individuals to the Hiroshima atomic bomb. *Pediatrics*, **18**, 1.

Miller, R.W. and Mulvihill, J.J. 1976: Small head size after atomic irradiation. *Teratology*, **14**, 355–7.

Mojsilovic, J. and Zecevic, N. 1991: Early development of the human thalamus: Golgi and Nissl study. *Early Human Development*, **27**, 119–44.

Morriss-Kay, G.M. and Crutch, B. 1982: Culture of rat embryos with beta-D-xyloside: evidence for a role for proteoglycans in neurulation. *Journal of Anatomy*, **134**, 491–506.

Mullick, F.G. 1973: Hexachlorophene toxicity: human experience at the Armed Forces Institute of Pathology. *Pediatrics*, **51**, 395–9.

Nagele, R.G., Bush, K.T., Kosciuk, M.C., Hunter, E.T., Steinberg, A.B. and Lee, H.Y. 1989: Intrinsic and extrinsic factors collaborate to generate driving forces for neural tube formation in the chick: a study using morphometry and computerized three-dimensional reconstruction. *Developmental Brain Research*, **50**, 101–11.

Nation, R.L. and Hotham, N. 1987: Drugs and breast-feeding. *Medical Journal of Australia*, **146**, 308–13.

Needleman, H.L., Schell, A., Bellinger, D., Leviton, A. and Ailred, E.N. 1990: The long-term effects of exposure to low doses of lead in childhood: an 11-year follow-up report. *New England Journal of Medicine*, **322**, 83–8.

Nicholson, J.L. and Altman, J. 1972: The effects of early hypo- and hyperthyroidism on the development of the rat cerebellar cortex. II. Synaptogenesis in the molecular layer. *Brain Research*, **44**, 25–36.

Nieminen, L., Bjondahl, K. and Mottonen, M. 1973: Effect of hexachlorophene on the rat brain during ontogenesis. *Food Cosmetic Toxicology*, **11**, 635–9.

Norman, R.M. 1967: Malformations of the nervous system, birth injury, and diseases of early life. In *Greenfield's Neuropathology*, Blackwood, W., McMenemy, W.H., Meyer A. *et al.* (eds). Baltimore, MD: Williams & Wilkins.

Null, D.H., Gartside, P.S. and Wei, E. 1973: Methyl mercury accumulation in brains of pregnant, nonpregnant and fetal rats. *Life Sciences*, **12**, 65–72.

Nzelibe, C.G., Knight, E.M. and Adkins, J.S. 1986: Effect of carbohydrates on lead absorption and retention in weaning rats. *Environmental Research*, **41**, 458–65.

Ong, C.N., Phoon, W.O., Law, H.Y., Tye, C.Y. and Lim, H.H. 1985: Concentrations of lead in maternal blood, cord blood, and breast milk. *Archives of Disease in Childhood*, **60**, 756–9.

Ono, K., Shimada, M. and Yamano, T. 1990: Reorganization of the corticospinal tract following neonatal unilateral cortical ablation in rats. *Brain Development*, **12**, 226–36.

Ono, K., Yamano, T. and Shimada, M. 1991: Formation of an ipsilateral corticospinal tract after ablation of cerebral cortex in neonatal rat. *Brain Development*, **13**, 348–51.

Oppenheim, R.W. 1991: Cell death during development of the nervous system. *Annual Review Neuroscience*, **14**, 453–501.

Oppenheim, R.W., Schwartz, L.M. and Shatz, C.J. 1992: Neuronal death, a tradition of dying. *Journal of Neurobiology*, **23**, 1111–5.

O'Rourke, N.A., Dailey, M.E., Smith, S.J. and McConnel, S.K. 1992: Diverse migratory pathways in the developing cerebral cortex. *Science*, **255**, 373–6.

Otake, M. and Schull, W.J. 1984: *In utero* exposure to a-bomb radiation and mental retardation: a reassessment. *British Journal of Radiology*, **57**, 409–14.

Otake, M., Schull, W.J., Fujikoshi, Y. and Yoshimaru, H. 1988: *Effect on school Performance of Prenatal Exposure to Ionizing Radiation in Hiroshima: a Comparison of the T65DR and DS86 Dosimetry Systems, TR 2-88*. Hiroshima: Radiation Effects Research Foundation.

Parsons, M.P., Worthen, G.S., Moore, E.E., Tate, R.M. and Henson, P.E. 1989: The association of circulating endotoxin with the development of the adult respiratory distress syndrome. *American Review of Respiratory Diseases*, **140**, 294–301.

Patterson, P.H. and Nawa, H. 1993: Neuronal differentiation factors/cytokines and synaptic plasticity. *Neuron*, **10**, 123–37.

Petit, T., Alfano, D. and LeBoutillier, J. 1983: Early lead exposure and the hippocampus: a review and recent advances. *Neurotoxicology*, **4**, 79–94.

Petit, T. and LeBoutillier, J. 1979: Effects of lead exposure during development on neocortical dendritic and synaptic structure. *Experimental Neurology*, **64**, 482–92.

Petit, T.L., LeBoutillier, J.C., Alfano, D.P. and Becker, L.E. 1984: Synaptic development in the human fetus: a morphometric analysis of normal and Down's syndrome neocortex. *Experimental Neurology*, **83**, 13–23.

Plummer, G. 1952: Anomalies occurring in children exposed *in utero* to the atomic bomb in Hiroshima. *Pediatrics*, **10**, 687.

Powell, H., Swarner, O., Gluck, L. and Lampert, P. 1973: Hexachlorophene myelinopathy in premature infants. *The Journal of Pediatrics*, **82**, 976–81.

Purpura, D.P. 1975: Dendritic differentiation in human cerebral cortex: normal and aberrant developmental patterns. In *Advances in Neurology*, Kruetzberg, G.W. (ed.), pp 91–134. New York: Raven Press.

Purves, D. and Lichtman, J.W. 1980: Elimination of synapses in the developing nervous system. *Science*, **210**, 153–7.

Purves, D. and Lichtman, J.W. 1985: In *Principles of Neural Development*. Sutherland, MA: Sinauer Associates.

Rabacchi, S., Bailly, Y., Delhaye-Bouchaud, N. and Mariani, J. 1992: Involvement of the *N*-methyl-D-aspartate (NMDA) receptor in synapse elimination during cerebellar development. *Science*, **256**, 1823–5.

Rabinowitz, M., Leviton, A. and Needleman, H. 1985: Lead in milk and infant blood: a dose-response model. *Archives of Environmental Health*, **40**, 283–6.

Raine, C.S. 1984: Morphology of myelin and myelination. In *Myelin*, Morell, P. (ed.), p 1. New York: Plenum Press.

Rakic, P. 1975a: Timing of major ontogenetic events in the visual cortex of the rhesus monkey. UCLA Forum. *Medical Science*, **18**, 3–40.

Rakic, P. 1975b: Cell migration and neuronal ectopias in the brain. *Birth Defects*, **11**, 95–129.

Rakic, P. 1988a: Specification of cerebral cortical areas. *Science*, **241**, 170–6.

Rakic, P. 1988b: Defects of neuronal migration and the pathogenesis of cortical malformations. *Progress Brain Research*, **73**, 15–37.

Rakic, P. 1990: Principles of neural cell migration. *Experientia*, **46**, 882–91.

Rakic, P. and Yakovleu, P.I. 1968: Development of the corpus callosum and cavum septi in man. *Journal of Comparative Neurology*, **132**, 45–72.

Raper, J.A. and Grunewald, E.B. 1990: Temporal retinal growth cones collapse on contact with nasal retinal axons. *Experimental Neurology*, **109**, 70.

Regan, C.M., Cookman, G.R. and Keane, G.J. 1989: The effects of chronic low-level lead exposure on the early structuring of the central nervous system. In *Lead Exposure and Child Development: an International Assessment*, Smith, M.A., Grant, L.D., and Sors, A.I. (eds), Vol. 450, p 52. Dordrecht: Kluwer Academic.

Reichardt, L.F. and Tomaselli, K.J. 1991: Extracellular matrix molecules and their receptors. *Annual Review of Neuroscience*, **14**, 531–70.

Riordan, J. and Riordan, M. 1984: Drugs in breast milk. *American Journal of Nursing*, **84**, 328–32.

Robaye, B., Mosselmans, R., Fiers, W., Dumont, J.E. and Galand, P. 1991: Tumor necrosis factor induces apoptosis (programmed cell death) in normal endothelial cells *in vitro*. *American Journal of Pathology*, **138**, 447–53.

Robbins, D.S., Shirazi, Y., Drysdale, B.E., Lieberman, A., Shin, H.S. and Shin, M.L. 1987: Production of cytotoxic factor for oligodendrocytes by stimulated astrocytes. *Journal of Innumology*, **139**, 2593–7.

Rogan, W.J. 1996: Pollutants in breast milk. *Archives of Pediatrics and Adolescent Medicine*, **150**, 981–90.

Rogan, W.J., Gladen, B.C., Hung, K.L. *et al.* 1988: Congenital poisoning by polychlorinated biphenyls and their contaminants in Taiwan. *Science*, **241**, 334–6.

Rogan, W.J., Gladen, B.C., McKinney, J.D. *et al.* 1986: Neonatal effects of transplacental exposure to PCBs and DDT. *Journal of Pediatrics*, **109**, 335–41.

Rossi, D.J. and Slater, N.T. 1993: The developmental onset of NMDA receptor-channel activity during neuronal migration secondary to abnormality of Bergmann glia. *Proceedings National Academy of Science of the United States of America*, **70**, 240–4.

Reuhl, K.R. and Cranmer, J.M. 1984: Development neuropathology of organotin compounds. *Neurotoxicology*, **5**, 187–204.

Ruel, J., Raire, R. and Dussault, J.H. 1985: Regional distribution of nuclear T3 receptors in rat brain and evidence for preferential localization in neurons. *Journal of Endocrinology Investigations*, **8**, 343–8.

Rustam, H. and Hamdi, T. 1974: Methyl mercury poisoning in Iraq. A neurological study. *Brain*, **97**, 500–10.

Rutishauser, U., Acheson, A., Hall, A.K., Mann, D.M. and Sunshine, J. 1988: The neural cell adhesion molecules (NCAM) as a regulator of cell–cell interactions. *Science*, **240**, 53–7.

Rye, J.E., Ziegler, E.E., Nelson, S.E. and Fomon S.J. 1983: Dietary intake of lead and blood lead concentration in early infancy. *American Journal of Disease in Children*, **137**, 886–91.

Safe, S. 1984: Polychlorinated biphenyls (PCBs) and polybrominated biphenyls (PBBs): biochemistry, toxicology, and mechanism of action. *CRC Critical Reviews in Toxicology*, **13**, 319–95.

Sawyer, D.B. and Andersen, O.S. 1989: Platelet-activating factor is a general membrane perturbant. *Biochimica et Biophysica Acta*, **987**, 129–32.

Schade, J.P. and Groenigen, W.B. 1961: Structural organization of the human cerebral cortex. I. Maturation of the middle frontal gyrus. *Acta Anatomica*, **47**, 79–111.

Schapiro, S., Vukovich, K. and Globus, A. 1973: Effects of neonatal thyroxine and hydrocortisone administration on the development of dendritic spines in the visual cortex of rats. *Experimental Neurology*, **40**, 286–96.

Schlaggar, B.I., Fox, K. and O'Leary, D.M. 1993: Postsynaptic control of plasticity in developing somatosensory cortex. *Nature*, **364**, 623–6.

Schmitt, T.J., Zawia, N. and Harry, G.J. 1996: GAP-43 mRNA expression in the developing rat brain: alterations following lead-acetate exposure. *Neurotoxicology*, **17**, 407–14.

Schramel, P., Lill, G., Hasse, S. and Klose, B.-J. 1988: Mineral and trace element concentrations in human breast milk, placenta, maternal blood, and the blood of the newborn. *Biological Trace Elemental Research*, **16**, 67–75.

Schull, W.J. and Otake, M. 1986: *Effect on Intelligence of Prenatal Exposure to Ionizing Radiation, TR 7–86*. Hiroshima: Radiation Effects Research Foundation.

Schwartz, H.L. and Oppenheimer, J.H. 1978: Nuclear triiodothyronine receptor sites in the brain: probable identity with hepatic receptors and regional distribution. *Endocrinology*, **103**, 267–73.

Selmaj, K., Raine, C.S., Path, F.R. and Cross, C. 1988: Tumor necrosis factor mediates myelin and oligodendrocyte damage *in vitro*. *Annals of Neurology*, **23**, 339–46.

Shannon, M. and Graef, J. 1989: Lead intoxication. From lead-contaminated water used to reconstitute infant formula. *Clinical Pediatrics*, **28**, 380–2.

Sheppard, A.M., Hamilton, S.K. and Pearlman, A.L. 1991: Changes in the distribution of extracellular matrix components accompany early morphogenetic events of mammalian cortical development. *Journal of Neuroscience*, **11**, 3928–42.

Shuman, R.M., Leech, R.W. and Alvord, E.C. Jr 1975: Neurotoxicity of hexachlorophene in humans. II. A clinicopathologic study of 46 premature infants. *Archives of Neurology*, **32**, 320–5.

Sidman, R.L. and Rakic, P. 1973: Neuronal migration, with special reference to developing human brain: a review. *Brain Research*, **62**, 1–35.

Sikorski, R., Paszkowski, T. and Milart, P. 1988: Intrapartum levels of trace metals in maternal blood in relation to umbilicial cord blood values: lead, iron, copper, zinc. *International Journal of Gynecology and Obstetrics*, **26**, 213–21.

Silbergeld, E.K., Schwartz, J. and Mahaffey, K. 1988: Lead and osteoporosis: mobilization of lead from bone in postmenopausal women. *Environmental Research*, **47**, 79–94.

Sim, M.R. and McNeil, J.J. 1992: Monitoring chemical exposure using breast milk: a methodological review. *American Journal of Epidemiology*, **136**, 1–11.

Smart, I.H.M. and Smart, M. 1982: Growth patterns in the lateral wall of the mouse telencephalon. I. Autoradiographic studies of the histogenesis of the isocortex and adjacent areas. *Journal of Anatomy*, **134**, 273–98.

Snow, D.M., Watanabe, M., Letourneau, P.C. and Silver, J. 1991: A chondroitin sulfate proteoglycan may influence the direction of retinal genglion cell outgrowth. *Development*, **113**, 1473–85.

Snyder, R.D. 1971: Congenital mercury poisoning. *New England Journal of Medicine*, **284**, 1014–6.

Spyker, J.M. 1975: Assessing the impact of low-level chemicals on development: behavioral and latent effects. *Federation Proceedings*, **34**, 1835–44.

Sternowsky, H.J. and Wessolowski, R. 1985: Lead and cadmium in breast milk: higher levels in urban vs rural mothers during the first three months of lactation. *Archives of Toxicology*, **57**, 41–5.

Stipp, C.S., Litwack, E.D. and Lander, A.D. 1994: Cerebroglycan: an integral membrane heparan sulfate proteoglycan that is unique to the developing nervous system and expressed specifically during neuronal differentiation. *Journal of Cell Biology*, **124**, 149–60.

Takashima, S. and Mito, T. 1985: Neuronal development in the medullary reticular formation in sudden infant death syndrome and premature infants. *Neuropediatrics*, **16**, 76–9.

Takashima, S., Mito, T. and Becker, L.E. 1990: Dendritic development of motor neurons in the cervical anterior horn and hypoglossal nucleus of normal infants and victims of sudden infant death syndrome. *Neuropediatrics*, **21**, 24–6.

Tarleton, J.C. and Saul, R.A. 1993: Molecular genetic advances in fragile-X syndrome. *Journal of Pediatrics*, **122**, 169–85.

Tilson, H.A., Jacobson, J.L. and Rogan, W.J. 1990: Polychlorinated biphenyls and the developing nervous system: cross-species comparisons. *Neurotoxicology and Teratolology*, **12**, 239–48.

Tilson, H.A. and Sparber, S.B. (eds) 1987: *Neurotoxicants and Neurobiological Functions: Effects of Organo Heavy Metals*. New York: Wiley Press.

Toews, A.D., Blaker, W.D., Thomas, D.J. et al. 1983: Myelin deficits produced by early postnatal exposure to inorganic lead or triethyltin are persistent. *Journal of Neurochemistry*, **41**, 816–22.

Tracey, K.J., Fong, Y., Hesse, D.G. et al. 1987: Anticachectin/TNF monoclonal antibodies prevent septic shock during lethal bacteremia. *Nature*, **330**, 662–4.

Truska, P., Rosival, L., Balazova, G. et al. 1989: Blood and placental concentrations of cadmium, lead, and mercury in mothers and

their newborns. *Journal of Hygenic Epidemiolology Microbiolology Immunology*, **33**, 141–7.

Tyrala, E.E., Hillman, L.S., Hillman, R.E. and Dodson, W.E. 1977: Clinical pharmacology of hexachlorophene in newborn infants. *Journal of Pediatrics*, **91**, 481–6.

Unsicker, K., Grothe, G., Ludecke, G., Otto, D. and Westermann, R. 1993: Fibroblast growth factors: their roles in the central and peripheral nervous system. In *Neurotrophic Factors*, Loughlin, E.E. and Fallon, J.H. (eds), pp 313–26. New York: Academic Press.

US Environmental Protection Agency 1986: *Air Quality Criteria for Lead*, Office of Health and Environmental Assessment, Environmental Criteria and Assessment Office, EPA Report EPA-600/8-83-028aF-dF. Research Triangle Park, North Carolina: Environmental Protection Agency.

Valois, A.A. and Webster, W.S. 1987: Retention and distribution of cadmium in the mouse brain: an autoradiograph and gamma counting study. *Neurotoxicology*, **8**, 463–9.

van Straaten, H.W., Hekking, J.W., Beursgens, J.P., Terwindt-Rouwenhorst, E. and Drukker, J. 1989: Effect of the notochord on proliferation and differentiation in the neural tube of the chick embryo. *Development*, **107**, 793–803.

Veronesi, B. and Bondy, S. 1986: Triethyltin-induced neuronal damage in neonatally exposed rats. *Neurotoxicology*, **7**, 69–79.

Viny, M.J., Takahashi, Y. and Lorscheider, F.L. 1990: Maternal-fetal distribution of mercury (^{203}Hg) released from dental amalgam fillings. *American Journal of Physiology*, **258**, R939.

Volpe, J.J. 1977: Normal and abnormal human brain development. *Clinical Perinatology*, **4**, 3–30.

Volpe, J.J. 1995: *Neurology of the Newborn*, 3rd edn. Philadelphia, PA: W.B. Saunders.

Walsh, C. and Cepko, C.L. 1990: Cell lineage and cell migration in the developing cerebral cortex. *Experientia*, **46**, 940–7.

Walsh, C. and Cepko, C.L. 1993: Clonal dispersion in proliferative layers of developing cerebral cortex. *Nature*, **362**, 632–5.

Warren, M.A. and Bedi, K.S. 1982: Synapse-to-neuron ratios in the visual cortex of adult rats undernourished from about birth until 100 days of age. *Journal of Comparative Neurology*, **210**, 147–53.

Webster, H.deF. 1975: Peripheral nerve structure. In *The Peripheral Nervous System*, Hubbard, J.E. (ed.), p 3. New York: Plenum Press.

Weil, W.B., Spencer, M., Benjamin, D. and Seagull, E. 1981: The effect of polybrominated biphenyl on infants and young children. *Journal of Pediatrics*, **98**, 47–51.

Wellicome, S.M., Thornhill, M.H., Pitzalis, C. et al. 1990: A monoclonal antibody that detects a novel antigen on endothelial cells that is induced by tumor necrosis factor, IL-1, or lipopolysaccharide. *Journal of Immunology*, **144**, 2558–65.

Wiesel, T.N. 1982: Postnatal development of the visual cortex and the influence of environment. *Nature*, **299**, 583–91.

Wilson, J.T. 1983: Determinants and consequences of drug excretion in breast milk. *Drug Metabolism Review*, **14**, 619–52.

Wilson, J.T., Brown, R.D., Cherek, D.R. et al. 1980: Drug excretion in human breast milk: principles, pharmacokinetics and projected consequences. *Clinical Pharmacokinetics*, **5**, 1–66.

Wisniewski, K.E. 1990: Down's syndrome children often have brain with maturation delay, retardation of growth, and cortical dysgenesis. *American Journal Medical Genetics*, **7**, 274–81.

Yamaguchi, T., Yoshimura, T. and Kuratsune, M. 1971: A survey of pregnant women having consumed rice oil contaminated with chlorobiphenyls and their babies. *Fukuoka Acta Medicine*, **62**, 117–22.

Yamashita, F. and Hayashi, M. 1985: Fetal PCB syndrome: clinical features, intrauerine growth retardation and possible alteration in calcium metabolism. *Environmental Health Perspectives*, **59**, 41–5.

3

Environmental causes of psychiatric and behavioral disease

MALCOLM LADER

INTRODUCTION

The brain is a sensitive organ. It has a rich blood supply, a high metabolic rate, and is highly complex both anatomically and physiologically. Environmental insults can lead to a wide variety of temporary and permanent damage. Among the effects of such damage are psychiatric disturbances which can occur on their own or as complications of neurological disabilities.

Despite the importance of such reactions, the literature on this topic is patchy at best and downright uninformative at worst. The implications for psychiatric health are often overlooked, methods of treating toxic reactions remain inchoate or unexplored, and the long-term outcome of the condition, treated or untreated, remains unclear. Increase in public concern, for example, over organophosphate insecticide 'sheep-dip' poisoning, has led to more research activity, although psychiatric and behavioral aspects are often relatively neglected or inexpertly investigated. Finally, the burgeoning of legal actions for personal injury resulting from negligence has focused the attention of medico-legal circles.

The purpose of this chapter is to review the psychiatric and psychological effects of acute and chronic exposure to a range of environmental toxic chemicals used in agriculture and industry. These include heavy metals, organic solvents and inhalants, carbon monoxide, and organophosphate insecticides. Some mention is made of substance misuse where this is of general interest, for example, toxic effects of 'Ecstasy,' but this is not intended to be a comprehensive review of illicit drug-induced psychiatric disorders, nor are prescribed drugs discussed except when useful parallels can be drawn. It is hoped that this review will constitute a useful reference source for doctors and others exploring this fascinating topic of 'psycho-toxicology.'

THE PSYCHIATRIC AND BEHAVIORAL DISORDERS

In much of the literature on disturbances induced by environmental toxins, reports of psychiatric and psychological disturbances are woefully inadequate, frequently to the point of being uninformative. Phrases such as 'anxiety and depression,' and 'memory disturbance' abound, and obsolescent diagnoses such as 'neurasthenia' and 'cerebral decline' persist. Some of this, admittedly, reflects the inchoate nature of psychiatric diagnostic schemata until about 1980 but the subject of psychiatry is now on a much more rational footing. Other problems relate to changes in how psychologists codify behavioral, cognitive, and emotional functions, so that the interpretation of standard research instruments may shift. However, the main reason is the lack of expertise on the part of many medical practitioners in the assessment and diagnosis of psychiatric disorders and psychological abnormalities, compounded by a reluctance of investigators to seek expert advice when needed.

Psychiatric sequelæ to environmental toxins can occur at the symptomatic, the syndromal or the disorder level. A very wide range of symptoms are encountered in psychiatry, both psychological and somatic. Many are exaggerations of normal. For example, anxiety is an ubiquitous emotion, experienced by us all, and has an important survival value. Only when it becomes too severe, too frequent or too all-pervasive for the individual to tolerate can it be regarded as a symptom. Elicitation of symptoms is not as easy as it may appear. The interviewer is dependent on the verbal skills of the interviewee and on the 'labeling' ascribed to a particular feeling. There are no validating criteria for a complaint of 'feeling tense' or 'down-in-the-dumps.' It is important to probe what is meant by a word or phrase, to get the patient to re-express it in different terms. Sometimes the symptom is outside normal experience and only experienced under the influence of a drug or toxin. Lysergic acid diethylamide (LSD)-induced states are the most notorious example. However, non-drugged states may result in abnormal experiences. One example is 'derealization' when the patient feels detached from the environment, insulated by an invisible barrier. The term 'spaced out' may be used to describe this but can refer to other types of feeling, even to vertigo. Consequently, it can never be assumed that a patient is necessarily describing the same state as the interviewer would describe, even though the same word is used.

The bodily symptoms induced by a toxin can be primary or secondary. Primary symptoms are directly induced, for example, sweating or anorexia with organophosphate pesticides. Secondary symptoms are those which accompany central emotional states, for example, sweating as a symptom of anxiety or loss of appetite with depression.

At the syndromal level, a recognizable constellation of symptoms and signs is encountered. The syndrome of 'delirium' is characterized by clouding of consciousness, disorientation in time and space, anxiety and agitation, and frightening visual hallucinations. There is usually partial or complete amnesia for the episode. Delirium is a non-specific syndrome and can be induced by a wide variety of substances such as alcohol, cannabis, hallucinogens, inhalants, sedatives, anticholinergic agents and digitalis, by head injury, various toxins, and in the course of other conditions such as thyroid deficiency and severe infections.

Many other syndromes can be induced by environmental toxins. Amnesic syndromes may be severe and global, or subtle and localized, the latter requiring expert testing (see Chapter 16). The deficits themselves may be restricted to memory function or be part of a wider deterioration with dementia. In the latter case, tests for aphasia, apraxia, agnosia, and executive functions are needed to establish the profile of impairments. Even the dementia can be part of a more general syndrome with emotional flattening or lability, sleep rhythm inversion, and behavioral disturbances such as aggressive outbursts and nocturnal wanderings.

The highest level of diagnosis involves well-specified disorders such as major depressive disorder and Alzheimer's-type dementia. The distinction between syndrome and disorder is often an artificial one in psychiatry but, generally speaking, epidemiological studies will have supported the status of disorder for a well-defined condition. Nevertheless, the high rate of co-morbidity in psychiatric disorders should leave no room for complacency. For example, two main forms of depressive disorder are distinguished in the Diagnostic and Statistical Manual (DSM)-IV: major depressive disorder and dysthymic disorder. The former is an acute episode, the latter a chronic condition of at least two years' duration. Commonly, however, dysthymic individuals develop an episode of major depressive disorder, so-called 'dual diagnosis.' The entire psychiatric diagnostic schema is constantly being revised as new research data accrue. Nevertheless, it is important to use a generally accepted system such as DSM-IV (1994) or International Classification of Diseases (ICD)-10 (1992) in order to facilitate communication between researchers and clinicians. The headings of the section of the ICD-10 dealing with disorders secondary to psychoactive substance use are set out in Table 3.1.

The lack of objective validating criteria is a major handicap in psychiatry. Symptoms are subjective, signs are secondary and often 'soft' or non-specific. Syndromes are clusters of symptoms and signs established by frequency. Disorders are elaborate value judgements of experts, albeit increasingly informed by empirical data. There are very few objective tests and those that exist relate to some primary condition, for example, a hormonal dysfunction. Others are non-specific, for example, measurement of heart rate or sweat-gland activity in states of arousal such as anxiety, aggression, and embarrassment.

With behavioral and cognitive abnormalities, controlled observation and formal testing is routine and highly informative. However, personnel administering these tests must be properly trained. In the UK, this usually means the involvement of a Chartered Clinical Psychologist.

Reactions induced by environmental toxins are typically non-specific in psychiatric or psychological terms with anxiety, depression, memory disturbances, and so on at the symptomatic or syndromal level. Sometimes, however, specific defined disorders are

Table 3.1 *Mental and behavioral disorders due to psychoactive substance use. Source: ICD-10, WHO, 1992*

Acute intoxication
  Uncomplicated
  With trauma or other bodily injury
  With other medical complications
  With delirium
  With perceptual distortions
  With coma
  With convulsions
  Pathological intoxication
Harmful use
Dependence syndrome
  Currently abstinent
  Currently abstinent, but in a protected environment
  Currently on a clinically supervised maintenance or
replacement regime (controlled dependence)
  Currently abstinent, but receiving treatment with aversive
or blocking drugs
  Currently using the substance (active dependence)
  Continuous use
  Episodic use (dipsomania)
Withdrawal state
  Uncomplicated
  With complications
Withdrawal state with delirium
  Without convulsions
  With convulsions
Psychotic disorder
  Schizophrenia-like
  Predominantly delusional
  Predominantly hallucinatory
  Predominantly polymorphic
  Predominantly depressive symptoms
  Predominantly manic symptoms
  Mixed
Amnesic syndrome
Residual and late-onset psychotic disorder
  Flashbacks
  Personality or behavior disorder
  Residual affective disorder
  Dementia
  Other persisting cognitive impairment
  Late-onset psychotic disorder
Other mental and behavioral disorders
Unspecified mental and behavioral disorder

introduced which closely resemble spontaneously occurring conditions. Perhaps the best example is amphetamine-induced paranoid psychosis which is almost indistinguishable from schizophrenic disorders of the paranoid type. Even in this instance, the amphetamine abuse precipitates the schizophrenic-type psychosis in individuals at risk of developing schizophrenia anyway, thereby accelerating the onset of the illness.

Predisposition to psychiatric disorders is an important factor in the induction of reactions to environ-mental toxins. A detailed previous psychiatric history and assessment of previous psychological and other functioning is essential in assessing reactions to environmental insults. Often psychological symptoms have occurred chronically or sporadically prior to the exposure. Ascription of causation can then become very difficult particularly when multiple agents and a complex response are involved. As well as psychological predispositions, physical predispositions are operative, for example, polymorphisms in metabolizing enzymes for organic chemicals. Similar polymorphisms are suspected of influencing susceptibility to psychiatric disorders.

METALS

Many of these elements are associated with significant psychiatric and psychological morbidity. They can be ingested in inorganic form or as organic derivatives, and the toxic effects may differ accordingly. Psychological consequences vary greatly in importance, both in terms of frequency of poisoning and severity of effects (Reinicke, 1982). Various metals are reviewed in turn below (in alphabetical order).

Aluminum

Aluminum is a widespread metallic element used in packaging materials, utensils, and the aviation and car industries. It is generally regarded as a non-toxic element but concerns about its toxicity in certain usages and contexts have led to a continuing reappraisal. In the context of this chapter, the possibility that some neurodegenerative diseases might be related to exposure to aluminum needs examination.

The element can be absorbed from food, drinking water, and drugs given by mouth. The process is complex depending on the form of the aluminum, factors relating to local conditions in the gut, and the physiological state of the individual, for example, renal function. Many organs contain aluminum but the concentrations are relatively low in the brain. It is mainly excreted via the urine.

Neurotoxic effects of aluminum are well established as in dialysis encephalopathy. The main effect is an aberration of cytoskeletal proteins with the formation of neurofibrillary tangles in neurones. Predisposing factors include: renal disorders; treatment with aluminum-contaminated parenteral preparations; oral exposure to aluminum-containing drugs or to milk. Dialysis encephalopathy is characterized by speech and coordination difficulties, twitching, myoclonic jerks, anxiety and depression, personality changes, and, ultimately, global dementia. The psychiatric abnormalities may progress to paranoid and suicidal behavior, and to hyperactivity and clouding of consciousness with delirium. Visual and auditory hallucinations are common. The dementia is fairly typical with disturbances of attention, concentration and motivation, and then disturbances of memory, followed by confusion and behavioral deterioration. Marked electroencephalogram (EEG) abnormalities occur early, with bursts of high-voltage slow-wave activity, with spike and wave discharges.

The dementia in dialysis encephalopathy and the neurotoxic changes in the brain have led to suggestions that aluminum toxicity is implicated in some way in Alzheimer's dementia (Alfrey et al., 1976). Thus, neurofibrillary tangles are found in both conditions as are senile plaques and granulovacuolar degeneration. Some early studies claimed to detect focal accumulations of aluminum in the brains of Alzheimer's patients (Candy et al., 1986; Ganrot, 1986). However, a more recent study using nuclear microscopy failed to show aluminum in the plaque cores of Alzheimer's patients (Landsberg et al., 1992).

Epidemiological studies have attempted to relate the prevalence of Alzheimer's disease to aluminum in the local environment. Some studies have claimed such a link (Martyn et al., 1989; Neri and Hewitt, 1991) whereas others have failed to establish any connection (Flaten et al., 1991; Wettstein et al., 1991). The evidence is thus inconclusive.

Another neuropsychiatric condition related to aluminum is parkinsonism/dementia found in some parts of south-east Asia and northern Australia. It is believed to be related to high levels of aluminum in the soil (Garruto et al., 1984, 1985).

Aluminum neurotoxicity can be minimized in dialysis patients by keeping aluminum levels as low as possible in the dialysis medium. Toxicity itself can be treated and reversed using the chelating agent, desferrioxamine (DFO) (McLachlan et al., 1991).

Arsenic

Arsenic has long enjoyed a nefarious reputation as a favored means of homicide by poisoners (Bednarczyk and Matusiak, 1982). Outbreaks of acute arsenic poisoning have also been described (Roses et al., 1991). Most exposure, however, is through chronic low-level exposure through the environment (Kreiss et al., 1983). Some pharmaceutical compounds used to contain arsenic and some unofficial preparations still do. Arsenic is used in the manufacture of insecticides and wood preservatives. The brewing of beer in the nineteenth century (Kelynack, 1990) and of 'moonshine' liquor in the twentieth century (Gerhardt et al., 1980) has been associated with arsenical contamination and syndromes which contain 'fatigue' as a prominent symptom. Arsenic is widely spread in the environment so that low-grade exposure is inevitable.

Arsenic is absorbed to a variable degree depending on its chemical form. It passes the blood–brain barrier with difficulty but accumulates in hair, nails, and skin.

Acute arsenic poisoning results in nausea and vomiting, and a condition resembling cholera. An odor resembling garlic in the breath may be noted. Chronic exposure may induce a peripheral neuropathy with tingling sensations, numbness in the limbs, and symmetrical muscular weakness (Chhuttani et al., 1967).

Barium

Barium derivatives are widely used in paints, glassmaking, and in the oil, rubber and sugar industries. The free barium ion is readily absorbed from gut or lung and it accumulates in the skeleton and eye. The ion is a muscle poison and causes nausea and vomiting, followed by loss of tendon reflexes and ultimately paralysis. No direct psychiatric effects have been described other than anxious reactions to the bodily symptoms, particularly muscular paralysis.

Bismuth

Bismuth is widely used in medicinal preparations but its industrial use is increasing as it replaces lead in some applications. Inorganic bismuth compounds are prescribed for a range of gastrointestinal symptoms such as peptic ulcer, flatulence, diarrhea and cramps, and in many countries compounds are available over the counter (Bradley et al., 1989). Bismuth can be absorbed from the gastrointestinal tract but bioavailability is very low. It can penetrate the brain but its concentrations there are lower than those in kidney, lung, and spleen.

Bismuth poisoning has an insidious onset with several weeks of prodromata such as memory impairment, insomnia, anxiety, depression, excitation, and hallucinations. This is followed by the sudden onset of an encephalopathy with clouding of consciousness and cerebellar signs such as ataxia and dysarthria (Mattle et al., 1982). Complete disorientation for time and place may lead on to coma. Terrifying visual hallucinations may be experienced, as may auditory hallucinations, agitation, and lowered arousal (de Mol et al., 1979). Sleep may be disrupted and about one-third of patients become depressed. A similar proportion show intellectual impairment with poor concentration, distractibility, and difficulty recalling recent events. The encephalopathy is usually reversible but after intoxication some patients have persisting intellectual difficulties, particularly affecting memory, together with severe insomnia and affective disorders (Buge et al., 1977).

Cobalt

This metal can be toxic and induce a cardiomyopathy but psychiatric effects have not been documented.

Gold

Gold compounds are used as slow-acting anti-rheumatic drugs. However, their efficacy has never been firmly established. The gold compounds are complex salts and are administered by injection but also orally, although they tend to be poorly absorbed. Because of the insolubility of gold, industrial poisoning is not usually encountered.

Nervous system reactions include neuropathies and the Guillain–Barré syndrome. Psychiatric symptoms vary from mild depression to frank confusional psychosis, the latter being part of a toxic encephalopathy (Sundelin, 1941).

Lead

This is a common element but has no known biological function. Nevertheless, it is toxic and lead poisoning has long been known to be an occupational hazard. Chronic plumbism was recognized in craftsmen, such as miners and painters, and comprised pallor, colics, joint pains, headaches, and neuropathies. The commonest current use is as an additive to petrol with concern that children could suffer ill-effects from both lead pollution in the atmosphere and contamination from household lead in tap-water pipes. The removal of lead from the environment proceeds apace.

Lead is taken into the body through the gastrointestinal tract, skin, and lungs. It is distributed widely in the body including brain and bones. It is excreted through most body fluids and waste products. Children absorb lead more extensively than do adults. In the central nervous system (CNS), lead tends to accumulate in the cerebellum, hippocampus, and cortex, followed by brain stem. Lead inhibits heme synthesis but its pathological actions in the CNS remain obscure.

Lead poisoning (plumbism) has many rather vague psychological features. Fatigue is one of the first features, coming on at the end of the day at first but then earlier and earlier. Anxiety and insomnia develop, together with loss of appetite and libido, and a 'masked' depressive illness may be suspected. Headaches, tremor, and abdominal colic then appear. Neuropsychological testing may reveal increasing impairments. Polyneuropathy is common, especially in adults.

Acute lead poisoning presents with lethargy, intense headaches and vomiting, ataxia, and even seizures. Psychiatric symptoms include anxiety and memory impairment. Alternating stupor and lucid intervals can present a confusing picture to the diagnostician. Untreated, coma and death may occur.

The more chronic forms of plumbism also present diagnostic problems. Lead encephalopathy develops insidiously with subtle personality changes, with fatigue, intellectual impairment, and sometimes psychotic phenomena, such as hallucinations, often in the context of clouding of consciousness (Cullen et al., 1983; Balestra, 1991). The EEG is, however, usually within normal limits (Sachs et al., 1979). The psychiatric abnormalities are typically accompanied by neurological and neuropathological abnormalities.

The cognitive–behavioral impairments associated with lead poisoning in children led to a longstanding controversy often conducted with vigor and verbal assertiveness bordering on vituperation. As it seemed that the nervous system of infants and children was more susceptible to lead poisoning than that of adults, studies were set in motion to detect any possible deleterious effects of low lead exposure. To do this, a variety of neuropsychological tests were used of varying sensitivity, reliability, and relevance to children's intellectual functioning.

The data from the studies were neither consistent nor conclusive. For example, Landrigan et al. (1975) reported a mean reduction of 10% in the IQ of children exposed to lead, whereas Pueschel (1974) found motor but no IQ impairment. The data relating to finger-wrist tapping speed are displayed in Figure 3.1. After reviewing the literature, Chisholm and Barltrop (1979) concluded that children with high levels of exposure to lead might run some risk of subtle neuropsychological impairments but that the evidence was by no means conclusive. Unfortunately, such words of caution became lost in exaggerated claims that permanent damage could occur at low levels of exposure, claims which environmentalists used to demand major and often unrealistic reductions in lead exposures.

Yule et al. (1981) tested 166 children whose blood lead levels had previously been measured. A battery of psychometric tests was used including the Wechsler Intelligence Scale, Neale Analysis of Reading Ability, and tests of spelling and arithmetic. There were significant associations between blood lead levels and some attainment scores, which remained even when social class was taken into account, although such measures were crude.

In the UK, several reports addressed this issue after review of the mass of often contradictory evidence (Department of Health and Social Security, 1980; Rutter, 1980; Medical Research Council 1983; 1988). The various reports came to a consensus best summed up in the words of Smith (1989, p. 42):

> Studies of the effects of lead on children are, for necessary ethical reasons, non-experimental in

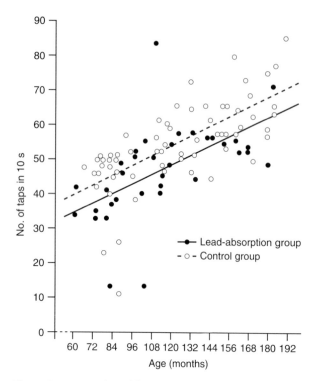

Figure 3.1 *Regression of finger-wrist tapping speed (dominant hand) by age and study group. (From Landrigan et al., 1975, with permission.)*

design. Such studies, particularly when they involve multivariate social data, pose problems in drawing causative inferences, and lead studies are no exception. Despite the wealth of data, and including data from experimental studies with animals, it is still not possible to conclude with any certainty that lead at low levels is affecting the performance or behavior of children. It is clear, however, that any differences in a measure such as IQ, which might be attributed to lead, are likely to be small, accounting for about 1 or 2% of the variance. The educational significance of even a small difference when applied to a total population is substantial, so the implication is not that such differences are unimportant: merely that they are difficult to detect amid the much larger influences of a number of interacting variables. Thus, it would seem that raised blood lead levels (above $40 \mu g/100 ml$) are probably associated with mild cognitive impairment and may possibly increase the likelihood of behavioral problems (Rutter, 1980). However, low-level lead exposure is probably a very minor and clinically unimportant factor in child development. In reality lead is ubiquitous and although measures such as encouraging the use of lead-free petrol and removing lead pipes in houses can be taken to reduce its concentration in the environment, it is

unrealistic to demand its almost complete elimination, even for children. Indeed although much progress has been made to lower lead concentrations in tap water, one recent survey in Glasgow showed that an estimated 13% of infants were exposed via bottle feeds to tap water lead concentrations above the WHO's guideline of $10 \mu g/l$ (Watt *et al.*, 1996).

Lithium

This element has been a component of various medicines for over a century. Its biological activities were rediscovered almost 50 years ago and it gradually became established for the treatment and prevention of affective disorders. It is now the standard medication for these conditions despite its known toxic and unwanted effects, and lingering doubts about its efficacy.

The acute toxic effects of lithium include nausea, vertigo, muscle weakness, tremor, ataxia, tinnitus, blurred vision, dysarthria, and drowsiness. They are listed in the data sheets of the various formulations available for medical prescription. More severe features are increasing disorientation, seizures, coma, and death. Chronic toxic effects are often subtle and insidious. These comprise polyuria with eventual changes in kidney structure and function, hypothyroidism, and memory impairment.

Acute episodes of toxicity may result in irreversible neuropsychiatric deficits, particularly cerebellar ataxia and dementia (Kores and Lader, 1997). Co-prescription of antipsychotic medication is a predisposing factor. Hemodialysis may be needed to reduce toxic lithium levels as rapidly as possible and the need for this should reflect the clinical state of the patient rather than serum lithium levels which may even appear within the normal range.

Manganese

Manganese is a common element used in metal industries. It has a biological function as part of a cofactor for some enzymes. It is poorly absorbed from the gut but passes the blood–brain barrier. Manganese intoxication can result in a form of parkinsonism, with degeneration of the basal ganglia, and psychiatric abnormalities are common in the earlier stages. These include a range of subjective symptoms (Figure 3.2) and mood changes with emotional lability and uncontrollable laughter (Roels *et al.*, 1987). In more severe cases, hallucinations and hyperactivity may occur (Chandra *et al.*, 1974). This psychosis then progresses to a clinical picture dominated by movement disorders. Neuropsychological testing shows impaired psychomotor

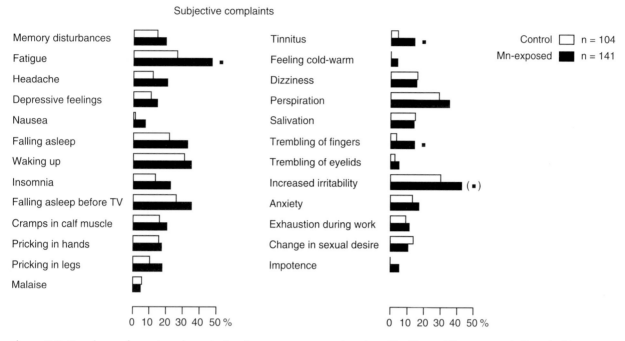

Figure 3.2 *Prevalence of symptoms in control and manganese-exposed workers. Significant differences are indicated with squares. (From Roels et al., 1987, by permission of Wiley-Liss, a subsidiary of John Wiley & Sons.)*

ability (Roels *et al.*, 1987), reflecting basal ganglia damage but also impaired cognitive functioning (Hua and Huang, 1991).

Mercury

The toxicity of mercury and its sulfide, cinnabar, was known to the ancients. Paracelsus described mercury poisoning as an industrial disease but also introduced its treatment for syphilis. Some ointments and dental amalgams still contain it. Industrial use is much less but it is still employed to refine gold.

Traditionally, mercury poisoning was associated with the making of hats, with the use of mercury in nitric acid as a stiffening agent for felt, producing 'hatters' shakes.' Methyl mercury poisoning has been seen on a large scale in Japan. This occurred when inorganic mercury was discharged into enclosed volumes of water in bays and was converted by bacteria to methyl mercury, becoming concentrated into the food chain (Clarkson, 1992). Methyl mercury in fish is much more toxic than inorganic mercury.

One of the earliest signs of inorganic (elemental) mercury poisoning is so-called erethism. This is characterized by irritability and difficulty in concentration, insomnia, and then by hallucinations and agitation (Gowers, 1893). More subtle changes include

marked timidity, social phobias, apathy, loss of confidence, and anhedonia. The mood can progress to a more obvious depression, accompanied by marked memory loss (Hamilton and Hardy, 1949). Neuro-psychological testing, used extensively in recent times to evaluate outbreaks of mercury poisoning, showed impairment of cognitive function and subjective fatigue, depression, and dysphoria. Older people were particularly affected (Bluhm *et al.*, 1990; Liang *et al.*, 1993).

Numerous neurological features can be seen including ataxia, tremor, acrodynia (see below), neuro-myasthenia, Guillain–Barré syndrome, and a progressive neuropathy. Some of the features may be atypical or rather bizarre and, together with the personality changes, may lead to the individual's complaints being dismissed as 'hysterical.'

Acrodynia is a form of chronic inorganic mercury poisoning in infants and children and was recognized in the first decades of this century (Warkany, 1966). The commonest causes were teething powders and worming powders containing mercury compounds. Acrodynia has an insidious onset with a change in behavior in the child. Irritability, apathy, insomnia, and anorexia lead to physical deterioration. Epidemiological data suggested that only a small minority of children exposed to mercury develop acrodynia but the predisposing factors are unknown.

Thallium

Thallium is a heavy metal used to kill insects and rodents, and is used in the jewelry industry. A cardinal feature of poisoning is hair-loss but gastrointestinal disturbances can include nausea, vomiting, and even hemorrhage. Neurological signs comprise neuropathies, ataxia, choreic movements, and fits (Prick, 1979).

The psychiatric features comprise a major disturbance of sleep rhythm. The patient is fatigued during the day but cannot sleep at night because of dysregulation of the sleep/wake cycle. The patient becomes disoriented, often severely, and speech becomes incoherent. Fits can occur with peculiar emotional and behavioral concomitants. Instinctive forms of behavior such as chewing and sniffing predominate. Hyperemotionality is seen in less severe cases, together with apathy at other times. Dementia is a common sequela (Reed et al., 1963).

Tin

Tin is a common metal used as an alloy in bronze. It is generally regarded as innocuous in the elemental form. However, organotin compounds can be highly toxic (Foncin and Gruner, 1979). The first symptom is severe headache radiating to face and neck. Photophobia and vomiting may occur imitating meningitis. Drowsiness or paradoxical insomnia, clouding of consciousness, anxiety, fear of dying, fatigue, and weakness are subsequent psychiatric symptoms. The condition is usually reversible but memory disturbances may persist.

Zinc

Zinc is an essential element, a constituent of several enzymes. Metal fume fever can occur in the metal industry such as in galvanizing processes. It is mainly respiratory in nature, together with nausea and vomiting, but weakness and fatigue may occur (Langham Brown, 1988).

CARBON MONOXIDE

Carbon monoxide (CO) is a product of incomplete combustion of carbon-containing substances, such as petrol. It combines with hemoglobin with an affinity several hundred times that of oxygen. At sufficient concentrations of carboxyhemoglobin (COHb), tissue anoxia results. The commonest causes of carbon monoxide poisoning are poorly ventilated heating systems. It can be a cause of suicidal poisoning, usually by attaching a hose-pipe to the car exhaust. When coal gas contained CO, it was commonly used, especially by women, to attempt suicide but natural gas has insufficient CO to be toxic.

Acute intoxication is accompanied by a variety of symptoms attributable to cerebral anoxia including headache, fatigue, malaise, nausea and vomiting, and dizziness (Lowe-Ponsford and Henry, 1989). The sufferer may be confused and lethargic and lapse into coma. In one large-scale poisoning of 184 people at a high school in Ann Arbor, Michigan, the commonest symptom was headache (90%), then dizziness (82%), and weakness (53%) (Burney et al., 1982). The symptoms are exposure-related and related to the COHb in the blood. Thus, 0.2% in the atmosphere is rapidly fatal (Table 3.2) (Winter and Miller, 1976).

Permanent damage can follow acute CO intoxication. Dementia is common, often accompanied by a confusional psychosis and movement disorders such as chorea and parkinsonism (Klawans et al., 1982; Schwartz et al., 1985; Davous et al., 1986). Obsessive–compulsive behavior may be noted with obvious parallels to a postencephalitic state (Laplane et al., 1982). Gilles de la Tourette's syndrome has been reported as an extreme form of obsessive disability following CO poisoning (Pulst et al., 1983). As with

Table 3.2 *Symptoms associated with varying levels of carbon monoxide poisoning. Source: Winter and Miller, 1976, p 1503, with permission*

CO in atmosphere, %	COHb in blood, %	Physiological and subjective symptoms
0.007	10	No appreciable effect, except shortness of breath on vigorous exertion; possible tightness across the forehead; dilation of cutaneous blood vessels
0.012	20	Shortness of breath on moderate exertion; occasional headache with throbbing in temples
0.022	30	Decided headache; irritable; easily fatigued; judgement disturbed; possible dizziness; dimness of vision
0.035–0.052	40–50	Headache; confusion; collapse; fainting on exertion
0.080–0.122	60–70	Unconsciousness; intermittent convulsions; respiratory failure; death if exposure is long continued
0.195	80	Rapidly fatal
0.195	80	Immediately fatal

other forms of brain damage, the patient may be inert and passive, but can be disturbed with aggressive outbursts.

Some patients appear to recover completely from acute CO poisoning only to succumb to delayed poisoning 3–28 days after exposure (Sawa *et al.*, 1981; Myers *et al.*, 1985). Following apparent recovery ('pseudorecovery'), the patient, usually elderly, suddenly deteriorates despite a normal Hb concentration (Norris *et al.*, 1982). Neuropsychiatric symptoms predominate (Roos, 1994), of which the psychiatric components include lethargy, memory disturbances, dementia, and bizarre behavioral upsets to the point of psychosis. Less severe symptoms are emotional lability, anxiety, and depressive phases. The condition may remit, but often slowly, or it may progress to severe dementia and death (Smith and Brandon, 1973). Even in those who apparently remit, neuropsychological tests will still reveal some deficits, particularly of memory and of personality changes.

Chronic intoxication with CO occurs with long-term low-grade exposure, for example, from a poorly ventilated gas fire. The symptoms are similar to those of acute poisoning but fluctuate, related to the usage of the appliance. Typically, the symptoms such as headache and depression resolve when the sufferer is away from home or in the summer. Anorexia and weight loss, anxiety, mood swings, and personality changes may all occur. These deficits may become permanent.

ALCOHOLS AND GLYCOLS

In this section, psychiatric features of acute and chronic poisoning, and the sequelæ thereof, of various alcohols and glycols are summarized. The exception is ethanol which would warrant a volume on its own and reference should be made to standard textbooks of psychiatry.

Methanol

Methanol is widely used as a solvent in the paint industry, as an antifreeze, and elsewhere. It is metabolized to formaldehyde, then to formic acid, carbon dioxide, and water. Methanol itself is non-toxic; it is the metabolites that cause the neurological damage including optic atrophy.

The initial effects of methanol poisoning are mild CNS depression without the disinhibition and euphoria seen with ethanol. After a further 12–24 h, gastrointestinal disturbances, ocular abnormalities, and metabolic acidosis set in. Among the symptoms are headache and weakness. Subjective complications of diminished light

perception, with yellow or gray spots or flashes, may be misdiagnosed as hysterical phenomena, but fundal changes eventually become apparent. CNS symptoms may intensify and include confusion with disorientation to time and place, irritability, and amnesia. Convulsions and death may follow.

Late sequels in those who survive the acute phase are a frontal lobe syndrome with lack of initiative and dementia (McLean *et al.*, 1980; Anderson *et al.*, 1987; 1989). In the most severe cases, a vegetative state may occur.

Isopropanol

This is an industrial solvent which is about twice as potent as ethanol in causing CNS depression.

Ethylene glycol

Ethylene glycol (1,2-ethanediol) is widely used as a coolant, antifreeze, and solvent. Intoxications result from both accidental and deliberate ingestion, and sometimes from adulteration, for example, in white wine. The toxic metabolites are glycoaldehyde, glycolic acid, glyoxylic acid, and oxalic acid.

Neurological and psychiatric symptoms usually supervene within 12 h of ingestion. The latter include intoxication, slurred speech, irritability, and stupor. Residual effects are usually neurological, with cranial polyneuropathy, although renal damage may also occur.

OTHER SOLVENTS AND INHALANTS

This rubric covers a group of liquid volatile compounds which include trichloroethylene, toluene, xylene, styrene, benzene, acetone and petroleum products, and hundreds of others. Their use is widespread in industry with millions of workers worldwide exposed to them. The main method of absorption is by inhalation; absorption through the skin is of minor importance. Many of these compounds are also abused. Both acute and chronic toxicity have been described and both syndromal groups have psychiatric and cognitive components.

Acute effects comprise drowsiness, fatigue, dizziness, light-headedness, and headache. Tolerance to these effects is usual although a few people exposed to organic solvents remain intolerant either chronically or on re-exposure, for example, on returning to work after the weekend. Some individuals seek out the intoxicant effects of these substances and may be in a mildly euphoric or exhilarated state for much of their work time.

The long-term effects of these solvents have given rise to much debate and some controversy. A range of studies has been carried out, mainly case-control epidemiological in type, to ascertain whether neuropsychiatric syndromes and cognitive deficits are associated with long-term exposure to organic solvents (Baker, 1994). Despite some difficulties, three groups of symptoms have been delineated.

The first is an organic affective syndrome with subjective features only. These include depression, fatigue, loss of interest, and irritability. The second has cognitive elements as well as mood disturbances and more closely resembles a mild chronic toxic encephalopathy. There are memory and attention deficits and also some psychomotor impairments. The third syndrome is a rare severe chronic toxic encephalopathy with irreversible CNS damage. Personality changes, impaired judgment, explosive outbursts, and cognitive deficits may severely limit the patient's occupational and social capacity.

The personality disturbances in the second syndrome were described in detail by Morrow et al. (1989). Using the Minnesota Multiphasic Personality Inventory (MMPI), they noted increased rates of depression, anxiety, difficulties in thinking and concentration, and feelings of unreality. The similarity to post-traumatic stress disorder (PTSD) was commented upon.

Sleep apnoea has been suggested as a feature of chronic solvent abuse, presumably due to chronic poisoning of the respiratory centers with insensitivity to carbon dioxide. In one small series, half the patients with solvent exposure showed this feature (Monstad et al., 1987). Nevertheless, most of the neuropsychiatric features in workers exposed to solvents are non-specific. For example, Axelson et al. (1976), in a case-referent study, used data from a regional Swedish support fund. They calculated a risk ratio of 1.8 for non-specific psychiatric disorders among solvent-exposed workers as compared with those not so exposed. The longer the exposure, the higher the risk. The diagnoses were made according to the International Classification of Diseases for 1965 and they are difficult to translate into current categories. 'Neurasthenia' and alcoholism were the commonest afflictions in the exposed subjects followed by anxiety and 'dementia.'

A similar study was carried out among Danish furniture and wood workers who were pensioned off due to disability (Olsen and Sabroe, 1980). Former employees such as cabinet makers with high levels of exposure to lacquers and glues had a higher risk of being in receipt of a disability pension for a neuropsychiatric condition than carpenters who in turn had a higher risk than non-exposed individuals. 'Neuroses' were especially common. A Finnish study of car painters with long-term exposure to mixtures of organic solvents reported symptoms of excessive tiredness, poor memory, impaired concentration, and

disturbances in vigilance at a higher rate than the control groups of train drivers (Husman, 1980). A symptom questionnaire and standardized psychiatric interview were conducted in a comparison of 80 car or industrial spray painters with long-term low-level exposure to organic solvents in comparison to two groups of unexposed workers (Elofsson et al., 1980). Eight of the 52 psychiatric symptom questions in the questionnaire were answered positively at a significantly higher rate in the exposed than non-exposed groups. They were: strong (sic) fatigue after work, feelings of exhaustion, notes needed for remembrance (sic), mixing things up in mind, help needed for recollection, absentmindedness, feelings of distress, and nightmares. A wide range of complaints were elicited at interview relating to short-term memory problems, headache, lability of mood, and difficulties with precise movements.

A most unusual syndrome has been described in one group of solvent-exposed workers (Ryan et al., 1988). These people described hypersensitivity to smells ('cacosmia') such as petrol, perfumes or ordure, and developed dizziness, nausea and feelings of weakness. Cognitive performance was also impaired in these patients.

Neuropsychological performance

A relatively large number of studies have used neuropsychological tests to attempt to detect continuing impairment in workers exposed to industrial solvents. A whole range of solvents have been involved, both singly and in mixtures. The topic is a complex one, most comprehensively reviewed by Baker (1994) following two important international conferences in 1985 which evaluated the whole area.

A large number of studies have been carried out within many industries and only a sample of the findings can be given. However, the literature on neuropsychological deficits in workers exposed to solvents is not entirely consistent. The study of Elofsson et al. (1980), cited earlier, found statistically significant differences between solvent-exposed and unexposed workers with respect to manual dexterity, perceptual speed, and short-term memory. Tests of verbal and spatial skills and of reasoning were unaffected, suggesting fairly specific solvent-related effects. Neuropsychological testing of Finnish car painters suggested impairment of verbal skills, both intelligence and memory (Hänninen et al., 1976).

More recent studies suggest that short-term memory, visuospatial ability, psychomotor speed and precision, and attentional processes are most often impaired in solvent-exposed workers (Baker, 1994). Dose and/or duration effects are apparent in some of the larger studies. For example, Spurgeon et al. (1992) detected a significant effect on cognitive functioning in workers exposed to organic solvents for more than 30 years.

One ingenious study used identical twin-pairs, one exposed to solvents, the co-twin not exposed (Hänninen *et al.*, 1991). Cognitive but not psychomotor function was impaired in the exposed twin group as compared with the control twins. The data for the Stroop test are shown in Figure 3.3.

The long-term prognosis in workers with previously diagnosed chronic solvent intoxication due to trichloroethylene was examined in a study from Helsinki (Lindström *et al.*, 1982). No clear-cut trends were found.

Overall, the burgeoning literature on organic solvent neuropsychiatric toxicity points to changes in mood and personality on chronic exposure, with anxiety, depression, and irritability. Feelings of unreality and disturbances in thinking are also common. Neuropsychological deficits involve short-term memory and psychomotor function.

Volatile substance abuse (VSA) remains a problem among adolescents (Flanagan and Ives, 1994). The lay term 'glue-sniffing' refers to VSA and the commonest substances involved are toluene, petroleum products, halogenated solvents, and volatile hydrocarbons. Small doses lead to euphoria, higher doses may induce hallucinations and delusions, often paranoia.

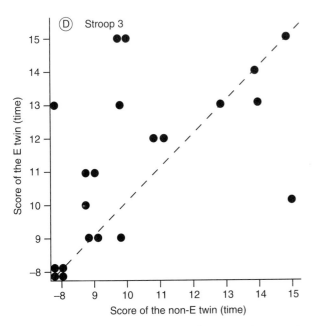

Figure 3.3 *Scores for Stroop test of twins exposed to organic solvents plotted against those of non-exposed co-twins (performance time in seconds). (From Hänninen et al., 1991, with permission of BMJ Publishing Group.)*

ORGANOCHLORINE COMPOUNDS (OCS)

These compounds were once extensively used as insecticides but are largely replaced by the organophosphates. They comprise three general classes: (a) dichlorodiphenylethanes (for example, dicophane (DDT)); (b) chlorinated cyclodienes (aldrin/dieldrin); (c) hexachlorocyclohexanes (lindane). The function of several neurotransmitters is altered by the OCs.

Poisoning in humans is accompanied by CNS excitation with dizziness and confusion. Individuals exposed to Agent Orange in Vietnam or to dioxin after an explosion in a chemical factory in Seveso, Italy, or in other incidents experienced irritability, fatigue, problems with memory, inability to concentrate, and sleep disturbances (Pazderova-Vejlupková *et al.*, 1981; Levy, 1988).

ORGANOPHOSPHATES (OPS)

These compounds are extensively used as pesticides, for example, in spraying crops and in dipping sheep. They act by inhibiting the enzyme cholinesterase, thereby permitting the accumulation of acetylcholine in the synaptic cleft and neuromuscular junction, and thus prolonging its effect. Much controversy has accompanied the use of these compounds, particularly as sheep-dips. As compulsory measures were introduced in some countries to enforce annual dipping of sheep, any resulting toxicity could be blamed on the agricultural agencies and ultimately the governments. Consequently, establishing the link between possible neurological damage and the use of organophosphate pesticides has become an important medico-legal issue. It is, however, also important to establish whether any link exists between such usage and psychiatric/neuropsychological dysfunction.

The acute effects of exposure to OPs are well known. The first symptoms are mainly psychological with anxiety, tension, irritability, restlessness, emotional lability, and insomnia with excessive dreaming. Other non-specific symptoms include drowsiness, headaches and dizziness, and tremor may be marked. Disturbances of attention, concentration, and memory are noted both subjectively and on formal testing. Less common psychiatric symptoms are depression and withdrawal.

Some neuropsychological test procedures have been conducted on workers exposed acutely to OPs. The first was that of Durham *et al.* (1965). They used various tests of 'mental alertness,' including complex reaction time and paced vigilance tests. The study group was crop sprayers of varying degrees of exposure, the controls had no history of exposure. Immediately after exposure, decrements in performance were noted but these did not persist beyond the period of exposure. No dose–effect relationships were uncovered.

Abnormalities of memory, signal processing, vigilance, semantic performance, and proprioceptive feedback were tested in 23 workers exposed to OP pesticides (Rodnitzky et al., 1975). Compared with unexposed individuals, no deficits were detected, leading the authors to the conclusion that higher CNS functions are relatively resistant to the acute effects of OPs.

The OP, diazinon, was used by 99 pest control workers who were tested before and after their work shift using a computerized battery of tests (Maizlish et al., 1987). Again, no unequivocal decrements in performance were detected but it does seem that the diazinon exposure was fairly low level.

Delayed effects of OP exposure have been described and the syndrome is termed the organophosphorous-induced delayed (poly) neuropathy (OPIDP or OPIDN) or the intermediate syndrome. Symptoms begin one to three weeks after acute exposure and generally resemble those of acute exposure itself. Psychiatric symptoms have not been described other than those in reaction to the physical symptoms such as pain, numbness, and limb weakness.

Attempts have been made to discover any chronic sequelæ resulting from one or more episodes of undoubted acute toxicity. Savage et al. (1988) compared 100 individuals with previous acute exposure to OPs with carefully matched individuals not so poisoned. A physical examination with neurological evaluations, EEG recordings, and various neuropsychological and personality tests were incorporated in the battery. No differences between the groups were found with respect to special sense function or the EEG. However, the poisoned subjects were worse than the controls on four out of five summary measures – memory, abstraction, depressed mood, and motor reflexes. More specifically, deficits were found with respect to widely differing abilities such as intellectual functioning, academic skills, flexibility of thinking, and simple motor skills. The authors concluded that their careful matching of cases and controls and the exclusion of other possible sources of neuropsychological impairment 'make it likely that the excess deficits recorded in the poisoned subjects are due to their previous OP poisoning.' However, close analysis of their data shows that pre-morbid intelligence, as assessed by verbal IQ, was significantly higher in the controls but was not used as a co-variate in analyzing the other variables. This criticism can be leveled at some other studies as well.

A retrospective study of agricultural workers in Nicaragua compared 36 men previously poisoned with OPs with men without episodes of poisoning, although possibly exposed to OP use (Rosenstock et al., 1991). A WHO neuropsychological core test battery was used and differences were found in the digit span, digit

vigilance, Benton visual retention, digit symbol, trails A, block design, pursuit aiming and dexterity tests. Again, the poisoned groups had lower vocabulary scores than the non-poisoned group but including this in the analysis of the other variables only lessened the contrast to a minor degree. No psychiatric symptoms were reported.

Duffy et al. (1979) used both clinical and computer-analyzed EEG to seek persistent brain abnormalities following acute exposure to the OP compound, sarin. Some differences were found both during waking and sleeping, and may be interpreted to reflect long-term sequelæ. In another study, 235 individuals reported as having been poisoned by an OP were interviewed (Tabershaw and Cooper, 1966). About one-third reported persistent effects including unspecified neuropsychiatric symptoms.

Neurological effects after acute and subacute OP exposure are well documented (Baker and Sedgwick, 1996) but the effects of chronic exposure to low OP levels are more difficult to detect (Beach et al., 1996). Psychiatric abnormalities on chronic exposure have long been believed to occur. In 1961, Gershon and Shaw (1961) reported on 16 cases in Australia in whom psychiatric sequelæ to chronic OP exposure were claimed. Of these, 11 had experienced acute episodes of schizophrenic and depressive-type symptoms, as well as more chronic symptoms. Psychological symptoms included severe impairment of memory and difficulty in concentration. By 12 months postexposure 'almost all reverted to normal.' An epidemiological study, also in Australia, carried out in response to the Gershon and Shaw report evaluated the incidence of psychiatric admissions in Victoria (Stoller et al., 1965). No relationship to sales of OP pesticides was found, although patients with OP-related symptoms not admitted to hospital would have been missed.

Another early study involved two crop-spraying pilots who developed psychiatric symptoms such as depression, phobia, and acute anxiety (Dille and Smith, 1964). It is interesting to note that it was common practice at that time for such pilots to take atropine to suppress the acute symptoms of exposure in order to continue work.

The study by Davignon et al. (1965) compared 441 apple-growers exposed to OP pesticides with 170 persons living in the same environment and 162 other people with no OP exposure. Some neurological but no psychiatric differences were found.

An index of chronic exposure levels to OPs was developed and used to dichotomize 59 male workers (Korsak and Sato, 1977). Outcome measures included tests from a neuropsychological test battery and power-spectral analyzed EEG. Plasma cholinesterase estimates were also made. Visuo-spatial impairment was detected in the trail making test and the Bender visual motor Gestalt test, with respect to the high- and low-exposure groups. Some EEG differences were also noted. The authors concluded that left frontal lobe function was particularly vulnerable to OPs.

A cross-sectional comparison was made of neuropsychological performance in 146 sheep farmers exposed to OP during sheep-dipping and 143 non-exposed quarry workers (Stephens *et al.*, 1995). The General Health Questionnaire (GHQ) was used to assess 'vulnerability to psychiatric disorder' and a battery of eight neuropsychological tests was used. Exposed subjects were 1.5 times more likely to reach criteria for 'caseness' on the GHQ ($p = 0.035$). The farmers performed significantly worse than controls on tests of sustained attention and speed of information processing (see Figure 3.4). Co-varying out pre-existing differences with respect to numerous inter-group differences still left test performance differences, but this posthoc procedure is less rigorous than very careful matching. Another criticism is that time-of-day and place-of-test effects may have acted differently on the two groups as the farmers were visited at home in the evening and the quarrymen were tested during the day at work. Furthermore, despite reluctance to wear adequate protective clothing, sheep farmers usually manage to avoid significant OP toxicity (Rees, 1996).

It is probable that neuropsychological and psychiatric effects can occur after OP poisoning (Eyer, 1995). The most frequent symptoms are listed in Table 3.3. However, the same reviewer concluded that 'the presently available data do not indicate that asymptomatic exposure to organophosphates is connected with an increasing risk of neuropsychopathological sequelæ.' This is essentially the conclusion of a team of psychologists who also reviewed the topic and called for more sophisticated and complex research (Mearns

Table 3.3 *Most frequent long-term symptoms following acute OP poisoning (Eyer, 1995)*

Impaired vigilance and reduced concentration
Reduced information processing and psychomotor speed
Memory deficit
Linguistic disturbances
Depression, anxiety, and irritability

et al., 1994). Factors such as individual predisposition, type of compound, use of alcohol, or concurrent illness or disability have not been explored. Longitudinal studies would be invaluable (Steenland, 1996), together with meticulous neurophysiological investigations.

Thus, the question as to possible psychiatric and neuropsychological effects of low-level OP exposure remains unresolved. Despite long-standing interest in the topic (Kraybill, 1969), a recent conference involving doctors, farmers and others was unable to reach a conclusion backed by any adequate data (National Farmers' Union, 1995).

Organophosphate nerve agents comprise a group of rapidly acting cholinesterase inhibitors. Many of the features of acute and sub-acute poisoning resemble these of OP pesticide poisoning but very few data are available. As with the pesticides, the possibility that chronic low-level exposure might result in psychiatric and neuropsychological pathology has not been excluded (for review, see Marrs and Maynard, 1994).

EOSINOPHILIA-MYALGIA SYNDROME (EMS) AND L-TRYPTOPHAN

L-Tryptophan is a naturally occurring amino acid, the precursor of 5-hydroxytryptamine, serotonin. It is used as an adjunct to antidepressants and was available either on prescription or in health-food shops. An unusual symptom-complex comprising intense myalgia and blood eosinophilia was identified and seemed to be associated with the use of L-tryptophan (Kaufman and Philen, 1993). Eventually, it became highly probable that the syndrome was due to a contaminant, perhaps an ethylidene derivative, introduced during the manufacture of the L-tryptophan. Similarities to the 'toxic oil syndrome' have also been noted.

Among the neuropsychiatric features of the EMS are memory and concentration disturbances, and psychomotor slowing (Krupp *et al.*, 1993).

LSD AND MDMA

A wide range of licit and illicit drugs can induce psychiatric and behavioral toxicity. Space precludes a

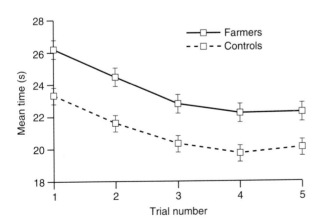

Figure 3.4 *Symbol-digit substitution in five blocks of nine items in OP-exposed farmers and controls. (From Stephens et al., 1995, with permission.)*

systematic evaluation and text books of therapeutics and drug abuse cover this topic in some depth. However, LSD and MDMA ('Ecstasy') poisoning incorporate some interesting features which it is interesting to consider, particularly with respect to long-term effects.

LSD

The use of natural substances such as mushrooms and cacti to induce abnormal mental states goes back to antiquity. However, the discovery in 1943 by the Swiss pharmacologist, Albert Hoffmann, of the hallucinogenic properties of the ergot derivative, LSD, facilitated systematic study of these substances. As well as numerous research investigations, LSD was also used in the clinical context to try and reproduce psychotic phenomena ('psychotomimetic'), to loosen inhibitions during various forms of psychotherapy ('psycholytic'), and to provide an ineffable mind-expanding experience ('psychedelic'). In none of these uses was the efficacy of LSD ever established but the dangers quickly became apparent (Report by the Advisory Committee on Drug Dependence, 1970).

For the purpose of describing the adverse reactions described with LSD, the classification suggested by Cohen (1966) will be used, excluding accidental overdose, illicit use, and chromosomal abnormalities.

PSYCHOTIC DISORDERS

Elkes et al. (1955) warned as early as this date of possible dangers, including harm during intoxication, delayed and severe response, and aggravation of early psychotic conditions. By 1959, Klee and Weintraub were referring to the 'well-known' paranoid reaction following LSD and described four such reactions in previously normal individuals. They warn about the possible chronicity of such reactions.

Probably the most influential publication on the adverse effects and complications of LSD was that by Cohen (1960) who gave the results of a questionnaire survey of 62 investigators who had used LSD or mescaline. Data on almost 5000 individuals given these drugs on more than 25 000 occasions were available. Adverse reactions were commoner at doses of LSD over 75 μg. Immediate reactions included excessive sympathetic responses (rapid heart beat, flushing, etc.), one case of convulsion, panic episodes, and severe physical reactions. The LSD psychosis-like state could be prolonged for 'another day or two.' Prolonged psychotic breakdowns were reported in a few patients, with occasional incomplete recovery. The rate of such reactions was about 2/1000 patients. A later publication described some more cases of prolonged psychosis but Cohen and Ditman (1963) conclude that

such serious complications 'are infrequent.' Persistent hallucinosis is one particular form of these prolonged reactions (Rosenthal, 1964).

Further reports focused on prolonged psychotic reactions in patients with pre-existing psychoses. Fink et al. (1966) found an incidence of 2% of such reactions, 10 times that of Cohen. These authors considered that the hazard of LSD therapy lay not in precipitating a schizophrenic-like state but rather in decreasing emotional controls. Manifestly, it is much more difficult to evaluate a psychosis persisting or worsening in a psychotic patient than the apparent induction of a psychosis in a neurotic individual. Illicit use of LSD was also associated with psychiatric complications. Freedman (1968) from his extensive experience on the campus of Chicago University was of the opinion that 'users who end up in hospitals with prolonged and serious psychoses are initially a quite unstable group.' Similar experiences at the University of California, Los Angeles, led Ungerlieder et al. (1966) to raise concerns about the widespread, unsupervised use of LSD.

In Malleson's survey (1971), 37 cases of psychosis were reported in the 4300 subjects, an incidence of 8/1000. Of these at least 10 were chronic and failed to recover, although in some cases the clinician thought they would have become psychotic anyway. The remaining 19 cases recovered completely but some took several months to do so.

FLASHBACKS

The spontaneous recurrence of LSD-induced visual phenomena has been termed 'flashback.' The flashbacks can be of three types – perceptual distortions, heightened imagery, and recurrent unbidden images (Horowitz, 1969). The definitive review is that by Abraham (1983). Abraham studied 123 persons with a history of LSD use, comparing them with 40 control subjects. A variety of visual disturbances were reported, and in half the users such flashbacks tended to persist, at least for the five years of follow-up. Some individuals developed flashbacks after single exposure to LSD, others only after several hundred exposures. Flashbacks could be delayed for up to six years after the LSD episode. Benzodiazepine tranquilizers lessened the intensity and frequency of flashbacks. In neither Cohen's (1960) nor Malleson's (1971) surveys is flashback mentioned.

DEPRESSIVE DISORDERS AND SUICIDE

This third major category is an important one as it underlines the dangers of LSD therapy even under supervised administration. Cohen's (1960) survey focused on attempted and completed suicides in patients and came up with an incidence of 1.2/1000 for the former and 0.4/1000 for the latter. No such reactions were reported in normal subjects given LSD experimentally. However, the literature on the dangers of illicit LSD use makes frequent mention of this complication (Ungerlieder *et al.*, 1966; Freedman, 1968). McGlothlin and Arnold (1971) found seven of their 247 subjects to believe that LSD had contributed to increased anxiety and/or depression. Malleson (1971) reported three suicides which 'appeared to have a temporal relationship to LSD' (a rate of 0.7/1000). There were also nine cases of definite attempted suicides and 11 further cases with insufficient data.

Other adverse reactions include paranoid reactions, chronic anxiety, panic states, dyssocial behavior, antisocial behavior, convulsions (Cohen, 1960), disinhibition (Cohen and Ditman, 1963), and multiple somatic complaints.

It is always difficult to set into perspective the incidence of adverse effects when these effects can often be part and parcel of the underlying condition for which the drug was given. It is impossible to be sure that a patient presenting with neurotic complaints of anxiety or obsessive symptoms is not already in the prodromal phase of a psychosis or a depressive disorder. Every psychiatrist can recall patients with apparently minor symptoms who steadily and inexorably lapse into a severe, chronic, and unremitting psychosis. Attempted and completed suicide is a known risk of depression and of schizophrenia, with about 10% of sufferers from these conditions ending their lives this way. Temporal sequences of drug and then a putative reaction do not equate to a causal relationship. It is therefore difficult to be certain that psychotic reactions and depression are caused by the use of LSD. Flashbacks, which are not a feature of mental illness, except for post-traumatic stress disorder, can be much more confidently attributed to LSD use.

MDMA ('Ecstasy')

MDMA is 3,4-methylenedioxymethamphetamine, known on the 'street' as Ecstasy. It was synthesized at the beginning of this century but only came into vogue about 10 years ago. It is widely taken on a sporadic basis to induce feelings of euphoria and tirelessness, and is firmly embedded in the 'rave scene,' parties of teenagers who congregate at the weekend for prolonged dancing sessions. As with many drugs of abuse, acute toxicity can occur.

The acute effects of MDMA are probably related to the release of dopamine and serotonin. However, evidence from animal experiments suggests that it can cause degeneration of serotonergic neurones (Green and Goodwin, 1996). Evidence in humans is not yet compelling but the possibility of long-term neuronal damage in habitual users cannot be dismissed. Thus, serotonin metabolites in the cerebrospinal fluid (CSF) are lowered in Ecstasy users (McCann *et al.*, 1994). Psychiatric abnormalities including depression have also been described (McGuire *et al.*, 1994). The severe, irreversible form of parkinsonism induced by the meperidine analogue, MPTP (1-methyl-4-phenyl-1,2,3,6-tetrahydropyridine), is proof that neurotoxicity of a highly specific nature can occur in humans (Langston *et al.*, 1993).

CONCLUSIONS

An extremely wide range of chemical and other environmental insults can impinge on the brain to cause psychiatric and behavioral disorders. These abnormalities can be mild, such as anxiety, depression, fatigability, and minor disturbances of memory; major, such as dementia, confusional or paranoid psychosis, and severe personality change. As well as these nonspecific syndromes, a few specific conditions have been described.

The development of psychiatry recently has provided the framework for the careful description of these toxin-induced psychiatric syndromes. Diagnostic and severity rating scales are available and are useful both for research and clinical purposes. The symptoms, psychiatric and behavioral syndromes, and disorders induced by environmental toxins should be as carefully studied as are the neurological consequences of exposure. In particular, long-term studies will help set the entire topic into perspective.

REFERENCES

Abraham, H.D. 1983: Visual phenomenology of the LSD flashback. *Archives of General Psychiatry*, **40**, 884–9.

Alfrey, A.C., LeGendre, G.R. and Kaehny, W. 1976: The dialysis encephalopathy syndrome. *New England Journal of Medicine*, **294**, 184–8.

American Psychiatric Association 1994: *Diagnostic and Statistical Manual-IV: Diagnostic Criteria from DSM-IV*. Washington, DC: American Psychiatric Association.

Anderson, T.J., Shuaib, A. and Becker, W.J. 1987: Neurologic sequelæ of methanol poisoning. *Canadian Medical Association Journal*, **136**, 1177–9.

Anderson, T.J., Shuaib, A. and Becker, W.J. 1989: Methanol poisoning: factors associated with neurologic complications. *Canadian Journal of Neurological Sciences*, **16**, 432–5.

Axelson, O., Hane, M. and Hogstedt, C. 1976: A case-referent study on neuropsychiatric disorders among workers exposed to solvents. *Scandinavian Journal of Work Environment and Health*, **2**, 14–20.

Baker, D.J. and Sedgwick, E.M. 1996: Single fiber electromyographic changes in man after organophosphate exposure. *Human and Experimental Toxicology*, **15**, 369–75.

Baker, E.L. 1994: A review of recent research on health effects of human occupational exposure to organic solvents. A critical review. *Journal of Occupational Medicine*, **36**, 1079–92.

Balestra, D.J. 1991: Adult chronic lead intoxication. *Archives of Internal Medicine*, **151**, 1718–20.

Beach, J.R., Spurgeon, A., Stephens, R. *et al.* 1996: Abnormalities on neurological examination among sheep farmers exposed to organophosphorous pesticides. *Occupational and Environmental Medicine*, **53**, 520–5.

Bednarczyk, L.R. and Matusiak, W. 1982: Case report: an arsenic murder. *Journal of Analytical Toxicology*, **6**, 260–1.

Bluhm, R.E., Welch, L.W., Bobbitt, R.G., Bonfiglio, J.F., Wood, A.J.J. and Branch, R.A. 1990: Acute elemental mercury exposure induces dose-related persistent neuropsychological sequelæ in man. *Veterinary and Human Toxicology*, **32**, 364.

Bradley, B., Singleton, M. and Li Wan Po, A. 1989: Bismuth toxicity – a reassessment. *Journal of Clinical Pharmacy and Therapeutics*, **14**, 423–41.

Buge, A., Rancurel, G. and Dechy, H. 1977: Encéphalopathies myocloniques bismuthiques formes évolutives, complications tardives durables ou définitives. *Revue de Neurologie (Paris)*, **133**, 401–15.

Burney, R.E., Wu, S-C. and Nemiroff, M.J. 1982: Mass carbon monoxide poisoning: clinical effects and results of treatment in 184 victims. *Annals of Emergency Medicine*, **11**, 394–9.

Candy, J.M., Klinowski, J., Perry, R.H. *et al.* 1986: Aluminosilicates and senile plaque formation in Alzheimer's disease. *Lancet*, **i**, 354–6.

Chandra, S.V., Seth, P.K. and Mankeshwar, J.K. 1974: Manganese poisoning: clinical and biochemical observations. *Environmental Research*, **7**, 374–80.

Chhuttani, P.N., Chawla, L.S. and Sharma, T.D. 1967: Arsenical neuropathy. *Neurology*, **17**, 269–74.

Chisolm, J.J. and Barltrop, D. 1979: Recognition and management of children with increased lead absorption. *Archives of Disease in Childhood*, **54**, 249–62.

Clarkson, T.W. 1992: Mercury: major issues in environmental health. *Environmental Health Perspectives*, **100**, 31–8.

Cohen, S. 1960: Lysergic acid diethylamide: side effects and complications. *Journal of Nervous and Mental Disease*, **130**, 30–40.

Cohen, S. 1966: A classification of LSD complications. *Psychosomatics*, **7**, 182–6.

Cohen, S. and Ditman, K.S. 1963: Prolonged adverse reactions to lysergic acid diethylamide. *Archives of General Psychiatry*, **8**, 475–80.

Cullen, M.R., Robins, J.M. and Eskenazi, B. 1983: Adult inorganic lead intoxication: presentation of 31 new cases and a review of recent advances in the literature. *Medicine*, **62**, 221–6.

Davignon, L.F., St-Pierre, J., Charest, G. and Tourangeau, F.J. 1965: A study of the chronic effects of insecticides in man. *Journal of the Canadian Medical Association*, **92**, 597–602.

Davous, P., Rondot, P., Marion, M.H. and Guegen, B. 1986: Severe chorea after acute carbon monoxide poisoning. *Journal of Neurology, Neurosurgery, and Psychiatry*, **49**, 206–8.

de Mol, J., Loseke, N. and Leleux, C. 1979: Mental troubles in bismuth encephalopathy. *Acta Psychiatrica Belgica*, **79**, 185–97.

Department of Health and Social Security 1980: *Lead and Health. The Report of a DHSS Working Party on Lead in the Environment*, B615, Vol. 739, pp 15–99. London: HMSO.

Dille, J.R. and Smith, P.W. 1964: Central nervous system effects of chronic exposure to organophosphate insecticides. *Aerospace Medicine*, **6**, 475–8.

Duffy, F.H., Burchfiel, J.L., Bartels, P.H., Gaon, M. and Sim, V.M. 1979: Long-term effects of an organophosphate upon the human electroencephalogram. *Toxicology and Applied Pharmacology*, **47**, 161–76.

Durham, W.F., Wolfe, H.R. and Quinby, G.E. 1965: Organophosphorus insecticides and mental alertness. Studies in exposed workers and in poisoning cases. *Archives of Environmental Health*, **10**, 55–66.

Elkes, C., Elkes, J. and Mayer-Gross, W. 1955: Hallucinogenic drugs. *Lancet*, **i**, 719.

Elofsson, S-A., Gamberale, F., Iregren, T.A. *et al.* 1980: Exposure to organic solvents. A cross-sectional epidemiologic investigation on occupationally exposed car and industrial spray painters with special reference to the nervous system. *Scandinavian Journal of Work and Environmental Health*, **6**, 239–73.

Eyer, P. 1995: Neuropsychopathological changes by organophosphorus compounds – a review. *Human and Experimental Toxicology*, **14**, 857–64.

Fink, M., Simeon, J., Haque, W. and Itil, T. 1966: Prolonged adverse reactions to LSD in psychotic subjects. *Archives of General Psychiatry*, **15**, 450–4.

Flanagan, R.J. and Ives, R.J. 1994: Volatile substance abuse. *Bulletin on Narcotics*, **46**, 49–78.

Flaten, T.P., Glattre, E., Viste, A. and Søreide, O. 1991: Mortality from dementia among gastroduodenal ulcer patients. *Journal of Epidemiology and Community Health*, **45**, 203–6.

Foncin, J.F. and Gruner, J.E. 1979: Tin neurotoxicity. In *Handbook of Clinical Neurology*, Vinken, P.J. and Bruyn, G.W. (eds), pp 279–89. Amsterdam: North-Holland.

Freedman, D.X. 1968: On the use and abuse of LSD. *Archives of General Psychiatry*, **18**, 330–47.

Ganrot, P.O. 1986: Metabolism and possible health effects of aluminum. *Environmental Health Perspectives*, **65**, 363–441.

Garruto, R.M., Fukatsu, R., Yanagihara, R., Gajdusek, D.C., Hook, G. and Fiori, C.E. 1984: Imaging of calcium and aluminum in neurofibrillary tangle-bearing neurons in parkinsonism dementia of Guam. *Proceedings of the National Academy of Sciences of the United States of America*, **81**, 1875–9.

Garruto, R.M., Swyt, C., Fiori, C.E., Yanagihara, R. and Gajdusek, D.C. 1985: Intraneuronal deposition of calcium and aluminum in amyotropic lateral sclerosis of Guam. *Lancet*, **ii**, 1353.

Gerhardt, R.E., Crecelius E.A. and Hudson, J.B. 1980: Moonshine-related arsenic poisoning. *Archives of Internal Medicine*, **140**, 211–3.

Gershon, S. and Shaw, F.H. 1961: Psychiatric sequelæ of chronic exposure to organophosphorus insecticides. *Lancet*, **i**, 1371–4.

Gowers, W.R. 1893: Mercurial poisoning. In *A Manual of Diseases of the Nervous System*, Gowers, W.R. (ed.), 2nd edn, Vol. 2, pp 968–970. London: Churchill.

Green, A.R. and Goodwin, G.M. 1996: Ecstasy and neurodegeneration. *British Medical Journal*, **312**, 1493.

Hamilton, A. and Hardy, H.L. 1949: *Industrial Toxicology*, 2nd edn. New York: P.B. Hoeber.

Hänninen, H., Antti-Poika, M., Juntunen, J. and Koskenvuo, M. 1991: Exposure to organic solvents and neuropsychological dysfunction: a study on monozygotic twins. *British Journal of Industrial Medicine*, **48**, 18–25.

Hänninen, H., Eskelinen, L., Husman, K. and Nurminen, M. 1976: Behavioral effects of long-term exposure to a mixture of organic solvents. *Scandinavian Journal of Work Environment and Health*, **4**, 240–55.

Horowitz, M.J. 1969: Flashbacks: recurrent intrusive images after the use of LSD. *American Journal of Psychiatry*, **126**, 565–9.

Hua, M-S. and Huang, C.C. 1991: Chronic occupational exposure to manganese and neurobehavioral function. *Journal of Clinical and Experimental Neuropsychology*, **13**, 495–507.

Husman, K. 1980: Symptoms of car painters with long-term exposure to a mixture of organic solvents. *Scandinavian Journal of Work Environment and Health*, **6**, 19–32.

Kaufman, L.D. and Philen, R.M. 1993: Tryptophan. Current status and future trends for oral administration. *Drug Safety*, **8**, 89–98.

Kelynack, T.N., Kirby, W., Delépine, S. and Tattershall, C.H. 1990: Arsenical poisoning from beer drinking. *Lancet*, **ii**, 1600–3.

Klawans, H.L., Stein, R.W., Tanner, C.M. and Goetz, C.G. 1982: A pure Parkinsonian syndrome following acute carbon monoxide intoxication. *Archives of Neurology*, **39**, 302–4.

Klee, G.D. and Weintraub, W. 1959: Paranoid reactions following lysergic acid diethylamide (LSD-254). In *Neuropsychopharmacology. Proceedings of the First International Congress of Neuropsychopharmacology*, Bradley, P.B., Deniker, P. and Radouco-Thomas, C. (eds), pp 457–60. Amsterdam: Elsevier.

Kores, B. and Lader, M.H. 1997: Irreversible lithium neurotoxicity: an overview. *Clinical Neuropharmacology*, **20**, 283–9.

Korsak, R.J. and Sato, M.M. 1977: Effects of chronic organophosphate pesticide exposure on the central nervous system. *Clinical Toxicology*, **11**, 83–95.

Kraybill, H.F. 1969: Biological effects of pesticides in mammalian systems. *Annals of the New York Academy of Sciences*, **160**, 1–422.

Kreiss, K., Zack, M.M., Feldman, R.G. *et al.* 1983: Neurologic evaluation of a population exposed to arsenic in Alaskan well water. *Archives of Environmental Health*, **38**, 116–21.

Krupp, L.B., Masur, D.M. and Kaufman, L.D. 1993: Neurocognitive dysfunction in the eosinophilia-myalgia syndrome. *Neurology*, **43**, 931–6.

Landrigan, P.J., Baloh, R.W., Barthel, W.F., Whitworth, R.H., Staehling, N.W. and Rosenblum, B.F. 1975: Neuropsychological dysfunction in children with chronic low-level lead absorption. *Lancet*, **i**, 708–12.

Landsberg, J.P., McDonald, B. and Watt, F. 1992: Absence of aluminum in neuritic plaque cores in Alzheimer's disease. *Nature*, **360**, 65–8.

Langham Brown, J.J. 1988: Zinc fume fever. *British Journal of Radiology*, **61**, 327–9.

Langston, J.W., Ballard, P.A., Tetrud, J.W. and Irwin, I. 1993: Chronic parkinsonism in humans due to a product of meperidine-analog synthesis. *Science*, **219**, 979–80.

Laplane, D., Baulac, M., Pillon, B. and Panayotopoulou-Achimastos, I. 1982: Perte de l'auto-activation psychique. Activité compulsive d'allure obsessionnelle. Lésion lenticulaire bilatérale. *Revue de Neurologie (Paris)*, **138**, 137–41.

Levy, C.J. 1988: Agent Orange exposure and post-traumatic stress disorder. *Journal of Nervous and Mental Disease*, **176**, 242–5.

Liang, Y., Sun, R., Sun, Y., Chen, Z-Q. and Li, L-H. 1993: Psychological effects of low exposure to mercury vapor: application of a computer-administered neurobehavioral evaluation system. *Environmental Research*, **60**, 320–7.

Lindström, K., Antti-Poika, M., Sakari, T. and Hyytiäinen, A. 1982: Psychological prognosis of diagnosed chronic organic solvent intoxication. *Neurobehavioral Toxicology and Teratology*, **4**, 581–8.

Lowe-Ponsford, F.L. and Henry, J.A. 1989: Clinical aspects of carbon monoxide poisoning. *Adverse Drug Reactions and Acute Poisoning Review*, **8**, 217–40.

Maizlish, N., Schenker, M., Weisskopf, C., Seiber, J. and Samuels, S. 1987: A behavioral evaluation of pest control workers with short-term, low-level exposure to the organophosphate diazinon. *American Journal of Industrial Medicine*, **12**, 153–72.

Malleson, N. 1971: Acute adverse reactions to LSD in clinical and experimental use in the United Kingdom. *British Journal of Psychiatry*, **118**, 229–30.

Marrs, T.C. and Maynard, R.L. 1994: Neurotoxicity of chemical warfare agents. In *Handbook of Clinical Neurology: Intoxications of the Nervous System*, de Wolff, F.A. (ed.), Vol. 20, pp 223–38. Amsterdam: Elsevier.

Martyn, C.N., Osmond, C., Edwardson, J.A., Barker, D.J.P., Harris, E.C. and Lacey, R.F. 1989: Geographical relation between Alzheimer's disease and aluminum in drinking water. *Lancet*, **i**, 59–62.

Mattle, H., Henn, V. and Baumgartner, G. 1982: Akutes Delir bei Wismut-intoxikation. *Schweizerische Medizinische Wochenschrift*, **112**, 1308–11.

McCann, U.D., Ridenour, A., Shaham, Y. and Ricaurte, G.A. 1994: Seronergic neurotoxicity after (±)3,4-methylenedioxymethamphetamine (MDMA; 'Ecstasy'): a controlled study in humans. *Neuropsychopharmacology*, **10**, 129–38.

McGlothlin, W.H. and Arnold, D.O. 1971: LSD revisited. A ten-year follow-up of medical LSD use. *Archives of General Psychiatry*, **24**, 35–49.

McGuire, P.K., Cope, H. and Fahy, T.A. 1994: Diversity of psychopathology associated with use of 3,4-methylenedioxymethamphetamine ('Ecstasy'). *British Journal of Psychiatry*, **165**, 391–5.

McLachlan, D.R.C., Dalton, A.J., Kruck, T.P.A. *et al.* 1991: Intramuscular desferrioxamine in patients with Alzheimer's disease. *Lancet*, **337**, 1304–8.

McLean, D.R., Jacobs, H. and Mielke, B.W. 1980: Methanol poisoning: a clinical and pathological study. *Annals of Neurology*, **8**, 161–7.

Mearns, J., Dunn, J. and Lees-Haley, P.R. 1994: Psychological effects of organophosphate pesticides: a review and call for research by psychologists. *Journal of Clinical Psychology*, **50**, 286–94.

Medical Research Council 1983: *The Neuropsychological Effects of Lead in Children. A Review of Recent Research, 1979–1983*. London: Medical Research Council.

Medical Research Council 1988: *The Neuropsychological Effects of Lead in Children. A Review of the Research, 1984–1988*. London: Medical Research Council.

Monstad, P., Nissen, T., Sulg, I.A. and Mellgren, S.I. 1987: Sleep apnoea and organic solvent exposure. *Journal of Neurology*, **234**, 152–4.

Morrow, L.A., Ryan, C.M., Goldstein, G. and Hodgson, M.J. 1989: A distinct pattern of personality disturbance following exposure to mixtures of organic solvents. *Journal of Occupational Medicine*, **31**, 743–6.

Myers, R.A.M., Snyder, S.K. and Emhoff, T.A. 1985: Subacute sequelæ of carbon monoxide poisoning. *Annals of Emergency Medicine*, **14**, 1163–7.

National Farmers' Union 1995: *Organophosphate Sheep-dips and Human Health*. London: National Farmers' Union.

Neri, L.C. and Hewitt, D. 1991: Aluminum, Alzheimer's disease, and drinking water. *Lancet*, **338**, 390.

Norris, C.R., Trench, J.M. and Hook, R. 1982: Delayed carbon monoxide encephalopathy: clinical and research implications. *Journal of Clinical Psychiatry*, **43**, 294–5.

Olsen, J. and Sabroe, S. 1980: A case-reference study of neuropsychiatric disorders among workers exposed to solvents in the Danish wood and furniture industry. *Scandinavian Journal of Social Medicine*, **16**, 44–9.

Pazderova-Vejlupková, J., Nemcova, M., Písková, J., Jirásek, L. and Lukás, E. 1981: The development and prognosis of chronic intoxication by tetrachlordibenzo-p-dioxin in men. *Archives of Environmental Health*, **36**, 5–11.

Prick, J.J.G. 1979: Thallium poisoning. In *Handbook of Clinical Neurology*, Vinken, P.J. and Bruyn, G.W. (eds), pp 239–78. Amsterdam: North-Holland.

Pueschel, S.M. 1974: Neurological and psychomotor functions in children with an increased lead burden. *Environmental Health Perspectives*, **7**, 13–6.

Pulst, S-M., Walshe, T.M. and Romero, J.A. 1983: Carbon monoxide poisoning with features of Gilles de la Tourette's syndrome. *Archives of Neurology*, **40**, 443–4.

Reed, D., Crawley, J., Faro, S.N., Pieper, S.J. and Kurland, L.T. 1963: Thallotoxicosis. Acute manifestations and sequelæ. *Journal of the American Medical Association*, **183**, 516–22.

Rees, H. 1996: Exposure to sheep-dip and the incidence of acute symptoms in a group of Welsh sheep farmers. *Occupational and Environmental Medicine*, **53**, 258–63.

Reinicke, C. 1982: Metals. In *Side Effects of Drugs Annual Six. A Worldwide Yearly Survey of New Data and Trends*, Dukes, M.N.G. and Elis, J. (eds), pp 217–28. Amsterdam: Excerpta Medica.

Report by the Advisory Committee on Drug Dependence 1970: *The Amphetamines and Lysergic Acid Diethylamide*. London: HMSO.

Rodnitzky, R.L., Levin, H.S. and Mick, D.L. 1975: Occupational exposure to organophosphate pesticides. A neurobehavioral study. *Archives of Environmental Health*, **30**, 98–103.

Roels, H., Lauwerys, R., Buchet, J-P., Genet, P., Sarhan, M.J. and Hanotiau, I. 1987: Epidemiological survey among workers exposed to manganese: effects on lung, central nervous system, and some biological indices. *American Journal of Industrial Medicine*, **11**, 307–27.

Roos, R.A.C. 1994: Neurological complications of carbon monoxide intoxication. In *Intoxications of the Nervous System*, Part I, de Wolff, F.A. (ed.), pp 31–38. Amsterdam: Elsevier.

Rosenstock, L., Keifer, M., Daniell, W.E., McConnell, R., Claypoole, K. and the Pesticide Health Effects Study Group. 1991: Chronic central nervous system effects of acute organophosphate pesticide intoxication. *Lancet*, **338**, 223–7.

Rosenthal, S.H. 1964: Persistent hallucinosis following repeated administration of hallucinogenic drugs. *American Journal of Psychiatry*, **121**, 238–44.

Roses, O.E., García Fernández, J.C., Villaamil, E.C. *et al.* 1991: Mass poisoning by sodium arsenite. *Clinical Toxicology*, **29**, 209–13.

Rutter, M. 1980: Raised lead levels and impaired cognitive/behavioral functioning: a review of the evidence. *Developmental Medicine and Child Neurology*, **22**, 1–26.

Ryan, C.M., Morrow, L.A. and Hodgson, M. 1988: Cacosmia and neurobehavioral dysfunction associated with occupational exposure to mixtures of organic solvents. *American Journal of Psychiatry*, **145**, 1442–5.

Sachs, H.K., McCaughran, D.A., Krall, V., Rozenfeld, I.H. and Yongsmith, N. 1979: Lead poisoning without encephalopathy. *American Journal of Diseases of Children*, **133**, 786–90.

Savage, E.P., Keefe, T.J., Mounce, L.M., Heaton, R.K., Lewis, J.A. and Burcar, P.J. 1988: Chronic neurological sequelæ of acute organophospate pesticide poisoning. *Archives of Environmental Health*, **43**, 38–45.

Sawa, G.M., Watson, C.P.N., Terbrugge, K. and Chiu, M. 1981: Delayed encephalopathy following carbon monoxide intoxication. *Canadian Journal of Neurological Sciences*, **8**, 77–9.

Schwartz, A., Hennerici, M. and Wegener, O.H. 1985: Delayed choreoathetosis following acute carbon monoxide poisoning. *Neurology*, **35**, 98–9.

Smith, J.S. and Brandon, S. 1973: Morbidity from acute carbon monoxide poisoning at three-year follow-up. *British Medical Journal*, **1**, 318–21.

Smith, M. 1989: The effects of low-level lead exposure on children. In *Lead Exposure and Child Development*, Smith, M.A., Grant, L.D. and Sors, A.I. (eds), pp 3–47. Dordrecht: Kluwer Academic.

Spurgeon, A., Gray, C.N., Sims, J. *et al.* 1992: Neurobehavioral effects of long-term occupational exposure to organic solvents: two comparable studies. *American Journal of Industrial Medicine*, **22**, 325–35.

Steenland, K. 1996: Chronic neurological effects of organophosphate pesticides. *British Medical Journal*, **312**, 1312–3.

Stephens, R., Spurgeon, A., Calvert, I.A. *et al.* 1995: Neuropsychological effects of long-term exposure to organophosphates in sheep-dip. *Lancet*, **345**, 1135–9.

Stoller, A., Krupinski, J., Christophers, A.J. and Blanks G.K. 1965: Organophosphorus insecticides and major mental illness. An epidemiological investigation. *Lancet*, **i**, 1387–8.

Sundelin, F. 1941: Goldbehandlung der chronischen Arthritis unter besonderer Berücksichtung der Komplikationen. *Acta Medica Scandinavica*, **67**, 1–191.

Tabershaw, I.R. and Cooper, W.C. 1966: Sequelæ of acute organic phosphate poisoning. *Journal of Occupational Medicine*, **8**, 5–20.

Ungerleider, J.T., Fisher, D.D. and Fuller, M. 1966: The dangers of LSD. *Journal of the American Medical Association*, **197**, 389–92.

Warkany, J. 1966: Acrodynia – postmortem of a disease. *American Journal of Diseases of Children*, **112**, 147–56.

Watt, G.C.M., Britton, A., Gilmour, W.H. *et al.* 1996: Is lead in tap water still a public health problem? An observational study in Glasgow. *British Medical Journal*, **313**, 979–81.

Wettstein, A., Aeppli, J., Gautschi, K. and Peters, M. 1991: Failure to find a relationship between mnestic skills of octogenarians and aluminum in drinking water. *International Archives of Occupational and Environmental Health*, **63**, 97–103.

Winter, P.M. and Miller, J.N. 1976: Carbon monoxide poisoning. *Journal of the American Medical Association*, **236**, 1502–4.

World Health Organization 1992: *The ICD-10 Classification of Mental and Behavioral Disorders*, pp 70–1. Geneva: World Health Organization.

Yule, Y., Lansdown, R., Millar, I.B. and Urbanowicz, M-A. 1981: The relationship between blood-lead concentrations, intelligence and attainment in a school population: a pilot study. *Developmental Medicine and Childhood Neurology*, **23**, 567–76.

4

Special senses – the eye and visual system

JOHN W HOWE AND DON GR JAYAMANNE

INTRODUCTION

The eyes and visual system can be affected by a wide variety of toxic agents. Liquids, solids, gases, vapors, and dust can readily affect the eyelids, cornea and conjunctiva causing damage as a result of direct contact. Alternatively, many agents may be systemically absorbed and affect the internal ocular structures such as the uveal tract, lens, retina, and optic nerve. The net effect of such exposure may therefore be mild consisting of initial irritation, which soon resolves, or may be quite extensive and sight threatening. A wide variety of drugs have also been documented as causing a range of ocular effects. These are usually administered orally and identification of the toxic agent needs to be made quickly in the hope that cessation of administration can prevent further toxic damage occurring. The purpose of this chapter is to outline some of the pathological mechanisms involved and give some indication with regard to the potential visual outcome following such exposure.

THE CORNEA AND CONJUNCTIVA

Accidental splashing of liquids into the eye is probably the commonest type of toxic eye injury. Chemically inert solvents usually produce an immediate conjunctival vasodilatation. This may be accompanied by a variable degree of chemosis. The patient immediately becomes aware of a stinging or burning sensation in the eye. The visual acuity may be normal although the patient usually experiences some degree of blurring as a result of reflex epiphora. Minor degrees of punctate epithelial corneal loss are compatible with normal standards of vision although more extensive loss of epithelium may be associated with a reduced level of acuity. Bowman's membrane, which lies immediately beneath the epithelium, usually remains intact and under these circumstances there is likely to be a rapid return of epithelialization over two to three days without any long-term corneal scarring. During the time the epithelium is healing there may be some mild corneal edema producing a slight haziness of the cornea but once epithelialization is complete this rapidly resolves.

Surfactants and detergent agents tend to produce similar problems to those seen with solvents. Occasionally damage to the corneal and conjunctival epithelium may not become apparent until several hours after exposure. Many surfactants have local anaesthetic properties and exposure to such agents may produce only minimal levels of discomfort while at the same time exhibit widespread corneal and conjunctival damage on slit-lamp examination.

The most serious ocular injuries encountered following exposure to toxic agents are those from caustic chemicals (Escapini, 1965). Although weaker acids and alkalis may produce only superficial damage with rapid recovery, the effects of stronger concentrations on the ocular tissues can be overwhelming.

Alkalis are potentially more damaging to the ocular tissues than acids because of their more rapid tissue penetration (Hughes, 1946). In the experimental situation ammonium chloride has been recovered from the aqueous within 5 s of the application of the chemical to the cornea (Lemp, 1974). In the cornea, the epithelium and endothelium form barriers to water soluble substances while the stroma constitutes a barrier to lipid soluble agents. Substances therefore that possess both water and lipid soluble phases (for example ammonium hydroxide) will penetrate the fastest. If the epithelium is damaged then the rates of penetration of a wide variety of alkalis is approximately equal, although ammonium hydroxide remains the fastest. The damaging effect of alkalis lies in the fact that they destroy both enzymatic and structural proteins. In general the higher the pH then the greater the tissue damage with the most significant damage occurring at about pH 11 (Paton and Goldberg, 1976).

Acids have much less ability to penetrate ocular tissues and tend to cause less severe and more localized damage than do alkalis. The corneal epithelium appears to show resistance against weaker acids, the most severe damage occurring when the pH is 2.5 or less. By precipitating tissue proteins, acids tend to localize the damage occurring to the ocular tissues. The major exceptions to the general rule that acids penetrate the ocular tissues poorly are acids containing heavy metals. These tend to penetrate the cornea quite rapidly. Both weak acids and weak alkalis produce a similar clinical picture. Conjunctival hyperemia is associated with chemosis, epithelial erosions, and mild corneal clouding. Slit-lamp examination may reveal a mild flare in the aqueous with an occasional cell being visible.

Attempts have been made by a number of authors to grade the severity of caustic injuries to the eye in order to arrive at a clinically valid visual prognosis (Roper Hall, 1965). It is now established that the most critical factor in determining the severity of damage is the degree of ischemia to the limbal area of the eye (Figure 4.1, below and in color plate section). When there is simply corneal epithelial damage (Figure 4.2, above and in color plate section), with no significant conjunctival ischemia, then the visual prognosis is good and the return of a satisfactory level of acuity can be anticipated. In more severe burns the cornea may be

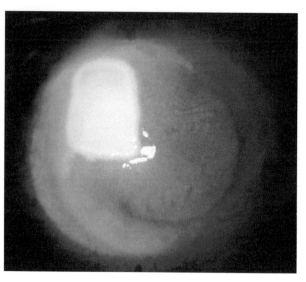

Figure 4.2 *Epithelial erosion following caustic burn.*

hazy but provided there is less than one-third of the limbus ischemic then the prognosis is again, in general, good. When over one-third of the limbus is ischemic however there is usually total epithelial loss associated with stromal haze and the vision invariably remains reduced as a result of development of corneal vascularization (Figure 4.3, below and in color plate section). In the most severe forms of chemical burn the cornea is invariably opaque and there are no details of the iris visible on examination. When more than half of the limbus is ischemic the prognosis for return of useful vision is very poor and the eye is usually the site of chronic irritation.

The two most important repair processes occurring within the cornea and conjunctiva as the result of chemical burns are re-epithelialization and vascularization. Epithelialization may take many weeks to occur in the more severe cases as a result of occlusion to the peri-limbal blood supply. Epithelial loss of the conjunctiva may lead to eventual symblepharon formation (Figure 4.4, opposite and in color plate section) as a result of adhesion between the bulbar and tarsal

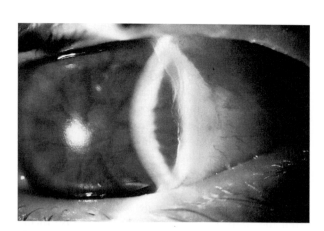

Figure 4.1 *Limbal ischemia.*

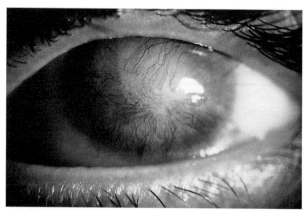

Figure 4.3 *Severe corneal vascularization following alkali burn.*

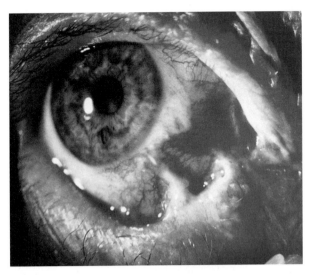

Figure 4.4 *Symblepharon formation in lower fornix.*

conjunctiva. The healthy cornea is quite avascular but following stromal oedema new blood vessels may grow in from the limbal region, changes which can be accentuated by limbal ischemic edema. Vascularization is associated with the in-growth of fibroblasts leading to an increased degree of corneal scarring. If the endothelium has been damaged by the caustic agent this may be replaced eventually by fibroblasts which secrete a collagenous membrane. In the most severe cases symblepharon formation can limit the movement of the globe and eyelids, and vision is severely impaired as a result of corneal vascularization and opacification. Recurrent corneal ulceration is a significant problem in these patients.

Given the potential for severe and catastrophic ocular complications which may be caused by caustic chemicals, rapid first-aid treatment is essential and may have a significant bearing on the eventual visual outcome. The most appropriate treatment is copious irrigation with distilled water. It is usually recommended that several liters of water be instilled into the eye in the immediate postaccident phase. Specialized ophthalmic referral is then essential in order to form an opinion with regard to the long-term prognosis and also to institute topical treatment in order to minimize complications.

Drugs can cause corneal deposition which may or may not affect vision. The anti-malarial drug chloroquine has been reported to cause decreased corneal sensitivity, the exact mechanism of which is uncertain. Corneal sub-epithelial deposits which appear as fine gray, brown multi-focal granules in a vortex pattern have been described with amiodarone, chloroquine, hydroxychloroquine and indomethacin. Patients with this distinctive corneal appearance, which is known as cornea verticillata, may complain of glare, especially at night. Chlorpromazine can cause corneal pigment

deposition usually in a location in the corneal stroma near Descemet's membrane. Calcium deposits within the cornea in a specific pattern known as band-shaped keratopathy is documented with vitamin D toxicity. Chlorambucil has been reported to cause minor corneal epithelial erosions, while Butazolidin (phenylbutazone) and gold salts can cause a severe ulcerative keratitis. Beta blockers, such as Practolol, when given systemically can cause corneal thinning, pacification, and ulceration. Colchicine may cause stromal oedema.

Abnormalities in copper metabolism such as those seen in Wilson's hepatolenticular degeneration may be associated with corneal abnormalities. The Kayser–Fleischer ring is a discoloration of the peripheral cornea by copper. Retained copper intraocular foreign bodies can also be associated with corneal changes. Slit-lamp examination under these circumstances may reveal a blue/green appearance in the deeper corneal layers. The cornea is rarely discolored in the presence of iron containing foreign bodies but when it is, fine rust-brown dots are visible in the deeper corneal layers.

Patients who complain of a gritty irritation effect of the eyes or experience altered sensitivity to glare or photophobia and are taking drugs known to cause corneal changes should have a careful slit-lamp examination of the cornea and conjunctiva in order to identify any lesions. If they are confirmed to be present then drug therapy should be discontinued.

The conjunctiva may be discolored during absorption of acute hemorrhages in arsine poisoning and has also been described from discoloration of the blood in methemoglobinemia in aniline and nitrobenzene poisoning. Mepacrine may cause a yellow discoloration and a gray discoloration is seen in silver poisoning either from chronic industrial exposure or from ingestion of silver containing drugs over a prolonged period of time. Conjunctival hyperemia may be seen following exposure to dibenzyline, or ethylene glycol. Adrenergic agents applied topically for the management of glaucoma may also be associated with an intense reactive hyperemia.

THE LENS

The human lens is a biconvex structure approximately 9 mm in diameter and up to 5 mm across in this thickest part. It is derived embryologically from the surface ectoderm and because it is enclosed within the developing optic vesicle before immunological tolerance develops the lens proteins are never recognized as self-proteins and are thus capable of initiating a severe immunological response. Damage to the lens with release of lens proteins into the aqueous is associated with a severe form of uveitis (phacoanaphylactic uveitis) (Luntz, 1964).

The most common reaction to toxic damage in the lens however is a loss of transparency as a result of cataract formation. The normal lens comprises of about 65% water and 35% protein (Throft and Kinoshita, 1965). The electrolyte composition of the lens resembles that of other single cells within the body having a high potassium concentration and a low sodium and chloride concentration.

There appears to be a potassium pump mechanism located primarily in the membranes of the epithelial cells and this requires energy to operate (Kinsey and Mcleon, 1970). This mechanism actively pumps potassium into the cell and sodium outwards, and requires the activity of the enzyme sodium/potassium-activated adenosine triphosphatase (ATPase). Glucose is the primary substrate metabolized for energy production and since the supply of oxygen is restricted in the lens most of the metabolism of glucose is through anerobic glycolysis.

Following toxic damage to the lens there is an initial increase in water content with swelling of the lens fibers which is eventually followed by a decrease in hydration as the cataract becomes mature. There is a significant potassium loss from the lens during cataract formation as the presumed result of interruption of the potassium pump within the cell membrane. In the experimental situation glutathione disappears and the ascorbic acid concentration also falls. Finally there is also a decrease in the total protein content within the lens as the cataract develops (Francois *et al.*, 1965). It appears most likely that toxins cause cataract formation by direct toxic damage to the enzymes within the lens. Galactose and xylose have been used to produce experimental cataracts in animals. The mechanism of production of cataract appears to be the diversion of the excess sugar to sorbitol (Chylack and Kinoshita, 1969). In this pathway glucose is converted to sorbitol with the aid of the enzyme aldose reductase. When this pathway is utilized there is an accumulation of polyhydric alcohol through the action of the aldose reductase enzyme. The insolubility of the accumulated polyhydric alcohol results in an increased osmolarity with subsequent over hydration and swelling of the lens fibers.

Steroids can be associated with the development of lens opacities (Skalka and Prchal, 1980) usually in the posterior subcapsular region (Figure 4.5, above and in color plate section). These lens opacities may be a complication of the administration of either systemic or topical steroids. Characteristically, although the lens opacities may be relatively insignificant, as a result of their site of origin near the nodal point of the lens, they produce quite marked visual deterioration and may require early surgery. The mechanism suggested for steroid-induced cataracts includes increased ion permeability and inhibition of ribonucleic acid (RNA) synthesis due to elevation of glucose in the aqueous.

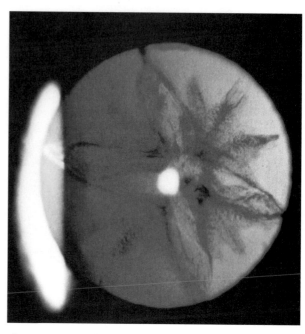

Figure 4.5 *Posterior subcapsular cataract induced by steroids.*

Busulphan can effect lens epithelial mitosis and cause cataracts. Chlorpromazine has been noted to cause pigment deposition on the crystalline lens. Other medication associated with cataract formation include: allopurinol, dinitrophenol, haloperidol, naphthalene, nimosine and ergot.

Miotic agents such as diisopropy fluorosphase (DFP), Echothiophate (phospholine iodide), paraoxon (Mintacol), demecarium bromide (Tosmilen), and pilocarpine, used in the treatment of chronic glaucoma, have been reported on occasion to produce lens opacities. Reports have also suggested that oral contraceptives may also have a similar effect, at least in the experimental situation (Lee *et al.*, 1969).

In the early stages of cataract development there may be quite marked fluctuations in vision. This is particularly the case in diabetic cataract in which changes in lens hydration correlate to blood sugar concentration (McGuiness, 1967). Hyperglycemia is generally associated with increased lens hydration and a refractive shift towards increased myopia. On the other hand, hypoglycemia is associated with reduced lens hydration and a shift towards hypermetropia. Normalization of the blood sugar can result in stabilization of hydration within the lens but in many patients progressive opacities occur. Cataracts tend to present at an earlier stage in the diabetic population as opposed to the general population.

Naphthalene and its derivatives have been reported to cause cortical cataracts while benzol and its nitro-compounds may be associated with anterior subcapsular changes. Lens opacities have also been reported from lead, mercury, gold, and silver. The most profound opacities due to metal intoxication are, however, seen as the result of iron or copper containing intraocular foreign bodies. Siderosis is the name given to iron toxicity and in the lens the first change seen is a yellow discoloration which later becomes a rusty brown, Multiple brown dots may be seen on the anterior lens surface and eventually a mature cataract develops. Copper causes so-called chalcosis. In the lens a typical sun flower opacity is seen in the posterior subcapsular region and this may be associated with multiple lenticular deposits.

Since most forms of toxic cataract result in over hydration of the lens, a tendency towards increasing myopia is common. As the lens opacities increase then the patient may become photophobic as a result of an irregular scatter of light. Lens opacities are also one of the commoner causes of monocular diplopia. As the cataract increases in severity, then the visual acuity progressively drops but even in advanced cases of cataract formation the patient is always able to distinguish light from darkness provided the underlying retina and optic nerve remain healthy.

THE UVEAL TRACT

The uveal tract comprises the iris, ciliary body, and choroid. The iris and ciliary body are liberally supplied with nerve fibers from the autonomic nervous system. The parasympathetic supply is from the third cranial (oculomotor) nerve and the sympathetic supply is via the superior cervical ganglion. Stimulation of the parasympathetic system causes pupillary constriction (myosis) as the result of contraction of the sphincter pupillae muscle. Agents which block the release of acetylcholine from the parasympathetic nerves will result in pupillary dilation (mydriasis) as the result of the unopposed activity of the dilator pupillae muscle which is innervated by the sympathetic system. Conversely any agent which results in a blockage of the release of non-adrenaline from sympathetic fibers will result in a reflex myosis. When both the sphincter and dilator muscles contract simultaneously, as may be seen in iridocyclitis, then the net result is usually a miotic pupil as the sphincter muscle is the stronger of the two.

Accommodation is the mechanism by which an object of regard is brought to a point of focus on the retina and thus seen clearly over a large range of distances. Contraction of the ciliary muscle, supplied by the parasympathetic system, results in an increased curvature and hence dioptric power of the lens as the result of the elastic recoil of the lens capsule which is attached to the ciliary body by the zonular fibers. The greatest degree of accommodation is undertaken when near objects are viewed and hence any agent which causes a paralysis of accommodation will severely affect the ability to undertake close work. The most commonly used agents causing a paralysis of accommodation (cyclopedia) are the anti-cholinergic drugs. At the same time these agents are usually associated with mydriasis. Many of the short-acting agents, such as tropicamide and cyclopentolate are used in ophthalmology as an aid to the ophthalmoscopic examination of the fundus. The effects of these drugs last only a few hours but when atropine is used in the eye drop or ointment form, then these effects may last for 10 days or more.

While parasympathomemtic and parasympatholytic agents usually have an effect on both pupil size and accommodation, most sympathomimetic agents such as phenylephrine and hydroxyamphetamine have little if any cycloplegic action but rather cause primary mydriasis. The exception to this rule is cocaine which can affect both the iris and ciliary body equally.

A potentially serious complication of any agent causing mydriasis is the development of an episode of acute angle closure glaucoma. Patients at most risk from developing this complication are those with pre-existing narrow angles associated with shallow anterior chambers. This situation is seen most commonly in hypermetropic patients who should therefore be given drugs which may cause pupillary dilation with some caution. Symptoms associated with acute glaucoma are ocular pain associated with blurring of vision. As the result of increased intraocular pressure there is over hydration of the corneal stroma. Fluid collects within the stroma as tiny droplets each of which acts as a biconvex lens. The effect on incident white light is to bring shorter wavelengths (i.e. at the blue end of the spectrum) to a point focus before those colors of longer wavelength (i.e. the red end of the spectrum). Subjectively, the patient becomes aware of colored halos around lights in which the full spectrum is visible, the blue being placed centrally and the red end of the spectrum peripherally. The associated painful eye along with colored halos is therefore very suggestive of acute glaucoma and prompt treatment is necessary in order to prevent long-term visual complications developing as the result of optic nerve head ischemia.

Agents which may cause mydriasis include haloperidol levadopa, monoaminoxodae inhibitors, tricyclic antidepressants, atropine and chlorpropamide. Steroids, particularly when applied topically to the eye, can also cause a raised intraocular pressure. Steroid-induced glaucoma is typically painless and of the open angle variety. This susceptibility to arise in intraocular pressure after the administration of steroids occurs in about 2% of the population and is believed to be due to an alteration in the metabolism of glycosaminoglycans within the trabecular meshwork. Typically the rise in intraocular pressure appears after several weeks of application of steroids and therefore those patients using topical steroids over a prolonged period of time require regular assessment of intraocular pressure along with visual field analysis. Cessation of steroid administration is usually associated with a return to normal of the intraocular pressure within a matter of weeks.

Carbonic anhydrase inhibitors, frusemide and barbiturates can cause a reduction in intraocular pressure as the result of reduced secretion of aqueous from the ciliary body epithelium. Neostigmine and carbachol can also reduce intraocular pressure by altering aqueous drainage via the uveo-sclera out-flow mechanism. Haloperidol, salicylates and cannabis have also been associated with reduced intraocular pressure and the possible risk of hypotony.

Transient blurring of vision as a result of changes within the lens are also seen with a variety of drugs which interfere with accommodation. Accommodation is achieved by contraction of the radial component of the ciliary muscle within the ciliary body. These fibers are stimulated by cholinergic agents and relax the pull of the zonular fibers on the lens. Under these circumstances the lens assumes are a more spherical shape as a result of contraction of the elastic component of the lens capsule (Moses, 1981). Anticholinergic drugs and ganglion blocking agents can cause a paralysis of accommodation and this is usually associated with pupillary dilatation. Botulinum toxin, used in the management of orbicularis spasm and some forms of squint, can cause paralysis of accommodation and mydriasis as a result of long-lasting interference with the release of acetylcholine.

The capillaries in the ciliary body normally have so called 'tight junctions' which have the effect of preventing large molecular weight proteins gaining access to the aqueous humor. On slit-lamp examination the aqueous therefore appears optically clear. When an inflammation reaction occurs then these tight junctions break down and proteins gain access to the aqueous which now has an opalescent appearance on slit-lamp examination. This constitutes a so-called aqueous flare and this is a characteristic feature of iridocyclitis. Along with aqueous flare, white cells gain access to the anterior chamber and these are easily seen on slit-lamp examination. They may accumulate on the endothelial surface of the cornea as keratic precipitates (KP) (Figure 4.6, above and in color plate section).

Iridocyclitis may be seen as a toxic reaction to any chemical gaining access to the anterior chamber. A mild aqueous flare and cellular profileration are typically seen in alkali injuries to the eye which have been discussed previously.

Retained intraocular foreign bodies, particularly iron- and copper-containing solids, can produce an intense iridocyclitis with extensive synechia formation and alterations in intraocular pressure. With copper-containing foreign bodies the iridocyclitis may be particularly severe with intense flare and cells, and a

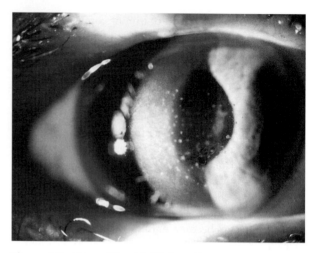

Figure 4.6 *Iridocyclitis with KP formation.*

severe plasmoid aqueous response. The iris may develop a slightly greenish color due to deposition within the iris tissue itself. Classically the discoloration tends to be more intense towards the pupillary margin of the iris. With iron-containing foreign bodies on the other hand, the iris is discolored yellowish green to brown as the result of hemosiderin deposition. Toxic effects on the uveal tract have been noted with some topically administered drugs, such as Metapranolol, a beta blocker used in the management of glaucoma (Akingbehin and Villada, 1991). The condition has only been described with the stronger 0.6% solution and not with the 0.1% and 0.3% solutions. For this reason the stronger formulation has been discontinued.

THE RETINA

Embryologically the retina develops as an out-pouching of neuroectoderm in the primitive forebrain. These so-called optic vesicles are connected to the forebrain by the optic stalks which eventually develop into the optic nerve. The optic vesicle invaginates to produce the optic cup so that the outer wall of the optic vesicle becomes approximated to its inner wall. The outer wall remains one cell thick and constitutes the retinal pigment epithelium. On the other hand, the inner wall shows massive cellular proliferation and comes to comprise the photoreceptors, bipolar cells, the retinal ganglion cells, and their associated neuronal components. Although the retinal pigment epithelium and neural retina are closely attached to each other, there remains a potential space between the pigment epithelium and the photoreceptors, and this is known as the subretinal space. It is this area which opens up during the formation of retinal detachment.

Toxic damage to the retina may primarily affect the pigment epithelium or the neuroretina, most commonly the photoreceptors. In practice the majority of retinotoxic agents appear to primarily affect the pigment epithelium which then leads to secondary photoreceptor malfunction. Under normal circumstances light falling on the photoreceptor causes a breakdown of photopigment. This results in the generation of an electrical potential which is then amplified and integrated by the bipolar, horizontal, and amacrine cells and the signal is then transmitted via the ganglion cells to the optic nerve. The retinal pigment epithelium provides a nutritional basis for the regeneration of photoreceptor visual pigment and is involved in the removal of waste products from the outer layer of the retina. Interference with this function can rapidly lead to secondary photoreceptor damage. Whether the primary site of the interaction of the toxic molecule is within the cell membrane, an enzyme or other special protein has, in many cases, yet to be identified.

Clinically, retinal function can be tested by recording the visual acuity, by perimetry, color vision testing and by electrophysiological tests such as the electroretinogram (ERG) and the electro-oculogram (EOG).

The ERG is generated at the level of the photoreceptors and bipolar cell region, and gives useful clinic information regarding toxic damage to the outer two-thirds of the retina (Brown, 1968). The initial negative 'a' wave is thought to be generated by the photoreceptors and the subsequent positive 'b' wave by the Müller cells in the bipolar region. There is no contribution to the ERG from the retinal ganglion cells. The EOG, on the other hand, represents the standing potential generated by the retinal pigment epithelium (Taumer, 1976) and may show attenuation in the early stages of pigment epithelial toxicity.

Fluorescein angiography can also be valuable in detecting abnormalities within the pigment epithelium and within the retinal and choroidal circulation. Reduced level of visual acuity is a common clinical manifestation of retinal toxicity and is particularly severely impaired when the central retinal photoreceptors (the cones) have been involved. As well as being responsible for high levels of visual discrimination, the cones are also necessary for normal color perception. Typically red/green color defects can be demonstrated in patients suffering from retinal phototoxicity. It should be noted in using color discrimination as a means of assessing potential retinal toxicity that approximately 8% of the male population show some degree of red/green color defect. Such a finding is extremely rare in the female population.

Retinal toxicity has been reported following the ingestion of a wide variety of drugs. Iodine-containing compounds have been demonstrated to be retinotoxic and, in the early pioneering work on the electroretinogram, it was demonstrated (Noell, 1951) that sodium iodo-acetate caused the retinal potentials to be extinguished. This was thought to be due to inhibition of glycolysis, although this is yet to be proven conclusively.

Chloroquine was initially developed for the treatment of malaria but is also used in the treatment of a wide variety of diseases including rheumatoid arthritis, systemic lumpus erythematosus and photosensitivity disorders. Retinal toxicity from this drug was originally described in 1959 (Hobbs et al., 1959) and there are now a large number of patients who have been found to be affected. In general, toxicity is usually found when in excess of 600 g have been ingested over several years. This author has, however, observed a patient in whom a total dosage as small as 20 g has been associated with typical retinopathy. Chloroquine has a particular affinity for pigmented structures throughout the body (Bernstein et al., 1963). Studies on pigmented rats have shown concentrations of the drug in the iris and retinal pigment can be up to 80 times that seen in other non-pigmented structures after a loading dose of the drug (Abraham and Hendy, 1970). Excretion from pigmented tissues is extremely slow and may take several years to complete. Experience indicates that once toxic damage has developed then it is unlikely to regress even when the drug has been discontinued. Indeed there are numerous cases on record in which the severity of visual loss increases for several years. Under these circumstances, it is clearly important that patients taking this drug should be monitored very carefully, including recordings of electrophysiological function particularly the electro-oculogram. Ideally, such tests should be carried out prior to treatment with chloroquine. The classical ophthalmoscopic appearance of chloroquine toxicity is the development of a so-called bull's-eye maculopathy (Figure 4.7, below and in color plate section) in which pigment is scattered throughout the posterior pole with relative sparing of the fovea. The retinal arterioles show some attenuation but there is little or no perivascular pigment clumping.

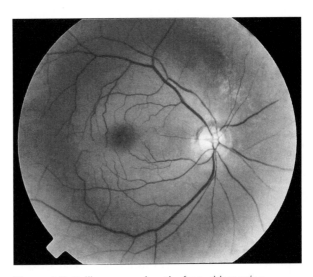

Figure 4.7 *Bull's-eye maculopathy from chloroquine.*

Pathological specimens tend to show a loss of pigment from the retinal pigment epithelium along with migration of pigment into the inner nuclear layer of the retina. Extensive destruction of the photoreceptors and outer nuclear layer are seen.

Phenothiazines, originally developed as analgesics and subsequently as antiseptic agents, are now most commonly used for their psychotropic properties. Piperidylchlorophenothiazine hydrochloride was initially developed for clinical use, but was found to be extremely toxic and to produce pigmentary retinal changes. Thioridazine is much more widely used but in 1960 reports of pigments retinopathy consisting of pigment deposits scattered between the posterior pole and the equator after use of this drug were made (May et al., 1960). Again, as with chloroquine, these changes have been reported to be dose related and are rarely seen in patients who are receiving less than 800 mg daily of the drug. Unfortunately, there is no specific treatment available.

Digitalis can be associated with a wide variety of visual symptoms, including photopsiae, scintillating scotomas, and hazy or 'unclear' vision (Robertson et al., 1966). Visual symptoms do not appear to be dose related and can occur after a variable period of ingestion of the drug. The mechanism of toxicity is uncertain and may be either at the retinal level (particularly since entopic phenomena are thought to originate in this area) or at the level of the visual cortex.

Indomethacin is widely used as an analgesic, particularly in the treatment of arthritic disorders, and has been reported to be associated with reduced ERG values. Ophthalmoscopic changes include macular pucker, central serous retinopathy and macular pigmentary degeneration.

Tamoxifen is a non-steroidal antiestrogen agent widely used for the medical treatment of breast cancer (Kaiser-Kupfer and Lippman, 1978). Retinal toxicity consisting of tiny white refractile lesions at the posterior pole have been reported in patients using the drug for over a year, in doses ranging from 90 mg to 160 mg twice daily. Fluorescein angiography may show the presence of cystoid macular edema.

Adrenaline eye drops, used in the management of glaucoma, may be associated with macular edema in aphakic patients and this is frequently reversible following discontinuation of the drug (Kolker and Becker, 1968). Since most patients now have intraocular implants at the time of cataract surgery, this complication is now only rarely encountered.

Oxygen therapy given to premature infants may lead to the development of the retinopathy of prematurity (formally known as retrolental fibroplasia) (Ashton et al., 1953). The effect of the oxygen is to cause retinal arteriolar constriction which is eventually associated with severe fibrotic changes in the retina and vitreous cavity. Careful monitoring of the fundus by an experienced ophthalmologist is essential for premature infants undergoing oxygen therapy so that early signs of vessel closure can be observed and oxygen concentrations altered accordingly.

Methoxyfluorane is an anaesthetic agent which has been associated with a flecked retina. Autopsy studies have demonstrated crystalline calcium oxalate to be present in the retinal pigment epithelium (Albert et al., 1975).

Although the systemic use of antibiotics has not been associated with retinal toxicity, the use of intravitreal antibiotics used in the treatment of bacterial endophthalmitis has been demonstrated to have harmful effects (Stainer et al., 1977). Cephaloridine, gentamicin, chloramphenicol, tobramycin and clindamycine have all been shown to be retinotoxic in large doses. Safety levels for the use of these drugs by intravitreal injection have been established and should not be exceeded.

Retinopathy can be seen in individuals involved in illicit drug abuse. The toxic effects are not usually related to the drug but rather to the route and means of administration. The communal use of needles in intravenous drug abusers has contributed to the spread of acquired immune deficiency syndrome (AIDS). Severe visual loss in patients affected is usually associated with cytomegalovirus retinitis (Skolnik et al., 1991). Occasionally septic emboli associated with subacute bacterial endocarditis may be seen.

A retinopathy may be associated with the intravenous injection of crushed tablets of amphetamine or amphetamine-like agents. In this situation smaller yellow crystalline deposits are seen in the paramacular region. These changes are not due to deposition of the drug within the retina but are due to the insoluble 'fillers' and 'binders' used in formulating the tablets for oral ingestion (Atlee, 1972).

Acute intoxication with stimulant drugs such as cocaine can result in a hypertensive crisis. This may be associated with transient papilloedema and retinal nerve fiber hemorrhages which resolve once the crisis has settled.

Retained intraocular foreign bodies containing either iron or copper may have a disastrous effect on visual function as the result of severe retinal degeneration. Because such injuries are caused by high-impact foreign bodies, they are rarely associated with intraocular infection. In general, foreign bodies within the anterior segment of the eye cause a more intense initial reaction while those within the posterior segment or lens can produce a more chronic inflammation. Siderosis is the name given to the changes seen with iron-containing foreign bodies. Degeneration of the external and internal nuclear layers along with proliferation of the pigment epithelium is seen in the early stages (Cibis et al., 1959). Eventually complete degeneration of the retina with retrograde atrophy of the optic nerve is seen. Changes in the ERG may occur at an early stage and suggest a poor visual prognosis. A reduced amplitude response indicates photoreceptor damage and makes removal of the intraocular foreign body mandatory. Even following removal however, there may be progressive reduction in visual function. It appears that ferrous forms of iron have a greater toxic effect than ferric forms. The toxic effects within the ocular tissues are secondary to the iron being oxidized by the intraocular fluids.

Copper-contained foreign bodies including brass, bronze, and aluminium alloys may cause severe toxic damage to the eye (chalcosis). There is a severe ocular inflammation with an intense iridocyclitis. Clouding of the vitreous with inflammatory cells may prevent an adequate view of the retina. Subsequent contraction of the vitreous body can be associated with retinal detachment. The retinal photoreceptors are damaged at an early stage and the ERG is likely to be severely subnormal. As with the ERG changes in siderosis, attenuation of response should be an indication for early removal of the intraocular foreign body in order to hopefully preserve eyesight, although this may not always be possible.

OPTIC NERVE AND HIGHER VISUAL PATHWAYS

The term 'toxic amblyopia' is usually taken to imply that toxic damage has occurred within the optic nerve. Although this is frequently the case, occasionally the damage is within the retinal ganglion cells with secondary optic nerve atrophy or even within the higher visual pathways. The diagnosis may occasionally be made on the basis of the ophthalmoscopic recognition of disc pallor (Figure 4.8, above and in color plate section) but frequently other investigations, particularly those of color vision, visual field assessment, and recording of the visual evoked potential, are required to confirm the nature of the visual disturbance. Acquired color defects are usually the result of retinal or optic nerve disease. Retinal pathology is usually associated with defects at the blue end of the spectrum while optic nerve pathology is frequently associated with defects of perception at the red end of the spectrum.

The visual evoked potential will show characteristic delay and attenuation of the signal with lesions affecting the retinal ganglion cells, optic nerves, and higher visual pathway (Weinstein, 1978). Under these circumstances it is a non-specific response which cannot identify the exact pathological site of toxic damage. It will however give confirmatory evidence that these foregoing structures have been damaged and may be of value when occasionally a patient is thought to be malingering.

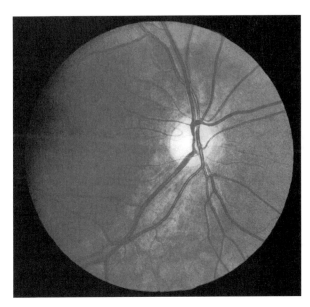

Figure 4.8 *Optic atrophy.*

Visual fields characteristically show either central or peripheral defects in the toxic amblyopias and indeed they may be used as a basis for the classification of toxic amblyopia. Central or centro-caecal defects usually imply that the papillo-macular bundle of fibers is unduly susceptible to the toxic agent whereas more peripheral defects suggest that this bundle is more resistant to the toxic agent. Table 4.1 lists some of those agents in which central defects are more common and Table 4.2 lists those agents which are more usually associated with peripheral defects. It should be noted however that such a distinction is not hard and fast, and indeed there are many instances where both central and peripheral defects are present although often with different degrees of intensity.

Table 4.1 *Some agents associated with central scotoma*

1 Alcohols – methyl and ethyl
2 Tobacco/nutritional
3 Lead
4 Drugs – adrenaline
     – digitalis
     – streptomycin
     – ethambutol
     – isoniazid
     – chloramphenicol
     – disulphiram
     – sulphonamides
5 Iodoform
6 Carbon disulfide

Considering the number of people who continue to smoke, tobacco amblyopia is a very uncommon disorder. It does not appear to be a problem associated with cigarette smoking but rather from pipe smoking of strong, dark tobacco. Reports indicating the value of hydroxycyanocobalmin suggest that this form of amblyopia may be a form of cyanide poisoning to the optic nerves although this is by no means conclusively proven (Fould *et al.*, 1970).

Toxic damage from alcohol may be seen with either methyl alcohol (methanol), or ethyl alcohol (ethanol). Methyl alcohol is widely used as a solvent, anti-freeze and fuel, and is extremely toxic to the eye. It may result from deliberate consumption but many cases have been described in which alcohol such as whiskey and gin have been criminally adulterated. Since methyl alcohol is very slowly metabolized, volumes as small as 10 ml may have serious consequences. Visual symptoms vary from blurring of vision to complete blindness. Frequently the patient is very ill and may even become comatosed (Benton and Calhoun, 1952). There is frequently a severe metabolic acidosis and widespread central nervous system involvement. It is thought that the ocular damage is due to the slow oxidation of methyl alcohol to formaldehyde which in turn affects oxidative enzyme systems. This then results in tissue anoxia, edema and retinal degeneration. There is a significant mortality with methyl alcohol poisoning but even when there is some degree of clinical recovery the visual defect is usually permanent.

Most cases of ethyl alcohol amblyopia are due to the chronic intake of high levels of alcohol. Most of these patients have an inadequate diet and indeed the total caloric intake maybe limited entirely to alcohol consumption. The etiology of the toxic amblyopia under these circumstances is therefore usually complex and may indeed be more accurately described as a nutritional amblyopia (Harrington, 1962). Typically the field defect is a small central scotoma extending no more than 5 degrees from fixation although occasionally this may enlarge temporally to form a centro-caecal scotoma. The field defects are characteristically bilateral with little or no defect in the peripheral field. Acute episodes of ethyl alcohol amblyopia are usually associated with a fairly large volume intake and low quality, impure and unregulated spirits. In view of the fact that other toxic agents may be involved in the production of the visual defect such acute episodes may not be entirely the result of ethyl alcohol ingestion. The visual symptoms that occur in this situation are complex and may result from damage to the higher visual pathways and resemble cortical blindness.

Lead poisoning is now very rare as a result of legislation reducing this as a potential hazard in industries. It may still rarely occur sporadically as an occupational disease in some plumbers, painters, workers in battery factories, and those who handle leaded petrol or petrol additives. Rarely it maybe seen in children who have eaten lead-based paints. Typically the visual loss is gradual and appears to result from toxic damage at the level of the retina, optic nerve, and higher visual pathways (Popoff *et al.*, 1963). Papilloedema may be observed in the early stages but eventually optic atrophy is present. Visual field examination may reveal both central and peripheral defects.

A variety of drugs (Table 4.1) may be associated with blurring of vision due to optic nerve or cortical effects. The incidence of toxicity with digitalis maybe as high as 25% and the most common symptoms of ocular toxicity are blurred vision and disturbed color perception. Visual field defects are commonly a central scotoma affecting both eyes and are thought to be due either to optic neuropathy or retinal ganglion cell toxicity. Typically the symptoms resolve completely within two weeks of cessation of drug therapy. Because of the risk of toxicity chloramphenicol is now rarely used as a systemic antibiotic but optic neuropathy has been described as a manifestation of its ocular toxic effect (Ramilo *et al.*, 1988). Bilateral central scotoma and optic nerve head swelling are characteristic features. Optic neuritis has been described as a manifestation of sulphonamide sensitivity, although it has been suggested that the optic nerve inflammation is the result of an idiosyncratic response rather than direct toxicity. Ethambutol and isoniazid have both been reported to be associated with blurring of vision and altered color perception (DeVita *et al.*, 1987). These agents may be used in combination for the treatment of tuberculosis and the toxic effects of both drugs can be synergistic. Streptomycin, which may also be used in the treatment of tuberculosis, has also been reported to produce an optic neuropathy, although the incidence of this complication seems to be very low.

Some of the agents which may be associated with peripheral field loss are shown in Table 4.2. Chloroquine retinopathy has already been discussed and produces a characteristic ring scotoma in which a large central scotoma is present but with a small island of lesser loss of sensitivity centrally.

Quinine may be used in the treatment of leg cramps or as an antimalarial prophylactic or occasionally large

Table 4.2 *Some agents associated with peripheral field defects*

1	Quinine
2	Chloroquine
3	Organic arsenicals
4	Gases – hyperbaric oxygen – carbon monoxide
5	Oral contraceptives
6	Thoridazine/piperidylchlorophenothiazine
7	Methyl mercury compounds

doses have been used to induce abortions. In the lower doses used to treat leg cramps ocular toxicity is thought to be due to an individual hypersensitivity (Barsky, 1961) but with larger doses toxic damage to the retina and optic nerve have been observed. Typically blurring is associated with contraction of the peripheral fields with only small central areas of the field remaining intact. Fundus examination in the early stages shows a marked attenuation of the retinal blood vessels but in later stages there is a secondary optic atrophy present. A quinine-induced optic nerve hypoplasia has been reported in infants whose mothers ingested large quantities of the drug during pregnancy (McKinna, 1966).

Inorganic arsenicals, used in industry as pesticides, seem to have little potential for causing ocular damage. On the other hand, organic arsenicals which were originally used in the treatment of syphilis prior to the development of appropriate antibiotics have been recorded as producing toxic optic nerve damage. Methyl mercury compounds are used for protecting wood or seeds, and poisoning may occur in the manufacturing process by inhalation. It may also develop as the result of eating treated seeds or contaminated food stuffs. Typically there is gross contraction of the field of vision and pathological studies have indicated that the major effect is on the visual cortex which may show severe atrophy in advanced toxic cases.

CONCLUSIONS

From this chapter it can be appreciated that a wide variety of agents can have a detrimental effect on the visual system. The cause of the visual disturbance may be quite obvious but occasionally further investigations are necessary in order to identify the exact site of damage. Once the toxic agent has been identified then avoidance is necessary in order to, hopefully, prevent further damage occurring, although in many instances progressive loss of vision may be observed.

REFERENCES

Abraham, R. and Hendy, R.J. 1970: Irreversible lysosomal damage induced by chloroquine in the retina of pigmented and albino rats. *Experimental Molecular Pathology*, **12**, 185.

Akingbehin, T. and Villada, Jr 1991: Metipranolol associated granulomatous uveitis. *British Journal of Ophthalmology*, **75**, 519–23.

Albert, D.M., Bullock, J.D., Lahav, M. and Caine, R. 1975: Flecked retina secondary to oxalate crystals from methoxyflurane anaesthesia. *Transactions of the American Academy of Ophthalmic Otolaryngologia*, **79**, 817.

Ashton, N., Ward, B. and Serpell, G. 1953: Role of oxygen in the genesis of retrolental fibroplasia. *British Journal of Ophthalmology*, **37**, 513

Atlee, W.E. Jr 1972: Talc and cornstarch emboli in eyes of drug abusers. *Journal of the American Medical Association*, **1**, 49.

Barsky, D. 1961: Quinine idiosyncrasy and optic-atrophy. *Journal of the Michigan Medical Society*, **60**, 612–3.

Benton, C.D. Jr and Calhoun, F.P. Jr 1952: Ocular effects of methyl alcohol poisoning. *Transactions of the American Academy of Ophthalmology and Otolaryngology*, **56**, 875

Bernstein, H., Zvaifler, N., Rubin, M. and Mansur, A. 1963: The ocular deposition of chloroquine. *Investigative Ophthalmology*, **2**, 384.

Brown, K.T. 1968: The electroretinogram. Its components and their origin. *Vision Research*, **8**, 633.

Chylack, L.T. Jr and Kinoshita, J.H. 1969: A biochemical evaluation of a cataract induced in a high glucose medium. *Experimental Eye Research*, **8**, 401.

Cibis, P.A., Yamashita, T. and Rodriguez, F. 1959: Clinical aspects of ocular siderosis and hemosiderosis. *Archives of Ophthalmology*, **62**, 180–7.

DeVita, E.G., Miao, M. and Sadun, A.A. 1987: Optic neuropathy in ethambutol-treated renal tuberculosis. *Journal of Clinical Neurology and Ophthalmology*, **7**, 77.

Escapini, H. 1965: Trauma to the cornea. In *The Cornea World Congress*, J.H. King Jr and J.W. McTigue (eds), pp 300–15. London: Butterworth.

Fould, W.S., Chisholm, I.A., Bronte-Stewart, J. and Reif, H.C.R. 1970: Investigation and therapy of the toxic amblyopias. *Transactions of the Ophthalmological Society of the United Kingdom*, **90**, 739.

Francois, J., Rabaey, M. and Stockmans, L. 1965: Gel filtration of the soluble proteins from normal and cataractous human lenses. *Experimental Eye Research*, **4**, 312.

Harrington, D. 1962: Amblyopia due to tobacco, alcohol and nutritional deficiency. *American Journal of Ophthalmology*, **53**, 967.

Hobbs, H.E., Sorsby, A. and Freedman, A. 1959: Retinopathy following chloroquine therapy. *Lancet*, **2**, 478.

Hughes, W.F. 1946: Alkali burns to the eye. *Archives of Ophthalmology*, **35**, 423–49.

Kaiser-Kupfer, M.I. and Lippman M.E. 1978: Tamoxifen retinopathy. *Cancer Treatment Report*, **3**, 315.

Kinsey, V.E. and McLeon, I.W. 1970: Studies on the crystalline lens. XVI. Characterization of active transport and diffusion of potassium, rubidium and cesium. *Investigative Ophthalmology*, **9**, 769.

Kolker, A.E. and Becker, B. 1968: Epinephrine maculopathy. *Archives of Ophthalmology*, **79**, 552.

Lee, P., Donovan, R.H. and Muskai, N. 1969: Effects of norethinodrel with mestranol on the rabbit eye. *Archives of Ophthalmology*, **81**, 89.

Lemp, M.A. 1974: Cornea and sclera. *Archives of Ophthalmology*, **92**, 158–70.

Luntz, M.H. 1964: Experimental endophthalmitis phacoanaphylactica. *Experimental Eye Research*, **3**, 166.

May, R.H., Selymes. P., Weekley, R.D. and Potts, A.M. 1960: Thioridazine therapy – results and complications. *Journal of New Mental Disease*, **130**, 230.

McGuiness, R. 1967: Association of diabetes and cataract. *British Medical Journal*, **2**, 416–18.

McKinna, A.J. 1966: Quinine-induced hypoplasia of the optic nerve. *Canadian Journal of Ophthalmology*, **1**, 261–6.

Moses, R.A. 1981: Accommodation. In *Adler's Physiology of the Eye*, F.H. Adler (ed.), 7th edn, pp 304–25. St Louis, MO: C.V. Mosby.

Noell, W.K. 1951: The effects of iodoacetate on the vertebrate retina. *Journal of Cellular Comparative Physiology*, **37**, 283.

Paton, D. and Goldberg, M.F. (eds) 1976: Burns of the eye and adnexa. In *Management of Ocular Injuries*, pp 163–80. Philadelphia, PA: W.B. Saunders.

Popoff, N., Weinberg, S. and Feigin, I. 1963: Pathological observations in lead encephalopathy with special reference to vascular changes. *Neurology*, **13**, 101.

Ramilo, O., Kinane, B.T. and McCracken, G.H. 1988: Chloramphenicol neurotoxicity. *Pediatric Infectious Diseases Journal*, **7**, 358.

Robertson, D.M., Hollenhorst, R.W. and Callahan, J.A. 1966: Ocular manifestations of digitalis toxicity. *Archives of Ophthalmology*, **76**, 640.

Roper Hall, M.J. 1965: Thermal and chemical burns. *Transactions of the Ophthalmological Society of the United Kingdom*, **35**, 631–46.

Skalka, H.W. and Prchal, T.J. 1980: Effect of cortico steroids on cataract formation. *Archives of Ophthalmology*, **98**, 1773–7.

Skolnik, P.R., Pomerantz, R.J., De la Monte, S.M. *et al.* 1991: Dual infection of retina with human immunodeficiency virus type 1 and cytomegalovirus. *American Journal of Ophthalmology*, **107**, 361–72.

Stainer, G.A., Peyman, G.A., Meisels, H. and Fishman, G. 1977: Toxicity of selected antibiotics in vitreous replacement fluid. *Annals of Ophthalmology*, **9**, 615.

Taumer, R. 1976: Electro-oculography. Its clinical importance. *Bibliotheca Ophthalmol*, **85**.

Throft, R.A. and Kinoshita, J.H. 1965: The extracellular space of the lens. *Experimental Eye Research*, **4**, 287.

Weinstein, G.W. 1978: Clinical aspects of the visual evoked potential. *Ophthalmic Surgery*, **9**, 56.

5

Special senses – taste, smell, hearing and balance

THOMAS P NIKOLOPOULOS AND JOHN P BIRCHALL

INTRODUCTION

Chemical agents can damage the special senses of taste, smell, hearing, and balance by interactions at a cellular or molecular level. Understanding the mechanisms of taste and smell are less advanced than those of balance and hearing. Techniques for measuring hearing and its disorders are far more sophisticated than any of the other aforementioned three senses. This has resulted in a much larger volume of literature concerning ototoxicity. There are several excellent reviews about ototoxicity; however, they can be opaque to readers with little knowledge of otology. This chapter, therefore, focuses mainly on audiology to redress the balance. Dizziness is a very complex topic. Our understanding of this system is not as well understood as hearing, but still better than taste and smell.

All the aforementioned senses may be damaged or lost for no apparent reason, with clinical investigations failing to demonstrate a lesion. Against this background of sporadic cases one must exercise caution in attributing the cause to a drug or a chemical compound. The attribution of toxicity is often made from single case reports.

TASTE

Anatomy and physiology

Modified epithelial cells, the taste cells, together with other supporting cells constitute the taste receptors (taste buds). Most taste buds are located on nipple-like protuberances, called papillae, on the tongue surface, with a few on the epiglottis, soft palate, and pharynx. They range from $50-70\,\mu\mathrm{m}$ in diameter and open onto the surface of the tongue at the taste pore. Most taste buds are located on the sides of the vallate (circumvallate) papillae, which are found at the back of the tongue. Smaller fungiform and foliate papillae, on the sides and tip of the tongue, may also carry a few taste buds, whereas taste buds are not found on the numerous filiform papillae (Bray et al., 1994).

In adults, there are about 5000–10 000 taste buds and this number can vary significantly from person to person. In children, the number of taste buds is usually much larger and the distribution is different, being more on the tongue and on the insides of the cheeks. Taste buds contain several cell types. Besides the sensory taste cells and the supporting cells, there are also basal cells which give rise to the taste cells. The supporting cells can be divided into type 1 (dark) cells and type 2 (light) cells. It is not yet clear whether type 1 and type 2 cells are solely supporting cells, or simply represent different stages in the cycle of the taste cell (Bray *et al.*, 1994). Nevertheless, experiments with tritiated thymidine have shown that taste cells are produced by mitotic division of cells at the edge of the bud. These migrate to the center of the bud where they undergo apoptoses and disappear after a week (Emslie-Smith *et al.*, 1987).

The main nerves of taste are the lingual branch of the glossopharyngeal nerve for the posterior third of the tongue, including the vallate papillae; the anterior two-thirds are served by the chorda tympani branch of the facial nerve. All the nerve fibers pass centrally to the tractus solitarius, cross the midline and pass to the posterior ventral nucleus of the thalamus and then on to the lower part of the postcentral gyrus, and probably other areas nearby. It was noticed that after destruction of the postero-medial ventral nucleus, goats drunk strong solutions of quinine, acid or salt, which they had repeatedly refused before the operation. Stimulation of this area of the thalamus in intact unanaesthetized animals produces 'rejecting' movements of the jaw and tongue, exactly as seen when a solution of quinine is squirted into the mouth.

The lingual branch of the fifth nerve is the nerve of common sensibility for the anterior two-thirds of the tongue; the lingual branch of the glossopharyngeal nerve carries both taste and common sensibility fibers for the posterior third. Probably no true taste fibers pass into the brain stem via the fifth nerve, but tactile, pain, and thermal sensations conveyed by this nerve play an important part in the recognition of taste sensations. When the fifth nerve in humans is cut or destroyed the sense of taste is immediately lost in the front of the tongue but it returns in some cases after a few hours, in others after years. If the facial nerve is divided above its ganglion the sensation of taste is lost permanently on both the palate and the anterior part of the tongue; although the fifth nerve is intact, it is unable to provide a sensation of taste (Emslie-Smlth *et al.*, 1987).

Classically, four basic tastes are recognized: sweet, sour, salty and bitter. A fifth taste, umami, produced by compounds like monosodium glutamate, has also been described. All complex tastes are thought to be accounted for by combinations of these basic tastes; most of what the layperson calls 'taste' is a combination of taste and smell. Most sugars taste sweet; for example, glucose, sucrose, and lactose produce the sensation of sweetness, but so too do unrelated molecules like glycine, alanine, saccharine, and even certain proteins. The sensation of sourness is produced by acids and is related to the H concentration, but not all acids are equally sour at equivalent pH. Salty sensations are elicited mainly by cations such as Na^+ and Li^+, but different anions (Cl^-, SO_4^{2-}, NO_3^-) alter the taste quality. Many different organic compounds are described as bitter, for example, quinine, caffeine, nicotine, morphine, and strychnine (Bray *et al.*, 1994).

Substances act on the exposed microvilli in the taste pore of the taste buds to evoke generator potentials in the receptor cells, which generate action potentials in the sensory neurones. The way the molecules in solution produce generator potentials varies from one gustatory modality to another. Salt stimuli probably depolarize salt receptor cells by influx of Na^+ through passive, ungated apical channels. This is because in humans the application of the Na^+ channel-blocking diuretic amiloride directly to the tongue abolishes the ability to taste salt. Acids, which taste sour, probably depolarize receptor cells by H^+ blocking of apical K^+ channels. Substances that taste sweet appear to bind to membrane receptors and activate adenylate cyclase, with a resulting increase in intracellular cyclic AMP. The cyclic AMP acts via protein kinase A to reduce K^+ conductance by phosphorylating K^+ channels on the basolateral membranes of the taste cells. Substances that taste bitter appear to act in a different fashion. Unlike the others, they do not increase current flow in patch clamp preparations, and they probably act via G protein-coupled receptors and phospholipase C to trigger release of Ca^{2+} from the endoplasmic reticulum. A novel G protein (a subunit named a-gusducin) has recently been isolated and shown to occur in taste buds. It resembles the transducins (valuable proteins in vision). Another protein that binds taste-producing molecules has recently been cloned. It is produced by Ebner's glands, glands that secrete mucus into the cleft around vallate papillae, and probably has a concentrating and transport function similar to that of the odorant-binding proteins of olfaction. (Ganong, 1993).

Taste preferences mean simply that an animal will choose certain types of food in preference to others, and it automatically uses this to help control the type of diet it eats. Furthermore, its taste preferences often change in accord with the needs of the body for certain specific substances. For instance, adrenalectomized animals automatically select drinking water with a high concentration of sodium chloride in preference to pure water, and this in many instances is sufficient to supply the needs of the body and prevent death as a result of salt depletion. The phenomenon of taste preference almost certainly results from some mechanism located in the central nervous system and not from a mechanism in the taste receptors themselves. An important reason for believing taste preference to be mainly a central phenomenon is that previous experience with unpleasant or pleasant tastes plays a major role in determining one's different taste preferences. For instance, if a person becomes sick soon after eating a particular type of food, the person generally develops a negative taste preference, or taste aversion, for that particular food thereafter (Guyton, 1992).

Testing the taste function

If testing the olfactory function is difficult and subjective, the evaluation of taste is more limited since there are only four accepted basic tastes to discriminate: sweet, sour, bitter, and salt. As a consequence, clinical assessment of taste has usually involved detection of thresholds or recognition of thresholds. The detection threshold is the lowest concentration of a given tastant detected as different from a non-tastant, such as water. The recognition threshold is the most dilute concentration of solute that can be consistently recognized as bitter, sweet, salty, or sour. In theory, for both detection and recognition of thresholds, there are two ways to perform the evaluation of taste: local testing (involving cotton swabs dripped in solutions or drop techniques) and whole-mouth testing (involving bigger quantities of solution in the whole mouth imitating 'real-life' situations but sparing the fact that the disorder of taste can be in a certain area or due to a specific cranial nerve).

However, threshold measures in taste are not only subjective but prone to influences such as salivary adaptation, water tastes imparted by adaptation, or the size of the tongue area stimulated, and thus tend to be quite variable (Smith, 1991). Moreover, what is tested in threshold levels may be significantly different in a suprathreshold level. This is illustrated by the fact that patients can recover with regard to their taste function following radiation therapy and, in threshold testing, may score 'normal'. However, the same patients may still have significant loss in their ability in estimating the suprathreshold taste intensities (Bartoshuk, 1978). Therefore, category scaling has been introduced in suprathreshold tests asking the patient to rate the intensity of the taste into one of a series of various functional gradings. One significant disadvantage of this assessment is that it does not allow comparisons among different patients. This is because the grading is totally subjective and can be influenced even by psychological factors. In other words, what is extremely sweet to a certain individual can be slightly sweet to another person, when both have normal taste.

The most commonly used tests are: the Connecticut Chemosensory Clinical Research Center (CCCRC) test; the Monell Chemical Senses Center test (Monell); and the University of Pennsylvania Smell and Taste Center test (UPENN). These tests use both local and whole-mouth procedures. They can also be performed with the threshold or scaling method (series of nine gradings for the UPENN test, 10 gradings for the CCCRC test, and 13 gradings for the Monell test).

Overall, the evaluation of taste function is a very difficult and subjective task. This has an obvious implication in monitoring substances that have potential toxic effects and in giving objective answers when questions of medico-legal origin are raised.

SMELL

Anatomy and physiology

The sense of smell is a major determinant in the appreciation of taste. Odors must reach the neuro-epithelium of the olfactory nerve in the roof of the nose. Conditions which limit nasal airflow may result in diminished olfaction which is most commonly seen in patients with rhinitis and hypertrophic nasal mucosa, nasal polyposis, or less commonly it is a complaint of laryngectomees who do not nose breathe. The aforementioned all have normal olfactory pathways. Damage to the olfactory nerve or bulb due to trauma, head injury or surgical procedures of the skull base in the anterior cranial fossa and, uncommonly, meningioma cause a true sensory deficit.

Olfaction is the function of the first cranial nerve. However, some pungent substances such as ammonia may stimulate somatosensory nerve endings of the V cranial nerve in the nose, and cranial nerves IX and X in the oropharynx.

The olfactory epithelium consists of receptor cells with microvilli and supporting cells. There is a turnover of cells and immature receptor cells are also present. Unmyelinated fibers from the receptor cells project through the foramina of the cribriform plate and synapse in the olfactory bulb in the glomeruli. The second order neurones, mitral and tufted cells, run to the primary olfactory cortex. The neural pathways are complex and include the anterior olfactory nucleus, olfactory tubercle, piriform cortex, lateral entorhinal cortex, and the periamygdaloid cortex. Efferent fibers project to the olfactory bulb from the areas the afferents innervate. The olfactory bulbs and anygdala project to the hypothalamus. There are indirect connections to the hippocampus from the entorhinal cortex, which also supplies the orbitofrontal cortex via the thalamus.

PHYSIOLOGY

The idea that one receptor cell had one specific olfactory receptor has been considered for many years. Recent evidence that makes this appear to be the case. It has long been known that a receptor cell responds to a range of odors out of the possible millions of chemical configurations. There are hundreds of olfactory receptors (OR), and current thinking takes concepts from immunology: the first is that only one of the two alleles of the OR gene is expressed (allelic exclusion) and, second, only one OR gene is expressed (idiotype exclusion). For the latter to be the case then the OR would have to have multiple specificities rather than numerous genes being expressed by one receptor cell. It is also thought that locus exclusion is operating which would allow a great deal of genetic polymorphism and allow OR of different odor specificients to be expressed (Lancet, 1994).

Odorant binding processes (OBPs) are small water-soluble proteins found in the nasal mucus. They enhance the capture of odorants and facilitate the transport of hydrophobic odorants to the sensory cillia. They may also have a role in signal transduction.

Single cell recordings from olfactory neurones have shown that the receptor cells respond to a unique spectrum of odors and it follows that each odorant stimulates a defined population of receptor cells.

Medical aspects of olfaction

By analogy to hearing loss, olfaction loss can be considered as having three components: conductive, where the odorant is prevented from reaching the sensory epithelium; neural, where there is a fault in generating or transmitting the electrical message; and a cortical component responsible for identifying the odorant. The conductive element is the most common cause of olfactory dysfunction. A prerequisite of normal olfaction is a satisfactory nasal airway, the most common cause of obstruction being nasal polyposis. Nasal polyps arise usually from the ethmoidal air cells and grow into the nasal air passages causing complete nasal obstruction. This prevents the odorant-carrying air from reaching the sensory epithelium. Pathology of the nasal mucosa, commonly hypertrophy as found in rhinitis, may result in mechanical abnormalities around the sensory epithelium. Structural abnormalities may cause turbulence in the nasal airflow, causing drying of the nasal mucosa and squamous metaplasia, and resulting in the loss of the mucus blanket, which again could prevent odorants from reaching the receptor cells. There is also the possibility that some agents may block or destroy the OBPs.

The sensory element is most vulnerable in the roof of the nose, cribriform plate, and anterior cranial fossa. Fractures of the floor of the anterior cranial fossa, or neurosurgical access via the anterior cranial fossa may result in irreversible anosmia. Tumors of the nose and anterior cranial fossa may result in the destruction of the olfactory pathways with or without surgery. Pathology of the higher centers may present with olfactory hallucinations.

Symptoms and their prevalence

Patients complain of anosmia, hyposmia or a selective loss where certain odorants cannot be detected. The National Geographic magazine conducted a survey of its readership and 1.2% of the 1.5 million respondents reported olfactory dysfunction. The Panel of Communicative Disorders (1979) estimated that 2 million Americans had disorders of taste and smell. Around 20% of the population in Western Europe have rhinitis and 22.5% of patients with rhinosinusitis had olfactory dysfunction (Schiffman and Troy Nagle, 1992).

Testing olfactory function

Odorants used must not be pungent or irritant otherwise the trigeminal nerve will be stimulated. Subjective assessment of olfaction depends on the subject's ability to identify the odor, and presupposes they have been exposed to it in the past and can retrieve it from olfactory memory. The latter is not well developed in most humans and therefore forced alternative choice is used in the testing procedure. A widely used test is the University of Pennsylvania Smell Identification Test (UPSIT). This consists of scratch-and-sniff cards and the subject is asked to identify the odor from a choice of four options. The Connecticut Chemosensory Clinical Research Center (CCCRC) test also has a determination of olfactory threshold using different concentrations of 1-butamol. Robson et al. (1996) reported a combined olfactory test which incorporates the forced choice element of the UPSIT and the threshold element of the CCCRC test. Interestingly, some subjects, who claimed to be anosmic on testing, obtained olfactory scores that were in the normal range.

The above tests all rely on a subjective response. There is currently no technique that is clinically useful in determining an objective response. When the veracity of the subject's response is suspect, ammonia is employed on the basis that denial of being able to 'smell' it would indicate malingering.

CLASSIFICATION OF SMELL AND TASTE DISORDERS

The disorders of smell and taste can be classified into three functional groups with regard to: decrease of function; increase of function; and distortion of function.

Decrease of function

Anosmia and ageusia (Greek origin, meaning 'without smell' and 'without taste') define the loss of the ability to smell or taste, respectively.

Hyposmia and hypogeusia (Greek origin, meaning 'less smell' and 'less taste') define the decreased ability to smell or taste.

These disorders can be general (all stimuli), partial (some stimuli) or specific (one or a few specific stimuli).

Increase of function

Hyperosmia and hypergeusia (Greek origin, meaning 'excessive smell' and 'excessive taste') define the increased ability (sensitivity) of smell or taste. They can be general (all stimuli), partial (some stimuli) or specific (one or a few specific stimuli).

Distortion of function

According to Henkin (1993) the distortion of function can be subdivided into two categories which have three or four further subcategories.

ALIOSMIA AND ALIAGEUSIA

Aliosmia and aliageusia (Greek origin, meaning 'other smell' and 'other taste') define the unpleasant smell or taste of substances that are expected (or considered) to be pleasant. However, in some cases the smell or taste of the substance may not be unpleasant but different than expected. It has four subcategories:

1 Cacosmia and cacogeusia (Greek origin, meaning 'bad smell' and 'bad taste') define the 'decayed' or 'rotten' experience of substances that usually have a pleasant smell or taste.
2 Torquosmia and torquegeusia (torque in Latin means twisted metal) define the metallic (bitter) smell and taste of substances that usually have a pleasant smell and taste.
3 Mixed (combination of the above two subcategories).
4 Parosmia and parageusia (Greek origin, meaning 'different or wrong smell' and 'different or wrong taste') define the distortion of smell or taste of a substance to be experienced as another substance or as having other properties (for example, coffee can be identified as garlic and sugar as salt). This sensation is not necessarily unpleasant.

PHANTOSMIA AND PHANTOGEUSIA

Phantosmia and phantogeusia (from the word phantom that comes from old French fantosme, ultimately from Greek phantasma, meaning the illusion or the perception of something that does not exist) define the unpleasant smell or taste of substances that are not present when the patient has the respective experience. It has three subcategories:

1 cacosmia and cacogeusia ('decayed' or 'rotten' smell or taste);
2 torquosmia and torquegeusia (metallic or bitter smell and taste);
3 mixed (combination of the above two subcategories).

SMELL AND TASTE DYSFUNCTION DUE TO TOXIC EXPOSURE TO SUBSTANCES AND DRUGS

A toxic substance can affect the smell or taste function at three levels:

1 receptors;
2 neural pathways (from the receptors to the central nervous system);
3 specific centers and their connections in the central nervous system.

The damage may occur in one or any combination of the three levels. However, the most frequent level of toxic damage, especially in drug injury, is the receptor level. The impairment may be associated with histopathologic lesions, physiological changes, or both.

Histopathologic lesions associated with toxic-induced smell and taste loss

Many authors have described histopathologic changes secondary to exposure to toxic substances and drugs (Feron et al., 1986; Bogdanffy and Frame, 1994; Hastings and Miller, 1997).

The main histopathologic changes, observed mainly in experiments with animals, are: degeneration, necrosis, atrophy, hyperplasia, metaplasia, ulceration, production of pseudoglandular or cystlike structures, karyomegaly and cytomegaly of epithelial cells of Bowman's glands, reduced numbers or loss of Bowman's glands, inflammatory infiltration, development of fibrous tissue, iron accumulation, disorientation of sensory cells, osseous remodeling, loss of nerve bundles in the submucosa, adenocarcinoma, esthesioneuroepithelioma, and neuroepithelioma.

Physiological changes

The interference of toxic compounds and drugs in the physiology of smell and taste is difficult to assess as we know so little with regard to the physiology and pathophysiology of smell and taste, especially at the molecular level.

However, several authors (Schiffman and Troy Nagle, 1992; Witek, 1993; Henkin, 1994; Ackerman and Kasbekar, 1997) have proposed or reviewed pathophysiologic mechanisms related to smell and taste disorders due to toxic effects of substances and drugs. The main mechanisms proposed are the following: decreased mucosal blood flow, reduced mucus flow, impaired mucociliary clearance, alteration in the turnover of sensory cells, modification of energy production of these cells, disruption of the lipids in the cell membranes, modification of channels or second messenger systems, interaction with saliva, modification of saliva (quality and quantity), decreased dopamine metabolism, increased serotonin concentration, zinc displacement, chelation of zinc, ion channel disturbance, excess bradykinin accumulation, decreased calcium-mediated neurotransmission, binding to sodium channels, dopaminergic nerve depression, poisoning cyclic adenosine-3′,5′-monophosphate (cAMP) synthesis, chelation of copper, gustin inhibition, impairment of receptor-coupled on and off events, inhibition of receptor kinases, cAMP inhibition, alteration of catecholamine effects, inhibition of receptor action potentials, vitamin A inhibition, protein synthesis inhibition, mRNA misreading, DNA synthesis inhibition, cytochrome-P450 inhibition, isozymes inhibition, development of membrane leakage of small molecules, disruption of mitotic activity, prostaglandin inhibition, and inhibition of receptor-membrane activity. However, besides the effect on smell and taste, a toxic compound may cause a variety of other symptoms as well: stuffy nose, catarrhal rhinitis, rhinorrhea, sneezing, irritation, congestion, obstruction, nosebleeds, dryness, xerostomia, or itching (Leopold, 1994).

SUBSTANCES AND DRUGS WHICH CAN CAUSE SMELL AND TASTE DISORDERS

The medico-legal problems, that frequently arise from claims that a specific compound (usually workplace related) or a specific drug has caused a smell or taste disorder, are very difficult to be settled because:

1 the scientific reports that correlate a substance with a smell or taste disorder are usually case reports or describe a limited number of patients, are not double-blind or have no statistical confirmation;
2 experimental surveys usually concern animal models and their results may not be applicable to humans;
3 the concentration of a compound needed to cause an acute toxic effect in many cases is so high that it would only occur in an accident;
4 sub-acute and chronic toxic effects through many years of exposure are very difficult to assess and thereby establish a causal relationship, as many other confounding factors may be involved (smoking, alcohol consumption, use of drugs for therapeutic reasons, aging, viral infections, etc.).

The Occupational Safety and Health Administration (OSHA) has established guidelines and regulations with regard to threshold limit values (TLVs) for industrial human exposure to airborne chemicals. Chronic exposure to a substance at a concentration under the respective TLV is expected to be safe for the majority of the workers. However, the effect of long-term exposure

to a lot of chemicals has not yet been properly investigated. Moreover, TLVs are sometimes partially based on the calculation of a value of 0.03 times the concentration of a substance needed to cause a 50% decrease in the respiratory rate (RD_{50}) of mice, as this has been found to be a good estimate for human TLVs (Kane et al., 1979; Alarie, 1981).

Taking into consideration the above-mentioned limitations in defining a substance or a drug as toxic to smell and taste, Appendix 1 at the end of this chapter lists the compounds (and processes) that have been reported to be a potential cause of smell and/or taste disorders (Amoore, 1986; Alarie and Luo, 1989; Schiffman and Troy Nagle, 1992; Schiffman and Gatlin, 1993; Henkin, 1994; Ackerman and Kasbekar, 1997).

Surprisingly, the number of compounds and drugs, which may cause toxic effects on smell and taste, is enormous. However, with some substances, the toxic disorder may be associated with a quite prolonged exposure (40 years or more) and the incidence might be a small percentage of the workers or patients exposed. One could argue that in cases of widely used drugs, even if the incidence of toxic effect is low, the numbers of patients may be significant. For example, paracetamol is toxic (causing hypogeusia) in less than 1% of patients who take the drug (Needleman and Rez, 1976; Henkin, 1994). However, taking into consideration the number of patients who use this drug (millions), the moderate amount of drug required to give the toxic effect (1000–5000 mg daily), and the short period of time required to give the toxic effect (4–8 weeks), it could be assumed that a large number of patients worldwide may experience hypogeusia due to paracetamol. Another factor that complicates further the study of toxic exposure to compounds and drugs is that, in general, the degree of olfactory loss (which has been studied more thoroughly than the gustatory loss) depends on the individual person and is not necessarily associated with the exposure levels or time since last exposure (Schiffman and Troy Nagle, 1992). Therefore, before a causal relationship between a specific compound and a smell/taste disorder is established, thorough and detailed investigation is clearly needed.

OTOTOXICITY AND VESTIBULOTOXICITY

Anatomy and physiology

The inner ear is divided on functional grounds into the cochlea, responsible for hearing, and the vestibular system for balance. Both are in fact a single structure with their respective sensory epithelia bathed in endolymph. The cochlea sensory epithelium consists of hair cells, a single inner row innervated by afferent nerve cells on three rows of outer hair cells innervated by efferent nerve fibers, all lying in the organ of Corti. The sensory epithelium of the vestibular system is found in the saccule, utricle, and the ampullae of the semicircular canals. In essence, all the hair cells are electro-mechanical devices for converting mechanical energy to electrical energy; the outer hair cells do the reverse. Hair cells have a range of supportive cells and the potassium-rich endolymph is produced by the stria vascularis. All these components must be intact for normal function.

The afferent nerve fibers from the cochlea have cell bodies in the spiral ganglion, relay with the cochlear nucleus, and project to the auditory cortex by the superior olivary complex, lateral lemniscus, inferior colliculus, and medial genniculate body. The efferent fibers arise in the superior olivary complex and leave the brainstem in the VIIIth cranial nerve. They pass into the auditory nerve in the internal auditory meatus and then to the cochlea to innervate the outer hair cells. They are thought to be involved in feedback to the cochlea improving frequency resolution and are responsible for the production of the otoacoustic emissions. The efferent vestibular fibers have their cell bodies in Scarpa's ganglion; the proximal fibers then run as the superior and inferior vestibular nerves and join the cochlear nerve in the internal auditory meatus and then to synapse in the vestibular nuclei. Projections are made with cerebellum, vestibulo-spinal tracts, thalamus, cortex, reticular formation, autonomic nerve system, contralateral vestibular nuclei, and cranial nerves III, IV, and VI. The saccule and utricle have otolith organs which detect linear accelerations whilst the ampullae of the semicircular canals detect angular accelerations.

Detection of deafness

Although pure tone audiometry (PTA) is readily available, it is relatively insensitive and a deterioration in hearing may occur before it is apparent on the PTA. Speech discrimination is a better test and even better is speech presented in noise. This approximates better to the handicap that a patient experiences and these tests are available in most audiology departments. There are a range of psychoacoustic tests which can detect subtle changes in audition but many are research tools or only available in some centers.

Electric tests are used to measure the neural integrity of the auditory system. They are objective, requiring no active participation of the subject. Electro-cochleography (ECochG) can detect hair cell function (cochlear microphonic), the DC shift in the stimulated cochlea (summating potential), and the compound action potential generated by the auditory nerve. ECochG used in clinical practice is uncomfortable, but it is a very useful tool for animal models of ototoxicity.

Auditory brain stem responses (ABRs) are used to assess the integrity of the auditory pathway from the auditory nerve up to the inferior colliculus. This is done with surface electrodes and is therefore not uncomfortable.

Otoacoustic emissions

If a sound is presented to the ear this is followed by the cochlea emitting a sound; this cochlear echo is thought to be generated by the outer hair cells (OHCs) following stimulation by the cochlear efferent nerve fibers. This otoacoustic emission (OAE) can be detected by a very sensitive microphone in the ear canal. The analysis of the signal is complex but commercially available machines are readily available. The technique is simple, an ear plug with a small speaker and microphone is placed in the ear canal. The test is quick, taking 1–2 minutes to perform. In general OAE are not elicited if the hearing loss is greater than 30 dB. Frequency-specific information can be obtained if the distortion product variant of the test is used. This is a promising test for determining cochlea damage in patients on ototoxic drugs, providing a response is present at the outset of treatment, as it requires no subjective response from the patient and can be performed at the bedside.

Detection of vestibular dysfunction

These tests are less sensitive than auditory tests. The caloric test is used to assess vestibular function, largely of the lateral semicircular canal, by irrigating each ear in turn with water at 7°C above and below body temperature. If no response is detected (canal paresis) ice-cold water is then used which may or may not show a response, depending on the degree of vestibular damage. Other tests commonly used are the measurement of optokinetic nystagmus, pendulum tracking, gaze and positional nystagmus, and rotational chairs. Posturography measures the subject's ability to maintain a steady posture and is usually measured on force platforms.

Histopathology

To get good preparations of the inner ear for histology the tissue needs to be fixed as soon after death as possible. This is achieved by infusing with glutueraldyle via the oval window. Over the last two decades great improvements have occurred both in cutting sections and imaging, particularly with the scanning electron microscope. These techniques have allowed the precise location of cell damage, both in humans and animals, to be ascertained. Ototoxicity refers to reversible and non-reversible damage to the cochlea and vestibular system; cochleotoxic means damage to hearing; and vestibulotoxic to the balance system. Although the neuroepithelium of the inner ear is often the site of ototoxicity, neural connections, both peripheral and central, can give rise to some of the behavioral changes observed in patients. Therefore, more than one site of damage may be involved.

AMINOGLYCOSIDE OTOTOXICITY

The aminoglycosides are ototoxic and vestibulotoxic to different degrees. They are the most studied and serve as a good example as to how ototoxic drugs are investigated. The OHCs of the basal turn are most susceptible to damage, the first row then the middle and the third row, and then damage spreads to the cochlea apex. The inner hair cells (IHCs) appear to be damaged only after extensive OHC destruction (Matz, 1993). Hair cells do not regenerate. Loss of spiral ganglion nerve cells has been observed in most cases, and this is probably secondary to the hair cell loss. In the vestibular system, selective destruction occurs of the type I hair cells found in the cristae ampularis; type II hair cells are more resistant to damage.

Pharmacokinetics

How aminoglycocides leave the blood stream and reach the hair cells is unknown; the ototoxic effect is not simply related to the inner ear concentration (Henley and Schacht, 1988). There is also a delay in the ototoxic effect and a reversible element. Gentamicin has been shown to bind to the base of the OHCs, high affinity binding sites have been identified, and the dissociation constants show a four-fold higher affinity in the vestible compared with the cochlea (Tran Ba Huy and Deffrennes, 1988a, b). Isolated Guinea pig OHCs were not killed by gentamicin but were killed by a metabolite. Gentamicin is more slowly cleared from the perilymph than serum and the half-life in the perilymph is increased in animals with impaired renal function (Huy et al., 1981). Clinical studies show that higher perilymph levels of gentamicin are associated with impaired renal function and treatment duration (Matz and Lerner, 1981).

The initial ototoxic effect appears to be due to an interaction with the hair cell's cell membrane affecting phospholipids. This is demonstrated by the loss of the cochlear microphonic which can be reversed by the infusion of Ca^{2+} ions (Takada and Schacht, 1982). A reduced uptake of radio-labeled phosphate has been shown in the presence of gentamicin to be correlated with a loss of the cochlear microphonic but no structural damage to the hair cells could be demonstrated (Takada and Schacht, 1982).

Delayed toxicity in animal and humans is the norm, resulting in permanent damage, and is thought to be due to aminoglycosides accumulating in the inner ear. However, a study of rat inner ears over several months showed the concentration of gentamicin never exceeded peak serum levels, saturation of the inner ear occurred within three hours, and tissue levels did not correlate with ototoxicity. Ototoxicity, as measured by auditory brainstem responses, did not occur until three weeks into the treatment (Tran Ba Huy et al., 1986). It has therefore been hypothesized that gentamicin has been metabolized to an active ototoxic form. However, no mammalian enzyme has been found to act on the aminoglycosides and urinary recovery of injected drugs appears to be complete. Organ cultures of outer hair cells are not damaged by gentamicin unless the drug has first been incubated with a metabolizing liver fraction (Crann et al., 1992). Therefore metabolism of at least a small fraction of aminoglycoside is required to cause ototoxicity, but how and where this occurs is yet to be determined. Gentamicin has a very high affinity for phosphatidyl inositol 4,5-biophosphate which appears to be specific to the OHC and intracellular binding results in blocking the activation of protein kinase C. These intracellular events are probably responsible for the permanent damage. Sensorineural deafness may occur because of damage to the IHCs, or OHCs, disturbances of the inner ear biochemistry or neuronal damage. Depending on the site and severity of the insult, deafness may be temporary or permanent, partial or total. In general, it is the hair cells involved with the perception of high frequency, which lie at the basal end of the cochlea sounds, that are the most vulnerable. Different cells in the inner ear have different susceptibilities to toxic agents; for example, gentamicin is predominantly vestibulotoxic but will cause deafness.

PREVENTION OF OTOTOXICITY

Numerous protective agents from vitamin C to free radical scavengers have been tested. The effects of the latter have been patchy; WR-2721 attenuates kanamycin ototoxicity in guinea pigs, whereas N-acetylcysteine is ineffective. Glutathione attenuates gentamicin ototoxicity in malnourished or stressed animals but not in well-nourished ones (Lautermann et al., 1995). Unfortunately the type of free radical is not known, although it has been shown that an iron–gentamicin complex can form free radicals in vitro. Therefore, the protective effect of iron chelators has been studied in guinea pigs. Desferrioxamine and 2,3-dihydrobenzoate significantly reduced gentamicin hearing threshold shifts. In the same set of experiments moderate attenuation of ototoxicity was found with mannitol, 4-methylthio-benzoate, and WR-2721, but no protection was found with allopurinol, dimethyl sulfoxide, benzoate, and lazeroid U74389G (Song and Schact, 1996).

THERAPEUTIC VESTIBULOTOXICITY

Bouts of vertigo occur in most patients who suffer from Ménière's disease. In about 10% of cases traditional medical therapy (cinnarizine, betahistine, diuretics) fails to control the vertigo. Traditionally the treatment of incapacitated and intractable cases was labyrinthectomy, but this resulted in total deafness in the operated ear and, therefore, was not practicable in bilateral cases. Vestibular neurectomy is effective but is a neurosurgical procedure during which the auditory and facial nerve is at risk. Chemical vestibular neurectomy has attractions. Initially intramuscular streptomycin was evaluated and, although the treatment was effective in stopping vertigo in 95% of patients and no deafness occurred, 35% had persistent ataxia and 15% had persistent oscillopsia (Schuknect, 1991).

These side effects are due to the ablation of both vestibular systems but are so troublesome that this form of treatment has been abandoned, except in the most severe bilateral cases. Intratympanic delivery of gentamicin is now gaining popularity as this poses less risk to hearing, the effect is delayed, and unsteadiness appears two to five days after treatment, corresponding to the loss of the caloric response and nystagmus.

Hearing loss has occurred in about 15% of patients receiving up to seven days' treatment; in those receiving two days' treatment with gentamicin, no hearing loss was observed.

ANTINEOPLASTIC AGENTS

These are now the greatest cause of ototoxicity.

Platinum compounds

Cis-diamminedichloroplatinum II (CDDP, cisplatin, platinol, cis $(PtCl_2(NH_2))$ is the first generation of divalent platinum compounds. Cis-diammine-1,1-cyclobutane decarboxylate platinum II (BDCA, carboplatin; paraplatin) is the second generation compound. The first generation compounds are the most ototoxic.

The toxic effects of cisplatin are well recognized and include: ototoxicity, peripheral neuropathies, nephrotoxicity, myelosuppression, and gastrointestinal toxicity. With improvement in administration with respect to hydration, nephrotoxicity is no longer the dose-limiting factor but has been replaced by ototoxicity.

Cisplatin is primarily cochleo-toxic causing basal OHC degeneration, loss of supporting cells, damage to the stria vascularis of the auditory nerve, and, at high doses, total collapse of the membranous labyrinth. Clinically deafness is insidious in onset, affecting high frequencies first. It is usually irreversible and may progress following the cessation of treatment but usually follows the accumulation of several doses, although this is idiosyncratic.

Cisplatin is largely bound to serum proteins which are chemically reactive, as is the free form (Hegedus et al., 1987). The latter is thought to be responsible for the ototoxicity. Excretion is primarily renal, and nephrotoxicity correlates with the drug concentration in renal tissue.

The mechanism of cell damage in the inner ear is unknown. Cisplatic inhibits adenylate cyclase (Bagger-Sjoback et al., 1980), ATPase, and membrane-bound phosphatase (Tay, 1988). Cisplatin is not cytotoxic to outer hair cells and therefore a metabolic transformation is proposed.

Chemoprotection

The main thrust of this approach has been against superoxide radicals. Sulfur-containing compounds had been shown to give nephroprotection, and sodium thiosulfate and diethyl-dithiocarbamate (DDTC) provide otoprotection. Unfortunately, sodium thiosulfate interferes with tumoricidal action and DDTC increases mortality. D-Methionine (D-Met) is the most effective nephroprotectant and does not decrease anti-tumor activity; pre-administration to rats prior to cisplatin administration showed 'excellent' otoprotection and no adverse effects, all rats surviving the experiment (Campbell et al., 1996). Sulfur-containing drugs are thought to prevent cisplatin from interacting with intracellular target molecules, in particular methionine and glutathione groups in proteins (Lempers and Reedijk, 1990).

Carboplatin is a second-generation platinum compound, and is less oto- and nephrotoxic, as demonstrated in pigmented guinea pigs (Schweitzer et al., 1986). Myelosuppression is the primary dose-limiting effect.

Other antineoplastic agents

Evidence of ototoxicity, though present, is of much less and, often, not of clinical importance as other side effects limit treatment. Vincristine and vinblastine sulfate both damage the organ of Corti, the former also damages the spiral ganglion. Nitrogen mustard (2,2'-dichloro-N-methyldiethylamine hydrochloride) damages OHCs. Misonidazole, a radio-sensitizer, is highly toxic; 49% of patients develop a peripheral neuropathy and 9% had evidence of ototoxicity (Philips, 1981). Due to its toxicity at levels that might provide radio-sensitization, it is not marketed in the USA.

DL-α-difluromethyl ornithine (DFMO), as well as having antirenoplastic properties, is also an antiparasitic drug used in African trypanosomiasis. It is also effective against pneomocystitis carinii. Ototoxicity has been observed in less than 10% of cases.

DRUGS CAUSING REVERSIBLE OTOTOXICITY

These agents are often of more interest to those unraveling hearing physiology than clinicians using them therapeutically. However, any agent causing a reversible ototoxicity may in certain circumstances cause permanent hearing loss.

Loop diuretics

In animal models all loop diuretics have been shown to be ototoxic. However, this has been observed mainly with frusimide, ethyacrynic acid, and bumetanide. The reported cases of permanent hearing loss are so few, and no consistent relationship is seen in the mode of administration, which implies that idiosyncratic reactions of the patient are important.

Analgesics

Salicylate ototoxicity causes deafness and tinnitus at doses of 6–8 g per day. Recovery takes from 24–72 h, the tinnitus preceding the deafness. Otoacoustic emissions are reversibly lost and salicylate is thought to act directly on the outer hair cells.

MONITORING OTOTOXICITY

It does appear that many clinical trials, which are designed to determine the therapeutic efficiency of drugs, are blighted by inadequate monitoring of ototoxicity. This is because no standard protocol is in general use. This is particularly pertinent to the numerous trials of anti-neoplastic drugs.

Clearly some measure of hearing should be performed before the onset of treatment. Pure tone audiometry is the quickest and simplest physio-acoustic test. Clinical audiometry is accurate to about 5 dB, but test–retest error is also about 5 dB, so that a difference between two audiograms of 10 dB is not significant. The problem is worse at 8 kHz and most audiologists exclude 8 kHz in assessing hearing loss. The audio-

metric threshold is raised (hearing appears worse) in background noise, therefore audiometry should be performed in a sound-treated room not at the bedside or in the out-patient department. Ambient noise has its greatest effect on low frequencies. Clinical audiometers have a maximum frequency of 8 kHz, although children can hear up to 16 kHz and many ototoxic agents first affect the high frequencies, the very region which is not being monitored. The most important frequency range is 0.5–4 kHz, where most speech information is conveyed, and it is the loss of speech discrimination that causes greatest handicap and disability to the patient. Speech audiometry is the gold standard but takes longer to do than a PTA and requires greater concentration from the patient. Clearly a nauseated patient may not reach their optimal performance and this can make hearing loss appear worse than it is if a comparison is made between a pretreatment audiogram and one performed during treatment. A further refinement of speech audiometry is to perform the test in a standardized background noise environment, which approximates more closely to a real-life listening situation and, if available, is the test of choice.

Otoacoustic emission has the advantage of being quick (30–60 s) per ear and does not require a conscious response from the patient. It is therefore immune to a patient's general condition which might affect concentration, and can be used in children. Otoacoustic emissions provide a means of looking at cochlear physiology, in particular the OHCs, and can give frequent, specific information. The drawback is that emissions are not present if there is a hearing loss of around 30 dB or greater, or if there is an abnormal middle ear.

A combination of speech audiometry and OAE should be employed, the former would give the best evidence of a significant deterioration in hearing, the latter is ideal for frequent monitoring. If OAEs are absent prior to treatment, PTA could be substituted.

The timing and frequency of tests would vary according to the treatment regimen, so care should be addressed at detecting delayed effects of the ototoxicity and any reversible hearing loss. The critical analysis is the change in the pretreatment hearing level, the hearing level measured at a predetermined period post-treatment.

MONITORING VESTIBULAR TOXICITY

This is difficult in the bed-bound patient but more patients are receiving anti-tumor therapy and would be amenable for investigation. The onset of oscillopsia makes reading difficult or impossible and is readily testable (Longridge and Mallinson, 1987). Caloric tests and rotating chairs are impractical as both induce nausea and on occasions vomiting, and it would not be considerate to perform these tests on patients who were already nauseated. The Romberg test, with eyes closed, gives an indication of vestibular damage but this is subjective. Posturography, usually by force platform, gives a better measure of body stability and allows a numerical comparison between readings. The final measure following treatment is more problematical than with hearing. Central compensation for vestibular damage may occur in weeks or up to two years. Patients with bilateral total vestibular failure may never compensate.

SUMMARY

Most attributions of toxicity are based on unreliable information, such as case reports. Taste and smell have been underestimated with respect to toxic damage, but measuring the loss of these sensations is difficult. The estimation of safe levels of exposure is often based on animal models which can be misleading. The number of potentially toxic drugs and chemical substances is very large and may be beyond the knowledge of most clinicians.

Ototoxicity and vestibulotoxicity are much better documented. The fact that metabolites often cause toxicity suggests that care should be exercised when considering animal models. Therefore, proper monitoring of hearing and balance should be built into the drug trials. Chemoprotection is certainly an area that deserves further research, and detection of early vestibular damage in very sick patients is still a challenge.

REFERENCES

Ackerman, B. and Kasbekar, N. 1997: Disturbances of taste and smell induced by drugs. *Pharmacotherapy*, **17**, 482–96.

Alarie, Y. 1981: Dose-response analysis in animal studies: prediction of human responses. *Environmental Health Perspectives*, **42**, 9–13.

Alarie, Y. and Luo, J.E. 1989: Sensory irritation by airborne chemicals: a basis to establish acceptable levels of exposure. In *Toxicology of the Nasal Passages*, Barrow, C.S. (ed.), pp 91–100. Washington, DC: Hemisphere Publishing.

Amoore, J.E. 1986: Effects of chemical exposure on olfaction in humans. In *Toxicology of the Nasal Passages*, Barrow, C.S. (ed.), pp 155–90. Washington, DC: Hemisphere Publishing.

Bagger-Sjoback, D., Filiped, C.S. and Schacht, J. 1980: Characteristics and drug responses of cochlear and vesticular adenylate cyclase. *Archives of Otorhinolaryngology*, **228**, 217–22.

Bartoshuk, L.M. 1978: The psychophysics of taste. *American Journal of Clinical Nutrition*, **31**, 1068–77.

Bogdanffy, M. and Frame, S. 1994: Olfactory mucosal toxicity. *Inhalation Toxicology*, **6**, 205–19.

Bray, J., Cragg, P., Macknight, A., Mills, R. and Taylor, D. 1994: *Lecture Notes on Human Physiology*, 3rd edn, pp 187–9. Oxford: Blackwell Scientific.

Campbell, K.C.M., Rybak, L.P., Meech, R.P. and Hughes, L. 1996: D-Methionine provides excellent protection from cisplatin ototoxicity in the rat. *Hearing Research*, **102**, 90–8.

Crann, S.A., Huawy, M.Y., McClaren, J.D. and Schact, J. 1992: Formation of a toxic metabolite from gentamicin by hepatic cytosolic fraction. *Biochemical Pharmacology*, **43**, 1835–9.

Emslie-Smith, D., Paterson, C., Scratcherd, T. and Read, N. 1987: *Textbook of Physiology*, pp 234–5 and 486–8. Edinburgh: Churchill Livingstone.

Feron, V.J., Woutersen, R.A. and Spit, B.J. 1986: Pathology of chronic nasal toxic responses including cancer. In *Toxicology of the Nasal Passages*, Barrow, C.S. (ed.), pp 67–89. Washington, DC: Hemisphere Publishing.

Ganong, W.F. 1993: *Review of Medical Physiology*, pp 170–2. Connecticut: Lange Medical Publications.

Guyton, A.C. 1992: *Human Physiology and Mechanisms of Disease*, 5th edn, pp 398–400. Philadelphia, PA: W.B. Saunders.

Hastings, L. and Miller, M.L. 1997: Olfactory loss secondary to toxic exposure. In *Taste and Smell Disorders*, Seiden, A.M. (ed.), pp 88–106. New York: Thieme.

Hegadus, L., Van derVijgh, W.J.F. and Klein, I. 1987: Chemical reactivity of cisplatin bound to human plasma protein. *Cancer Chemotherapy and Pharmacology*, **20**, 211–2.

Henkin, R. 1994: Drug-induced taste and smell disorders. *Drug Safety*, **11**, 318–77.

Henkin, R.I. 1993: Evaluation and treatment of human olfactory dysfunction. In *Otolaryngology*, English, C. (ed.), Vol. II, pp 1–86. Philadelphia, PA: Lippincott.

Henley, C.M. and Schacht, J. 1988: Pharmacokinetics of aminoglycoside antibiotics in blood, inner ear fluids and tissues and their relationship to ototoxicity. *Audiology*, **27**, 137–46.

Huy, P.T.B., Manuel, C. and Meulemans, A. 1981: Kinetics of aminoglycoside antibiotics and loop-inhibiting diuretics in the guinea pig. In *Aminoglycoside Ototoxicity*, Lerner, S.A., Matz, G.J. and Hawkins, J.E. Jr (eds). Boston, MA: Little Brown.

Kane, L.E., Barrow, C.S. and Alarie, Y. 1979: A short-term test to predict acceptable levels of exposure to airborne sensory irritants. *American Industrial Hygiene Association Journal*, **40**, 207–29.

Lancet, D. 1994: Exclusive receptors. *Nature*, **372**, 321–2.

Lautermann, J., McClaren, J. and Schoct, J. 1995: Glutathione protection against gentamicin ototoxicity depends on nutritional status. *Hearing Research*, **86**, 15–24.

Lempers, E.L.M. and Reedijk, J. 1990: Reversibility of cisplatin-methionne in proteins by di-ethyl drithiocarbanate of thionnea: a study with model adducts. *Inorganic Chemistry*, **29**, 217–22.

Leopold, D.A. 1994: Nasal toxicity: end points of concern in humans. *Inhalation Toxicology*, **6**, 23–9.

Longridge, N.S. and Mallinson, A.I. 1987: The dynamic illegible E (DIE) test: a simple technique for assessing the ability of the vestibulo-ocular reflex to overcome vestibular pathology. *Journal of otolaryngology*, **16**, 97.

Matz, G.J. 1993: Aminoglycoside cochlear ototoxicity. In *Ototoxicity*, Rybak, L.P. (ed.), Vol. 26, pp 705–13. Otolaryngology Clinics of North America.

Matz, G.J. and Lerner, S.A. 1981: Prospective studies of aminoglycoside ototoxicity in adults. In *Aminoglycoside Ototoxicity*, Lerner, S.A., Matz, G.J. and Hawkins, J.E. Jr (eds). Boston, MA: Little Brown.

Needleman, M. and Rez, A. 1976: Thromboxanes: selective biosynthesis and distinct biological properties. *Journal of Clinical Investigation*, **193**, 163–5.

Phillips, T.L. 1981: Final report on the United States phase I clinical trial of the hypoxia cell radiosensitizer misonidazole. *Cancer*, **48**, 1697.

Robson, A.K., Woollons, A.C., Ryan, J., Horrocks, C., Williams, S. and Dawes, P.J.D. 1996: Validation of the combined olfactory test. *Clinical Otolaryngology*, **21**, 512–18.

Schiffman, S.S. and Gatlin, C.A. 1993: Clinical physiology of taste and smell. *Annual Review of Nutrition*, **13**, 405–36.

Schiffman, S.S. and Troy Nagle, H. 1992: Effect of environmental pollutants on taste and smell. *Otolaryngology Head and Neck Surgery*, **106**, 693–700.

Schuctnect, H.F. 1991: Ablation of vestibular function with intramuscular streptomycin. *Otolaryngology Head and Neck Surgery*, **21**, 38–40.

Schweitzer, V.G., Rarey, K.E. and Dolan, D.F. 1986: Ototoxicity of cisplatin vs platinum analogus CBDCA (JM-8) and CHIP (JM-9). *Otolaryngology Head and Neck Surgery*, **94**, 458–70.

Smith, D.V. 1991: Taste and smell dysfunction. In *Otolaryngology*, Paparella, M.M. and Shumrick, D.A. (eds), Vol. III, pp 1915–20. Philadelphia, PA: W.B. Saunders.

Song, B-B. and Schact, J. 1996: Variable efficacy of radical scavengers and iron chelators to attenuate gentamicinotototoxicity in guinea pig in vitro. *Hearing Research*, **94**, 87–93.

Takada, A. and Schacht, J. 1982: Calcium antagonism and reversibility of gentamicin-induced loss of cochlear microphonics in the guinea pig. *Hearing Research*, **8**, 179–86.

Tay, L. 1988: Effects of cisplatin on rabbit kidney in vivo and on rabbit renal proximal tubular cells in culture. *Cancer Research*, **48**, 2538–43.

Tran Ba Huy, P., Barnard, P. and Schact, J. 1986: Kinetics of gentamicin uptake and release in the rat. Comparison of inner ear tissues and fluids and other organs. *Journal of Clinical Investigation*, **77**, 1492–500.

Tran Ba Huy, P. and Deffrennes, D. 1988a: Aminoglycoside-binding sites in the inner ears of guinea pigs. *Antimicrobial Agents and Chemotherapy*, **32**, 467.

Tran Ba Huy, P. and Deffrennes, D. 1988b: Aminoglycoside ototoxicity influence of dosage regimen on drug uptake and correlations between membrane binding and some clinical features. *Acta Otolaryngology*, **105**, 511.

Witek, T.J. Jr 1993: The nose as a target for adverse effects from the environment: applying advances in nasal physiologic measurements and mechanisms. *American Journal of Industrial Medicine*, **24**, 649–57.

APPENDIX: CHEMICAL COMPOUNDS, PROCEDURES, AND DRUGS ASSOCIATED WITH SMELL AND TASTE DISORDERS

Drugs

Acetazolamide
Acetylcholine substances
Alcohol
Allicin
Allopurinol
Alprazolam
Amfebutamone
Amiloride
Amiodarone
Amiodipine
Amitriptyline
Amoxapine
Amoxicillin
Amphetamines
Amphotericin B
Ampicillin
Amrinone
Aspirin
Auranofin
Azathioprine
Baclofen
Bamifylline
Bamifylline hydrochloride
Beclomethasone
Benzocaine
Biguanides
Bleomycin
β-Blockers
Bretylium
Bromocriptine
Butorphanol
Captopril
Carbamazepine
Carbimazole
Carboplatin
Carmustine
Cefacetrile
Cefadroxil

Cefalexin
Cefamandole
Cefem agents
Cefpodoxime
Ceftriaxone
Chlomezanone
Chlorhexidine mouth wash
Chlormezanone
Chlorpheniramine
Chlorthalidone
Chlorxexidine
Cholestyramine
Choline magnesium trisalicylate
Cimetidine
Ciprofloxacin
Cisplatin
Clarithromycin
Clofibrate
Clomipramine
Cocaine
Colchicine
Corticosterones
Cyclobenzaprine
Cytarabine
Cytosine arabinoside
Dantrolene
Desipramine
Dexamphetamine
Diazepam
Diazoxide
Diclofenac
Dicyclomine
Didanosine
Diltiazem
Dipyridamole
Disulfiram
Doxazosin
Doxorubicin

Drugs continued

Doxycycline
EDTA
Enalapril
Enoxacin
Ergocalciferol
Estazolam
Ethacrynic acid
Ethambutol
Ethchlorvynol
Ethionamide
Etidronate
Etidronic acid
Etodolac
Etretinate
Famotidine
Felbamate
Felodipine
Fenfluramine
Flecainide
Flunisolide
5-Fluorouracil
Fluphenazine
Flurazepam
Flurbripofen
Foscarnet
Fosinopril
Furosemide
Gallium
Gemfibrozil
Gentamicin
Germine monoacetate
Glipizide
Glycopyrrolate
Gold
Granisetron
Griseofulvin
Hydralazine
Hydrochlorothiazide
Hydrocortisone
Hyoscyamine
Ibuprofen
Idoxuridine
Imipramine
Indomethacin
Insulin
Interferon-α
Interferon-γ
Interleukin-2
Iodine
Iron sorbitex
Isosorbide nitrates
Isotretinoin
Kanamycin
Ketoprophen
Ketorolac
Labetatol
β-Lactam antibiotics
Levamisole
Levodopa
Lidocaine
Lincomycin
Lisinopril
Lithium
Lomefloxacin
Lomustine
Loratadine
Losartan

Lovastatin
Mazindol
Mefenamic acid
Methimazole
Methocarbamol
Methotrexate
Methyl methacrylate
Methyldopa
Methylthiouracil
Metoclopramide
Metolazone
Metronidazole
Mexiletine
Minocycline
Misoprostol
Moracizine
Morphine
Nabumetone
Nicotine polacrilex
Nifedipine
Niridazole
Nitroglycerin
Ofloxacin
Opiates
Oxaprozin
Oxazepam
Oxyfedrine
Oxymetazoline
Paracetamol
Paroxetine
Penicillamine
Pentamidine
Pergolide
Phendimetrazine
Phenindione
Phenormin
Phentermine
Phenylbutazone
Phenylephrine
Piperacillin
Pirbuterol
Piroxicam
Pravastatin
Procainamide
Procaine penicillin
Promethazine
Propafenone
Propranolol
Propylthiouracil
Pseudoephedrine
Psilocybin
Rifabutin
Rimantadine
Risperidone
Scopolamine
Selegiline
Sertraline
Sodium fluoride
Spironolactone
Streptomycin
Strychnine
Sucralfate
Sulfafurazole (suifisoxazole)
Sulfasalazine
Sulindac
Sultasalazine
Sumatriptan

Drugs continued

Terbinafine
Terfenadine
Tetracycline
Thiamazole
5-Thiopyridoxine
Thiouracil
Tocainide
Tolbutamide
Trazodone
Triamterene
Triazolam

Trichlormethiazide
Trifluoperazine
Trihexyphenidyl
Trimipramine
Tyrothricin
Venlafaxine
Vincristine
Zalcitabine
Zidovudine
Zolpidem

Chemical compounds
Processes (manufacturing and metallurgical)

Acids
Aluminum fumes
Arsenic
Chromium
Chromium fumes
Chromium plating
Coal tar fumes
Copper fumes
Cutting oils (machining)
Fragrances
Isopropyl alcohol
Lead
Magnet production
Manganese fumes
Mercury
Nickel plating
Nickel refining (electrolytic)
Paint (lead)
Paprika
Pavinol (sewing)
Peppermint
Potash dust

Rubber vulcanization
Silver plating
Spices
Steel production
Styrene
Sulfuric acid
Sulfuric compounds
Sulfuric dioxide
Sulfuric dioxide with ammonia
Tanning
Tetrachloroethane
Tin fumes
Tobacco
Toluene
Trichloroethane
Trichloroethylene
Varnishes
War gases (WWI)
Wastewater (refinery)
Zinc chromate
Zinc fumes
Zinc production

Chemical substances

Acetaldehyde
Acetic acid
Acetone
Acetonitrile
Acetophenone
Acid chlorides
Acrolein
Alum
Ammonia
Amyl acetate
Arsenic compounds
Asphalt (oxidized)
Benzaldehyde
Benzine
Benzine with ethyl and butyl
acetate
Benzoic acid
Benzoquinone
Benzylchloride
Blasting powder
Bromine
2-Butoxyethanol
n-Butyl alcohol
Butylene glycol
Cadmium compounds
Cadmium oxide
Cadmium oxide with nickel
hydroxide
Carbon disulfide

Carbon monoxide
Carbon tetrachloride
Cement dust
Chloracetophenone
Chlorine
Chlorobenzene
Chlorobenzylidene
malononitrile
Chloroform
Chloromethanes
Chloropicrin
Chlorovinylarsine chlorides
Chromate salts
Chromic acid
Coke dust
Copper arsenite
Cotton dust
Cyanide dust
Cyclohexanone
o-Dichlorobenzene
Dichromates
Dimethyl sulfate
Dimethylamine
Epichlorohydrin
Ethyibenzene
Ethyl acetate
Ethyl acrylate

Chemical substances continued

Ethyl alcohol
Ethyl ether
Flax dust
Flour dust
Flue gas
Fluorine compounds
Formaldehyde
Fufural
Grain dust
Halogen compounds
Hardwood dust
Hydrazine
Hydrogen chloride
Hydrogen fluoride
Iodoform
Isoamyl alcohol
Isocyanates
Isophorone
Isopropylbenzene (cumene)
Lime dust
Lye (caustic soda)
Menthol
Methyl alcohol
Methyl ethylketone

Methylisobutyl ketone
Nitric acid
Nitro compounds
Nitrogen dioxide
Nitrogen dioxide with ammonia
Nitrogen dioxide with sulfur
dioxide
Osmium tetroxide
Phenol
Phenylene diamine
Phosgene
Potassium sulfide
Printing dust
n-Propyl alcohol
Selenium compounds
Selenium dioxide
Sewer gas
Silicosis dust
Silver nitrate
Strontium sulfate
p-Tert-butyltoluene
2,4-Toluene dilsocyanate
m-Xylene
o-Xylene

6

Environmental causes of disorders of movement

NIALL EF CARTLIDGE

INTRODUCTION

This chapter is concerned with those motor syndromes which result, or are thought to result, from the effects of environmental influences, most commonly exogenous toxins, on those systems within the central nervous system that are concerned with the control of movement. A classification of such disorders is difficult because many exogenous toxins affect multiple neuronal populations within the central nervous system involving functions other than the control of movement. At the same time they may involve the peripheral nervous system and non-neurological organs. Although this chapter is primarily concerned with environmental causes of movement disorders, a good knowledge of drug-induced problems is extremely important as it helps in the identification of other environmental causes.

Particular interest in environmental influences on disorders of movement has increased in recent years for the following reasons:

1 There is increasing evidence that neurodegenerative disorders such as motor neurone disease and Parkinson's disease might be caused by environmental influences.
2 It is recognized that a specific toxin, namely 1-methyl-4-phenyl-1,2,3,6-tetrahydropyridine (MPTP), may produce a syndrome clinically and pathologically almost identical to idiopathic Parkinson's disease (Langston, 1985).

Historical introduction

The nervous system is particularly susceptible to toxic insult and some of the clinical effects of chemical attack on the nervous system were even known to ancient civilizations. The neurological sequelæ of lead poisoning were described by the Greek poet physician, Nikander, before the birth of Christ (Major, 1945).

It has been suggested that mercurial encephalopathy was immortalized in the character of the Mad Hatter in the Alice in Wonderland stories, although doubt has been cast on this (Waldron, 1983).

Scattered throughout medical history may be found other examples of the effects of toxins upon the nervous system in general, and motor function in particular, and these will be dealt with in the appropriate sections.

Acute and chronic effects

The effect of exogenous toxins upon the nervous system in general, and motor function in particular, may be divided into acute and chronic effects; although these two obviously merge to some extent into one another.

A good example is the effect of ethyl alcohol. The most obvious acute effect is the encephalopathy which is almost too familiar to merit further discussion. Larger doses of alcohol produce the so-called drunken state where a clear effect upon motor function is seen in the form of slurring of speech and unsteadiness. This almost certainly results from the toxic effects of ethyl alcohol upon neurones within the vestibulocerebellar system (Kubo *et al.*, 1990).

Chronic alcohol abuse produces a similar effect upon the cerebellum with permanent damage and loss of cerebellar neurones (Victor *et al.*, 1956). There remains some doubt as to whether or not chronic alcoholism is associated with permanent encephalopathy in the form of dementia.

In general the acute effects upon motor function of a toxin mirror the chronic effects, although there are some notable exceptions to this such as the neuroleptic-induced movement disorders. In this group of disorders the acute effects of a neuroleptic drug producing, for example, an acute dystonia may differ very significantly clinically from the chronic effect which, in many instances, manifests itself as a parkinsonian syndrome (Tarsy, 1983).

In each section an attempt will be made to differentiate the acute effects of a particular toxin from the chronic effects.

Classification

The central nervous system structures concerned with the control of movement are quite complex and may be found in any standard neuroanatomy textbook.

For the purpose of this review the systems are simplified to the following:

1 the main descending motor pathway – the corticospinal tract;
2 the cerebellum;
3 the basal ganglia.

DISORDERS OF THE CORTICOSPINAL TRACT

Although the corticospinal tract is not the only descending motor pathway concerned with voluntary movement it is certainly the most important and traditionally damage to this tract produces the clinical picture of the so-called upper motor neurone syndrome.

Lathyrism

INTRODUCTION

The term 'lathyrism' was first applied by Contani in 1873 in Italy to a neurological disease characterized by loss of muscular control leading to the development of a spastic paraplegia. It is primarily a degenerative disorder of the central motor pathway caused by excessive consumption of the grass or chickling pea (*Lathyrus sativus*) or the seed of other potentially neurotoxic lathyrus species. These legumes typically make up a component of the diet of poor people in regions endemic for the disease and usually appear when adverse environmental conditions, such as floods or droughts, result in dependency on the hardy grass pea for food (Spencer, 1995).

HISTORY

Lathyrism was known to ancient Hindus, to Hypocrates, Plinney the elder and Galen. Hypocrates wrote 'At Ainos? all men and women, who ate continuously peas, became impotent in the legs.'

During the seventeenth, eighteenth, nineteenth, and twentieth centuries outbreaks of lathyrism occurred throughout Europe, northern Africa, the Middle East, Afghanistan, Russia, and India (Proust, 1883; Stockman, 1929; Selye, 1957; Barrow *et al.*, 1974).

CLINICAL PICTURE

All ages may be affected by the disease although it most commonly is seen in young adults. Males are more commonly and more severely affected than females, and females tend to develop the disorder before puberty, during pregnancy or after the menopause.

The disease displays a constant clinical picture consisting of varying degrees of spastic paraparesis involving the lower limbs almost exclusively (Tekle-Haimanot *et al.*, 1990). In almost all patients cramp in the legs is the earliest symptom resulting from spasmodic contractions in the calf muscles. Back and leg pain develops in as many as three-quarters of patients.

About 50% of the patients have the acute onset of symptoms with rapidly developing difficulty in walking due to a spastic paraparesis. Pain is a prominent feature in these patients.

In about 40% of cases there is a sub-acute onset of the condition with no pain.

In a smaller percentage of patients the condition is of insidious onset with a slowly progressive spastic paraparesis. Sensory symptoms are often present but bladder involvement is unusual (Haimanot *et al.*, 1990; Misra *et al.*, 1993).

The tendon reflexes are exaggerated, associated with spasticity, and the feet are often plantar flexed. Ankle clonus may be elicited and extensor plantar responses are commonly seen. Abdominal reflexes are often preserved. Impotence is common.

DIAGNOSIS

There are no specific clinical or laboratory tests for lathyrism and the diagnosis relies on obtaining a history of the heavy ingestion of an appropriate species for some weeks prior to the onset of neurological symptoms and signs.

TREATMENT

A prompt change of diet in the early stages of the development of the disorder may bring about recovery but persistent eating of the offending legume causes progression. Once the neurological signs are established recovery is unlikely. No specific treatment will reverse the neurological deficit.

NEUROPATHOLOGY

Most neuropathological studies have focused on the spinal cord which shows a predominantly distal symmetrical degeneration of the lateral and ventral corticospinal tracts (Streifler *et al.*, 1977).

PREVENTION

The grass pea and related species have formed an inexpensive component in the diet of people since time memorial and lathyrism is thus an important public health problem. Effective preventive measures include educating the people living in endemic areas about the harmful effects of consumption of *Lathyrus sativus*.

PATHOGENESIS (SPENCER, 1995)

There now appears to be good evidence that the agent responsible for lathyrism is a particular free excitatory amino acid found in the grass pea, beta-*N*-oxalylamino-L-alanine (BOAA).

The neurotoxic properties of BOAA have been shown in birds and mammals (Parker *et al.*, 1979; Spencer *et al.*, 1986). In primates BOAA produces motor system dysfunction but this is not so common in optimally nourished primates.

A major unsolved problem is how BOAA traverses the blood–brain barrier to produce its effect. Signs of impending lathyrism in the prodromal phase probably result from widespread BOAA-induced synaptic over-excitation of central nervous system (CNS) motor neurones. This accounts for the muscle spasms. The precise site of action of BOAA on motor neurones is uncertain although it seems more likely that the effect is on the cell body rather than the axons. The reason for the selective involvement of the corticospinal tracts to the legs rather than the arms remains uncertain.

At any event lathyrism can be regarded as a model motor system disease in the experimental laboratory with its probable effect being through excitotoxicity.

Skeletal fluorosis

INTRODUCTION

Flourine or fluoride have no direct toxic effect on the nervous system but excessive fluoride intake may affect the spinal skeleton and produce a secondary effect on the spinal cord and corticospinal tracts.

HISTORY

Fluorosis in humans was first mentioned as an occupational disease by Feil in 1930 and was recorded as a disease endemic in the Madras Presidency of India shortly thereafter (Shortt *et al.*, 1937).

EPIDEMIOLOGY

In most instances skeletal fluorosis results from excessive fluoride intake in natural water supplies. In tropical countries like India, where the high temperatures promote the ingestion of large quantities of water, fluoride intake may be high if the natural water supply contains significant quantities of fluoride. About 96–99% of the fluoride retained in the body combines with mineralized bones and the increase in fluoride content stimulates osteoblastic activity resulting in periosteal new bone formation, as well as calcification of ligaments and tendons.

CLINICAL FEATURES (REDDY, 1979)

There is a high degree of uniformity in the clinical manifestations of skeletal fluorosis. As the bones become remodeled pain and stiffness in the neck develops with increasing restriction of spinal movements. The stiffness thereafter spreads to various joints in the limbs resulting from involvement of joint capsules and ligaments.

The neurological sequelæ in skeletal fluorosis are those of a radiculomyelopathy arising principally because of the mechanical compression of the spinal cord and nerve roots. In the later stages compression of radicular vessels in the intervertebral foramina produce secondary vascular complications in the spinal cord and spinal roots.

Only about 10% of cases of skeletal fluorosis go on to neurological complications.

The cervical rather than the dorsal cord is most commonly affected and the cauda equina is less commonly damaged.

The most common clinical signs and symptoms are those of a progressive myelopathy with a spastic paraparesis. Radicular signs and symptoms in the upper limbs with muscle wasting, depression of tendon reflexes, pain, and sensory changes may be seen.

INVESTIGATIONS

The radiographic changes are usually quite striking with the bones showing increased density with over-growth.

TREATMENT

Whilst it is possible to create a negative fluoride balance by reducing fluoride intake this rarely has an effect upon the skeletal changes and any neurological manifestations. Decompressive surgery may be of value in those with significant spinal cord or spinal root compression, although surgical decompression of the spine is, in most instances, extensive (Reddy *et al.*, 1974).

IATROGENIC (DRUG-INDUCED) SPINAL DISORDERS

Intrathecal injections of certain drugs may be complicated by infective or aseptic meningitis, adhesive arachnoiditis, or toxic effects of the drug on the spinal cord. Intrathecal injection of corticosteroid preparations, such as Depo-Medrone, causes an acute meningeal reaction that is thought to be due to the polyethylene glycol detergent in the preparation and is associated with back and leg pain, paraesthesiae, bladder dysfunction, and a CSF pleocytosis with elevation of the protein level (Bernat, 1981).

Epidural injections, which are often used in the treatment of patients with chronic lumbar radicular pain, are not associated with such reactions unless there is inadvertent penetration of the dura. Spinal anesthesia is associated with a low incidence of lower limb numbness, paraesthesiae or weakness which has been attributed to the toxic effects of the anesthetic agent on the lumbosacral roots (Steen and Michenfelder, 1979). Symptoms usually develop immediately after operation and may persist for several months. The incidence of such complications is even lower following epidural anesthesia.

Intrathecal chemotherapy with methotrexate or cytosine arabinoside may cause a transient or permanent paraplegia (Hahn *et al.*, 1983). An acute transverse myelopathy may also occur in heroin addicts and has been attributed to ischemia of the cord due to vasculitis (Ell *et al.*, 1981).

A spinal cord syndrome similar if not identical to sub-acute combined degeneration of the cord has been described in dentists after prolonged exposure to nitrous oxide (Blanco and Peters, 1983). The condition is thought to be due to the inhibitory effects of nitrous oxide on vitamin B_{12} utilization. Recovery usually occurs after exposure to nitrous oxide is stopped.

Spinal cord compression attributed to increased extradural adipose tissue has been reported rarely in patients on prolonged corticosteroid therapy (Guegan *et al.*, 1982).

MOTOR NEURONE DISEASE-LIKE SYNDROMES

The term motor neurone disease is used in a somewhat unselective manner as an umbrella term referring to those diseases in which there is selective loss of function of the lower and/or upper motor neurones which control the voluntary muscles of the bulbar region or limbs. There is a wide range of such disorders (Table 6.1) yet the term motor neurone disease is often seen as synonymous with the specific disorder of amyotrophic lateral sclerosis, the most common and serious of this group of disorders.

Lathyrism can be regarded as being a motor neurone disease-like syndrome with the clinical features as indicated above.

Conzo is a similar disorder characterized by a symmetrical spastic paraparesis occurring in Africa. It may occur in epidemics at times of famine and appears to result from high blood cyanide levels from the cyanogens of ingested casseva flour (Tylleskar *et al.*, 1992).

The recognition that exogenous toxins cause a motor neurone disease-like syndrome has led to a search for possible environmental influences as a cause for an amyotrophic lateral sclerosis.

Table 6.1 *Classification of the motor neuron diseases*

Combined upper and lower motor neuron involvement
  Amyotrophic lateral sclerosis
  Sporadic
  Familial adult onset
  Familial juvenile onset
Pure lower motor neuron involvement
  Proximal hereditary motor neuronopathy
  Acute infantile form (Werdnig–Hoffmann)
  Chronic childhood form (Kugelberg–Welander)
  Autsomal recessive: adult onset
  Autosomal dominant
  Hereditary bulbar palsy
  With deafness (Fazio–Londe)
  X-linked bulbospinal neuronopathy
  Hexosaminidase deficiency
  Multifocal motor neuropathies
  Postpolio syndrome
  Postirradiation syndrome
  Monomelic, focal or segmental spinal musclular atrophy
Pure upper motor neuron involvement
  Primary lateral sclerosis
  Hereditary spastic paraplegia
  Lathyrism
  Konzo

MOTOR NEURONE DISEASE (AMYOTROPHIC LATERAL SCLEROSIS) AND ENVIRONMENTAL TOXINS

The cause of amyotrophic lateral sclerosis (ALS) is unknown but several environmental influences have been suggested as possible causes.

Metals and minerals

There have been many studies into the role of metals in the pathogenesis of ALS (Tandan and Bradley, 1985). Increased exposure to lead, mercury, or heavy metals as a group has been reported in ALS patients (Roelofs-Iverson et al., 1984; Yase, 1984), although not by all investigators (Kurtzke and Beebe, 1980). However, significant exposure to lead can sometimes be unknown, overlooked, or denied. Increased lead content in blood and cerebrospinal fluid (CSF) has been demonstrated in ALS patients as compared with controls, but this has not been noted universally (Mantan and Cook, 1979). The initial observation of markedly increased lead levels in the spinal cord of both lead-exposed and unexposed ALS patients has since been duplicated (Kurlander and Patten, 1979). A positive correlation has been achieved between cord lead level and duration of the disease. However, the report by Petkau and colleagues (1974) of elevated levels of lead in skeletal muscle remains unconfirmed. The precise mechanism underlying lead-induced neurotoxicity is unclear, but interference with synaptic activity, intracellular calcium homeostasis, and cholinergic function have been suggested (Singhal and Thomas, 1980). The exact mode of entry of lead into the nervous system is also obscure, but may involve initial capillary endothelial damage or retrograde axonal and trans-synaptic transport (Baruah et al., 1981).

A motor neurone disorder resembling ALS has followed outbreaks of organic mercury intoxication caused by use of fungicides, and after brief but intense exposure to elemental mercury (Barber, 1978). In some autopsied cases in which there was exposure to organic mercury, motor neuronal and pyramidal tract degeneration has been demonstrated. A significant reduction in neuronal ribonucleic acid (RNA) seen in experimental mercury intoxication suggests that selective inhibition of protein synthesis may be the basis of mercury neurotoxicity (Chang, 1980).

Experimental aluminum-induced neurofibrillary degeneration in susceptible laboratory animals shares the topographic and morphological characteristics of axonal swellings encountered in some ALS patients (Carpenter, 1968). Neutron activation analysis has detected aluminum in values that are higher than controls in the spinal cords of Chamorro ALS (Yoshimasu et al., 1980) and Parkinson's disease patients, and Japanese patients with ALS. Electron-probe X-ray microanalysis has demonstrated significant amounts of aluminum in the nucleoli of lumbar AHCs from some ALS patients and has also shown perivascular deposits of calcium, aluminum, and manganese in ALS cervical spinal cords (Yoshida, 1977). The relevance of these observations to the etiology of ALS is currently unknown.

Several observations suggest that manganese is involved in the pathogenesis of ALS. Chamorro miners in Guam who had had heavy exposure to manganese were more likely to develop the endemic ALS–parkinsonism–dementia complex (Yase, 1972). ALS has been reported following manganese intoxication in miners in another study (Voss, 1939). Relatively high concentrations of manganese and aluminum, and low concentrations of calcium and magnesium exist in water and soil samples from Guam, the Kii peninsula of Japan, and west New Guinea, three high-incidence foci of ALS (Gajdusek and Salazar, 1982). However, the determination of manganese in spinal cord tissue has revealed conflicting results. Skeletal muscle manganese levels were not different from controls in one study (Pierce-Ruhland and Patten, 1980).

There are similar discordant results of copper levels in ALS spinal cord. The report of ALS cases in a small community in South Dakota where affected subjects excreted abnormal amounts of urinary selenium could not be confirmed by other investigators (Norris, 1978). The wide range of selenium levels in spinal cords from ALS patients and controls probably represents a difference in dietary intake (Kurlander and Patten, 1979).

The discrepancies in these studies make it difficult to assign an etiopathogenetic role to metals in ALS. Inconsistent control levels of tissue metals reported by different investigators cause concern about reliability, and may depend on the analytical techniques employed. Moreover, the increased concentration of some metals in ALS tissues could be a consequence of atrophy, or could represent a phenomenon secondary to cellular damage or alteration in the blood–brain barrier. Nevertheless, further research is needed in this area to elucidate the involvement of metals and minerals in the pathogenesis of ALS.

Trauma and surgery

Back or limb trauma, prior skeletal disease or fracture, 'mechanical injuries' before onset of ALS, and exposure to electric shock or lightning have all been more frequently encountered in ALS patients than in controls (Rosati et al., 1977; Kurtzke and Beebe, 1980; Patten and Engel, 1982; Gowel *et al.*, 1983). The exact importance of this relationship is unknown, but may reflect a vulnerability to injury in the preclinical phase of ALS or suggest an etiological role for injury in precipitating the disease. However, no significant increase in prior trauma in cases of ALS was identified by Murros and Fogelholm (1983).

An increased incidence of previous surgical operations has been observed in ALS patients, although Kondo (1979) noted no predisposition to ALS following gastrectomy, and Murros and Fogelholm (1983) were unable to demonstrate more frequent prior surgery in ALS patients than in controls.

All these epidemiological retrospective analyses depend on adequate recall of events by ALS patients and controls, and on correct selection of the control population.

Other factors

Increased exposure to household pets, farm animals, animal carcasses and hides, and pneumatic tools have all been reported, but the role of these factors in the causation of ALS is unclear (Tandan and Bradley, 1985).

A syndrome resembling motor neurone disease follows irradiation of the lumbar spinal cord in the field used for the para-aortic lymph nodes in males with germ-cell tumors of the testes (Maier *et al.*, 1969). It can also occur after radiation to the head and neck region, mediastinum, or the whole neuraxis (Sadowsky *et al.*, 1976).

Further interest in a role of environmental influences are forthcoming from animal models of amyotrophic lateral sclerosis where a number of experimental neurotoxic disorders in animals have been identified as appropriate models of human motor neurone diseases (Ghetti, 1980; Griffin *et al.*, 1982, Spencer and Schaumburg, 1982; Troncoso *et al.*, 1982).

DISORDERS OF THE BASAL GANGLIA

Iatrogenic (drug-induced) extrapyramidal syndromes

INTRODUCTION

A number of groups of drugs may induce involuntary movements or abnormalities of postural muscle tone that resemble those associated with naturally occurring extrapyramidal disorders. There appears to be a marked individual variability in the susceptibility to these extrapyramidal reactions in that some patients develop side effects even after small doses of the drug, whereas many others take much higher doses and are unaf-

Table 6.2 *Clinical syndromes*

Drug-induced extrapyramidal disorders
Acute dytonic/dyskinetic reactions
Akathisia
Tardive dyskinesia
Chorea and choreoathetosis
Drug-induced parkinsonism
Neuroleptic parkinsonism
Neuroleptic malignant syndrome
Tremor
Tics
Myoclonus

fected. The factors responsible for this variable susceptibility are not fully understood, but there is some evidence that age, gender, and genetic factors play a part (Rawlins, 1986).

HISTORY

The recognition of this group of disorders occurred early during the clinical use of the first neuroleptic drug, chlorpromazine. Delay *et al.* (1952) initially demarcated chlorpromazine's affect of producing parkinsonian features and Fluegel (1956) was the first to suggest the significance of obtaining the 'psychological signs of parkinsonism' in psychiatric patients being treated with neuroleptic agents.

By the mid-1950s other signs of parkinsonism were being recognized in patients treated with these agents and since then a wide range of extrapyramidal side effects of these drugs has been recognized.

A classification of drug-induced extrapyramidal disorders is presented in Table 6.2.

ACUTE DYSTONIC/DYSKINETIC REACTIONS

An acute dystonic syndrome is a well-recognized complication of treatment with many neuroleptic drugs, such as the phenothiazines and butyrophenones, as well as with the tricyclic antidepressants, metoclopramide, and less frequently phenytoin, carbamazepine, propranolol, chlorzoxazone (Bateman *et al.*, 1985; Blain and Lane, 1998), and the calcium channel blockers, flunarizine and cinnarizine (Micheli *et al.*, 1987). The onset is usually within the first few days of starting treatment and may be abrupt and alarming. The dystonia may be confined to the muscles of the head and neck, causing facial grimacing, trismus, abnormal movements and spasms of the tongue, oculogyric crises, orofacial dyskinesias, torticollis, and retrocollis; or it may be more generalized with slow, writhing movements of the limbs and more prolonged tonic contractions of the axial and limb muscles, leading to opisthotonos, lordosis, tortipelvis, and a bizarre gait. The bizarre and protean nature of the manifestations may lead to a mistaken diagnosis of hysteria, tetanus, tetany, or epilepsy. The incidence of this type of extrapyramidal reaction has been estimated to be of the order of 2.5% in patients treated with neuroleptic drugs (Rupniak et al., 1986) and is considerably lower in patients treated with metoclopramide, prochlorperazine, and haloperidol (Bateman et al., 1986). Despite their dramatic and at times alarming nature, the acute dystonias are usually self-limiting and remit once the drug is ceased. Particularly severe reactions may be terminated by the intravenous administration of benztropine and diazepam.

Acute dyskinetic reactions involving the lips, face and tongue, and at times the limbs and trunk, occur commonly in parkinsonian patients treated with levodopa, and these are dose-related. These dyskinesias may develop early during the course of treatment with levodopa (or with various dopamine agonists) when the patient responds to a reduction in dose. With prolonged treatment dyskinesias become an increasing problem, tending to occur at times of maximal response to the levodopa and alternating with periods of akinesia and severe rigidity (the 'on-off' phenomenon). The administration of small, frequent doses of levodopa or a reduction in the overall dose and the introduction of dopamine agonists is sometimes helpful in alleviating this common complication of prolonged levodopa therapy.

Reversible forms of dyskinesia involving the face, mouth and tongue, and at times the limbs and trunk, have also been reported in patients treated with phenytoin (Reynolds and Trimble, 1985), flunarizine (Chouza et al., 1986) and the antimalarials, chlorquine and amodiaquine (Osifo,1979).

AKATHISIA

Akathisia is a state of motor restlessness characterized by an inability to be still and an urge to constantly move about, to pace, or even to run incessantly (Ball, 1985). The condition is seen particularly after the administration of phenothiazine derivatives (for example, fluphenazine, trifluoperazine, and prochlorperazine), and less frequently with the butyrophenones, reserpine, tricylic antidepressants, levodopa, and monoamine oxidase inhibitors. It may also occur with amoxapine and oxazepam withdrawal (Chase and Kopin, 1977; Blain and Lane, 1998). The reported incidence of akathisia in groups of patients treated with antipsychotic drugs has ranged from 12.5 to 45% (Ball, 1985). Akathisia may be associated with other extrapyramidal manifestations such as parkinsonism, tremor, and dystonia. The pathophysiological basis for akathisia is uncertain. Experimental work in the rat has produced evidence linking the phenomenon with a disturbance of the mesocortical dopaminergic system (Ball, 1985).

Akathisia usually remits within days or weeks of withdrawal of the neuroleptic drug, although in some cases it persists for several months or occasionally is even permanent (Ball, 1985). Anticholingergic drugs such as benztropine or diphenhydramine are usually effective in controlling akathisia when given by the intramuscular or intravenous route. Amantadine and propranolol have also been reported to be effective (Ball, 1985).

TARDIVE DYSKINESIA

The distinctive involuntary movement disorder called tardive dyskinesia occurs most frequently after prolonged treatment with dopamine antagonists, particularly the antipsychotic drugs, but also with antiemetic drugs such as metoclopramide and prochlorperazine (Table 6.3) (Burke, 1984; Barnes, 1988). Some studies have found tardive dyskinesia in up to 50% of patients treated with antipsychotic drugs (Barnes, 1988).

In contrast to the acute dystonic/dyskinetic syndrome, tardive dyskinesia usually develops after more than 12 months of continuous therapy, although it has been reported with periods as short as three months (Burke, 1984); it occasionally develops after cessation of therapy (Chase and Kopin, 1977). The condition is more common and more severe in the elderly and is less likely to remit in these patients than in younger individuals (Burke, 1984; Barnes, 1988).

The condition typically takes the form of an orofaciolingual dyskinesia with lip smacking and pursing, sucking, jaw opening and closing, protrusion, side-to-side, or writhing movements of the tongue, and facial grimacing. The movements tend to be rather stereotyped and, when severe, may interfere with speech or swallowing. In some cases more generalized choreoathetotic movements of the limbs and trunk, and repetitive foot tapping are present, and the

Table 6.3 Drugs associated with the development of tardive dyskinesia

Phenothiazines	Dibenzapines
Chlorpromazine	Loxapine
Triflupromazine	**Diphenylbutylpiperidines**
Fluphenazine	Pimozide
Perphenazine	**Indolones**
Trifluoperazine	Molindone
Pericyazine	**Antiemetics**
Promazine	Metoclopramide
Thiopropazate	Phenothiazines
Thioridazine	Prochlorperazine
Mesoridazine	Thiethylperazine
Thioxanthines	Promethazine
Thiothixene	Chlorprothixene
Butyrophenones	Droperidol
Haloperidol	

condition may resemble Huntington's chorea. Less frequently, dystonic posturing of the neck and myoclonic jerking of the distal extremities are also present, and concomitant akathisia or parkinsonism may also occur (Chase and Kopin, 1977; Jankovic, 1981; Burke, 1984). A related syndrome ('withdrawal emergence' syndrome) characterized by choreoathetoid and myoclonic movements of the limbs, trunk, and mouth has been described after sudden withdrawal of antipsychotic drugs in children (Burke, 1984).

The pathophysiological basis for tardive dyskinesia has not been clearly established. The most widely held theory is that, as a result of prolonged dopamine receptor blockade in the corpus striatum, a state of hypersensitivity to endogenous dopamine develops because of changes in receptor properties or numbers (Burke, 1984).

The severity of tardive dyskinesia is variable, and the condition is not often disabling. It remits in up to 40% of cases, even those on continued therapy (Burke, 1984). In cases where it is possible to withdraw the offending drug, there is usually gradual resolution of the dyskinesia over a period of several weeks or months, although in some cases the condition persists. Occasionally a remission occurs even several years after withdrawal of antipsychotic drugs (Burke, 1984). Interruption of therapy when dyskinesia first develops may be beneficial, but there is some evidence that repeated interruption may lead to an increased prevalence and persistence of dyskinesia (Burke, 1984; Casey and Gerlach, 1986).

Although many pharmacological agents have been used to treat tardive dyskinesia, none has proved to be consistently beneficial. The drugs used include, on the one hand, agents with an effect on dopaminergic transmission (for example, reserpine, tetrabenazine, bromocriptine, and levodopa) and, on the other hand, drugs with a cholingergic action, including deanol, choline, and lecithin. Other drugs reported to be beneficial in some cases include baclofen, propranolol, diazepam, α-tocopherol, sodium valproate, and the calcium channel blockers verapamil and diltiazem (Ames and Webber, 1984; Burke, 1984; Barnes, 1988).

CHOREA AND CHOREOATHETOSIS

A number of drugs may produce chorea, which is characterized by irregular multifocal, non-stereotyped, semipurposive 'fidgety' or jerky movements (Blain and Lane, 1998). At times chorea is associated with the slower, more sinuous movements of athetosis or with dystonia. These involuntary movements are thought to result from dopamine overactivity or cholinergic underactivity in the basal ganglia. Chorea or choreoathetosis has been reported with phenytoin intoxication and clonazepam withdrawal (O'Flaherty et al., 1985; Blain and and Lane, 1998), long-term treatment

with benzhexol (Blain and Lane, 1998), and treatment with amphetamines, methadone, methylphenidate, amoxapine, pemoline, ciimetine, neuroleptics, the androgenic steroid oxymetholone, and oral contraceptives (Tilzey et al., 1981). Contraceptive-induced chorea, although rare, may occur with high- or low-dose estrogen preparations (Nausieda et al., 1979). Some patients who develop the condition have a history of rheumatic chorea and may be more susceptible (Nausieda et al., 1979). The occurrence of contraceptive-induced chorea is followed by the development of chorea gravidarum in some women (Yiannikas, 1984).

It is not uncommon for the dyskinsia that occurs in parkinsonian patients treated with levodopa to have a choreic quality (Marsden et al., 1982). Similarly, the orofacial and other involuntary movements of tardive dyskinesia may also resemble chorea, although in general they tend to be more repetitive and stereotyped (Jankovic, 1981).

PARKINSONISM

Parkinsonism can occur at all ages but is more frequent in the elderly and is probably the most common form of drug-induced movement disorder (Chase and Kopin, 1977). The condition closely resembles naturally occurring Parkinson's disease; bradykinesia is usually the most prominent feature, with a variable degree of rigidity, tremor, facial masking, and abnormal gait. Although tremor has been said to be less prominent than in idiopathic Parkinson's disease, in some series the incidence of tremor has been as high in cases of drug-induced parkinsonism as in the naturally occurring variety (Stephen and Williamson, 1984). The drugs more frequently implicated are the neuroleptics, including almost all of the phenothiazeines (the most frequent being prochlorperazine), haloperidol, the tricyclic antidepressants, methoclopramide, methyldopa, lithium, and perhexiline (Blain and Lane, 1998). The condition is usually reversible after drug withdrawal or dose reduction. In a group of 48 cases, Stephen and Williamson (1984) found that the condition resolved over a mean period of seven weeks (1–36 weeks). Five patients who initially improved subsequently developed idiopathic parkinsonism after an interval of 3–18 months, suggestive that the drug had unmasked a latent form of idiopathic parkinsonism.

Anticholinergic agents such as benzhexol or benztropine may reverse parkinsonian symptoms in patients who need to continue on neuroleptic therapy. In some cases spontaneous improvements occur even if the causative agent is continued (Chase and Kopin, 1977). Prophylactic treatment with anticholinergic agents may predispose to the development of an irreversible form of tardive dyskinesia and is not advocated; treatment with levodopa may aggravate an underlying psychotic disorder (Blain and Lane, 1998).

NEUROLEPTIC MALIGNANT SYNDROME

The neuroleptic malignant syndrome, a serious and potentially lethal complication of treatment with antipsychotic drugs, is characterized by hyperpyrexia, severe rigidity, bradykinesia, tremor, and autonomic manifestations (Gibb and Lees, 1985). The serum creatine kinase activity is typically elevated, levels of up to 15 000 IU/l being recorded. The drugs most frequently implicated are haloperidol, fluphenazine, chlorpromazine and other phenothiazeines, and thioxanthenes, or combinations of these drugs with each other or with lithium, and less frequently metoclopramide or loxapine (Gibb and Lees, 1985). The condition may develop after commencing neuroleptic therapy, after an increase in dose, or following introduction of a second more potent drug. A similar syndrome has been reported after abrupt levodopa withdrawal in patients with Parkinson's disease (Gibb and Lees, 1985). The syndrome of 'lethal catatonia,' which has been described in patients on long-term antipsychotic therapy, may be related to the neuroleptic malignant syndrome (Blain and Lane, 1998).

Although in mild cases complete recovery may occur within days or weeks of stopping the causative drug, severe cases may develop various complications, including metabolic acidosis, acute myoglobinuria with renal failure, coagulation defects, respiratory failure, shock, seizures and coma, with a mortality rate of 20% in some series (Gibb and Lees, 1985; Ingall and Tennant, 1986). Persisting neurological sequelæ occur in as many as 10% of survivors (Ingall and Tennant, 1986).

The pathophysiological mechanism responsible for the neuroleptic malignant syndrome is uncertain. The current view is that the condition is due to profound dopamine receptor blockade in the corpus striatum as well as in thermoregulatory and vasomotor centers in the hypothalamus (Knezevic et al., 1984; Gibb and Lees, 1985; Blain and Lane, 1998). Treatment involves discontinuation of the causative drug(s), together with vigorous cooling and correction of fluid, electrolyte balance and other complications. Specific measures that may be beneficial in reversing the rigidity and akinesia include the use of amantadine, bromcriptine, levodopa, pancuronium, or dantrolene sodium, or a combination of these drugs, for example dantolene with small doses of bromocriptine or levodopa (Gibb and Lees, 1985).

TREMOR

A number of drugs may aggravate physiological or essential tremor, including sympathomimetic agents, theophyline, doxapram, levodopa, corticosteroids, thyroxine, tricylic antidepressants, caffeine, phenothiazeines, butyrophenones, amphetamines, hypoglycemic agents, amiodarone, and adriamycin, as well as benzodiazepine or alcohol withdrawal (Bateman, 1979; Jankovic and Fahn, 1980; Koller and Musa, 1985; Koller et al., 1987; Blain and Lane, 1998). A postural or resting tremor resembling essential tremor and involving the hands, head, and trunk is not uncommon in patients treated with sodium valproate. The tremor usually develops over a period of several months and remits when the drug is stopped or the dose is reduced (Reynolds and Trimble, 1985). Treatment with propranolol or amantadine may alleviate the tremor (Karas et al., 1983). Cimetidine may induce a severe postural and action tremor by aggravating physiological or essential tremor (Tyrer et al., 1981). Postural or action tremor is an early manifestation of lithium intoxication and is common in patients taking therapeutic doses of the drug (Tyrer et al., 1981). Tremor with cerebellar ataxia may occur in patients on cyclosporin (Thompson et al., 1984).

Asterixis ('flapping tremor') occasionally occurs in patients treated with phenytoin, phenobarbital, carbamazepine, sodium valproate (Reynolds and Trimble, 1985), lithium (Newman and Saunders, 1979), or tocainide (Vincent and Vincent, 1985). Asterixis and bobbing that failed to recover have been reported following metrizamide myelography (Davis et al., 1982).

TICS

A syndrome resembling Gilles de la Tourette syndrome has been reported following the administration of dextroamphetamine, methylphenidate, pemoline, or haloperidol in children (Blain and Lane, 1998).

MYOCLONUS

Drug-induced myoclonus is rare but may occur in patients treated with antipsychotic and tricylic antidepressant drugs or lithium carbonate. Myoclonus has been reported in patients treated with amitriptyline and in imipramine toxicity (Koller and Musa, 1985). A clinical picture resembling that of Creutzfeldt–Jakob disease with myoclonus, coarse tremor, cerebellar and extrapyramidal manifestations, cognitive impairment, and periodic sharp wave complexes in the electroenecphalogram (EEG) has been reported in patients with lithium toxicity (Smith and Kocen, 1988). Complete resolution of the clinical and EEG changes occurred in these cases after withdrawal from the drug. Posturally induced myoclonic jerks in the upper limbs have been described in patients on long-term antipsychotic drug therapy and in a component of tardive dyskinesia in some patients (Buchman et al., 1987). Myoclonus may also occur in some patients with

Parkinson's disease who are treated with levodopa or bromocriptine (Tominaga *et al.*, 1987).

Manganese poisoning

INTRODUCTION

At present chronic manganese poisoning is identified as an industrial risk for manganese miners, workers in manganese mills and foundaries, and voltaic cell factories. The highest incidence appears to be in the mining villages of Chile (Mena *et al.*, 1967) and it is also not uncommon in Indian manganese miners (Goswami *et al.*, 1968).

HISTORY

Industrial manganese poisoning was first described by Couper in 1837 in five workers in a manganese mill. Couper described typical extrapyramidal symptoms and signs and further descriptions were provided in the early part of the twentieth century (Emden, 1901). Subsequently further cases were reported where manganese was being mined and there are now case descriptions from Russia, Chile, Mexico, Italy, India, and the former USSR.

CLINICAL FEATURES (FELDMAN, 1994)

The hallmarks of chronic manganese poisoning are the signs and symptoms of a progressive parkinsonian syndrome associated with an abnormality of gait and speech, and akinesia and rigidity in the limbs.

Sialorrhea and impotence are common. Usually abnormalities become permanently established within one or two years after the onset of the disease. Occasionally dystonia is a feature.

Very occasionally spontaneous regression of symptomatology after cessation of exposure has been reported (Penalver, 1957).

PATHOGENESIS

Manganese enters the human body by inhalation and is thereafter distributed through a variety of tissues.

There is some evidence to suggest that manganese accumulates in mitochondria and in the nuclei of cells rather than in other cellular structures.

PATHOLOGY

Damage to various structures within the basal ganglia have been shown to be features of manganese encephalopathy (Table 6.4).

The pathological features differ from Parkinson's disease in that there is relatively more damage to the sub-thalamic and caudate nuclei and putamen compared to the substantia nigra.

TREATMENT

Treatment with antiparkinsonian drugs in the form of levodopa appears to produce improvement (Mena, 1979). The use of chelating agents to remove the excess manganese has been tried but prevention is likely to be a more satisfactory therapeutic avenue (Cook *et al.*, 1974).

Carbon monoxide poisoning

INTRODUCTION

Carbon monoxide poisoning remains an important cause of death or disability even today, although is less common in western countries than it was, largely due to changes that have been made in combustion systems and heating fuels. Nonetheless, in the USA there are still more than 3500 deaths every year as a result of carbon monoxide intoxication. It also has a high incidence in South Korea where coal is widely used for cooking. Carbon monoxide intoxication remains one of the major ways of committing suicide (Roos, 1994).

Table 6.4 *Neuropathological findings of manganese encephalopathy (Barbeau et al., 1976)*

Authors	Age at death	Pallidum	Caudate nucleus	Putamen	Substantia nigra	Other lesions
Ashizawa (1927)	33	+++	++	++	+	Pons, internal capsule, thalamus, corpus luysi, red nucleus
Canavan *et al.* (1934)	69	+++	+++	++?		Thalamus
Stadler (1936)	46	+++	+++	+++	N	Frontal and parietal cortex
Voss (1939)	37	+	+	+	N	Pyramidal tract, anterior horn (amyotrophic lateral sclerosis)
Parnitzke and Pfieffer (1954)	43	+++	++?	++?	N	Subthalamic nucleus
Bernheimer *et al.* (1973)	67	++?		++?	+++	Red nucleus

Intensity of degeneration: +++ marked; ++ moderate; + slight; N normal; ? description doubtful.

HISTORY

In 1957 Claude Bernard first described the toxic effects of tissue hypoxia and in 1895 Haldane described the underlying mechanism of carbon monoxide toxicity (Haldane, 1895). Since then there have been more than 3000 bibliographic references to carbon monoxide intoxication (Lilienthal, 1950; Fink, 1966).

PATHOGENESIS

After inhalation carbon monoxide becomes bound to hemoglobin making oxygen transport progressively impossible and the predominant effect of carbon monoxide poisoning is that of generalized hypoxia which shows itself most obviously as an effect upon the brain.

There may be other effects of carbon monoxide in that it has been shown to have a direct histotoxic effect by binding to intracellular mitochondrial cytochrome oxidases (Penney, 1990). The central nervous system damage is probably a function of blood and tissue acidosis more than impaired energy metabolism. In the acute stage a decreased dopamine turnover has been measured, an effect that can be lasting. The pathophysiological mechanism of damage to the brain in acute carbon monoxide intoxication can be summarized as follows: reduced oxygen delivery resulting in hypoxia; general hypotension with decreased intracerebral blood flow; metabolic acidosis and inhibited intracellular metabolism by binding of carbon monoxide to mitochondrial enzymes. There is some evidence to suggest that there is a selective decrease in blood flow to the globus pallidus in acute carbon monoxide intoxication and this may be relevant to the delayed neurological effects (Song et al., 1983).

PATHOLOGY

Carbon monoxide intoxication induces parenchymal necrosis in selective areas of gray matter and white matter. Bilateral necrosis of the globus pallidus, caudate nucleus, putamen, substantia nigra, hippocampus, cerebellum, dentate nucleus, and hypothalamus has been seen (Lapresle and Fardeau, 1967). In patients with delayed neurological sequelæ confluent patchy demyelination is present in the central white matter with sparing of axons. These abnormalities are comparable to changes seen after other forms of hypoxic ischemia.

CLINICAL FEATURES

The main features of acute intoxication with carbon monoxide include headache, dizziness, lethargy, and coma. Epilepetic seizures may be seen and muscle rigidity may be present from an early stage. Chorea, dystonia, and tremor are reported (Jellinger, 1968).

Permanent sequelæ are seen and mirror the changes of any hypoxic insult to the brain. Some parkinsonian features in such patients are relatively common, although such cases usually have a variety of psychiatric symptoms (Klawans et al., 1982).

A recent review (Lee and Marsden, 1994) has described the outcome in 31 patients who survived carbon monoxide poisoning. Eight progressed into an akinetic mute state and 23 had a delayed relapse after initial recovery period.

DELAYED NEUROLOGICAL SEQUELÆ AFTER CARBON MONOXIDE INTOXICATION

Motor disorders are a prominent feature seen in those patients who recover from the acute effects of carbon monoxide intoxication and who then deteriorate. Typically the patients recover from the acute effects within a few days but some one to four weeks later deteriorate with the development of a variety of neuropsychiatric symptoms.

The syndrome develops in 10% of hospitalized patients (Choi, 1983) and is more common in patients with severe forms of acute carbon monoxide intoxication and in the elderly patients. Three-quarters of patients show improvement but in some the neurological syndrome persists. In those who recover this is complete within a year.

Computerized tomography (CT) scans performed in such patients often show white matter low-density lesions and low-density lesions in the globus pallidus. Typically as the syndrome deteriorates new abnormalities are seen on CT scans and the development of these abnormalities appears to indicate a bad prognosis (Lee and Marsden, 1994).

It has been suggested that hyperbaric oxygen therapy in the early stages might prevent the development of delayed sequelæ, although there is no good evidence for this, and currently there appears to be no effective strategy to prevent this delayed deterioration.

TREATMENT

Oxygen is the treatment of choice for acute carbon monoxide intoxication and there is some evidence to support the use of hyperbaric oxygen (Raphael et al., 1989). There is no evidence that any specific treatment prevents or delays the delayed neurological sequelæ.

In those patients who have developed the delayed parkinsonian syndrome there is a poor response to levodopa or other forms of dopaminergic therapy (Pooter et al., 1991).

MPTP

INTRODUCTION

Probably the most familiar synthetic neurotoxicant is 1-methyl-4-phenyl-1,2,3,6-tetrahydropyridine (MPTP).

In humans and a wide variety of animal species this compound produces a parkinson-like syndrome which shares many clinical, behavioral, neuropathological, and biochemical features of idiopathic Parkinson's disease (Irwin and Langston, 1993).

The actual discovery of MPTP as a nigrostriatal neurotoxicant was related to the clandestine production of so-called designer drugs. The term designer drugs was introduced to describe chemical modifications of existing, often naturally occurring, psychoactive drugs.

HISTORY

In the early 1980s a chemist in northern California attempted to synthesize an opioid analgesic called 1-2-methyl-4-phenyl-4-proprio-oxypiperydine (MPPP), a meperadine (pethidine) analogue with potent narcotic effects. Preparations containing MPTP were subsequently distributed on the street and sold to young addicts. Within a short period of time in the summer of 1982 four young heroin addicts developed full-blown parkinsonian syndrome with a remarkable clinical resemblance to Parkinson's disease (Langston et al., 1983). Further cases were subsequently discovered and analysis of the street preparations used by these addicts revealed that they had injected themselves with a batch of MPPP contaminated with MPTP.

Soon after these effects were discovered it was shown that parkinsonian features could be reproduced in primates by systemic administration of MPTP (Langston and Ballard, 1984).

Exposure to MPTP producing parkinsonism has been noted in subjects not addicted to drugs. Langston and Ballard (1983) described a chemist of a pharmaceutical industry who developed parkinsonian features at aged 37 after working with compounds containing MPTP. Other such cases have been described (Barbeau et al., 1985).

CLINICAL FEATURES

In the Californian patients who had used high quantities of MPTP persistent parkinsonian features developed within days to two weeks after exposure (Ballard et al., 1985). The clinical features of these severely affected patients showed a dramatic resemblance to those commonly seen in advanced Parkinson's disease. The classic features of akinesia, rigidity, and postural instability were present in all patients. An asymmetrical resting tremor was noted in four of the seven severely affected cases. All patients exhibited additional typical parkinsonian features such as flexed posture, short-stepped shuffling gait with loss of associated movements, monotonous speech, reduced eye blinking, and loss of facial expression. Dystonic features were present in two patients (Tetrud and Langston, 1993). Facial seborrhoea, drooling, and micrographia were also present. There were no signs of involvement of other areas of the nervous system in any of these patients.

Although detailed mental status examination revealed slight changes in intellectual function, there was no evidence of severe cognitive impairment in any patient (Stern and Langston, 1985). Any such changes noted on detailed neuropsychological investigations were similar to those seen in advanced Parkinson's disease. Depression occurred in three of the seven patients.

PATHOLOGY

Neuropathological analysis shows destruction of the substantia nigra pars compacta with moderately severe neuronal loss, neuromelanin accumulation in microglial cells, and gliosis (Davis et al., 1979). Typical Lewy bodies are not seen. Other parts of the central nervous system which are commonly affected in Parkinson's disease, such as locus ceruleus, may be affected in certain experimental animals (Forno et al., 1986).

TREATMENT

Of interest is the response of MPTP parkinsonian patients to treatment with levodopa. The clinical features can be effectively corrected with levodopa alone or in combination with dopamine agonists. Shortly after initiation of therapy, severe and often dose-limiting side effects, similar to those seen after several years of such therapy in parkinsonian patients, are noted (Ballard et al., 1985). Virtually the complete spectrum of side effects has been noted including end-of-dose deterioration, on-off fluctuations, peak dose dyskinesias, and severe psychiatric complications.

PARKINSON'S DISEASE AND ENVIRONMENTAL TOXINS

The cause of Parkinson's disease is unknown but the recognition of the MPTP model has led to a hunt for evidence that an environmental influence might be the cause of the condition.

Prevalence data

The prevalence of Parkinson's disease varies considerably, higher rates being described in northern Europe, the USA and Bombay, with lower prevalence rates shown in Japan, China, Sardinia, and Nigeria (Tanner and Langston, 1990). The most striking difference between these groups is that industries are more common in the group with a higher prevalence of Parkinson's disease, suggesting that an industrial toxin may be responsible.

Further support comes from the fact that no integrated description of Parkinson's disease existed before James Parkinson's description at a time when there was increasing industrialization in England. Further evidence is from US death records (1959–1961) which show a higher prevalence in the more industrialized northern regions of the USA (Tanner and Langston, 1986).

The search for geographical or time-specific clusters may also provide evidence for the industrial toxin theory; a higher prevalence in a distinct area or at a certain time suggesting a higher level of exposure.

Barbeau *et al.* (1986) studied Parkinson's disease prevalence rates in hydrographic regions in Quebec by four distinct selection methods, all identifying the region where commercial vegetable production associated with pesticide use occurred to have the highest prevalence rate. Another study in Sweden described a relationship between saw and paper mills and steel alloy industries and an increased prevalence rate of Parkinson's disease (Koller *et al.*, 1990).

MPTP shows structural similarities to agricultural chemicals such as paraquat, which was widely used as a herbicide in the past. There are reports of parkinsonism occurring in a citrus farmer who had worked with paraquat (Semchuk *et al.*, 1992) and lesions of the substantia nigra are seen in some survivors of acute lethal paraquat poisoning. However, there are no animal models of paraquat-induced parkinsonism and an epidemiological study of paraquat workers failed to reveal any parkinsonian cases (Semchuk *et al.*, 1992).

The increasing evidence supporting an environmental cause for the amyotrophic lateral sclerosis–parkinsonism–dementia complex in Guam has led to a series of case-control studies looking at a variety of potentially toxins (Table 6.5).

In most studies an increased risk of developing Parkinson's disease appears to be associated with rural living and where drinking water is taken from a well. A study of non-parkinsonian cases found at autopsy that the substantia nigra cell counts of residents in rural areas were lower than urban residence of the same age.

Whilst the environmental toxin theory of Parkinson's disease remains interesting other data strongly supports genetic factors (Duvoisin, 1986; Zweig *et al.*, 1992).

Implications for Parkinson's disease

The accidental discovery of the potent ability of MPTP to induce parkinsonism in unfortunate drug addicts has led to an unprecedented increase in interest in Parkinson's disease and has given us, for the first time, an animal model. The effects of MPTP in humans has emphasized the possibility that either man-made or naturally occurring toxins could at some point trigger the series of events that could ultimately result in the development of Parkinson's disease. This theory, attractive though it is, remains unproven.

CEREBELLAR SYNDROMES

The cerebellum seems particularly sensitive to the acute effects of a wide variety of exogenous drugs or toxins, and unsteadiness and slurring of speech are commonly seen as an acute effect of any such substance producing an effect upon the central nervous system. Such effects may be non-specific and clear data to support the view that such abnormalities are a definite manifestation of cerebellar dysfunction are not available.

There are, however, some clear cerebellar disorders which result from specific intoxications and these will be dealt with within this section.

Iatrogenic (drug-induced) cerebellar disorders

Various drugs may cause ataxia, incoordination, and other manifestations of cerebellar dysfunction. Sedatives (for example, chloral hydrate, barbiturates, benzodiazepines, paraldehyde) and anticonvulsants (for example, phenytoin, carbamazepine, primidone,

Table 6.5 *Case-controlled studies of Parkinson's disease, rural home, well-water drinking, farming, and chemicals (Liou et al., 1997)*

	Cases/controls	Rural home	Well-water drinking	Farming	Chemicals (industrial, herbicides, pesticides)
China	100/200	↓	not studied	↓	↑
Hong Kong	35/105	↑	↔	↑	↑
Kansas	150/150	↑	↑	not studied	not studied
New Jersey	106/106	↑	not studied	not studied	↑
Chicago	78/78	not studied	not studied	↑	not studied
Madrid	81/162	↔	↑	↔	↑
Quebec	42/42	↔	↑	↔	↑
Calgary	130/260	↔	↔	↑	↑

↑ increased risk of PD; ↓ decreased risk of PD; ↔ not significant.

ethosuximide, methosuximide) are most often responsible, their effects being dose dependent (Chase and Kopin, 1977). Individual tolerance to these drugs varies considerably, but in general symptoms are most likely to develop when high doses are administered too quickly. This is particularly important in the case of carbamazepine, which should be commenced in a low dose and then slowly increased over a period of at least a week. Ataxia and drowsiness may occur during administration of high doses of most tranquilizers, including diazepam, chlordiazepoxide, and meprobamate; and signs of cerebellar dysfunction may be caused more rarely by phenothiazines, monoamine oxidase inhibitors, reserpine, thioxanthenes, and lithium salts. The latter may cause an isolated cerebellar ataxia or a more diffuse encephalopathy, even with blood levels within the therapeutic range (Chase and Kopin, 1977; Peiffer, 1981; Jacome, 1987). These disorders are usually reversible when the causative agent is withdrawn or the dose adjusted, although there are occasional reports of permanent cerebellar dysfunction in patients treated with phenytoin or lithium (Peiffer, 1981; Crombie, 1985). Cerebellar ataxia has also been reported in bone marrow transplant recipients treated with cyclosporin A and has been associated with hypomagnesemia (Thompson et al., 1984).

A reversible cerebellar syndrome has been described in patients with leukemia or lymphoma treated with high doses of cytosine arabinoside; in some patients the drug causes irreversible cerebellar degeneration (Winkelman and Hines, 1983). Cerebellar dysfunction has also been reported in cancer patients treated with high- or low-dose fluorouracil (Goldberg et al., 1982; Shaprio and Young, 1984) or in those with impaired renal function receiving colistin. It may be associated with a peripheral neuropathy in certain patients taking nitrofurantoin or perhexiline (Graebner and Herskowitz, 1973, Chase and Kopin, 1977; Argov and Mastaglia, 1979).

Ethyl alcohol

INTRODUCTION

The early signs of acute ethyl alcohol intoxication include as prominent features ataxia, nystagmus and dysarthria, and these almost certainly result from an effect upon the cerebellum. Measurable impairment of co-ordination occurs with blood concentrations of ethanol of between 30 and 60 mg/dl in non-alcoholics.

A wide variety of neurological complications are seen in alcoholics, although the precise etiology of these in most instances is unknown. There is certainly no clear relationship between the amount of alcohol consumed and the likelihood of neurological complications (Estrin, 1987).

ALCOHOLIC CEREBELLAR DEGENERATION

Some alcoholic patients develop a chronic cerebellar syndrome that, like the Korsakoff amnestic syndrome, may represent a long-term sequel of Wernicke's encephalopathy (Victor et al., 1956). In common with the Wernicke and Korsakoff syndromes, alcoholic cerebellar degeneration is generally attributed to nutritional deficency and specifically to depletion of thiamine (Victor et al., 1956, Mancall and McEntee, 1965). However, it has also been suggested that the disorder may result from a direct toxic effect of alcohol on the cerebellum or from electrolyte abnormalities associated with alcoholism (Kleinschmidt-DeMasters and Norenberg, 1981).

The neuropathology of alcoholic cerebellar degeneration consists of loss of cerebellar cortical neurons, especially Purkinje cells, with particular predilection for the anterior and superior vermis; the anterior and superior cerebellar hemispheres are affected less often (Victor et al., 1956). This distribution of cerebellar pathology is strikingly similar to that seen in Wernick's encephalopathy (Malamud and Skillicorn, 1956; Victor et al., 1971), providing an important clue that the two disorders may be pathophysiologically linked.

The natural history of alcoholic cerebellar degeneration is variable (Victor et al., 1956). The syndrome usually occurs in the setting of chronic alcoholism of 10 years' or more duration. The most frequent mode of onset is with ataxia of gait that progresses steadily for weeks to months. A more gradually progressive disorder that evolves over years is also common. Less often, a mild and stable deficit that has been present for years may become suddenly worse.

Although gait ataxia is the most prominent manifestation of both alcoholic cerebellar degeneration and Wernicke's encephalopathy (Victor et al., 1956; Victor et al., 1971), the pattern of involvement in the two disorders may otherwise differ. Limb ataxia, which is absent in most patients with Wernicke's syndrome, is usually detectable in alcoholic cerebellar degeneration. Examination of such patients typically discloses severe involvement of the arms. Dysarthria, which is usually mild, is also more frequent in alcoholic cerebellar degeneration. In contrast, nystagmus is present far less often than in Wernicke's encephalopathy.

Uncommon manifestations of alcoholic cerebellar degeneration include hypotonia, ocular dysmetria, and postural tremor (Victor et al., 1956). Patients with alcoholic cerebellar degeneration may also exhibit signs of polyneuropathy (see below).

Alcoholic cerebellar ataxia is a clinical diagnosis. The CT scan or magnetic resonance imaging (MRI) may show cerebellar cortical atrophy, but laboratory findings are generally helpful only for excluding other causes of ataxia. Conditions that must be considered in the differential diagnosis of subacute or chronic cerebellar ataxia in middle life include multiple sclerosis, hypothyroidism, paraneoplastic cerebellar degeneration, idiopathic cerebellar or olivopontocerebellar atrophies, Creutzfeldt–Jakob disease, and posterior fossa tumors. Like alcoholic cerebellar degeneration, many of these disorders can produce ataxia preferentially affecting the gait.

Ataxia due to alcoholic cerebellar degeneration often stabilizes or improves with cessation of drinking and improved nutritional status (Victor *et al.*, 1956; Diener *et al.*, 1984), although the relative importance of these two factors is uncertain. Patients with this condition should receive parenteral thiamin.

Toluene

Toluene is a volatile, aromatic hydrocarbon used in the production of adhesives, glues, laquers, paints, rubber, and thinners. The main routes of absorption are inhalation and percutaneous absorption, although the latter is minimal.

It produces an ethanol- and barbiturate-type of intoxication which explains its abuse potential (Rees *et al.*, 1985). The acute effects in humans have been studied experimentally and include impairment of memory functions and manual dexterity (Echeverria *et al.*, 1989).

There is conflicting evidence on the chronic effects of long-term low-level exposure to toluene (Cherry *et al.*, 1984).

Many authors report that toluene is a substance of choice for sniffers. Its regular use over a prolonged period of time induces both neurological and neuro-psychological deficits. The neurological lesions most frequently reported include cerebellar encephalopathy (King, 1983). Individuals develop a progressive cerebellar syndrome characterized by dysarthria, nystagmus and incoordination, and this is often accompanied by intellectual and memory impairment.

Pathologically there is cerebral, cerebellar, and brain stem atrophy (King, 1983). The clinical effects once developed have a poor prognosis and do not recover.

Mercury intoxication

The clinical spectrum of the different types of mercury poisoning nicely illustrates the difficulties of the attempted classification used in this chapter. Mercury poisoning to a large extent depends on the type of mercury involved, inorganic mercury intoxication differing significantly from organic mercury intoxication. The problem is compounded further by the differing clinical syndromes and the mixed pattern of motor abnormalities that may be seen.

INORGANIC MERCURY INTOXICATION

History
The variety of mercury intoxication syndromes have been known for at least 20 centuries. Pliny implies that it was common knowledge in the Roman empire that mercury made people sick. Plutarch and Galan recognized the intoxication and the fact that mercury produced slow death in men working the rich metallic mercury mines in Spain (Hamilton and Hardy, 1949). Despite this, mercury and its salts were used during the seventeenth and eighteenth centuries as medicines although thankfully nowadays only eye ointments, dental amalgams, dermatological antiseptics, and hemorrhoidal sclerotics are still common medicinal sources of mercury.

Mercury still produces iatrogenic disease but the most serious epidemic of mercury poisoning is among people working in, or living near, the Clandestine goldmines of Brazil (Erikson *et al.*, 1992).

Although mercury does leak from amalgam fillings there is no definite evidence that inorganic mercury intoxication has resulted from this.

Clinical features
Chronic elemental mercury poisoning is the classical disease of miners, goldsmiths, mirror makers, hatters, and workers in thermometer factories (Williams *et al.*, 1968).

The clinical picture was described by Paracelsus (1567) and numerous others including Gowers (1893).

The initial symptoms differ from case to case although the typical motor feature is tremor (Kark, 1994). This is often accompanied by irritability and difficulty with concentration. In the early stages the tremor is a fine action tremor affecting eye lids, tongue, and the outstretched hand and, if the intoxication progresses, then the tremor adopts the features of a cerebellar intention tremor. Thereafter incoordination of speech, gait, and limbs develops, ultimately associated with head titubation.

Few pathological studies have been made in such patients, although in 1934 Wolf *et al.* described a case where the Purkinje cells of the cerebellum were swollen. In other cases no neuropathological changes were noted (Taylor, 1901). Using histochemical stains it has been shown that mercury is found in many large neurones including Purkinje cells (Takahata *et al.*, 1970).

The pathogenesis is uncertain although mercury is known to inhibit a large number of enzymes (Kark, 1994).

Treatment
The major treatment for mercury toxicity is to remove the patient from the source of the metal and in addition treatment with chelating agents may be of value. Sadly all too often the illness does not improve (Gowers, 1893). There is a need for active treatment in any case

of inorganic mercury intoxication that does not respond quickly to removal from exposure to mercury by using chelating agents. So far there is only weak scientific evidence that any chelating agent is of value as there have been no good controlled trials of such treatment (Kark, 1994).

ORGANIC MERCURY

Organic mercury compounds exist in a variety of forms although toxicologically the most important of these are the methyl mercury compounds.

Clinical features

The first detailed account of the neurological syndrome induced by methyl mercury appeared in 1940 when Hunter *et al.* described four men who developed a neurological syndrome characterized particularly by ataxia of gait and dysarthria. Other neurological signs and symptoms were present and this constellation of symptoms and signs became known as the Hunter–Russell syndrome. Pathologically these cases showed cortical atrophy within the cerebellum and cerebrum.

A mass outbreak of methyl mercury poisoning occurred in the Minamata area of Japan and subsequently became known as Minamata disease. Cerebellar ataxia was a prominent feature of those affected although, again, other features including sensory symptoms, emotional lability, and mental impairment were present (Eto, 1989).

The main target for methyl mercury is the brain and in those brains studied of affected individuals there is invariably gross atrophy of the cerebral cortex, particularly the calcarine cortex and the cerebellum (Takeuchi, *et al.*, 1989).

A high frequency of cerebral palsy was observed in the Minamata area amongst children born during the relevant period and methyl mercury poisoning was probably responsible (Marsh *et al.*, 1987).

MIXED MOTOR SYNDROMES

Methanol intoxication

INTRODUCTION

Methanol intoxication is seen most commonly in those who cannot afford marketed ethyl alcohol drinks and purchase substitutes, the contents of which have been adulterated by methyl alcohol.

The toxic effects of methanol upon the nervous system are most commonly centered on the optic nerves (see above). Acute intoxication is associated with impairment of consciousness and marked cerebral edema underlies a severe deficit with deep coma and flaccid tetraplegia.

In those who survive, a wide variety of motor deficits may be seen apart from the blindness. These include parkinsonian signs (Pelletier *et al.*, 1992), dystonia (Chen *et al.*, 1991), a pyramidal syndrome (Betta and Forno, 1980) and transverse myelopathy (Anderson *et al.*, 1989).

The pathological changes within the brain are similar to those of hypoxic ischemic encephalopathy (Ginsberg *et al.*, 1976).

Aluminum neurotoxicity

INTRODUCTION

The most clearly identified syndrome of aluminum neurotoxicity became recognized in the mid-1970s as dialysis encephalopathy (Kerr *et al.*, 1992). Subsequently there have been claims that aluminum might be involved as a causative factor in Alzheimer's disease based on the presence of aluminum, the senile plaques which are such a characteristic histological feature of the disease (Candy *et al.*, 1986). This association remains unproven.

CLINICAL FEATURES

A number of motor features are seen in patients with dialysis encephalopathy. These include an ataxia of gait, dysarthria, and myoclonic jerks. Other florrid clinical features of the condition include psychiatric abnormalities, dementia, and seizures (Kerr *et al.*, 1992).

Bismuth

INTRODUCTION

The mixed picture of signs and symptoms occurring as the result of bismuth neurotoxicity became recognized in the 1970s, although pathological studies in such patients have been few and far between.

CLINICAL FEATURES

Bismuth produces a mixed picture of neurotoxicity with impairment of gait and slurring of speech as prominent features. Myoclonic jerks, memory disturbances, and seizures are also seen (Reinicke, 1982). One patient who died of bismuth neurotoxicity showed lamina necrosis of the cerebral and cerebellar cortex (Buge *et al.*, 1979).

Heat stroke

Heat stroke is a complex clinical syndrome caused by extreme increases in body temperature. Neurological manifestations are common in the early stages and include coma, convulsions, pupillary abnormalities, spasticity, muscle rigidity, and opisthotonius (Malamud et al., 1946; Shibolet et al., 1967).

Transient neurological signs are not infrequent during convalescence and include disturbed mental function, slurring of speech, and unsteadiness.

The most characteristic chronic disability after heat stroke is a cerebellar syndrome in combination with mild corticospinal tract signs, with hyperreflexia, and extensor plantar responses (Stewart, 1918).

Bee stings

There are occasional reports of delayed neurological complications occurring after hymenoptera stings and these are probably immunological in nature (Means et al., 1973).

Jellinger and Spunda (1953) reported a 70-year-old man who developed a progressive radicular myelopathy after a hornet's sting on the leg. The patient died and at autopsy there was demyelination of the lower thoracic and lumbar rootlets as well as areas of demyelination in the spinal cord.

Means et al. (1973) described a 52-year-old woman who developed a progressive quadraplegia one week after a yellow jacket sting on the shoulder. She died and at autopsy there were multiple foci of demyelination in the spinal cord.

Clinically and pathologically the cases are similar to acute disseminated encephalomyelitis.

SUMMARY

There are a wide variety of known environmental influences, most commonly toxins, which may damage the central nervous system structures involved in the control of movement.

Some of these syndromes resemble motor disorders such as motor neurone disease and Parkinson's disease, which are of unknown cause. There is good but not compelling evidence that environmental influences may be important in causation of these two neurological disorders, and this is an important area for continued research.

REFERENCES

Ames, D. and Webber, J. 1984: Sodium valproate and tardive dyskinesia. Medical Journal of Australia, **140**, 350

Anderson, T.J., Shuaib, A. and Becker, W.J. 1989: Methanol poisoning: factors associated with neurologic complications. Canadian Journal of Neurological Sciences,**16**, 432–5.

Argov, Z. and Mastaglia, F.L. 1979: Drug-induced peripheral neuropathies. British Medical Journal, **1**, 663.

Ball, R. 1985: Drug-induced akathisia: a review. Journal of the Royal Society of Medicine, **78**, 748.

Ballard, P.A., Tetrud, J.W. and Langston, J.W. 1985: Permanent human parkinsonism due to 1-methyl-4-phenyl-1,2,3,6-tetrahydropyridine (MPTP): seven cases. Neurology, **35**, 949–56.

Barbeau, A., Cloutier, R.T., Plasse, L. and Paris, S. 1986: Environmental and genetic factors in the etiology of Parkinson'sdisease. In Advances in Neurology, Yahr, M.D. and Bergmann, K.J. (eds), Vol. 45, pp 299–306. New York: Raven Press.

Barbeau, A., Inoue, N. and Cloutier, T. 1976: Role of manganese in dystonia. In Advances in Neurology, Eldridge, R. and Fahn, S. (eds), Vol. 14. New York: Raven Press.

Barbeau, A., Roy, M. and Langston, J.W. 1985: Neurological consequence of industrial exposure to 1-methyl-4-phenyl-1,2,3,6-tetrahydropyridine. Lancet, **1**, 1747.

Barber, F.E. 1978: Inorganic mercury intoxication reminiscent of amyotrophic lateral sclerosis. Journal of Occupational Medicine, **20**, 667–9.

Barnes, T.R.E. 1988: Tardive dyskinesia. British Medical Journal, **296**, 150.

Barrow, M.V., Simpson, C.F. and Miller, E.J. 1974: Lathyrism: a review. Quarterly Review of Biology, **49**, 101–28.

Baruahm, J.K., Rasool, C.G., Bradley, W.G. and Munsat, T.L. 1981: Retrograde axonal transport of lead in rat sciatic nerve. Neurology, **31**, 612–16.

Bateman, D.N. 1979: Drug-induced movement disorders. Adverse Drug Reactions Bulletin, **79**, 284.

Bateman, D.N., Rawlins, M.D. and Simpson, J.M. 1985: Extrapyramidal reactions with metoclopramide. British Medical Journal, **291**, 930.

Bateman, D.N., Rawlins, M.D. and Simpson, J.M. 1986: Extrapyramidal reactions to prochlorperazine and haloperidol in the United Kingdom. American Journal of Medicine, **59**, 549.

Bernat, J.L. 1981: Intraspinal steroid therapy. Neurology, **31**, 168.

Betta, P.G. and Forno, G. 1980: Necrosi emorragica del putamen da intossicazione acuta da alcool metilico. Patologica (Roma), **80**, 215–18.

Blain, P.G. and Lane, R.J.M. 1985: Neurological disorders. In Textbook of Adverse Drug Reactions, Davides, D.M. (ed.), 3rd edn. Oxford: Oxford University Press.

Blanco, G. and Peters, H.A. 1983: Myeloneuropathy and macrocytosis associated with nitrous oxide abuse. Archives of Neurology, **40**, 416.

Buchman, A.S., Bennett, D.A. and Goetz, C.G. 1987: Bromocriptine-induced myoclonus. Neurology, **37**, 885

Buge, A., Supino-Viterbo, V., Rancurel, G., Metzber, J., Dechy, H. and Gardeur, D. 1979: Correlations evolutives: cliniques electro-encepahlographiques, tomodensitometriques et toxicologiques, dans cinq cas d'encephalopathies bismutiquews. Sem Hop Paris, **55**, 1466–72.

Burke, R.E. 1984: Tardive dyskinesia: current clinical issues. Neurology, **34**, 1348.

Candy, J.M., Oakly, A.E., Klinowski, J. et al. 1986: Aluminosilicates and senile plaque formation in Alzheimer's disease. Lancet, **i**, 354–7.

Carpenter, S. 1968: Proximal axonal enlargement in motor neuron disease. Neurology (Minneapolis), **18**, 842–51.

Casey, D.E. and Gerlach, J. 1986: Is tardive dyskinesia due to dopamine hypersensitivity? Clinical Neuropharmacology, **9**, 134.

Chang, L.M. 1980: Mercury. In Experimental and Clinical Neurotoxicology, Spencer, P.S. and Schaumburg, H.H. (eds), pp 508–26. Baltimore, MD: Williams & Wilkins.

Chase, T.N. and Kopin, I.J. 1977: Drug-induced disorders of movement. In Scientific Approaches to Clinical Neurology, Goldensohn, E.S. and Appel, S.H. (eds), p 1190. Philadelphia, PA: Lea & Febiger.

Chen, J.C., Schneiderman, J.F. and Wortzman, G. 1991: Methane poisoning: bilateral putaminal and cerebellar cortical lesions on CT and MR. Journal of Computer Assisted Tomography, **15**, 522–4.

Cherry, N.M., Hutchins, H., Pace, T. and Waldron, H.A. 1984: Neurobehavioral effects of repeated occupational exposure to toluene and paint solvents. British Journal of Industrial Medicine, **42**, 291–300.

Choi, I.S. 1983: Delayed neurologic sequelae in carbon monoxide intoxication. Archives of Neurology, **40**, 433–5.

Chouza, C., Scaramelli, A. and Caamano, J.L. 1986: Parkinsonism, tardive dyskinesia, akathisia and depression induced by flunarizine. Lancet, **1**, 1303.

Contani, A. 1873: Lathyrismo illustra de tre casi clinici II. Morgagni, **15**, 745.

Cook, D.G., Fahn, S. and Brait, K.A. 1974: Chronic manganese intoxication. *Archives of Neurology*, **30**, 59–64.

Couper, J. 1837: On the effects of black oxide of manganese when inhaled into the lungs. *British Annals of Medical Pharmacology*, **1**, 41–2.

Crombie, A.L. 1985: Eye disorders. In *Textbook of Adverse Drug Reactions*, Davies, D.M. (ed.), 3rd edn, p 516. Oxford: Oxford University Press.

Davis, C.E. Jr, Smith, C. and Harris, R. 1982: Persistent movement disorder following metrizamide myelography. *Archives of Neurology*, **39**, 128.

Davis, G.C., Williams, A.C. and Markey, S.P. 1979: Chronic parkinsonism secondary to intravenous injection of merperidine analogues. *Psychiatry Research*, **1**, 249–54.

Delay, J.P., Deniker, P. and Harl, J.M. 1952: Utilisation en therapeutique psychiatrique d'une phenothiazine d'action centrale elective. *Annals of Medicine and Psychology*, **110**, 112–7.

Diener, H.C., Dichgans, J., Bacher, M. and Guschlbauer, B. 1984: Improvement of ataxia in alcoholic cerebellar atrophy through alcohol abstinence. *Journal of Neurology*, **231**, 258.

Duvoisin, R.C. 1986: On heredity, twins and Parkinson's Disease. *Annals of Neurology*, **19**, 409–11.

Echeverria, D., Fine, L., Langolf, G., Schork, A. and Sampaio, G. 1989: Acute neurobehavioral effects of toluene. *British Journal of Industrial Medicine*, **46**, 483–95.

Ell, J.J., Uttley, D. and Silver, J.R. 1981: Acute myelopathy in association with heroin addiction. *Journal of Neurology, Neurosurgery and Psychiatry*, **44**, 448.

Emden, H. 1901: Uber eine Nervenkrankheit nach Manganvergifung. *Munch Medizinische Wochenschrift*, **48**, 1852–3.

Erickson, T., Aks, S., Branches, F.J., Naleway, C., Chou, H.N. and Hryhorszuk, D.O. 1992: Fractional mercury levels in Brazilian gold refiners and miners. *Veterinary and Human Toxicology*, **34**, 354.

Estrin, W.J. 1987: Alcoholic cerebellar degeneration is not a dose-dependent phenomenon. *Alcoholism, Clinical and Experimental Research*, **11**, 372.

Eto, K. 1989: Difference between clinical and pathological diagnosis in minamata disease. In *Proceedings of the International Forum on Minamata Disease 1988*, Tsuru, S., Suzuki, T., Shiraki, H., Miyamoto, K., Shimizu, M. and Harada, M. (eds), pp 276–8, Tokyo: Keiso, Shobo.

Eto, Y., Wiesmann, U. and Herschkowitz, N.N. 1974: Sulfogalactosylsphingosine sulfatase. Characteristics of the enzyme and its deficiency in metachromatic leukodystrophy in human cultured skin fibroblasts. *Journal of Biological Chemistry*, **249**, 4955–60.

Feil, A. 1930: Le Fluorisme professionel. Intoxication professionelle par l'acide fluorhydrique et les sels fluor. *Paris Medicine*, **2**, 242–8.

Feldman, R.G. 1994: In *Manganese. Handbook of Clinical Neurology*, 303–18.

Finck, P.A. 1966: Exposure to carbon monoxide: review of the literature and 567 autopsies. *Military Medicine*, **131**, 1513–39.

Fluegel, E. 1956: Therapeutique par medication neuroleptique obtenue en realisant systematiquement des etats parkinsoniformes. *Encephale*, **45**, 790–2.

Forono, L.S., Langston, J.W., Delanney, L.E., Irwin, I. and Ricaurte, G.A. 1986: Locus ceruleus lesions and eosinophilic inclusions in MPTP-treated monkeys. *Annals of Neurology*, **20**(4).

Gajdusek, D.C. and Salazar, A.M. 1982: Amyotrophic lateral sclerosis and parkinsonian syndromes in high incidence among the Auyu and Jakai people of West New Guinea. *Neurology*, **32**, 107–26.

Ghetti, B. 1980: Experimental studies on neurofibrillary degeneration. In *Aging of the Brain and Dementia*, Amaducci, L., Davison, A.N. and Antuono, P. (eds), Vol. 13, pp 183–98. New York: Raven Press.

Gibb, W.R.G. and Lees, A.J. 1985: The neuroleptic malignant syndrome – a review. *Quarterly Journal of Medicine*, **56**, 421.

Ginsberg, M.B., Hedley-Whyte, E.T. and Richardson, E.P. 1976: Hypoxic ischemia leukoencephalopathy in man. *Archives of Neurology*, **33**, 5–14.

Goldberg, I.D., Bloomer, W.D. and Dawson, D.M. 1982: Nervous system toxic effects of cancer therapy. *Journal of the American Medical Association*, 247–1437.

Goswami, S.L., Nigogi, T.P. and Gupta, R.K. 1968: Chronic manganese poisoning. *Clinical and Biochemical Studies*, Personal communication.

Gowel, M., Zaiwalla, Z. and Rose, F.C. 1983: Antecedent events in motor neuron disease. *Journal of Neurology, Neurosurgery and Psychiatry*, **46**, 1041–3.

Gowers, W.R. 1893: Mercurial poisoning. In *A Manual of Diseases of the Nervous System*, London, J. and Churchill, A. (eds), 2nd edn, Vol. 2, pp 968–70.

Graebner, R.W. and Herskowitz, A. 1973: Cerebellar toxic effects from nitrofurantoin. *Archives of Neurology*, **29**, 195.

Griffin, J.W., Cork, L.C., Adams, R.J. and Price, D.L. 1982: Axonal transport in hereditary canine spinal muscular atrophy (HCSMA). *Journal of Neuropathology and Experimental Neurology*, **41**, 370.

Guegen, Y., Fardoun, R., Launis, B. and Pecker, J. 1982: Spinal cord compression by extradural fat after prolonged corticosteroid therapy. *Journal of Neurosurgery*, **56**, 267.

Hahn, A.F., Feasby, T.E. and Gilbert, J.J. 1983: Paraparesis following intrathecal chemotherapy. *Neurology*, **33**, 1032.

Haimanot, R.T., Kidane, Y., Wuhib, E. *et al.* 1990: Lathyrism in rural north western Ethiopia: a highly prevalent neurotoxic disorder. *International Journal of Epidemiology*, 664–72.

Haldane, J. 1895: The relation of the action of carbonic oxide to oxygen tension. *Journal of Physiology*, **18**, 201–17.

Hamilton, A. and Hardy, H.L. 1949: Mercury. In *Industrial Toxicology*, pp 104–26. New York: Paul B. Hoeber.

Hunter, D., Bomford, R.R. and Russell, D.S. 1940: Poisoning by methyl mercury compounds. *Quarterly Journal of Medicine*, **35**, 193–213.

Ingall, T.J. and Tennant, C. 1986: Neuroleptic malignant syndrome. *Medical Journal of Australia*, **145**, 414.

Irwin, I. and Langston, J.W. 1993: MPTP and Parkinson's disease. In *Natural and Synthetic Neurotoxins*, Harvey, A.L. (ed.), pp 225–56, London: Academic Press.

Jacome, D.E. 1987: Cerebellar syndrome in lithium poisoning. *Journal of Neurology, Neurosurgery and Psychiatry*, **40**, 1722.

Jankovic, J. 1981: Drug-induced and other orofacial-cervical dyskinesias. *Annals of Internal Medicine*, **94**, 788.

Jankovic, J. and Fahn, S. 1980: Physiologic and pathologic tremors. *Annals of International Medicine*, **93**, 460.

Jellinger, K. 1968: Pallidostriatal degenerations and exogenous lesions. In *Handbook of Clinical Neurology*, Venken, P.J. and Bruyn, G.W. (eds), Vol. 6, Chap. 25, pp 654–7. Amsterdam: North-Holland.

Jellinger, K. and Spunda, C. 1953: Aufsteigene Neuritis nach Insektenstich. *Wiener Klinische Wochenschr*, **73**, 81–4.

Karas, B.J., Wilder, B.J., Hammond, E.J. and Bauman, A.W. 1983: Treatment of valproate tremors. *Neurology*, **33**, 1380.

Kark, P.R.A. 1994: In *Clinical and Neurochemical Aspects of Inorganic Mercury Intoxication: Handbook of Clinical Neurology*, vol. 64.

Kerr, D.N.S., Ward, M.K., Ellis, H.A., Simpson, W. and Parkinson, I.S. 1992: Aluminum intoxication in renal disease. In *Aluminum in Biology and Medicine* (Ciba Foundation Symposium 169), Chadwick, P.J. and Whelan, J. (eds), pp 123–41. Chichester: Wiley.

King, M. 1983: Long-term neuropsychological effects of solvent abuse. In *The Neuropsychological Effects of Solvent Exposure*, Cherry, N. and Waldron, H.A. (eds), pp 75–84. Havant, Hampshire: Colt Foundation.

Klawans, H.L., Stein, R.W., Tanner, C.M. and Goetz, C.G. 1982: A pure parkinsonian syndrome following acute carbon monoxide intoxication. *Archives of Neurology*, **39**, 302–4.

Kleinschmidt-DeMasters, B.K. and Norenberg, M.D. 1981: Cerebellar degeneration in the rat following rapid correction of hyponatremia. *Annals of Neurology*, **10**, 561.

Knezevic, W., Mastaglia, F.L., Lefroy, R.B. and Fisher, A. 1984: Neuroleptic malignant syndrome. *Medical Journal of Australia*, **140**, 28.

Koller, W.C. and Musa, M.N. 1985: Amitripytline-induced abnormal movements. *Neurology*, **35**, 1086.

Koller, W., Cone, S. and Herbster, G. 1987: Caffeine and tremor. *Neurology*, **37**, 169.

Koller, W., Vetere-Overfield, B., Gray, C. *et al.* 1990: Environmental risk factors in Parkinson's disease. *Neurology*, **40**, 1218–21.

Kondo, K. 1979: Does gastrectomy predispose to amyotrophic lateral sclerosis? *Archives of Neurology*, **36**, 586–7.

Kubo, T., Sakata, A. and Koshimune, P. 1990: Position nystagmus and body sway after alcohol ingestion. *American Journal of Otolaryngology*, **11**, 416–9.

Kurlander, H.M. and Patten, B.M. 1979: Metals in spinal cord tissue of patients dying of motor neuron disease. *Annals of Neurology*, **6**, 21–4.

Kurtzke, J.F. and Beebe, G.W. 1980: Epidemiology of amyotrophic lateral sclerosis: A case-control comparison based on ALS deaths. *Neurology*, **30**, 453–62.

Langston, J.W. 1985: Mechanism of MPTP toxicity: more answers, more questions. *Trends in Pharmacological Sciences*, **6**, 375–8.

Langston, J.W. and Ballard, P.A. 1983: Parkinson's disease in a chemist working with 1-methyl-4-phenyl-1,2,5,6-tetrahydropyridine (MPTP). *New England Journal of Medicine*, **209**, 309–10.

Langston, J.W. and Ballard, P. 1984: Parkinsonism induced by 1-methyl-4-phenyl-1,2,3,6-tetrahydropyridine (MPTP): implications for treatment and the pathogenesis of Parkinson's disease. *Canadian Journal of Neurological Sciences*, **11**, 160–5.

Langston, J.W., Ballard, P., Tetrud, J.W. and Irwin, I. 1983: Chronic parkinsonism in humans due to a product of meperidine analog synthesis. *Science*, **219**, 979–80.

Lapresle, J. and Fardeau, M. 1967: The central nervous system and carbon monoxide poisoning. II. Anatomical study of brain lesions following intoxications with carbon monoxide (22 cases). *Progress in Brain Research*, **24**, 31–74.

Lee, M.S. and Marsden, C.D. 1994: Neurological sequelae following carbon monoxide poisoning clinical course and outcome according to the clinical types and brain computed tomography scan findings. *Movement Disorders*, **9**, 550–5.

Lilienthal, J.L., Jr 1950: Carbon monoxide. *Pharmacological Review*, **2**, 324–54.

Liou, H.H., Tsai, M.C., Chen, C.J. *et al.* 1997: Environmental risk factors and Parkinson's disease: a case-controlled study in Taiwan. *Neurology*, **46**, 1583–8.

Maier, J.G., Perry, R.H., Saylor, W. and Syulak, M.H. 1969: Radiation myelitis of the dorsolumbar spinal cord. *Radiology*, **93**, 154–60.

Major, R.H. 1945: *Classic Descriptions of Disease*, 3rd edn. Springfield, IL: Charles C. Thomas.

Malamud, N., Haymaker, W. and Custer, R.P. 1946: Heat stroke; a clinicopathologic study of 125 fatal cases. *Military Surgery*, **99**, 397–449.

Mancall, E.L. and McEntee, W.J. 1965: Alterations of the cerebellar cortex in nutritional encephalopathy. *Neurology*, **15**, 303.

Manton, W.J. and Cook, J.D. 1979: Lead content of cerebrospinal fluid and other tissue in amyotrophic lateral sclerosis (ALS). *Neurology*, **29**, 611–12.

Marsden, C.D., Parkes, J.D. and Quinn, F. 1982: Fluctuations of disability in Parkinson's disease – clinical aspects. In *Movement Disorders*, Marsden, C.S. and Fahn, S. (eds), p 96. London: Butterworths.

Marsh, D.O., Clarkson, T.W., Cox, C., Myers, G.J., Amin-Zaki, L. and Al-Tikritti, S. 1987: Fetal methyl mercury poisoning. *Archives of Neurology*, **44**, 1017–22.

Means, E.D., Barron, K.D. and Van Dyne, B.J. 1973: Nervous system lesions after sting by yellow jacket. *Neurology*, **23**, 881–90.

Mena, I. 1979: Manganese poisoning. In *Handbook of Clinical Neurology*, Vinken, P.J. and Bruyn, G.W. (ser eds), Vinken, P.J., Bruyn, G.W., Cohen, M.M. and Klawans, H.L. (vol. eds), Vol. 36, pp 217–37. Amsterdam: North-Holland.

Mena, I., Marin, O., Fuenzalida, S. and Cotzias, G.C. 1967: Chronic manganese poisoning: clinical picture and manganese turnover. *Neurology*, **17**, 128–36.

Micheli, F., Pardal, M.F. and Gatto, M. 1987: Flunarizine and cinnarizine-induced extrapyramidal reactions. *Neurology*, **37**, 881.

Misra, U.K., Sharma, V.P. and Singh, V.P. 1993: Clinical aspects of neurolathyrism in Unnao, India. *Paraplegia*, **31**, 249–54.

Murros, K. and Fogelholme, R. 1983: Amyotrophic lateral sclerosis in middle Finland: an epidemiolgocial study. *Acta Neurologica Scandinavica*, **67**, 41–6.

Nausieda, P.A., Killer, W.C., Wiener, W.J. and Klawans, H.L. 1979: Chorea induced by oral contraceptives. *Neurology*, **29**, 1605.

Newman, P.K. and Saunders, M. 1979: Lithium neurotoxicity. *Postgraduate Medical Journal*, **55**, 701.

Norris, F.H. 1978: Amyotrophic lateral sclerosis and low urinary selenium levels (letter). *Journal of the American Medical Association*, **239**, 404.

O'Flaherty, S., Evans, M., Epps, A. and Buchanan, N. 1985: Chreoathetosis and clonazepam. *Medical Journal of Australia*, **142**, 453.

Osifo, N.G. 1979: Drug-related transient dyskinesias. *Clinical Pharmacology and Therapeutics*, **25**, 767.

Parker, A.J., Mehta, T., Zarghami, N.B., Pusick, P. and Haskell, B.E. 1979: Acute neurotoxicity of the *Lathyrus sativus* neurotoxin, L-3-oxalyl-2-amino-propionic acid, in the squirrel monkey. *Toxicology and Applied Pharmacology*, **47**, 135–43.

Patten, B.M. and Engel, W.K. 1982: Phosphate and parathyroid disorders associated with the syndrome of amotrophic lateral sclerosis. In *Human Motor Neuron Diseases*, Rowland, L.P. (ed.), pp 181–200. New York: Raven Press.

Peiffer, J. 1981: Clinical and neuropathological aspects of long-term damage to the central nervous system after lithium medication. *Archives of Psychiatrica Nervenkr*, **231**, 41.

Pelletier, J., Harib, M.H. and Khalil, R. 1992: Putaminal necrosis after methanol intoxication. *Journal of Neurology, Neurosurgery and Psychiatry*, **55**, 234–5.

Penalver, R. 1957: Diagnosis and treatment of manganese intoxication. *Archives of Industrial Health*, **16**, 64–6.

Penney, D.G. 1990: Acute carbon monoxide poisoning: animal models: a review. *Toxicology*, **123**, 160.

Petkau, A., Sawatzky, A., Hillier, C.R. and Hoogstraten, J. 1974: Lead content of neuromuscular tissue in amyotrophic lateral sclerosis. *British Medical Journal*, **31**, 275–87.

Pierce-Ruhland, R. and Patten, B.M. 1980: Muscle metals in motor neuron disease. *Annals of Neurology*, **8**, 193–5.

Pooter, M.C., Deleys, D., Godefroy, O., De Renck, J. and Petit, H. 1991: Syndrome parkinsonism postoxycarbone. *Revue Neurologique*, **147**, 399–403.

Proust, A. 1883: Du lathyrisme medulelaire spasmodique. *Bulletin de l'Academie de Medecine (Paris)*, **12**, 829.

Raphael, J.C., Elkharret, D., Jars-Guincestre, M.C. *et al.* 1989: Trial of normobaric and hyperbaric oxygen for acute carbon monoxide intocxication. *Lancet*, **ii**, 414–9.

Rawlins, M.D. 1986: Spontaneous reporting of adverse drug reactions. *Quarterly Journal of Medicine*, **59**, 531.

Reddy, D.R. 1979: Skeletal Fluorosis. In *Handbook of Clinical Neurology*, Vinken, P.J. and Bruyn, G.W. (eds), Vol. 36, pp 465–504. Amsterdam: North-Holland.

Reddy, D.R., Rao, B.D. and Subramanian, M.V. 1974: Results of surgery in spinal compression due to skeletal fluorosis. *Indian Journal of Surgery*, **36**, 30–2.

Rees, D.C., Coggeshall, E. and Balster, R.L. 1985: Inhaled toluene produces pentobarbital-like discriminative stimulus effects in mice. *Life Sciences*, **37**, 1319–25.

Reinicke, C. 1982: Bismuth. In *Side Effects of Drugs Annual 6*, Dukes, M.N.G. (ed.), pp 217–21. Amsterdam: Excerpta Medica.

Reynolds, E.H. and Trimble, M.R. 1985: Adverse neuropsychiatric effects of anticonvulsant drugs. *Drugs*, **29**, 570.

Roelofs-Iverson, R.A., Mulder, D.W. and Elveback, L.R. 1984: ALS and heavy metals: a pilot case-control study. *Neurology*, **34**, 393–5.

Roos, R.A.C. 1994: Neurological complications of carbon monoxide intoxication. In *Handbook of Clinical Neurology*, Vinken, P.J. and Bruyn G.W. (eds), Vol. 20, pp 31–8. Amsterdam: North-Holland.

Rosati, G., Pinna, L. and Granieri, E. 1977: Studies on epidemiological clinical and etiological aspects of als disease in Sardinia, Southern Italy. *Acta Neurologica Scandinavica*, **55**, 231–44.

Rupniak, N.M., Jenner, P. and Marsden, C.D. 1986: Acute dystonia induced by neuroleptic drugs. *Psychopharmacology*, **88**, 403.

Sadowsky, C.H., Sacks, E. and Ochoa, J. 1976: Postradiation mtoro neuron syndrome. *Archives of Neurology*, **33**, 786–7.

Selye, H. 1957: Lathyrism. *Revista Canadian Biology*, **16**, 1–82.

Semchuk, K.M., Love, E.J. and Lee, R.G. 1992: Parkinson's disease and exposure to agricultural work and pesiticide chemicals. *Neurology*, **42**, 1328–35.

Shapiro, W.R. and Young, D.R. 1984: Neurological complications of antineoplastic therapy. *Acta Neurologica Scandinavica*, **70**, 125.

Shibolet, S., Coll, R. and Gilat, T. 1967: Heatstroke: its clinical picture and mechanism in 36 cases. *Quarterly Journal of Medicine*, **36**, 525–48.

Shortt, H.E., McRobert, G.R., Barnard, T.W. and Nayar, A.M.S. 1937: Endemic fluorosis in Madras Presidency. *Indian Journal of Medical Research*, **25**, 553–68.

Sigerist, H.H. 1941: *Four Treatises of Theophrastus Von Hohenheim called Paracelsus*. Baltimore, MD: Johns Hopkins Press.

Singhal, R.L. and Thomas, J.A. (eds) 1980: *Lead Toxicity*. Baltimore, MD: Urban and Scwarzenberg.

Smith, S.J.M. and Kocen, R.S. 1988: A Creutzfeldt–Jakob-like syndrome due to lithium toxicity. *Journal of Neurology, Neurosurgery and Psychiatry*, **51**, 120.

Song, S.Y., Okeda, R., Funata, N. and Higashino, F. 1983: An experimental study of the pathogenesis of the selective lesion of the globus pallidus in acute carbon monoxide poisoning in cats. *Acta Neuropathologica*, **61**, 232–8.

Spencer, P.S. 1995: Lathyrism. In *Handbook of Clinical Neurology Intoxications of the Nervous System*, Vinken, P.J. and Bruyn, G.W. (eds), Part 2, Vol. 65. Amsterdam: North-Holland.

Spencer, P.S. and Schaumburg, H.H. 1982: The pathogenesis of motor neuron disease: perspectives from neurotoxicology. In *Human Motor Neuron Diseases*, Rowland, L.P. (ed.), pp 249–66. New York: Raven Press.

Spencer, P.S., Roy, D.N., Ludolph, A.C., Hugon, J., Dwivedi, M.P. and Schaumberg, H.H. 1986: Lathyrism: evidence for the role of the neuroexcitatory amino acid BOAA. *Lancet*, **ii**, 1066–7.

Steen, P.A. and Michenfelder, J.D. 1979: Neurotoxicity of anesthetics. *Anesthesiology*, **50**, 437.

Stephen, P.J. and Williamson, J. 1984: Drug-induced parkinsonism in the elderly. *Lancet*, **2**, 1082.

Stern, Y. and Langston, J.W. 1985: Intellectual changes in patients with MPTP induced parkinsonism. *Neurology*, **35**, 1506–9.

Stewart, R.M. 1918: Occurrence of a cerebellar syndrome following heatstroke. *Review of Neurological Psychiatry*, **16**, 78–90.

Stockman, R. 1929: Lathyrism. *Journal of Pharmacology and Experimental Therapeutics*, **37**, 43.

Streifler, M., Cohn, D.F., Hirano, A. and Schujman, E. 1977: The central nervous system in a case of neurolathyrism. *Neurology*, **27**, 1176–8.

Takahata, N., Hayashi, H., Watanabe, S. and Anso, T. 1970: Accumulation of mercury in the brains of two autopsy cases with chronic inorganic mercury poisoning. *Folia Psychiatrica and Neurologica*, **24**, 59–69.

Takeuchi, T., Morikawa, N., Matsumoto, H. and Shiraishi, Y. 1972: Pathological studies of Minamata disease in Japan. *Acta Pathologica*, **2**, 40–57.

Tandan, R. and Bradley, W.G. 1985: Amyotrophic lateral sclerosis: Part 2. Etiopathogenesis. *Annals of Neurology*, **18**, 419–31.

Tanner, C.M. and Langston, J.W. 1990: Do environmental toxins cause Parkinson's disease? A critical review. *Neurology*, **3**, 17–30.

Tarsy, D. 1983: Neuroleptic-induced expraymidal ractions: classification, description and diagnosis. *Clinical Neuropharmacology* **6**, 59.

Taylor, J.G. 1901: Chronic mercurial poisoning, with special reference to the danger in hatter's furriers' manufactories. *Guy's Hospital Report*, **40**, 171–90.

Tekle-Haimont, R., Kidane, Y., Wuhib, E. *et al.* 1990: Lathyrism in rural north-western Ethiopia: a highly prevalent neurotoxic disorder. *International Journal of Epidemiology*, **19**, 664–72.

Tetrud, J.W. and Langston, J.W. 1993: MPTP and Parkinson's disease: one decade later. In *Parkinsonian Syndromes*, Stern, M.B. and Koller, W.C. (eds), pp 173–93. New York: Marcel Dekker.

Thompson, C.B., June, C.H., Sullivan, K.M. and Thomas, E.D. 1984: Association between cyclosporin neurotoxicity and hypomagnesemia. *Lancet*, **2**, 1116.

Tilzey, A., Heptonstall, J. and Hamblin, T. 1981: Toxic confusional state and choreiform movements after treatment with anabolic steroids. *British Medical Journal*, **283**, 349

Tominaga, H., Fukuzako, H. and Izumi, K. 1987: Tardive myoclonus. *Lancet*, **1**, 322.

Troncos, J.C., Price, D.L., Griffin, J.W. and Parhad, I.M. 1982: Neurofibrillary axonal pathology in aluminum intoxication. *Annals of Neurology*, **12**, 278–83.

Tylleskar, T., Banea, M. and Bikangi, N. 1992: Cassava cyanogens and konzo, an upper motor neuron disease found in Africa. *Lancet*, **339**, 208–11.

Tyrer, P., Lee, I. and Trotter, C. 1981: Physiological characteristics of tremor after chronic lithium therapy. *British Journal of Psychiatry*, **139**, 59.

Victor, M., Adams, R.D. and Collins, G.H. 1971: *The Wenicke–Korsakoff Syndrome: A Clinical and Pathological Study of 245 Patients, 82 with Post-mortem Examinations*. Philadelphia, PA: F.A. Davis.

Victor, M., Adams, R.D. and Mancall, E. 1956: A restricted form of cerebellar cortical degeneration occurring in alcoholic patients. *Archives of Neurology*, **76**, 586.

Vincent, F.M. and Vincent, T. 1985: Tocainide encephalopathy. *Neurology*, **35**, 1804.

Voss, H. 1939: Progressive bulbarparalyse and amyotrophische lateralsklerose nach chronischer maganvergiftung. *Archives of Gewerbepathol Gewerbehyg*, **9**, 464–76.

Waldron, H.A. 1983: Did the Mad Hatter have mercury poisoning? *British Medical Journal*, **187**, 1961.

Williams, H.L., Majer, A.J., Custer, J.L. and Miller, F.C. 1968: A survey of mercury vapor hazards in hospitals. *American Industrial Hygiene Association Journal*, **29**, 186–8.

Winkelman, M.D. and Hines, J.D. 1983: Cerebellar degeneration caused by high-dose cytosin arabinoside: a clinicopathological study. *Annals of Neurology*, **14**, 520.

Wolf, I.J., Paterson, N.J. and Davison, C. 1934: Acrodynia (erythredema, polyneuritis, vegetative neurosis, pink, or Swift disease). A historpathologic study of the nervous system. *Journal of Pediatrics*, **4**, 498–506.

Yase, Y. 1972: The pathogenesis of amyotrophic lateral sclerosis. *Lancet*, **2**, 292–6.

Yase, Y. 1984: Environmental contribution to the amyotrophic lateral sclerosis process. In *Neuromuscular Disease*, Serratrice, G., Desnuelle, C., Pellissier, J-F. *et al.* (eds), pp 335–9. New York: Raven Press.

Yiannikas, C. 1984: Chorea gravidarum. *Medical Journal of Australia*, **140**, 631

Yoshida, S. 1977: X-ray microanalytic studies on amyotrophic lateral sclerosis. II. Relationship of calcification and degeneration found in cervical spinal cord of ALS. *Clinical Neurology and Chirurgia*, **19**, 641–52.

Yoshimasu, F., Yasui, M. and Yase, Y. 1980: Studies on amyotrophic lateral sclerosis by neutron activation analysis. Comparative study of analytical results on Guam PD, Japanese ALS, and Alzheimer's disease cases. *Folia Psychiatrica and Neurologica*, **34**, 75–82.

Zweig, R.M., Singh, A., Cardillo, J.E. and Langston, J.W. 1992: The familial occurrence of Parkinson's disease: lack of evidence for maternal inheritance. *Archives of Neurology*, **49**, 1205–7.

7

Toxic neuropathies and disorders of the neuromuscular junction

ASHOK VERMA AND WALTER G BRADLEY

INTRODUCTION

The peripheral nervous system (PNS) has long been the focus for research and interest in neurotoxicology. This is largely because peripheral neuropathy is the commonest chemical neurotoxic reaction in humans and laboratory animals. The vast majority of biological neurotoxins also target the excitable peripheral nerve membrane and other components of the neuromuscular apparatus (Adams and Swanson, 1996). Chemical and biological neurotoxins have traditionally been the valuable research tools to probe and investigate the function of neuronal ion channels and other peripheral nerve constituents (Adams et al., 1994; Lotti, 1996). The scientific interest in this area parallels the growing concern that exposure to environmental pollutants may be involved in the etiology of certain chronic neuropathies, which as a group are common in the elderly population and which often defy attempts to identify the etiologic basis. Many existing chemicals, as well as the large number of new ones introduced each year, have never been adequately evaluated for peripheral neurotoxicity. Low-dose chronic exposure to chemical toxins (Calne et al., 1992), ion channel dysfunction (Hong and Driscoll, 1994), and cellular toxicity (Corcoran et al., 1994) have all been implicated or speculated as potential factors in apoptotic decline in certain neuronal populations. Recent research interest in this field continues to be directed to increasing knowledge about the cellular and molecular basis of neuropathies (Tilson, 1990; MacPhail, 1992; Lotti, 1996).

A variety of peripheral neuropathies occur following exposure to industrial chemicals, agricultural products, heavy metals, pharmacologic agents, and biotoxins. These neuropathies occur despite the existence of a protective 'blood–nerve barrier' to prevent the entry of potential toxins into the PNS. The reasons for the frequent development of neurotoxicity are several. First of all, some parts of the PNS lie outside the blood–nerve barrier (Rechthand and Rapoport, 1987) and thus are unprotected by it. These structures include the dorsal root ganglia (DRG), autonomic ganglia, and the nerve terminals at the neuromuscular junction (NMJ). These unprotected loci represent areas of special vulnerability for the entry of toxic agents. For example, within a minute after intravenous injection, doxorubicin fluorescence can be found in the nuclei of the DRG neurons and their satellite cells, but not in other parts of the PNS (Sahenk and Mendell, 1979). Doxorubicin is also reported to enter at the sensory and motor nerve terminals and then be transported to the parent neurons, a process called suicidal axonal transport (Le Quesne, 1993). Toxic materials entering at these sites can spread to other parts of the nervous system through mechanisms such as antero- and retrograde axonal transport and trans-synaptic transfer. Tetanus toxin (tetanospasmin) is a prime example of an agent that affects the spinal cord and brain stem by retrograde axonal and trans-synaptic spread. Capsaicin affects sensory neurons by entering the cutaneous sensory (C-fiber) terminals and causing depletion of substance P, a peptide neurotransmitter, from the nerve endings.

Secondary nerve damage by toxins

Some neurotoxins can damage the PNS as a secondary effect. The site of primary action may, for example, be the vascular endothelium of the blood–nerve barrier. A primary disruption of the vascular endothelium and loss of the protective blood–nerve barrier would secondarily expose the neural tissue to the effects of toxicants. Certain heavy metals, such as lead and cadmium, appear to cause toxic neuropathies in this manner (Hopkins, 1970; Ohnishi et al., 1977; Myers et al., 1980; Paduslo et al., 1982; Windebank, 1993).

The mechanism and outcome of a toxic action on vascular endothelium may even depend on the species and the maturity of the animal. Chronic lead poisoning, for example, produces an almost pure demyelinating neuropathy in adult rats (Ohnishi et al., 1977), an encephalopathy in suckling rats (Pentschew and Garro, 1966), and a mixed neuropathy (demyelinating and axonal) in guinea pigs (Fullerton, 1966). Curiously, despite a 'high' lead burden sufficient to produce toxic encephalopathy, the PNS of the suckling rat continues to develop normally and the myelination in the PNS proceeds unabated. Cattle and baboons develop lead encephalopathy but are relatively resistant to lead neuropathy (Hopkins, 1970). Acute cadmium poisoning in adult experimental animals damages the vascular endothelial cells and produces the consequent bleeding into the dorsal root and gasserian ganglia. Lead, however, damages the developing cerebral and cerebellar capillaries (Pentschew and Garro, 1966).

Neurotoxicity of metabolic products

The main neurotoxic mechanism may depend on a metabolite of a putative neurotoxin rather than the toxin itself, i.e. the putative neurotoxin may be a protoxin. One example is n-hexane and methyl-n-butyl-ketone (MnBK) that undergo omega-1 oxidation to produce a metabolic intermediate, 2,5-hexanedione (2,5-HD), which is highly neurotoxic (Spencer and Schaumburg, 1975; Schaumberg and Berger, 1993). The other homologous aliphatic hydrocarbons, such as methyl-ethyl-ketone (MEK) and methyl-imino-butyl-ketone (MiBK), which do not produce similar toxic metabolic intermediates, are generally non-toxic. Dichloroethylene, a decomposition product of trichloroethylene, is known to cause trigeminal neuropathy.

Host factors in neurotoxicity

Metabolic idiosyncrasy, inherited enzyme abnormality, or a pre-existing nutritional deficiency state may produce or contribute to the PNS toxicity in certain individuals. Isoniazid and dapsone generally produce toxic neuropathies in slow acetylators. These people metabolize these drugs more slowly than normal, and hence have higher blood levels. Organophosphorus-induced delayed polyneuropathy appears to result from inhibition and aging of one form of esterase – neuropathy target esterase (Lotti et al., 1993). An immune-mediated mechanism has been implicated in neuropathies caused by zimeldine (Fagius et al., 1985) and gold compounds (Katrak et al., 1980; Windebank, 1993). Nitrous oxide impairs cobalamine metabolism and may produce neuropathy in (unsuspected) cobalamine-deficient individuals or in those using large amounts of nitrous oxide (Green and Kinsella, 1995).

A large number of drugs are known to precipitate attacks of acute intermittent porphyria (AIP) in individuals who have inherited a deficiency of porphobilinogen (PBG) deaminase. Although AIP is a well-known cause of acute neuropathy, porphyric neuropathy was practically unknown before the advent of modern pharmaceuticals. Virtually all drugs that induce a hepatic microsomal cytochrome P-450 system can provoke attacks of acute porphyria. The increased incorporation of hem into the P-450 system reduces the free pool of hem and therefore induces the synthesis of aminolevulinic acid (ALA) synthase. The underactive PBG deaminase then becomes a rate-limiting step in hem synthesis in AIP patients, and there occurs rapid accumulation of the preceding substrates, namely ALA and PBG. Since ALA and PBG are not metabolized further, they leak out of the hepatic cells, are taken up into other tissues, including the PNS, and cause toxic damage. The cellular mechanism of neurotoxicity in AIP is not fully understood but appears to occur at multiple levels (for review, see Windebank and Bonkovsky, 1993).

Neurotoxicity through action upon ion channels

Nerve axonal membranes are uniquely excitable and, to accomplish this excitability, are endowed with a rich array of ion channels (Chiu and Ritchie, 1980; Chiu et al., 1984; Black et al., 1990). The neural synapses and NMJ are similarly provided with ion channels and ligand receptors, and a complex process of chemical transmission across the synaptic junction. Many of the major biotoxins of animal and plant origin selectively target these ion channels or other components of the neuromuscular transmission system (Verma, 1996). During evolution poisonous animals have developed an amazing range of paralytic toxins, either to ward off predators or, in predators, to incapacitate the prey as a food source.

Toxicity to a wide range of neural targets

The enormous size and complex metabolic functions of different neuronal cell types (motor, sensory, autonomic) and their association with myelin and myelin-producing cells and other supporting tissue provide a large range of potential targets for action of one or other noxious agents (see Toxic targets section below). Finally, the neurotoxic damage is more likely to manifest clinically and persist indefinitely because, compared to other organ-systems, the capacity for replacement of the lost cells does not exist in the nervous system. Although the capacity to regenerate is better in the PNS than it is in the central nervous system (CNS), the deficit following partial loss of a certain motor neuron pool may become manifest early and more severely in the PNS. This is because it is the final common pathway connecting the CNS to the effector (muscle). In addition, parts of the peripheral motor and somatosensory neurons reside in the central neuraxis (spinal cord and brain stem) where regeneration is inherently poor.

This chapter will first consider the broad morphologic and functional features of peripheral neurons and their ensheathing cells, and the neuromuscular junction, including the features that provide the potential basis for their selective vulnerability to certain neurotoxins. The specific cell constituents or cell types that act as targets in neurotoxic disease processes will be presented. It is not our intention to describe every individual toxic neuropathy. The final part will summarize a composite clinical pattern of common toxic neuropathies and disorders of the neuromuscular junction.

MORPHOLOGICAL CONSIDERATIONS

The PNS includes all neural structures lying outside the pial membrane of the spinal cord and brain stem. The motor axons emerge from the anterior horn cells and motor nuclei of the brain stem, and terminate on muscle fibers at the NMJs. The sensory neurons of the PNS consist of the dorsal root ganglia and cranial ganglion cells, their central processes inside the spinal cord and brain stem, and the peripheral processes that form the sensory axons in peripheral nerve branches. In addition, some peripheral nerves contain sympathetic and parasympathetic fibers. The axons are enveloped in segments of myelin of variable length (0.25–1 mm); each such internode is formed by a Schwann cell and its

membrane. Unmyelinated fibers, arising from the neurons of the DRG and autonomic ganglia, are arranged in small bundles of axons, each bundle enveloped by one Schwann cell at each level. The peripheral nerve fibers are further ensheathed by protective and supporting connective tissue (endo-, peri-, and epineurium) and have a unique vascular supply through longitudinal arrays of richly anastomosing nutrient arteriolar and capillary branches.

As the motor axon approaches the surface of the skeletal muscle, it emerges from its myelin sheath and ends in an array of terminal branches that synapse upon an individual muscle fiber. The synapses at the neuromuscular junction are specialized for chemical (cholinergic) transmission. Although postganglionic parasympathetic synapses also utilize the cholinergic transmission, their postsynaptic muscarinic receptors differ from the nicotinic receptors at the NMJ.

BIOCHEMICAL CONSIDERATIONS

Membrane ion channels

The axon is a uniquely specialized part of the neuron that generates and propagates bioelectric currents. The action potential is generated at the initial segment and is then propagated down the axon from node to node (saltatory conduction). The axon at nodes of Ranvier differs from the internodal axon in that it is not covered by a myelin sheath and that the patch of membrane (nodal axolemma) has certain unique features not present at the inexcitable internodal regions (Quick and Waxman, 1977). Studies with [3H]tetrodotoxin (TTX) and [3H]saxitoxin (STX), molecules which specifically bind to the outer part of the neuronal (N-type) sodium channel, indicate that sodium channels are concentrated at nodes; the density of sodium channels is about 500-fold greater at nodes (1.2×10^4/mm^3) than at internodal regions (25/mm^3) (Ritchie and Rogart, 1977). This may explain how certain neurotoxins acting on a specific ion channel may selectively target a segment of axolemma resulting in conduction failure. There is a family of diverse but related sodium channels in excitable cellular membranes of mammalian species (Waxman, 1995). The main polypeptide building blocks of nodal axolemma also appear to differ from those of the internodal axolemma. Autoradiographic studies with [3H]fucosyl glycoproteins suggest that certain proteins are selectively inserted and retained in the nodal and paranodal axolemma (Ritchie and Rogart, 1977).

More than one type of potassium channel is located in the nodal and internodal regions (Chiu and Ritchie, 1980; Roper and Schwartz, 1989; Waxman, 1995). There are additional potassium-channel types in non-excitable neural (such as Schwann cells) and non-neural tissues. The diversity of voltage-sensitive potassium channels in excitable tissues, including nerve axon and dendrites, is to help set the resting potential, repolarize the membrane, hyperpolarize the cell, and shape voltage trajectories in the sub-threshold range for action potentials. Most axolemmal potassium channels open only after the membrane is depolarized, but some only after it is hyperpolarized. Some potassium channels open rapidly and some slowly. Some are strongly modulated by neurotransmitters or intracellular messengers.

There are also equally pronounced differences between the potassium channel toxins that selectively target the channel subtypes. For example, the slow-type axolemmal potassium channel is sensitive to triethyl-ammonium (TEA) blockade, while the delayed-type rectifier potassium channel is sensitive to 4-amino-pyridine.

Calcium channels are ubiquitous and of various types. Voltage-sensitive calcium channels are specially concentrated at the motor nerve terminals. Additionally, the inexcitable plasma membrane on Schwann cells possesses a variety of ion channels (Chiu et al., 1984; Shrager et al., 1985), the function of which is unknown. The axolemmal ion channels are instrumental in the transmission of impulses along axons and across synaptic membranes.

Neuromuscular transmission

At the NMJ, depolarization of the nerve terminal by an incoming impulse is followed by an influx of calcium ions into the nerve terminal via voltage-sensitive calcium channels, and it is this influx that mediates transmitter release. The details of the mechanism by which calcium ingress triggers exocytosis of the synaptic vesicles is still not fully understood. However, it is now clear that increased calcium concentration in the nerve terminal releases the synaptic vesicles from cytoskeletal constraints and affects the interaction of several proteins which, together, are known as the synaptic fusion complex.

The synaptic space at the NMJ is lined by basal lamina. Acetylcholinesterase (AChE) is distributed throughout the basal lamina at a density of 2500 sites/mm^2 (Salpeter et al., 1978). The acetylcholine receptor (AChR) is concentrated on the terminal expansions of the postsynaptic junctional folds. Each AChR molecule is composed of five polypeptide subunits and its packaging density on the postsynaptic membrane is close to 10^4 receptors/mm^2 (Grohovaz et al., 1982). The voltage-sensitive sodium and calcium channels of the motor nerve terminal, synaptic fusion proteins, the AChR, and AChE are each known to be the specific targets of chemical and biological neuro-toxins.

Axoplasmic transport

The unusual geometry and functional specialization of peripheral nerve cells present a daunting task in intracellular communication over great distances. Virtually all organelles, membrane and axonal constituents, and synaptic vesicle-associated proteins are synthesized in the cell body. The axons and nerve terminals depend on their parent cell bodies for the continuous supply of essential constituents to maintain their viability, to support the nerve impulses, and to effect the release of neurotransmitters. The efficient delivery of these materials from the cell body to the axonal terminals is accomplished by the anterograde axonal transport system.

Similarly, an elaborate retrograde transport (from nerve terminals, axons, and their microenvironment to the cell body) of a variety of endogenous and exogenous materials also exists in the peripheral axon. Although the function of retrograde transport is not so well defined, the system appears to be important in recycling the endogenous materials such as spent vesicles, some membrane components, and foreign substances, including neurotoxins. Advantage is taken of this retrograde transport to trace the course of nerve fibers to their cell body origins by using molecular tracers such as horseradish peroxidase. Some micro-organisms, such as polio and herpes viruses, also utilize the axonal conduit to reach the neuronal cell body. Finally, neurotrophic substances transported from the cell body to the axon and nerve terminals are released to modify the function of muscles and other cells. Other neurotrophic components taken up by the nerve terminals are carried by retrograde transport to the cell body to modify its function. This highly complex bi-directional axonal transport system has been further characterized depending on the rate of movement into fast, intermediate, and slow anterograde and retrograde transport (Schwartz, 1979).

Although the mechanisms underlying axonal transport are not yet fully characterized, the slow transport system (1–3 mm/day) has been linked with at least three different cytoskeletal systems – microtubules, neurofilaments, and microfilaments. In mammalian axons, rapid axonal transport carries materials at a velocity of about 400 mm/day, a rate which appears to be independent of the age and species of the animals, the cell type (motor or sensory neuron), and the diameter and myelination of axon (Ochs and Brimijoin, 1993). The rapid transport system predominantly carries the membrane-associated proteins, glycoproteins, glycolipids, lipids, cholesterol, and a variety of materials associated with synaptic vesicles that are important for chemical transmission at the NMJ and neuronal synapses. A substantial proportion of the rapidly transported membrane-associated proteins stays within the axon, mainly contributing to the renewal of the axolemma (Holtzman, 1977). A fraction of these proteins are selectively retained in the nodal and internodal axolemma, while others are transported and retained within nerve terminals. Here, they are associated with synaptic vesicles and presynaptic plasma membrane. Still other substances are released from the axolemma during their passage and from the nerve terminals after their arrival.

In nerve axons, there also appears a phenomenon of 'routing' with regard to the specific constituents destined to the dendritic terminals or to the terminal axons (Aletta and Goldberg, 1984). For example, some labeled proteins are transported at significantly different rates in the two branches of the axon from the DRG neuron. The concept of routing embraces the passage of special components into one or other branches of a neuron. In the DRG neuron, for example, the neurotransmitter-related proteins pass into the dorsal root fiber to their terminal synapses in the spinal cord. However, other specialized substances pass down the peripheral fiber branches for sensory transduction in their terminals.

It is now clear that to transport the membrane-bound organelles, rapid axonal transport requires specific transporter proteins (kinesins and cytoplasmic dyneins), a well-organized backbone of axonal cytoskeleton, calcium and other factors, and ATP as the energy source (Ochs and Brimijoin, 1993). Because rapid transport requires considerable energy and the process depends on local oxidative metabolism, it is highly sensitive to a number of physical and chemical insults. When nerves *in vitro* are made anoxic by depriving them of oxygen or by exposure to agents that block the oxidative metabolism (azide, 2,4-dinitrophenol, sodium cyanide), fast axoplasmic transport fails in 10–30 min. Blockade of glycolysis by iodoacetate, or the citric acid cycle by fluoroacetate, lead to transport failure in 1–2 h (Ochs and Smith, 1971).

TOXIC TARGETS IN THE PNS

Since the gross cellular structure of the PNS appears to be relatively simple and well understood, one might suppose that each toxin that affects PNS would be known to affect one or other cellular or sub-cellular site. This is unfortunately not the case. A neurotoxin can act at more than one primary site and there are only limited pathological mechanisms whereby the peripheral nerve can react to the toxins. Nonetheless, stratification of PNS toxins based on their cellular target sites serves several useful purposes. It arguably is

a logical way to systematically classify the otherwise confusing list of neurotoxins. Identification of the cellular or sub-cellular target site allows one to predict the clinical pattern of neurological deficit a particular toxin may produce. Also, knowledge about the early and predominant cellular site of toxic action may help the design of appropriate electrophysiological or pathological tests to detect sub-clinical deficits.

Finally, delineation of a specific target site of neurotoxic action provides a valuable research tool to investigate the function of the targeted sub-cellular organelle.

NERVE AXON (AXONOPATHIES)

Distal retrograde axonal degeneration

'Dying back' neuropathy is the commonest cellular response in neurotoxic disease (Table 7.1). Although the PNS is conventionally defined as structures lying outside the pia mater, it is important to emphasize that the peripheral neuron may in part lie in the CNS, for example, the lower motor neuron, or it may posses two axons, one of which projects into the CNS, for example, the central axons of the dorsal root ganglion neurons. This model provides the basis for a syndrome encompassing both central and peripheral manifestations in relation to neurotoxic exposure. Although considerable overlap does exist, the distal axonopathy can be predominantly peripheral distal (for example, isoniazid), predominantly central distal (for example, clioquinol), or central–peripheral distal (acrylamide, hexacarbons). This conceptual model also explains the relatively poor functional recovery in certain axonopathies in which the central axons have been involved; the recovery in central distal axonopathy is not as complete as in the peripheral distal axonopathy.

The precise reason for the length-dependent peripheral localization of the lesion in distal 'dying back' axonopathy remains to be established. Theoretically, a distal axonopathy may be initiated by an assault on the neuronal perikaryon, the axon, the nerve terminal, or by an injury simultaneously at several sites. Early concepts presumed a defect in neuronal perikaryal synthesis (Cavanagh, 1964), but this failed to explain the multifocal preterminal distribution of the lesions subsequently found to characterize the distal axonopathies. The possibility was raised that the distal lesions might be related to direct attack on axons and that axonal transport failure could be the main pathogenic mechanism in distal axonopathies (Prineas 1969; Schaumburg *et al.*, 1974; Spencer and Schaumburg, 1977). This view was later expanded to explain how certain toxic agents, by binding to the axonal transport enzymes or by combining with the axonal cytoskeletal

Table 7.1 *Classification of peripheral nerve toxins based on their major target sites*

Nerve cell body (neuronopathy)
Nucleus
    Doxorubicin
Cytosol
  Mercury, vinca alkaloids, taxoids (docetexal), colchicine
Soma-dendritic synapse
  Tetanospasmin, strychnine, capsaicin, cycasin, glutamate, L-BOAA (*Lathyrus sativus*), L-BMAA (*Cycas cercinalis*)
Nerve axon (axonopathy)
Proximal axonopathy
  Dimethylpropionitrile (DMPN)
Distal axonopathy
  Industrial chemicals: Acrylamide, hexacarbons, carbon disulfide, organophosphates, styrene, allyl chloride, methyl bromide, ethylene oxide
  Heavy metals: Arsenic, thallium, gold, *cis*-platinum
  Drugs: Isoniazid, phenytoin, vincristine, nitrofurantoin, metronidazol, dapsone, amytriptylene, clioquinol, chloramphenicol, disulfiram, trichloroethylene, almitrine, amiodarone, nitrous oxide, pyridoxine, ddl, ddC, thalidomide, suramine
Myelin sheath (Schwannopathy, myelinopathy)
Schwann cell
  Lead, cadmium, diphtheria, chloroquin
Myelin sheath
  Hexachlorophene, perhexilene, tellurium, buckthorn (toxic berry), cassava (*Manihot esculenta*)
Dys-immune
  Zimeldine, gold compounds
Ion channel (axonal channelopathy)
Sodium channel
  Blockade
    Tetrodotoxin, saxitoxin, some ciguatoxins, lidocaine
  Increased duration of opening
    Ciguatoxins, brevetoxins, pyrethrins
  Prevention of channel closure
    Batrachatoxin (poison dart frogs), μ- and β-scorpion toxins, sea anemone toxin, μ-conotoxin (snails), μ-agatoxin (funnel web spider), curtatoxin (grass spider)
  Increased permeability
    Tityustoxin (*Tityus serrulatus*)
Potassium channel
  Blockade
    Tetraethylammonium, 4-aminopyridine

L-BMAA (β-*n*-methylaminoalanine), L-BOAA (β-*n*-oxalylaminoalanine), ddC (2,3-dideoxycytidine), ddI (2,3-dideoxyinosine).

elements, could result in axonal transport failure and distal axonopathy.

Axonal transport in axonopathies

Axonal transport has been extensively studied in vincristine-, hexacarbon- and acrylamide-induced toxic neuropathies (Prineas, 1969; Bradley *et al.*, 1970; Bradley and Williams, 1973; Schaumburg *et al.*, 1974; Spencer and Schaumburg, 1975; Howland *et al.*, 1980; Jakobson and Sidenius, 1983; Moretto and Sabri, 1988). In 1973, an outbreak of peripheral neuropathy at a printed-fabrics plant occurred when one organic solvent (MnBK) was substituted for another (MiBK). No neurotoxic activity had been reported for the other commonly used homologous organic solvents such as

MEK and MiBK. This suggested that MnBK neurotoxicity might not be intrinsic and could arise from an active metabolite not formed by the other isomeric and homologous aliphatic ketones. Mammalian systems metabolize aliphatic ketones by a variety of metabolic pathways, including reduction, α-oxidation, decarboxylation, transamination, and omega-1 oxidation. A body of evidence now exists that the metabolic intermediates of omega-1 oxidation of *n*-hexane and MnBK, such as 2,5-HD and 2-HD, are the major neurotoxicants in hexacarbon neurotoxicity (Spencer and Schaumburg, 1975).

The pathogenic role of transport failure in hexacarbon-induced distal axonopathies has been investigated at physiological levels. 2,5-HD is reported to react directly with free amino groups of the neurofilament proteins, leading to pyrrole formation and extensive cross-linking (Spencer and Schaumburg, 1975). This mechanism explains the selective impairment of the transport of the neurofilament components. Chemical modification and cross-bridging of the neurofilament subunits may contribute to the development of axonal filamentous accumulation, a pathologic hallmark in hexacarbon-induced toxic neuropathies. Alternatively, a local energy deficit may be responsible for the transport failure, since the toxic metabolites of hexacarbons are known to inhibit glycolytic enzymes (Sabri and Spencer, 1980). The inhibition of glycolytic enzymes by the hexacarbons is slow and cumulative, and this probably explains why the neuropathy develops only after weeks of daily dosing. The initial localization of the pathological changes at the terminal nodes of Ranvier could result from the abnormally high metabolic demands at these sites or be due to the structural specialization at the nodes, as mentioned above. β,β-iminodipropionitrile (IDPN) neurotoxicity is another example of a nerve disease that results from the impairment of the axonal transport. In IDPN-induced neuropathy, structural alteration of neurofilaments and their consequent impaired entry into the axons causes ballooning of the cell bodies and giant, filament-packed swellings in the proximal axons.

Any retardation of the anterograde axonal transport process could potentially impair the delivery of the essential materials to the distant axonal sites. The reasons for the transport retardation and delivery failure can be several: inefficient initial loading of the substance at the proximal axon; premature reversal of the transport; accelerated metabolism during passage; or increased incorporation of the material into the excess fixed structure, such as the accumulated neurofilaments. Under any of these circumstances, the distal axon would suffer first and most. Other important consequences can also occur. For example, reduced delivery of neurofilaments that determine cross-sectional area would produce distal axonal atrophy. The loss or failure to renew axolemmal proteins and ion channels would compromise function and impulse conduction. Failure to replenish the peptide's neurotransmitters may quickly and dramatically alter the character of neurotransmission, while the depletion of synaptic vesicles may cause long-term deficits of transmission.

In acrylamide neuropathy, defect in re-circulation of the fast-transported proteins, either because of impaired turnaround or because of blockade of retrograde transport, has been reported (Jakobson and Sidenius, 1983; Moretto and Sabri, 1988). Since acrylamide reacts with sulfhydril groups, and since sulfhydril-containing glycolytic enzymes generate ATP for axonal transport, energy failure appears to be a major mechanism in acrylamide-induced axonal transport failure and the consequent neuropathy (Howland

et al., 1980). Abnormalities in turnaround of rapidly transported proteins have also been reported in the experimental neuropathies induced by zinc pyridinethione (Sahenk and Mendell, 1980) and p-bromophenolacetylurea (Jakobson and Brimijoin, 1981).

The ultimate cellular effects of a distal axonopathy depend upon the degree of the toxic exposure and the rate of the nerve fiber degeneration (Bradley and Williams, 1973). A rapidly dying axon could lead to the death of the supporting nerve cell body, i.e. secondary neuronopathy. In slow distal degeneration in hexacarbon intoxication, the distal axon may focally enlarge causing retraction of myelin (secondary demyelination) at nearby nodes of Ranvier and focal block of impulse transmission (Spencer and Schaumburg, 1977). Following removal of the noxious agent, the peripheral axon is able to regenerate with functional restoration because the nerve cell body is still intact. The persisting Schwann cell tube can guide regenerating sprouts to reinnervate the appropriate end organ. However, advanced damage may carry the 'dying back' process too far towards the cell body for terminal reconnection to occur on cessation of the toxic exposure. As mentioned before, axonal degeneration in the CNS has a poor prognosis; even though a regenerating end bulb may develop on central axons (Blakemore and Cavanagh, 1969), they may not elongate, possibly because of the lack of appropriate surface molecules or due to the intervening astroglial proliferation.

MYELIN SHEATH (MYELINOPATHY, SCHWANNOPATHY)

The Schwann cells in the PNS are traditionally classified as either myelin-forming or non-myelinating. However, within these two broad classes there are subtle phenotypes. For example, Schwann cells of motor and sensory fibers express slightly different surface epitopes (Martini et al., 1988). Similarly, the satellite cells of the DRG neurons, the autonomic ganglia, and the Schwann cells of the olfactory nerve are phenotypically distinct from the Schwann cells elsewhere in the PNS. Also, the enteric glial cells of the autonomic nervous system appear to be a distinct class in themselves. Nevertheless, at least in the peripheral nerves, non-myelinating and myelin-forming Schwann cells can be induced to be interchangeable in cross-union experiments (Aguayo et al., 1976).

The production of the myelin sheath by the Schwann cell depends on axonal factors. Conversely, Schwann cells are essential for the maintenance of axonal integrity. Some axonally transported components probably leave the axon all along its length. Although the details are unknown, this transmural passage of nerve factor(s) and its action on the Schwann cells is inferred from the changes that characterize Wallerian degeneration. Intrusion and internalization of myelin components into the axon and their subsequent retrograde transport to the cell bodies has been demonstrated (for review, see Ochs and Brimijoin, 1993). The bi-directional interaction between the axon and Schwann cell has been shown in nerve graft studies where axons are made to regenerate into differing Schwann cell environments (Aguayo et al., 1976).

A toxic agent may selectively affect the Schwann cell (Schwannopathy) resulting in failure to form or maintain the myelin sheath, or a toxicant may directly attack the myelin sheath (myelinopathy) leading to its disruption and loss. Although demyelination may be restricted to the paranodal region (paranodal demyelination), a primary toxic disease that damages the Schwann cell generally results in complete breakdown of the internodal myelin (segmental demyelination). The demyelinated axon shrinks as a secondary effect (Cammer, 1980). If the Schwann cell body remains intact and, if mitosis can occur, the daughter Schwann cells will envelop the denuded axon and attempt remyelination, even in the continued presence of the myelinotoxin. Remyelinated internodes are shorter, however, and the myelin is relatively thin in proportion to the axon diameter (Bradley, 1974).

Unlike the myelinating cell of the CNS, the oligodendrocyte, that envelops internodes of several axons, one Schwann cell myelinates one internode in the PNS. The functional effect of losing a myelinating cell in the PNS is therefore smaller than it is in the CNS.

The archetype toxins that cause segmental demyelination are diphtheria toxin, lead, hexachlorphene, perhexilene, and the toxins of the coyotillo fruit (*Karwinskia humboldtiana*) (Charlton et al., 1971).

Diphtheritic neuropathy

The outstanding pathologic feature in diphtheritic neuropathy is the demyelination with preservation of the axonal continuity and marked proliferation of the Schwann cells. Inflammatory cells are conspicuously absent in diphtheritic neuropathy. The demyelination ranges from paranodal demyelination to complete segmental demyelination. The diphtheria myelinotoxin is an extracellular polypeptide which is cleaved by proteases into fragments A and B. These fragments remain linked by a disulfide link. Fragment B binds specifically to the surface receptors of Schwann cells and the bound toxin is internalized by the receptor-mediated endocytosis. When factor A reaches the cytoplasm it binds to and inactivates the elongation factor-2 (EF-2). EF-2 in eukaryotes plays a major role during ribosomal translation of the genetic message from mRNA into protein. It catabolizes the translocation reaction that moves the ribosome one codon down

the mRNA (i.e. polypeptide chain elongation) during protein synthesis.

The incidence of neuropathy in diphtheria is about 20%. Severity of throat or extrafaucial diphtheria infection is the major determinant of the consequent neuropathy. In patients with severe throat infection, so called malignant diphtheria, a 'nasal twang' in the voice may be present during the first week of infection. More often, the paralysis of the soft palate and impairment of ocular accommodation appear in the third or fourth week after infection. Between the fifth and seventh week from the onset of throat infection the patient may develop paralysis of the pharynx, larynx, and diaphragm, with potentially severe bulbar and respiratory symptoms. Diffuse neuropathy usually makes its appearance in the eighth to twelfth week of illness. Improvement in diphtheritic neuropathy begins within days or weeks of onset of symptoms, leading eventually to a complete recovery in several months.

The latent period of days to weeks before the neuropathy of diphtheria sets in and the sequential topography of neurologic involvement after the primary infection are still unexplained. Early bulbar and ocular paralysis appear to be due to the action of locally produced toxins on nearby nerves. Studies of short-term metabolic effects of the toxin on Schwann cells suggest that the demyelination may be secondary to the failure of myelin synthesis during turnover of its constituents (Pleasure et al., 1973).

Myelinopathies

Unlike the direct effect of diphtheria toxin on Schwann cells, hexachlorophene toxicity is due to a direct effect on the myelin, producing striking intramyelin edema with spongiform myelinopathy in experimental animals. Schwann cell metabolism, as such, remains unaffected in hexachlorophene toxicity. Perhexilene may cause extensive segmental demyelination, with the presence of crystalline and lamelar inclusions within the Schwann cells.

Demyelination due to neurovascular toxins

In experimental plumbism, structural changes of blood vessels, particularly at the capillary level, have been a consistent observation in almost all morphological studies. In one study (Paduslo et al., 1982), endoneurial fluid from the sciatic nerves of rats who were fed 4% lead carbonate diet showed elevated lead levels and a 4.9-fold increase of albumin at 12 weeks. Nerve edema and a progressive increase in endoneurial pressure, in tandem with the extravasation of the osmotically active macromolecules, reflect an alteration of the blood–nerve barrier in lead neuropathy. How the entry of lead and other plasma components into the endoneurial compartment causes demyelination is not well understood. Tellurium also causes initial injury to the vasa nervorum, disrupting the blood–nerve barrier, resulting in plasma leakage, intramyelin edema, and segmental demyelination (Fullerton, 1966).

NERVE CELL BODY (NEURONOPATHY)

Toxic damage to the neuronal cell body results in secondary dendritic and axonal degeneration, with subsequent collapse of the myelin sheath surrounding the degenerating axon. Axonal breakdown under such conditions may progress from proximal to distal direction ('dying forward') or vice versa ('dying back'). In the motor axon, this would result in denervation of the NMJ and a corresponding muscle fiber atrophy over several months. If there is no functional reinervation, the muscle fiber itself may become incapable of accepting reinervation in a few years. In the CNS, in the case of the primary sensory axon, neuronal degeneration may be followed by disconnection to the second order sensory neuron and astrocyte proliferation. There is currently no possibility of neuronal regeneration in this situation.

Probably the best examples of documented toxic neuronopathies are those induced by methyl mercury and doxorubicin (see Chapter 10). In both humans and animals, the major toxic effect of methyl mercury is on the DRG neurons. In *in vitro* experiments with cultured DRG neurons, methyl mercury is demonstrated to be directly toxic to neurons at very low concentrations (Windebank, 1993). It probably combines with enzymatically and structurally important sulfhydril groups. Cellular metabolic changes related to defects in amino acid incorporation and protein synthesis have been demonstrated in methyl mercury poisoning.

Doxorubicin, an antimitotic agent that binds to DNA by intercalation between base pairs of the double helix, interferes with DNA-dependent mRNA transcription. Doxorubicin neurotoxicity in humans is rare because its dose is limited by other toxic effects on the hematopoietic system, kidney, and heart. In experimental animals, the selective toxicity of doxorubicin is related to the rapid entry of the drug into the DRGs following intravenous injection (Sahenk and Mendell, 1979). Doxorubicin can also be taken up by the nerve terminals and be transported retrogradely to the neuronal cell body.

Vincristine is predictably and uniformly neurotoxic to all who receive it, and this is the dose-limiting factor in its use in cancer chemotherapy (Bradley *et al.*, 1970). Other vinca alkaloids, vinblastine and vinadesine, are less neurotoxic but are also less potent therapeutically. Neuropathy improves rapidly when these drugs are discontinued or reduced in dosage. Vinca alkaloids combine with tubulin and impair the perikaryal and axonal cytoskeleton network and hence lead to impaired axonal transport as well as impaired neuronal export of cytoskeletal proteins from the nerve cell body.

Excitotoxic damage

Neuronal synaptic transmission is another complex mechanism. The peripheral NMJ transmission is referred to below. In the central components of the PNS (namely the anterior horn cell) the cell bodies and dendrites of spinal motor neurons receive a variety of inter- and intrasegmental synaptic inputs. Although considerable overlap exists between these inputs, studies have indicated that specific inputs are distributed in specific patterns on the soma-dendritic receptor surfaces. Glutamate and acetylcholine are the main neurotransmitters of the Ia excitatory system; glycine (Price *et al.*, 1976) is the major inhibitory transmitter in the ventral horn, which mediates inputs from Ia-inhibitory afferents and interneurons. The topography of these inputs is of particular importance with regard to the motoneuronal toxicity of tetanospasmin and excitotoxic motor neuronopathy caused by both exogenous excitatory amino acids (for example, β-oxalyl-amino-alanine (BOAA) *Lathyrus sativus*; β-methyl-amino-alanine (BMAA) *Cycas circinalis*) and endogenous excitatory amino acids (for example, glutamate, aspartate) (Brown, 1996). Since excitotoxins may have additive, if not synergistic, neurotoxic potential, they constitute a family of neurotoxicants of considerable interest to the neurotoxicologist.

The excitotoxic concept of neuronal death in motor neuron disease encompasses a set of three inter-related assumptions: first pertaining to the excitatory depolarization; second to the selective dendrosomatic locus of activity; and third to a chain of events leading eventually to cell death. The working hypothesis is as follows: excitatory amino acids, when present in toxic amounts in the peri-somadendritic microenvironment, effect a state of continuous depolarization and sustained increase in membrane permeability. This process consumes cellular energy stores in an (unsuccessful) effort to restore ionic balance and allows calcium entry that poisons mitochondria, leading to energy depletion and free radical accumulation. The cell finally dies when the energy resources are exhausted or a lethal alteration in the cellular internal milieu (calcium influx, etc.) has occurred. Some extremely powerful neuronal excitotoxins are known to occur in biological systems. In one study using rat brain slices (Pai *et al.*, 1993), L-BOAA of *L. sativus* was reported to be a billion-fold more toxic than another excitotoxin (L-BMAA of *C. cercinalis*). Both the L-BOAA and L-BMAA have been implicated in endemic motor neuron syndromes, namely lathyrism and amyotrophic lateral sclerosis – Parkinson's dementia complex of Guam.

ION CHANNELS (AXONAL CHANNELOPATHIES)

The ion channels in axons are membrane proteins that are degraded and replenished throughout the lifetime of mammals. The axolemmal channel proteins are synthesized in the cell body and transported axoplasmically to their destination, which could be of the order of several feet away, for insertion. The metabolic burden this places on the cell body depends in part on the turnover rate of the axolemmal channel proteins, about which little is known. However, this metabolic load appears substantial in view of the number of these channels. The load is obviously increased many fold during the process of demyelination and remyelination, when the number of nodes per unit length nearly doubles (Ritchie *et al.*, 1981), and during axonal regeneration.

There are a group of recently defined toxic peripheral nerve disorders with impressive electrophysiological impairment in which neither axonal structural abnormalities nor demyelination occurs (Waxman, 1995; Gutmann and Gutmann, 1996). The major changes in these disorders are in the axolemmal ion channels of peripheral nerves, most notably in sodium channels.

It is now well established that sensory and motor axons express sodium channels with different biochemical and pharmacological properties. Moreover, different types of sensory axons (for example, muscle versus cutaneous afferents) possess different types of sodium channels. The existence of these different sodium-channel types may provide a basis for selective toxicity of many neurotoxins that target the axolemmal sodium channels.

Neurotoxic effects on sodium channels could render neurons hyperexcitable by interfering with de- or inactivation. Biological toxins directed against the neuronal-type sodium channels can slow (for example, α-scorpion and sea anemone toxins) or block (batrachatoxin, BTX) inactivation, or can induce abnormal bursting (for example, ciguatoxin, brevetoxin), which results in repetitive firing in axons. Positive sensory and motor symptoms secondary to the increased axonal sodium currents are common in marine neurotoxic poisoning. Another consequence of the toxic action on the sodium channel could be a decreased sodium conductance, due to channel blockade (for example, TTX, STX), resulting in conduction failure. Rapid onset of nerve conduction slowing or block, with a time-course that cannot be accounted for by demyelination or other structural damage, is characteristic in these toxin-induced channelopathies.

Biological neurotoxins affecting ion channels

The use of venom by predators to capture prey is an adaptation that has arisen independently over a wide phylogenetic spectrum. Many neurotoxins of animal venom target axolemmal ion channels (Tables 7.1 and 7.2). Many biotoxins of predators are directed to highly specific subtypes of certain ion channels, for example, TTX, STX and μ-conotoxin of marine animals, BTX of the black widow spider, α- and β-scorpion toxins, and pyrethrins of the chrysanthemum flower target axolemmal-type N-1 sodium channels. In fact, even their sensitivity may vary for channels located at distinct sites on the axolemma of one type of nerve fiber. The cone snail omega-conotoxin GVIA binds specifically and blocks completely axonal-type N-1 calcium channels. At first glance, this seems surprising, since venomous animals might be expected to have evolved broad spectrum neurotoxins, making them more flexible with respect to the potential prey. However, a narrow subtype specificity could in fact be an advantage, particularly if the speed of prey paralysis is a major consideration. Subtype-specific use of toxin might be the most rapid and efficient use if only a few toxin molecules are available, i.e. toxin selectively binding to the most relevant channel subtype and not to any other less relevant subtype.

Ciguatoxins and brevetoxins are extremely potent, heat stable, non-proteinous, lipophilic sodium-channel toxins that are produced by dinoflagelletes associated with dead coral and algae (Ayyar, 1996). Ciguatoxins are passed up the fish food chain and their accumulation in predatory fish may result in human outbreaks of ciguatera poisoning (Swift and Swift, 1993). More than 400 species of edible and predominantly reef fishes have been implicated in ciguatera fish poisoning. Nausea, vomiting, diarrhea, paresthesias (beginning as oropharyngeal and acral paresthesias), and a list of more than 175 other manifestations have been compiled from the cases of ciguatera poisoning (Sims, 1987), including a sensation of temperature reversal two to five days after the ingestion of the ciguatera-contaminated fish. The ciguatera and brevetoxins bind to the α-subunit of the sodium channel, causing inhibition of their inactivation. A shift of voltage-dependent sodium channel to more negative potentials results in a repetitive firing in axons. Prolonged hypertension or persistent hypotension, probably related to another toxin acting on calcium channels, have been reported in chronic ciguatera poisoning.

STX, the primary neurotoxin in paralytic fish poisoning, is produced by another species of dino-flagelletes (*Gonyaulax* spp.). TTX is the main neurotoxin in Japanese puffer fish (*Fugus rubripes*) poisoning. Molas and gobies are the other main categories of tetrodotoxic fishes. STX and TTX are heterocyclic compounds that bind to the outer side of the sodium channel and block sodium flux through the channel, resulting in axonal conduction failure. An encyclopedic list of toxins that act on different ion channels is compiled elsewhere (Adams and Swanson, 1996).

NEUROMUSCULAR JUNCTION TRANSMISSION FAILURE

The NMJ is a site of particular importance in neurotoxicology. As has been stated, the complexity of the NMJ structure and the complicated series of chemical processes involved in neuromuscular transmission across the pre- and postsynaptic membranes make NMJ specially vulnerable to a variety of neurotoxins (Table 7.2). Additionally, ion channels in the nerve terminals at the NMJ may be specifically attacked by certain neurotoxins. Of note, the motor nerve terminals are located outside the protective blood–nerve barrier and can be potential sites for the entry of toxins into the nervous system.

Many toxins that act on the NMJ naturally occur in some animal, plant, or bacterial species. They may act either presynaptically, postsynaptically, or directly on the muscle membrane. Major components of some snake venoms either bind and block the postsynaptic AChR (for example, α-bungarotoxin, α-BTX) or bind to the presynaptic terminals (for example, β-bungarotoxin, β-BTX) and interfere with exocytosis of vesicular membrane and ACh release.

α-Conotoxin of marine snails, like α-BTX of snake venom, competitively blocks the muscle nicotinic AChRs, resulting in flaccid paralysis. One component of BTX, known as neuronal BTX, of banded krait competitively blocks the neuronal AChR, causing failure of neuronal cholinergic transmission. β-BTX is a covalently linked dimeric polypeptide (A and B chains). The B chain targets the specific presynaptic receptor and the internalized A chain exerts action from the inside of the nerve terminal. β-BTX action on the nerve terminal is triphasic: transient inhibition; facilitation of AChR release; and irreversible depression of ACh release.

Scorpion venom contains a range of peptides capable of a variety of actions, including liberation of ACh from the motor and autonomic nerve endings, and several effects on axolemmal ion channels. The clinical effects depend upon the offending scorpion species and the active ingredients in the venom.

Black widow spider venom acts on the presynaptic nerve terminals. The purified toxin (α-latrotoxin) causes increased release of the ACh quanta and consequent vesicular depletion; it also releases catecholamines from the adrenergic nerve endings.

Table 7.2 *Classification of some neuromuscular junction toxins based on their major target sites*

Voltage-gated calcium channel
Blockade
  Botulinum toxin (heavy chain), Mg^{2+} excess, aminoglycosides, omega-conotoxin (*Conus striatus*), agelenin (*Agelena opulenta*), funnel spider toxin (*Agelena aperta*)
Acetylecholine release
Blockade
  Botulinum toxin (light chain), tick venom (*Ixodidae* and *Argasidae* spp.)
Depletion by excessive release
  α-Latrotoxin (black widow spider, *Latrodectus mactans*)
Acetylecholeine receptor
Blockade
  d-Tubocurarine, μ- and kappa-bungarotoxins (*Naja* and *Bungarus* spp.), μ-conotoxins (*Conus* spp.), tityus toxin (*Tityus serrulatus*), histrionicotoxin (*Dendrobates histrionicus*), nereistoxin (*Lubriconereis heteropoda*), lophotoxin (*Lophogorgia* spp.), neosurugatoxin (*Babylonia aponica*)
Stimulatory effect
  Succinylcholine, anatoxin-A (*Anabaena flos-aquae*)
Acetylcholine re-uptake
Blockade
  Hemicholinium-3, vesamicol
Acetylcholinesterase
Blockade
  Organophosphate compounds, carbamates, physostigmine, neostigmine, edrophonium, fasciculin-2 (*Dendroaspis angusticeps*)
Unknown target site
Versutoxin and robustoxin (*Atrax robustus*), pymotes toxin (*Pymotes tritici*)

Tick paralysis is a toxin-mediated disorder caused by the female tick's saliva. The main blockage in tick paralysis involves the terminal part of the motor nerve fiber, due to impaired mobilization or release of the ACh. The toxin appears to be rapidly excreted or metabolized once the tick is removed.

Botulinum toxin is a large polypeptide which is proteolytically processed to form a heavy chain (100 kDa) and a light chain (50 kDa). The heavy chain binds to the presynaptic nerve terminal and facilitates entry of the light chain into the terminal. The light chain is a Zn-endopeptidase, which blocks synaptic transmission via specific cleavage of exocytosis machinery protein. Each of seven serotypes (A, B, C, D, E, F, G) of botulinum toxin probably cleaves the protein at a specific site, with consequent inhibition of depolarization-induced ACh release from the nerve terminal.

Several chemical toxins also produce neurotoxicity by interfering with the neuromuscular transmission (Table 7.2). For a detailed account of individual toxins, their source and mechanisms of action, and the clinical syndromes that they produce, the reader is referred to Chapters 8–10 in this book and elsewhere (Senanayake and Roman, 1992; Adams and Swanson, 1996).

CLINICAL PATTERNS AND DIAGNOSIS OF PNS TOXICITY

Neuromuscular junction toxins

The clinical syndrome of toxic NMJ transmission failure is usually characteristic, although the establishment of etiology and the precise site of toxic action may call for further laboratory investigations. Neuromuscular junctional toxins are mostly biotoxins of animal or plant origin, or are chemical insecticides (Senanayake and Roman, 1992), and many are potentially fatal in severe poisoning. A history of toxic exposure, the relatively rapid onset of the characteristic pure motor syndrome, equally rapid reversibility in most cases after removal of the individual from the toxic source and following specific pharmacotherapy, and the associated muscarinic cholinergic effects in many cases make the diagnosis of toxic NMJ transmission impairment straightforward. Nerve terminal damage from β-BTX and botulinum toxin is slower in recovery.

Toxic neuropathies

Human toxic neuropathies can occur in sporadic, community, or occupational settings. A mysterious case of toxic neuropathy can appear in the physician's waiting room at any time, usually masquerading as some less exotic neuropathy. More commonly, sporadic cases are iatrogenic and pharmacologic, and can be recognized readily when the neuromuscular illness is temporally related to the exposure to a known neurotoxic drug or neurotoxin. The exposure to a known agricultural, environmental or industrial toxin, and the resulting epidemic neuropathy in a group of individuals, is also readily recognizable if suspected, particularly when there is a constant clinical pattern among individuals who are similarly exposed. However, determination that an isolated neuropathic illness is due to a toxin is more difficult, even in an occupational setting, because the exposure history may go unrecognized, be felt to be irrelevant, or forgotten. The resulting illness may mimic some naturally occurring disease. An example illustrates this point. A 65-year-old smoker with neuropathy had a history of exposure to industrial organic solvents and was found to have an elevated blood glucose and glycosylated hemoglobin (HbA_{1c}) level – evidence that this patient also had diabetes mellitus. The judgment that the neuropathy was causally linked to a neurotoxic hexacarbon or to diabetes mellitus, or to still another etiology (such as a small cell carcinoma of the lung) depends on the clinical pattern of the neuropathy and the results of further investigations. Such clinical judgments are possible only when the physician is knowledgeable and experienced regarding the natural history and patterns of various neuropathies.

In a case of suspected toxic neuropathy, we think that the neurological history that focuses on the patient's clinical pattern of neuropathic symptoms and details of his physical environment at the work-place, home, and recreation may be of enormous help in arriving at the accurate etiologic diagnosis. Effort should be made to recognize the pattern of nerves affected (mononeuropathy, polyneuropathy, proximal, distal, etc.); the population of neurons (motor, sensory, autonomic, mixed) or nerve fibers (large diameter, small diameter) involved; major part of the peripheral nerve affected (axonal, demyelination, mixed), time-course (acute, sub-acute, chronic, monophasic, recurrent); and the other associated clinical features (skin and skin-appendages, hematopoietic system, etc.). Industrial or other toxin-induced neuropathies may not occur in several persons at one time. The importance of recognizing the neurotoxic etiology at the earliest possible stage can not be overemphasized because prompt removal from the exposure generally leads to complete clinical recovery. Regulation of further exposure should prevent its recurrence. Since neurotoxins, like thallium, are sometimes used in murder attempts; early identification of the cause of the neuropathy may be lifesaving.

Sensory symptoms in toxic neuropathies

Sensory impairment in toxic neuropathy usually begins in and is often dominant in the feet, suggesting pathological involvement of nerve fibers in a length-dependent fashion. With clinical progression, hands may become involved and eventually the numbness may spread to the mid-abdomen (distal parts of the inter-costal nerves). Further, one sensory modality may be selectively or disproportionately involved depending on the sensory neuronal type affected. Subtle or neglected sensory symptoms may be recognized by careful questioning and by physical examination with sensitive automated testing systems. In doubtful cases, measurements of sensory nerve action potentials should be pursued; these are invaluable in establishing dysfunction of sensory fibers distal to the DRG.

cis-Platinum, metronidazole, and pyridoxin in high doses cause a pure sensory neuropathy. Industrial hexacarbons (acrylamide, MnBK), vincristine, phenytoin, and hydralazine also cause a predominantly sensory neuropathy. In many other neuropathies caused by drugs, arsenic, thallium, organophosphates, and diphtheria toxin, the sensory symptoms coexist with the motor deficit.

Relatively few neurotoxins are selectively toxic to the cranial nerves. Generally, such specificity, when it occurs, tends to affect sensory (trigeminal and auditory) nerves. Trichloroethylene may cause selective trigeminal neuropathy, attributable to dichloroethylene, a decomposition product. Ototoxicity is mainly a drug-related (quinine, aminoglycoside antibiotics, loop diuretics, cis-platinum, salicylates) phenomenon.

Positive sensory phenomena such as spontaneous pain as seen with arsenic, paresthesias, and restless limb movements may be prominent in toxic neuropathies. Tingling, 'pins and needles,' cold, warm, burning, pressure, and other perverse sensations are common complaints. Paresthesias are speculated to be derived from the spontaneous impulses generated in abnormal nerve fibers. Immature sprouts from small fibers may generate spontaneous impulses and serve as possible sources of pain in toxic neuropathies

Motor symptoms in toxic neuropathies

Lower motor neuron symptoms and signs which begin and predominate in distal limb segments, if coupled with the associated sensory and reflex loss, are almost diagnostic of a peripheral neuropathy. Inorganic lead and dapsone generally cause a pure motor neuropathy. A predominantly motor neuropathy with asymmetrical wrist drop is almost diagnostic of lead neuropathy. Large doses of arsenic, hexacarbons, triorthocresylphosphate (TOCP), gold compounds, vacor, diphtheria, buckthorn (toxic berry), and AIP are known to cause a

syndrome similar to acute inflammatory demyelinating polyradiculoneuropathy (Asbury, 1991; Le Quesne, 1993; Schaumburg and Berger, 1993), if they do not cause death.

The distal predominance of motor signs and symptoms is traditionally attributed to the 'dying back' pattern of pathological involvement. Lead neuropathy is an important exception, however. In lead neuropathy, motor neurons of the upper limbs may preferentially be involved, particularly those of the seventh cervical segment, which produces the typical wrist drop. Wasting of small muscles of the hands and feet indicates chronic exposure to toxins, with the resulting denervation of distal limb muscles. A genuinely pure lower motor neuron syndrome is characteristic of a neuromuscular junction disorder and is rarely due to a peripheral neuropathy. Similarly, proximal muscle weakness is decidedly rare in toxic neuropathies and may indicate the presence of mononeuritis multiplex, chronic inflammatory demyelinating polyradiculoneuropathy, AIP, or a concomitant primary muscle disorder. In doubtful cases electromyographic examination and nerve conduction velocities may be of great diagnostic help.

Positive motor phenomenon, such as fasciculations and cramps, may occur in toxic neuropathies.

Tendon (stretch) reflexes in toxic neuropathies

Tendon reflexes are diminished or absent in most sensorimotor polyneuropathies. As for sensory and motor symptoms, the most distal stretch reflex (ankle jerk) is the first to be affected in toxic neuropathies. However, neuropathies affecting selectively small diameter nerve fibers may spare the tendon reflexes. Brisk tendon reflexes may be seen in cases of peripheral neuropathies when there is concurrent damage to the pyramidal tracts in the spinal cord, as for example in some cases of toxic neuropathy caused by TOCP. Brisk reflexes and signs of spinal cord damage may also be present following toxic exposure to nitrous oxide (Green and Kinsella, 1995).

Autonomic symptoms in toxic neuropathies

Toxic neuropathies (other than type B botulism) rarely affect the autonomic nervous system predominantly. However, autonomic impairment may be a significant component of some toxic neuropathies. In such neuropathies, small nerve fibers are predominantly affected and autonomic symptoms may result from damage of the afferent or efferent components of the sympathetic and parasympathetic system. The autonomic impairment may cause or contribute to a typical syncope, bladder and bowel dysfunction, and impotence. Paradoxically, dimethylaminopropionitrile (DMAPN) toxicity causes a proximal axonopathy and may produce urinary hesitancy, sexual dysfunction, and sacral sensory loss.

Other systemic symptoms in toxic neuropathies

Toxic neuropathy may be associated with toxic effects related to damage in other systems. Central nervous system involvement has already been mentioned, when it may be a manifestation of a central–peripheral distal axonopathy. Acrylamide, carbon disulfide, clioquinol, thallium, TOCP, metronidazole, thalidomide, and lead intoxication in children may involve the CNS. Optic neuropathy is characteristic of clioquinol-induced subacute myelo-opticoneuropathy. Visual involvement in organic mercury toxicity is believed to be due to the involvement of the visual cortex. As mentioned before, dysuria and impotence in males can occur with DMAPN toxicity.

Arsenic neuropathy may follow prominent gastrointestinal symptoms, if toxic exposure has been severe, and may be accompanied by nail changes (Mees' lines), hyperkeratosis of soles and palms, and skin pigmentation (rain-drop appearance). Liver damage, anemia, and nephropathy can also occur in arsenic poisoning. Red skin and brittle nails have been reported in thalidomide toxicity. Alopecia may be prominent in thallium toxic neuropathy. In the undiagnosed patient, any history of urine color change should raise suspicion of porphyria. Lead toxic neuropathy may be associated with prominent gastrointestinal symptoms (lead gumlines, constipation) and hematopoietic (anemia, reticulocytosis) dysfunction. Diphtheritic bulbar and ocular neuropathy characteristically occurs three to four weeks after pharyngeal infection, while the diffuse demyelinating neuropathy may follow eight to 12 weeks after the infection. Toxic cardiomyopathy may precede diphtheritic neuropathy.

Laboratory investigation in toxic neuropathies

In general, the search for a toxic etiology relies more on the clinical and epidemiological investigations rather than on the laboratory evaluation. Laboratory screening may fail to detect a neurotoxin for several reasons: the suspected agent may not have been a previously recognized neurotoxin or may not be detectable by the existing laboratory means; or the toxin might have been metabolized or excreted from the system.

Heavy metal screening in blood and urine should be complimented with assays of nail clippings and hair for arsenic in appropriate clinical setting. Both head and pubic hair should be tested and urinary excretion of arsenic should be measured before and after penicillamine injection. The urinary excretion of delta-ALA and coproporphyrin is increased in lead poisoning, and in AIP.

Minimal evaluation in a toxic neuropathy should include sensory and motor conduction studies in several nerves. This will enable neurotoxicologists to confirm and document the severity of the neuropathy, to determine the type of nerve fiber involved, and also to rule out acute or chronic inflammatory demyelinating polyradiculoneuropathies. Sensory nerve action potentials are much more sensitive and reproducible than the purely clinical measurements of sensation. Further, sensory nerve potentials can be measured sequentially to judge the progress of the disease. Delineation of a neuromuscular junction disorder may require repetitive nerve stimulation. Conventional electromyographic examination using concentric electrodes contributes little to the diagnosis of patients with a toxic neuropathy; mostly electromyography simply provides evidence of denervation consistent with the clinical and nerve conduction data. However, quantitative electromyography may be useful in delineating borderline cases (Ochoa, 1980). A sural nerve biopsy may show pathological changes in a sub-clinical toxic neuropathy.

REFERENCES

Adams, M.E. and Olivera, B.M. 1994: Neurotoxins: overview of an emerging research technology. *Trends in Neuroscience*, **17**, 151–5.

Adams, M.E. and Swanson, G. 1996: Neurotoxins. *Trends in Neuroscience (Neurotoxins Supplement)*, **19**, 1–36.

Aguayo, A.J., Epps, J., Charron, L., Terry, L.C. and Sweezey, E. 1976: Multipotentiality of Schwann cells in cross-anastomosed and grafted myelinated and unmyelinated nerves. *Brain Research*, **104**, 1–20.

Aletta, J. M. and Goldberg, J. 1984: Routing of transmitter and other changes in fast axonal transport after transaction of one branch of the bifurcate axon on an identical neuron. *Journal of Neurosciences*, **4**, 1800–8.

Asbury, A.K. 1991: Diseases of the peripheral nervous system. In *Harrison's Principles of Internal Medicine*, Wilson, J.D., Braunwald, E., Isselbacher, K.J. *et al.* (eds), 12th edn, pp 2096–108. New York: McGraw-Hill.

Ayyar, D.R. 1996: Marine neurotoxins. In *Neurology in Clinical Practice*, Bradley, W.G., Daroff, R.B., Fenichel, G.M. and Marsden, C.D. (eds), 2nd edn, pp 1419–23. Boston, MA: Butterworth-Heinemann.

Black, J.A., Kocsis, J.D. and Waxman, S.G. 1990: Ion channel organization of the myelinated fiber. *Trends in Neurosciences*, **13**, 48–54.

Blakemore, W.F. and Cavanagh J.B. 1969: 'Neuroaxonal dystrophy' occurring in an experimental 'dying-back' process in the rat. *Brain*, **92**, 789–804.

Bradley, W.G. 1970: The neuromyopathy of vincristine in the guinea pig: an electrophysiological and pathological study. *Journal of Neurological Sciences*, **10**, 133–62.

Bradley, W.G. 1974: *Disorders of Peripheral Nerves*. Oxford: Blackwell Scientific.

Bradley, W.G., Lassman, L.P., Pearce, G.W. and Walton, J.N. 1970: The neuromyopathy of vincristine in man. Clinical, electrophysiological and pathological studies. *Journal of Neurological Sciences*, **10**, 107–31.

Bradley, W.G. and Williams, M.H. 1973: Axoplasmic flow in axonal neuropathies. I. Axoplasmic flow in cats with toxic neuropathies. *Brain*, **96**, 235–46.

Brown, R.H. 1996: Superoxide dismutase and familial ALS: new insights into mechanisms and treatments. *Annals of Neurology*, **39**, 145–6.

Calne, D.B., Hochberg, F.H., Snow, J.B. and Nygaard, T. 1992: Theories of neurodegeneration. In *Neurotoxins and Neurodegenerative Diseases*, Langston, J.W. and Young, A. (eds). *Annals of New York Academy of Sciences*, **648**, 1–5.

Cammer, W. 1980: Toxic demyelination: biochemical studies and hypothetical mechanisms. In *Experimental and Clinical Neurotoxicology*, Spencer, P.S. and Schaumburg, H.H. (eds), pp 239–55. Baltimore, MD: Williams & Wilkins.

Cavanagh, J.B. 1964: The significance of the 'dying-back' process in experimental and human neurological disease. *International Reviews of Experimental Pathology*, **3**, 219–67.

Charlton, K.M., Claborn, L.D. and Pierce, K.R. 1971: A neuropathy of goats caused by experimental coyotillo (*K. humboldtiana*) poisoning. I. Clinical and neurophysiological studies. *American Journal of Veterinary Research*, **32**, 1381–9.

Chiu, S.Y. and Ritchie, J.M. 1980: Potassium channels in nodal and internodal axonal membrane of mammalian myelinated fiber. *Nature*, **284**, 170–71.

Chiu, S.Y., Shrager, P. and Ritchie, J.M. 1984: Neuronal-type Na$^+$ and K$^+$ channels in rabbit cultured Schwann cells. *Nature*, **311**, 156–7.

Corcoran, G.B., Fix, L., Jones, D.P. *et al.* 1994: Apoptosis: molecular control point in toxicity. *Toxicology and Applied Pharmacology*, **128**, 169–81.

Fagius, J., Osterman, P.O., Siden, A. and Wilholm, B.E. 1985: Guillian–Barré syndrome following zimeldine treatment. *Journal of Neurology Neurosurgery and Psychiatry*, **48**, 65–9.

Fullerton, P.M. 1966: Chronic peripheral neuropathy produced by lead poisoning in guinea-pigs. *Journal of Neuropathology and Experimental Neurology*, **25**, 214–36.

Green, R. and Kinsella, L.J. 1995: Current concepts in the diagnosis of cobalamine deficiency. *Neurology*, **45**, 1435–40.

Grohovaz, F., Limbrick, A.R. and Miledi, R. 1982: Acetylcholine receptor at the rat neuromuscular junction as revealed by deep etching. *Proceedings of the Royal College of London (Biology)*, **215**, 147–54.

Gutmann, L. and Gutmann, L. 1996: Axonal channelopathies: an evolving concept in the pathogenesis of peripheral nerve disorders. *Neurology*, **47**, 18–21.

Holtzman, E. 1977: The origin and fate of secretory packages, especially synaptic vesicles. *Neuroscience*, **2**, 327–55.

Hong, K. and Driscoll, M. 1994: A trans-membrane domain of the putative channel sub-unit MEC-4 influences mechanotransduction and neurodegeneration in *C. elegans*. *Nature*, **367**, 470–73.

Hopkins, A. 1970: Experimental lead poisoning in the baboon. *British Journal of Industrial Medicine*, **27**, 130–40.

Howland, R.D., Vyas, I.L., Lowndes, H.E. and Argentieri, T.M. 1980: The etiology of toxic peripheral neuropathies: *in vitro* effects of acrylamide and 2,5-hexanedione on brain enolase and other glycolytic enzymes. *Brain Research*, **202**, 131–42.

Jakobson, J. and Brimijoin, S. 1981: Axonal transport of enzymes and labeled proteins in experimental axonopathies induced by p-bromophenylacetylurea. *Brain Research*, **229**, 103–22.

Jakobson, J. and Sidenius, P. 1983: Early and dose-dependent decrease in retrograde axonal transport in acrylamide intoxicated rats. *Journal of Neurochemistry*, **40**, 447–54.

Katrak, S.M., Pollock, M., O'Brien, C.P. *et al.* 1980: Clinical and morphological features of gold neuropathy. *Brain*, **103**, 671–93.

Le Quesne, P.M. 1993: Neuropathy due to drugs. In *Peripheral Neuropathy*, Dyck, P.J., Thomas, P.K., Griffin, J.W., Low, P.A. and Poduslo, J.F. (eds), 3rd edn, pp 1571–81. Philadelphia, PA: W.B. Saunders.

Lotti, M. 1996: Neurotoxicology: the cindrella of neuroscience. *Neurotoxicology*, **17**, 313–22.

Lotti, M., Morreto, A., Capodicasa, E., Bertolazzi, M., Periaca, M. and Scapellato, M.L. 1993: Interactions between neuropathy target esterase and its inhibitors and the development of polyneuropathy. *Toxicology and Applied Pharmacology*, **122**, 165–71.

MacPhail, P.C. 1992: Principles of identifying and characterizing neurotoxicity. *Toxicology Letters*, **64/65**, 209–15.

Martini, R., Bollensen, E. and Schachner, M. 1988: Immunocytochemical localization of the major peripheral nervous system glycoprotein P$_o$ and the L2/HNK-1 and L3 carbohydrate structures in developing and adult mouse sciatic nerve. *Developmental Biology*, **129**, 330–38.

Moretto, A. and Sabri, M.I. 1988: Progressive deficits in retrograde axon transport precede degeneration of motor axons in acrylamide neuropathy. *Brain Research*, **440**, 18–24.

Myers, R.R., Powell, H.C., Shapiro, H.M., Costello, M.L. and Lampert, P.W. 1980: Changes in endoneurial fluid pressure, permeability and peripheral nerve ultrastructure in experimental lead neuropathy. *Annals of Neurology*, **8**, 392–401.

Ochoa, J. 1980: Criteria for the assessment of polyneuropathy. In *Experimental and Clinical Neurotoxicology*, Spencer, P.S. and Schaumburg H.H. (eds), pp 681–707. Baltimore, MD: Williams & Wilkins.

Ochs, S. and Brimijoin, W.S. 1993: Axonal transport. In *Peripheral Neuropathy*, Dyck, P.J., Thomas, P.K., Griffin, J.W., Low, P. A. and Poduslo, J.F. (eds), 3rd edn, pp 331–60. Philadelphia, PA: W.B. Saunders.

Ochs, S. and Smith, C.B. 1971: Fast axonal transport in mammalian nerve *in vitro* after block of glycolysis with iodoacetic acid. *Journal of Neurochemistry*, **8**, 833–43.

Ohnishi, A., Schilling, K., Brimijoin, W.S., Lambert, E.H., Fairbanks, V.F. and Dyck, P.J. 1977: Lead neuropathy 1. Morphometry, nerve conduction, and choline acetyltransferase transport: new finding of endoneurial edema associated with segmental demyelination. *Journal of Neuropathology and Experimental Neurology*, **36**, 499–518.

Poduslo, J.F., Low, P.A., Windebank, A.J., Dyck, P.J., Berg, C.T. and Schmelzer, J.D. 1982: Altered blood–nerve barrier in experimental lead neuropathy assessed by changes in endoneurial albumin concentration. *Journal of Neurosciences*, **2**, 1507–14.

Pai, K.S., Shankar, S.K. and Ravindranath, V. 1993: Billion-fold difference in toxic potencies of two excitatory plant amino acids, L-BOAA and L-BMAA: biochemical and morphological studies using mouse brain slices. *Neuroscience Research*, **17**, 241–8.

Pentschew, A. and Garro, F. 1966: Lead encephalomyelopathy of the suckling rat and its implications on the porphyrinopathic nervous disease. *Acta Neuropathologica*, **6**, 266–78.

Pleasure, D.E., Feldmann, B. and Prockop, D.J. 1973: Diphtheria toxin inhibits the synthesis of myelin proteolipid and basic proteins by peripheral nerve *in vitro*. *Journal of Neurochemistry*, **20**, 81–90.

Price, D.L., Stocks, A., Griffin, J.W., Young, A. and Peck, K. 1976: Glycine-specific synapses in rat spinal cord. *Journal of Cell Biology*, **68**, 389–95.

Prineas, J. 1969: The pathogenesis of dying-back neuropathies. I. An ultrastructural study of tri-ortho-cresyl phosphate intoxication in the cat. *Journal of Neuropathology and Experimental Neurology*, **28**, 571–97.

Quick, D.C. and Waxman, S.G. 1977: Specific staining of the axon membrane at nodes of Ranvier with ferric ion and ferrocyanide. *Journal of the Neurological Sciences*, **31**, 1–11

Rechthand, E. and Rapoport, S.I. 1987: Regulation of the microenvironment of peripheral nerve: role of the blood–nerve barrier. *Progress in Neurobiology*, **28**, 303–43

Ritchie, J.M., Rang, H.P. and Pellegrino, R. 1981: Sodium and potassium channels in demyelinated and remyelinated peripheral nerve. *Nature*, **294**, 257–9.

Ritchie, J.M. and Rogart, R.B. 1977: Density of sodium channels in mammalian myelinated nerve fibers and nature of the axonal membrane under the myelin sheath. *Proceedings of the National Academy of Science of the United States of America*, **74**, 211–5.

Roper, J. and Schwartz, J.R. 1989: Heterogeneous distribution of fast and slow potassium channels in myelinated rat nerve fiber. *Journal of Physiology (London)*, **416**, 93–110.

Sabri, M.I. and Spencer, P.S. 1980: Toxic distal axonopathy: biochemical studies and hypothetical mechanisms. In *Experimental and Clinical Neurotoxicology*, Spencer, P.S. and Schaumburg, H.H. (eds), pp 206–19. Baltimore, MD: Williams & Wilkins.

Sahenk, Z. and Mendell, J.R., 1979: Ultrastructural study of zink pyridinethione-induced peripheral neuropathy. *Journal of Neuropathology and Experimental Neurology*, **38**, 532–50.

Sahenk, Z. and Mendell, J.R. 1980: Axoplasmic transport in zink pyridinethione-induced peripheral neuropathy. *Brain Research*, **186**, 343–53.

Salpeter, M.M., Rogers, A.W., Kasprzak, H. and McHenry, F.A. 1978: Acetylcholine in the fast extraocular muscle of the mouse by light and electron microscope autoradiography. *Journal of Cell Biology*, **78**, 274–85.

Schaumburg, H.H. and Berger, A.R. 1993: Human toxic neuropathy due to industrial agents. In *Peripheral Neuropathy*, Dyck, P.J., Thomas, P.K., Griffin, J.W., Low, P.A. and Poduslo, J.F. (eds), 3rd edn, pp 1533–48. Philadelphia, PA: W.B. Saunders.

Schaumburg, H.H., Wisniewski, H.M. and Spencer, P.S. 1974: Ultrastructural studies of the dying-back process. I. Peripheral nerve terminals and axon degeneration in systemic acrylamide intoxication. *Journal of Neuropathlogy and Experimental Neurology*, **23**, 260–84.

Schwartz, J.H. 1979: Axonal transport: components, mechanisms, and specificity. *Annual Review of Neuroscience*, **2**, 467–504.

Senanayake, N. and Roman, G.C. 1992: Disorders of neuromuscular transmission due to natural environmental toxins. *Journal of the Neurological Sciences*, **107**, 1–13.

Shrager, P., Chiu, S.Y. and Ritchie, J.M. 1985: Voltage-dependent sodium and potassium channels in mammalian cultured Schwann cells. *Proceedings of National Academy of Science of the United States of America*, **82**, 948–52.

Sim, J.K. 1987: A theoretical discourse on the pharmacology of toxic marine ingestions. *Annals of Emergency Medicine*, **16**, 1006–15.

Spencer, P.S. and Schaumburg, H.H. 1975: Experimental neuropathy produced by 2,5H.D – a major metabolite of the neurotoxic industrial solvent methyl-*n*-butyl-ketone. *Journal of Neurology, Neurosurgery and Psychiatry*, **38**, 771–5.

Spencer, P.S. and Schaumburg, H.H. 1977: Ultrastructural studies of the dying-back process. III. The evolution of experimental peripheral giant axonal degeneration. *Journal of Neuropathology and Experimental Neurology*, **36**, 276–99.

Swift, A.E.B. and Swift, T.R. 1993: Ciguatera. *Clinical Toxicology*, **31**, 1–29.

Tilson, H.A. 1990: Neurotoxicology in the 1990s. *Neurotoxicology and Teratology*, **12**, 293–300.

Verma, A. 1996: Neurotoxins of animal and plant origin. In *Neurology in Clinical Practice*, Bradley, W.G., Daroff, R.B., Fenichel, G.M. and Marsden, C.D. (eds), 2nd edn, pp 1415–18. Boston, MA: Butterworth-Heinemann.

Waxman, S.G. 1995: Sodium channel blockade by antibodies: a new mechanism of neurological disease. *Annals of Neurology*, **37**, 421–3.

Windebank, A.J. 1993: Metal neuropathy. In *Peripheral Neuropathy*, Dyck, P.J., Thomas, P.K., Griffin, J.W., Low, P. A. and Poduslo, J.F. (eds), 3rd edn, pp 1549–70. Philadelphia, PA: W.B. Saunders.

Windebank, A.J. and Bonkovsky, H.L. 1993: Porphyric neuropathy, In *Peripheral Neuropathy*, Dyck, P.J., Thomas, P.K., Griffin, J.W., Low, P.A. and Poduslo, J.F. (eds), 3rd edn, pp 1160–8. Philadelphia, PA: W.B. Saunders.

8

Neurological problems caused by envenoming bites and stings, and the consumption of poisonous seafood

AJITH GOONETILLEKE AND JOHN B HARRIS

INTRODUCTION

The natural environment is a hostile one, and numerous animals have evoked the ability to synthesize or accumulate toxic substances that will either enhance their ability to capture prey or protect them against a predator.

The majority of the toxins act on the nervous or cardiovascular systems. Those acting on the nervous system typically paralyze the hapless victim. The neurologist or neurotoxicologist is obviously likely to be involved in the management or treatment of the victim at an early stage, and a good understanding of the nature of clinical poisoning by natural venoms and toxins is essential if adequate treatment is to be made available.

Although incidents of poisoning by natural toxins is generally thought to be most common in the poorer countries of tropical and sub-tropical regions, it would be a mistake to consider this an esoteric branch of neurology or neurotoxicology. Private and institutional collections of venomous animals are common throughout the world, and in Western Europe bites by exotic venomous snakes are more common than bites by the indigenous viper, *Vipera berus*.

Moreover, the expanding trade in tropical seafood has resulted in the appearance of tropical seafood poisoning (for example, ciguatera) in locations such as Britain and France normally considered unaffected by such problems.

In this chapter we consider some of the neurological problems associated with bites, stings, and the consumption of poisonous seafood.

SNAKEBITE

Snakes are found in most regions of the world; those regions that are free of venomous snakes include the Arctic and Antarctic, Chile, and most of the islands of the western Mediterranean, Atlantic and Caribbean, including Madagascar, New Caledonia, New Zealand, Hawaii, Ireland, and Iceland. Approximately 3000 species of snake are known, and these are distributed between 13 families. Of the 3000 species known, only around 500 are known to be venomous. The venomous snakes are found in only six families:

1 Elapidae – cobras, kraits, mambas, coral snakes, Australasian venomous snakes;
2 Hydrophiidae – sea snakes;
3 Viperidae – vipers;
4 Crotalidae – pit vipers, rattlesnakes;
5 Atractaspididae – burrowing asps or stiletto snakes (a very small family);
6 Colubridae – only a few members of which are venomous.

The venom is introduced into the victim through a groove or closed channel in one or more pairs of enlarged fangs in the upper jaw (Figure 8.1, below and in color plate section). The venom glands of Elapidae, Hydrophiidae, Viperidae and Crotalidae are situated behind the eye, surrounded by compressor muscles. A duct opens at the base of the fang, and venom is conducted to its tip through a canal. In the Colubridae, venom is secreted by Duvernoy's gland, a secretory gland in the rear of the mouth, and then tracks along grooves in the anterior surfaces of the back fangs into the bite site.

Snake venoms may contain 20 or more components. More than 90% of the dry weight of venom is protein. The components may be enzymes, non-enzymatic toxins, and non-toxic proteins.

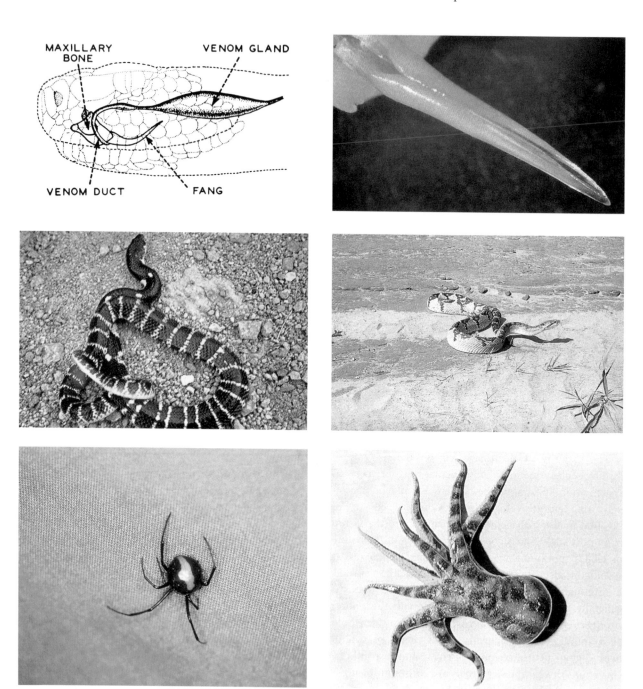

Figures 8.1–8.6 *(left–right). (1) Stylized head of viperid snake showing position of venom gland and fang folded against the roof of the mouth. (2) Fang of a typical venomous snake showing the opening at the tip of the fang. At the proximal end the venom duct connects the orifice of the fang to the venom gland. (3) Bungarus caeruleus, a typical elapid. Note the long, slender, light body. (4) Lachesis muta, a viperid snake of South America. Note the very heavy body typical of viperids and crotalids. (5) Latrodectus hasselti, the black widow spider of Australasia. (6) Octopus maculosa, the blue ringed octopus of Australia.*

Elapidae

All members of this family are venomous, but not all are dangerous to humans. The typical elapid snake is slender and agile and possesses short, immobile front fangs (Figure 8.3, opposite and in the color plate section). The African and Asian spitting cobras (for example, *Naja nigricollis, N. mossambica*) exhale as they eject their venom from the tips of the fangs. The fine spray of venom can be 'spat' for a distance of several meters into the eyes of their adversary. This results in local pain, swelling, blistering, and superficial necrosis, with painful enlargement of regional lymph nodes. In some instances corneal erosions have occurred.

The venom in elapid snakes is neurotoxic, and early symptoms of an envenoming bite by an elapid snake include recognized neurotoxic signs such as ptosis, blurred vision, hypersalivation, and piloerection ('goose-flesh'), in addition to more general effects such as headache, vomiting, perioral paraesthesia, hyperacusis, dizziness, vertigo, and congested conjunctivae. Ptosis and external ophthalmoplegia may appear as early as 15 min after the bite, but can be delayed for 120 h or more. Serious neuromuscular weakness may then become more widespread, respiratory failure occurring due to airway obstruction or, more commonly, paralysis of respiratory muscles.

Besides paralysis, envenoming bites by elapid snakes may be accompanied by defibrination, anticoagulation, hemolysis, rhabdomyolysis, and renal failure. Loin pain is a specific feature of envenoming bites by kraits and local necrosis, often very serious, is a common feature of envenoming bites by some species of cobra (especially *Naja kaouthia*).

Hydrophiidae

Sea snakes are closely related to the elapids, with which family they share many morphological features – slender agile bodies and short fixed fangs. They show considerable variation in the level of their adaptation to a marine environment, but all sea snakes possess salt glands, a paddle-shaped tail, eyes on the top of the head, and modified lungs. All sea snakes are venomous. They are relatively common throughout the tropical and warm temperate Pacific and Indian oceans. Envenoming appears to be declining in frequency, but whether this reflects declining numbers of snakes or a shift from manual to large-scale commercial fishing in the tropics is not clear.

Initial symptoms of envenomation include headache, thick feeling of the tongue, thirst, sweating, and vomiting. Generalized aching, stiffness, and muscle tenderness develops from between 30–200 min after the bite. Trismus is common. Later there is a generalized flaccid paralysis. Features of rhabdomyolysis and myoglobinuria may appear 3–8 h after the bite; myoglobin released from the damaged muscle may cause myoglobinuria and hyperkalemia, leading respectively to renal failure and cardiac arrest (Reid, 1979). It is not clear how commonly rhabdomyolysis occurs following an envenoming bite by a sea snake, and the absence of rhabdomyolysis following a putative sea-snake bite should not be considered counter-indicative of a positive diagnosis.

Viperidae and Crotalidae

These snakes possess long and curved fangs. The envenoming pair of fangs is mounted on a short maxillary bone that is capable of rotation. This ability to rotate allows the erection of the fang when the mouth is opened. When the mouth is closed the fangs are folded back against the roof of the mouth. Viperid and crotalid snakes tend to have a heavy head and body, a clear neck, and a short tail (Figure 8.4, opposite and in color plate section). The viperid snakes include the vipers and adders of Europe, Asia, and Africa. The crotalid snakes are pit vipers, possessing a heat-sensitive pit behind the nostril that is used to locate prey. The pit vipers include the rattlesnakes, moccasins, lance-headed vipers, and the Asian snakes of genus *Trimeresurus*. Viperid and crotalid snakes cause more human and animal deaths than any other group of snakes. Bites by Russell's viper probably kill more people in Asia than bites from the cobra, and the African puff adder is said to kill more people in Africa than deaths by all other animals put together.

Neurotoxicity is a significant and life-threatening feature of envenomation of only a few species of viperid or crotalid snakes, but envenoming bites by *Crotalus durrissus terrificus*, the Far Eastern *Agkistrodon sp.*, *Bitis atropos*, and Russell's viper of Sri Lanka can progress to respiratory or generalized paralysis. More typically envenomation by viperid or crotalid snakes produce the most severe local effects of all snakebites. Swelling spreads rapidly from the bite site, with associated pain and tenderness of local lymph nodes. If severe swelling occurs in a tight fascial compartment there may be ischemia leading to gangrene. Blistering and necrosis are particularly associated with bites by rattlesnakes, lance-headed vipers, Asian pit vipers, and African giant vipers. Hemostatic abnormalities are characteristic of envenomation by the crotalids, with spontaneous hemorrhages and persistent bleeding from puncture sites. If there is no swelling after 2 h of the bite it is often considered safe to assume there has been no envenomation, but fatal envenomation may occur in the absence of local effects, and all victims of snakebite should be observed for 24 h even in the absence of signs of envenoming.

Colubridae

This is the largest family of snakes containing within it about two-thirds of all known species of snake. Approximately 50% of colubrid snakes possess a Duvenoy's gland. This gland produces a secretion that is, in some species, toxic, and some of these snakes are potentially dangerous (for example, the boomslang (*Dispholidus typus*), the Japanese yamakagasi (*Rhabdophis tigrinus*), the south-east Asian red-necked keelback (*R. subminiatus*), and the Australasian brown tree snake (*Boiga irregularis*)).

Effects of envenomation may develop slowly over several days, and can range from local swelling and bruising to features of severe envenomation with repeated vomiting, abdominal colic, headache and widespread systemic bleeding, extensive ecchymoses, intravascular hemolysis, and renal failure. Only colubrids of the genus *Boiga* have been implicated in neurotoxic snake bite (Fritts *et al.*, 1990); bites by this snake can be fatal.

Atractaspididae

This small family includes the African and Middle Eastern burrowing asps or stiletto snakes (also known as burrowing or mole vipers, or adders). They strike sideways and impale their victims on a long front fang which protudes through a partially closed mouth.

Local effects include pain, swelling, blistering, necrosis, and tender enlargement of regional lymph nodes. Violent gastrointestinal effects (for example, nausea, vomiting, diarrhea), anaphylatic-like pathology (dyspnea, respiratory failure) and electrocardiogram (ECG) changes (AV block, ST- and T-wave changes) may occur after envenomation. Neurotoxic symptoms are rarely, if ever, reported.

Neurotoxic components of snake venoms

The primary objective of snake venom is to allow the envenoming snake to overcome the prey item and to initiate digestion. Snakes producing a neurotoxic venom achieve the first objective by causing neuromuscular weakness. The target sites involved are the acetylcholine receptors on the postjunctional membrane of the muscle fiber, and the motor nerve terminal. Myotoxic activity, which causes neuromuscular weakness by destroying motor axons and muscle fibers, is probably best considered an expression of the second objective, the initiation of the digestive process.

TOXINS TARGETING ACETYLCHOLINE RECEPTORS

The acetylcholine receptor at the vertebrate neuromuscular junction is a four subunit pentamer ($2 \times \alpha$, β, γ, δ). The two α-subunits contain the binding sites for the neurotransmitter, ACh. Each α-subunit possesses a number of alternative binding sites for neurotoxins targeting the receptor.

The postsynpatically active neurotoxins are relatively small polypeptides. There are two major groups of such toxins, those comprising 60–62 amino acids (short neurotoxins) and those comprising 64–74 amino acids (long neurotoxins). The short and long neurotoxins differ in certain aspects with respect to the number and positioning of disulfide bridges.

The toxins bind with very high affinity and very selectively to the α-subunits of the acetylcholine receptor, thus blocking access to the receptor by the natural transmitter. The onset of paralysis is rapid.

Postsynaptically active neurotoxins are ubiquitous components of the venoms of elapid and hydrophiid snakes, but are probably completely absent from the venom of snakes of other families.

THE PRESYNAPTICALLY ACTIVE NEUROTOXINS

The presynaptically active neurotoxins target a site or sites on the presynaptic nerve terminal. The precise target site is the subject of much controversy, and has not been properly identified. There are probably multiple sites, some involved in the depletion of transmitter and the destruction of the nerve terminal, some blocking transmitter release and some accelerating transmitter release.

The presynaptically active phospholipases of snake venoms are by far the most important of the presynaptically active neurotoxins. There are two major classes of toxic phospholipases. Class I phospholipases are constituents of elapid snake venoms. These toxins are homologues of pancreatic phospholipases and are probably derived from them. Structurally distinct but very similar toxic phospholipases (Class II phospholipases) in the venoms of viperid and crotalid snake venoms are homologues of cytosolic phospholipases (see Harris, 1997 for an introduction).

The presynaptically active phospholipases are important constituents of the elapid snakes of Australia, Irian Jaya/Papua New Guinea and the kraits of southeast Asia, and of a number of viperid and crotalid snakes including *Daboia russelli*, *Vipera ammodytes*, *Crotalus durrissus terrificus*, and *Bothrops asper*. It is probable that they are common constituents in a range of venoms. The toxicity of this large group of toxins is very variable. The most toxic have LD_{50} in the range of μg per mouse, and such high toxicity ensures that they are clinically important. Some, however, have much lower toxicity and their biological activity is likely to be overshadowed by other manifestations of envenomation including postsynaptic neurotoxicity and hematological disturbances.

It is commonly stated that the neurotoxic phospho-lipases either block transmitter release from the motor nerve terminal or block transmitter synthesis, thus effecting a failure of neuromuscular transmission. It now seems probable that their most common mode of action is first to deplete nerve terminals of stored transmitter and then to initiate the destruction of the motor nerve terminal and the intramuscular axons (Dixon and Harris, 1998).

Victims of envenoming bites by snakes whose venoms contain large quantities of highly toxic phospholipases – typical snakes include the taipans and kraits – would be expected to present with rapid onset, prolonged weakness, the prolonged phase only being resolved when the damaged axons regenerate and re-innervate the skeletal muscle.

Facilitatory toxins, that enhance the release of the transmitter, have been identified only in the venoms of the mambas, *Dendroaspis* sp. Their clinical significance is unclear.

MYOTOXIC TOXINS

The most important myotoxic toxins are the toxic phospholipases. Most of the presynaptically active neurotoxic phospholipases are myotoxic; β-bungaro-toxin from the venom of the snakes of the genus *Bungarus* (the kraits) is one of few exceptions, as a neurotoxic phospholipase without myotoxic activity. Myotoxic phospholipases are found principally in the venoms of the sea-snakes and the elapids of Australasia, but myotoxic phospholipases are found in the venoms of a number of viperid and crotalid snakes.

Many venoms of viperid and crotalid snakes contain non-hydrolytic phospholipase homologues that are myotoxic (for example, *Bothrops* sp.; *Ammodytes* sp.) and many crotalids elaborate small non-hydrolytic myotoxic polypeptides.

The mechanism of action of the myotoxic phospho-lipases is not well understood; the consequences of an envenoming bite by snakes whose venoms contain high levels of myotoxic toxins are the same, whichever myotoxin is inoculated – muscle pain, rhabdomyolysis, myoglobinuria and weakness that is resolved only by the regeneration of the muscle.

Other neurological signs

Bleeding into the central nervous system (CNS) is relatively uncommon, but bites by Russell's viper, *Daboia russellii*, in Burma (Myanmur) and Thailand can be associated with bleeding into the pituitary. The resulting neurological syndrome can develop several months after the bite (Warrell, 1991), presenting with coma and Addisonian crisis or panhypopituitarism. The toxins responsible for bleeding into the CNS have

not been identified. Such pathology has not been seen in experimental animals and is, therefore, very difficult to study.

Treatment of neurotoxic snake bite

It is important to understand that a serious envenoming bite results in the inoculation of a complex mixture of toxic and non-toxic, but foreign, polypeptides. The symptoms of an envenoming bite are, therefore, always complex, involving, in most cases, local pain, coagulation defects, swelling of the bitten limb, vomiting, hypotension, and shock. Local necrosis may follow and result in the loss of large areas of skin. Hemorrhage, involving bleeding from the gums, eyes, anus, nose, etc. can be life threatening, especially if much bleeding is internal and neurotoxic signs – especially ptosis, weakness and respiratory distress – will need urgent attention.

The 'typical' symptomology of envenoming bites by some major classes of snake are summarized in Table 8.1.

The rate of onset and the severity of an envenoming bite is dependent on a number of variables – the species of snake, the size of the victim, the location of the bite, the volume of venom inoculated are among the most obvious variables. Since venom is usually inoculated only into superficial soft tissues, systemic signs of envenoming can only become apparent as venom is absorbed from the bite site. This is usually a rapid process (i.e. a few minutes only) because venom may be distributed via both the vascular and the lymphatic systems, but uptake may be delayed, with consequential delays in the expression of envenoming.

Treatment may be conveniently considered in two parts: first aid and emergency treatment, and clinic-based care.

FIRST AID

The victim of a snake bite – even if the bite is by a non-venomous snake – will be fearful and anxious, and will often display signs not incompatible with an envenoming bite, for example anxiety, nausea, headache and possibly hypotension. The patient should be reassured and calmed, the bitten limb should be immobilized by a supportive bandage, bound as tightly as if the limb had been sprained, and splinted if possible. These measures may delay the distribution of venom.

The bite site should not be cut or sucked and no incisions should be made in areas around the bite site. No foreign materials (for example leaves, barks or mud) or chemicals (for example potassium permanganate) should be applied to the wound. The limb should not be frozen or packed with ice and a tourniquet should never be applied. All of these procedures are potentially

Table 8.1 *Major signs of systemic poisoning following an envenoming snake bite*

Sign	Viperid/crotalid	Elapid
Loss of coagulation	Common	Common
Bleeding	Common	Common
Hemorrhage	Common	Uncommon
Local blistering and necrosis	Common	Uncommon
Swelling of bitten limb	Common	Uncommon
Myonecrosis and rhabdomyolysis	Uncommon (except for crotalids and some viperids of N. and S. America)	Uncommon (except for elapids of Australasia)
Pain at bite site	Common	Common
Sudden collapse	Common	Common
Ptosis	Common	Common
Severe respiratory distress	Uncommon	Common
Intercranial bleeding	Uncommon	Uncommon

This guide to signs might allow the differentiation between an envenoming bite by a viperid and an elapid snake. Note, however, that this is a very broad generalization. Most snakebites result in a complex syndrome characterized by anxiety and fear, pain, local reactions, coagulopathies, and neuromuscular weakness.

dangerous. Cutting, for example, can introduce infection and may also lead to uncontrolled bleeding. Tourniquets may delay the onset of neurotoxic symptoms but can cause additional complications if an envenoming bite is associated with local necrosis. Improperly applied tourniquets, which comprise the majority applied in the field, probably cause more damage than the bite. A discussion on the use of tourniquets in the treatment of snakebite is available (Amaral *et al.*, 1998).

Pain should not be treated with narcotic analgesics because of the danger of depressing respiration; patients should be encouraged to stay conscious.

When possible, a clear description of the offending snake should be obtained. If the snake has been killed, it should be kept for formal identification. It is a common mistake to assume that local people can accurately differentiate between venomous and non-venomous snakes. In most surveys, 50–80% of victims of snakebite have been bitten by non-venomous snakes, or by lizards.

In many countries where snakebite is common, rural victims of snakebite are wary of the cost of medical treatment and doubt its efficacy. For these reasons, large numbers visit a local healer, whose arts may consist of the application of herbs and barks, the chanting of incantations or the performance of elaborate ceremonies. Details of their treatments are rarely disclosed. They may be dangerous, especially when cutting is involved and where tourniquets are applied; they may delay attendance of a seriously ill patient at a clinic; they may be harmless.

Once a patient has been transported to hospital or clinic, care should be conservative. Patients should be kept under constant supervision for 24 h and checked for sudden onset neuromuscular weakness or respirat-

ory or cardiac failure, changes in blood pressure, spontaneous bleeding from the gums, bite site or body orifices or other untoward signs.

Swabs of the bitten area and blood samples should be kept for the detection of venom antigens. This is usually done using immunological techniques, such as enzyme-linked immunosorbent assay (ELISA), and is the only definite way of identifying the offending snake in the absence of the actual animal.

Ptosis is the first sign of neurotoxicity, followed by aphonia, exophthalmoplegia, neuromuscular weakness, and respiratory distress. Muscle damage is associated with muscle pain and black urine as the result of loss of myoglobin.

Treatment should consist of the appropriate anti-venom (ideally an anti-venom designed to be active against the venoms of local snakes). The same dose should be given to children and adults (snakes do not modify the volume of venom inoculated according to the size of the victim). The anti-venoms should be given diluted in normal saline or similar, slowly and with cover available to control untoward immune reactions. Anti-venoms should not be inoculated into the bite site – it is an inefficient route of administration and may lead to additional local reactions.

Anticholinesterases are of potential value in the case of bites by snakes whose primary weapon is postsynaptically active toxins (for example many cobras).

Treatment can be difficult if presynaptically active or myotoxic toxins are present in the venom (for example kraits and taipans), and patients may require intensive care for several days. Artificial ventilation may be life saving in cases of elapid bites, but may be required for several hours. Manual ventilation (for example by using an Ambu bag) has been shown to be as effective as mechanical ventilation if the latter is unavailable.

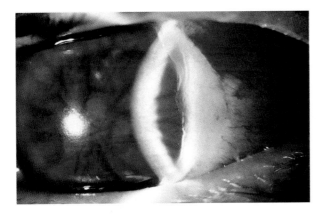

Figure 4.1 *Limbal ischemia.*

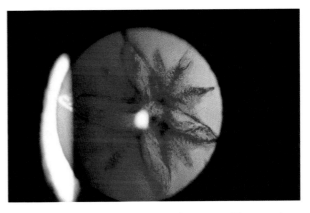

Figure 4.5 *Posterior subcapsular cataract induced by steroids.*

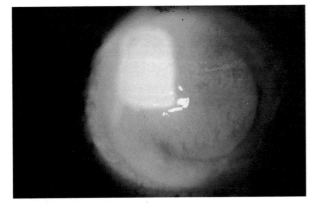

Figure 4.2 *Epithelial erosion following caustic burn.*

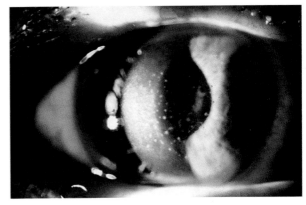

Figure 4.6 *Iridocyclitis with KP formation.*

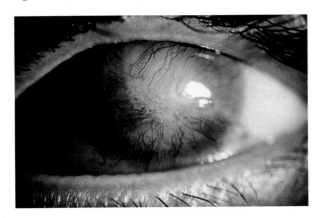

Figure 4.3 *Severe corneal vascularization following alkali burn.*

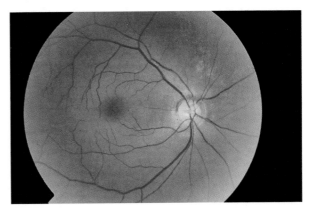

Figure 4.7 *Bull's-eye maculopathy from chloroquine.*

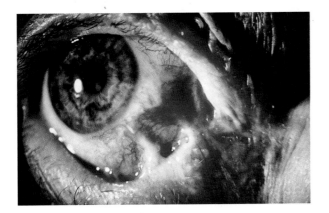

Figure 4.4 *Symblepharon formation in lower fornix.*

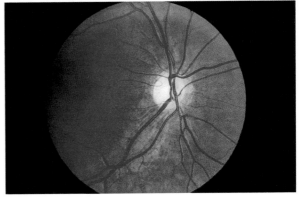

Figure 4.8 *Optic atrophy.*

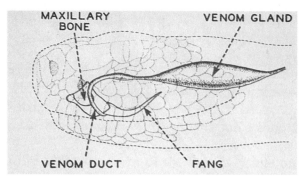

Figure 8.1 *Stylized head of viperid snake showing position of venom gland and fang folded against the roof of the mouth.*

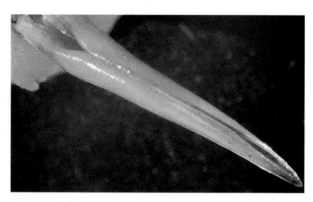

Figure 8.2 *Fang of a typical venomous snake showing the opening at the tip of the fang. At the proximal end the venom duct connects the orifice of the fang to the venom gland.*

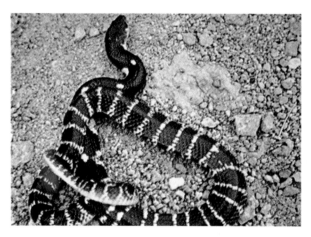

Figure 8.3 Bungarus caeruleus, *a typical elapid. Note the long, slender, light body.*

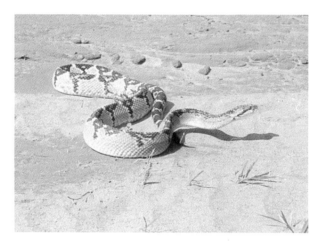

Figure 8.4 Lachesis muta, *a viperid snake of South America. Note the very heavy body typical of viperids and crotalids.*

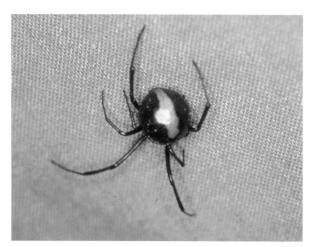

Figure 8.5 Latrodectus hasselti, *the black widow spider of Australasia.*

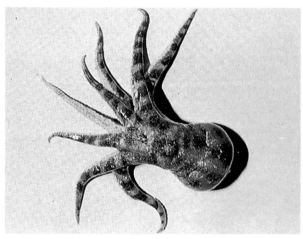

Figure 8.6 Octopus maculosa, *the blue ringer octopus of Australia.*

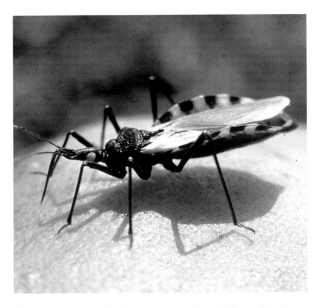

Figure 9.1 *A tsetse fly. (Courtesy of the The Wellcome Trust.)*

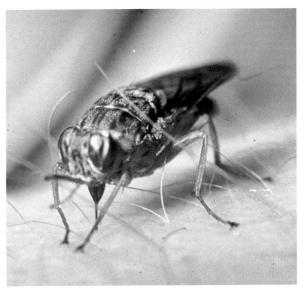

Figure 9.2 *The assassin bug. (Courtesy of the The Wellcome Trust.)*

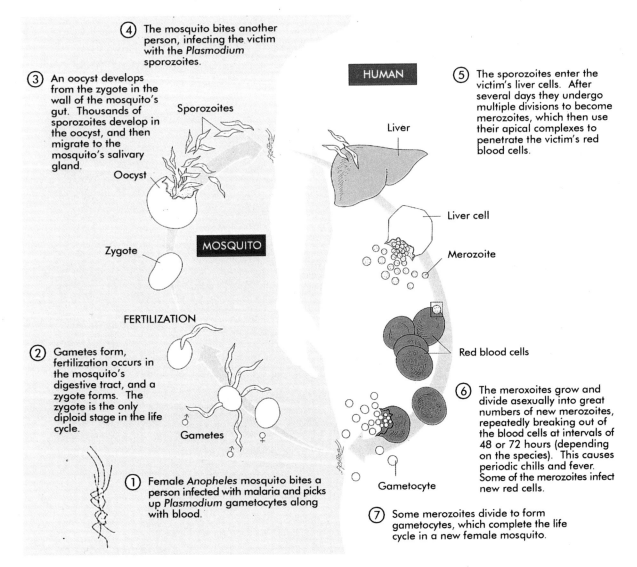

④ The mosquito bites another person, infecting the victim with the *Plasmodium* sporozoites.

③ An oocyst develops from the zygote in the wall of the mosquito's gut. Thousands of sporozoites develop in the oocyst, and then migrate to the mosquito's salivary gland.

Sporozoites

Oocyst

Zygote

MOSQUITO

FERTILIZATION

② Gametes form, fertilization occurs in the mosquito's digestive tract, and a zygote forms. The zygote is the only diploid stage in the life cycle.

Gametes

♂ ♀

♂

① Female *Anopheles* mosquito bites a person infected with malaria and picks up *Plasmodium* gametocytes along with blood.

HUMAN

⑤ The sporozoites enter the victim's liver cells. After several days they undergo multiple divisions to become merozoites, which then use their apical complexes to penetrate the victim's red blood cells.

Liver

Liver cell

Merozoite

Red blood cells

⑥ The meroxoites grow and divide asexually into great numbers of new merozoites, repeatedly breaking out of the blood cells at intervals of 48 or 72 hours (depending on the species). This causes periodic chills and fever. Some of the merozoites infect new red cells.

Gametocyte

⑦ Some merozoites divide to form gametocytes, which complete the life cycle in a new female mosquito.

Figure 9.3 *The life cycle of the malarial parasite. Amended from Campbell. Permission sought from Benjamin Cummings Inc.*

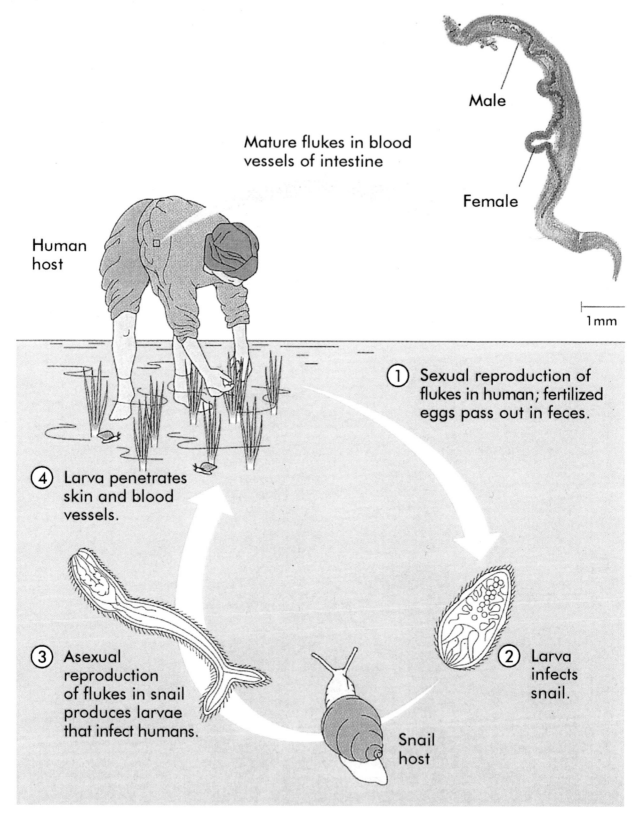

Male

Female

Mature flukes in blood
vessels of intestine

Human
host

1mm

① Sexual reproduction of
flukes in human; fertilized
eggs pass out in feces.

④ Larva penetrates
skin and blood
vessels.

③ Asexual
reproduction
of flukes in snail
produces larvae
that infect humans.

② Larva
infects
snail.

Snail
host

Figure 9.4 *The life cycle of the blood fluke Schistosome. Amended from Campbell. Permission sought from Benjamin Cummings Inc.*

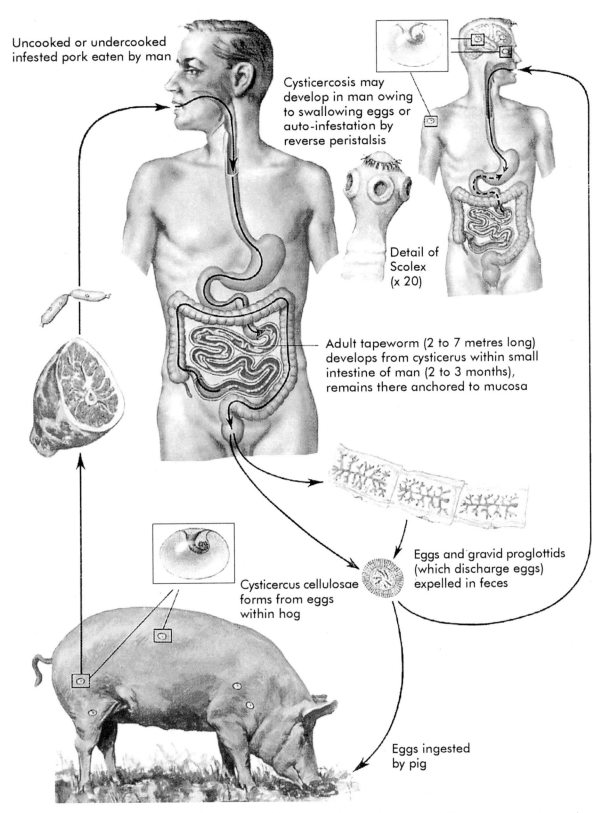

Uncooked or undercooked infested pork eaten by man

Cysticercosis may develop in man owing to swallowing eggs or auto-infestation by reverse peristalsis

Detail of Scolex (x 20)

Adult tapeworm (2 to 7 metres long) develops from cysticerus within small intestine of man (2 to 3 months), remains there anchored to mucosa

Eggs and gravid proglottids (which discharge eggs) expelled in feces

Cysticercus cellulosae forms from eggs within hog

Eggs ingested by pig

Figure 9.5 *The life cycle of the pork tapeworm. Reproduced from* The CIBA Collection of Medical Illustrations. *Permission sought from Novartis Pharmaceuticals Corp.*

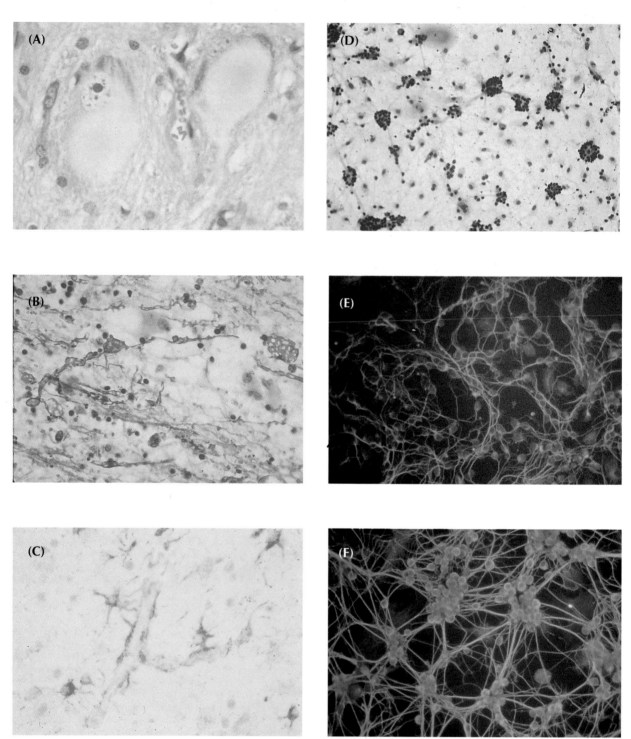

Figure 18.11 *(A) Central chromatolysis of neurons within the brain stem following trimethyllead intoxication. Note the balloon distension with eccentric nuclei, preserved nucleoli and loss of Nissl material from central region with preservation at the periphery H&E. (B) Solvent-induced leukoencephalopathy. Note the extensive demyelination throughout white matter with irregular myelin digestive chamber formation, some of which reveal fenestration. Hypertrophic astrocytes are present. Kluver–Barerra stain. (C) Reactive astrocytes aligned adjacent to capillary endothelium within cerebral cortex. Individual fibrillary fortive processes are apposed onto endothelium. Gliofibrillary acidic protein (GFAP) immunohistochemistry. (D) Rat cerebellar granule cell culture (14 DIV). Note the evenly separated neuronal aggregates with ill-defined connecting neurite bundles. Crystal violet. (E) Cytoskeletal microtubules revealed in neurites of developing cerebellar granule cell culture. The β-tubulin isoform has been selectively demonstrated with appropriate antibody using FITC immunofluorescence. (F) β-Tubulin immunofluorescence in cerebellar granule cell culture following 24 h incubation with 0.5 μM methyl mercury. Note the irregular neurite organization with thinning and fragmentation suggesting selective effect of a mercurial on microtubule structure during early morphogenesis. β-Tubulin FITC-immunofluorescence.*

Studies of the dynamics of antigen/antibody inter-actions have shown conclusively that multiple doses of anti-venom may be required to control circulating levels of venom. Anti-venom should therefore be used as often as necessary until the patient shows no sign of relapsing.

The use of anti-venom is relatively contraindicated in atopic patients and those who have reacted previously to equine antisera – these groups are at increased risk of developing severe reactions, and should only receive anti-venom if there are clear signs of severe systemic envenomation. Complications following the use of anti-venom include fever, which can result from contamination, but such reactions are becoming less common with the introduction of newer anti-venoms. Early anaphylactic-type reactions (for example itching, urticaria, cough, nausea, vomiting, fever, tachycardia) develop within 10–180 min of the injection; up to 40% with early reactions go on to develop systemic anaphylaxis with hypotension, bronchospasm, and angio-edema (Malasit *et al.*, 1986). Treatment of the anaphylactic reaction includes the use of adrenaline and antihistamines. Deaths from these reactions are rare. Late serum sickness-type reactions (for example fever, urticaria, arthralgia, lymphadenopathy, mononeuritis multiplex, encephalopathy) can develop 5–24 days after the use of antitoxin, and may be treated with steroids and antihistamines.

SCORPION STINGS

Scorpions are common throughout the tropical and sub-tropical world and in warmer temperate regions such as southern North America and southern Europe. Many scorpions are harmless to man or cause little more than a painful sting. Some, however, are very dangerous and have been implicated in fatal envenomations.

The systematics of scorpions is complex. Most of the dangerous species belong to the family Buthidae. This is a large family with two sub-families, the Old World Buthinae and the New World Titynae. Scorpions regularly involved in fatal neurotoxic envenoming are those of genera *Androctanus*, *Buthus*, *Buthacus*, and *Leirus* (north Africa and the Middle East), *Parabuthus* (South Africa), *Mesobuthus* (India), and *Tityus* and *Centruroides* (North, Central and South America and Trinidad).

The sting of a scorpion is attached to the last segment of the body. It consists of a bulbous base that contains two venom glands. On this base, and connected to the venom glands, is the hollow, curved sting. The entire structure is known as the telson.

The contractions of a muscular septum, which separates the pair of venom glands, forces out the venom from near the apex of the telson during the sting. The scorpion venoms stimulate the sustained and non-selective release of neurotransmitters such as acetylcholine and catecholamines from nerve terminals. It is commonly assumed that the initiation of transmitter release is responsible for most of the clinical problems associated with scorpion stings, but the accuracy of that view has not been critically tested.

Intense local pain is the commonest symptom following a scorpion sting, although on occasions this may be minimal or absent. The pain usually starts as a tingling or burning at the sting site, and may progress proximally. Mild local edema and tender enlargement of lymph nodes may occur. The onset of systemic effects may vary from a few minutes up to 24 h. Initial systemic effects tend to be predominantly cholinergic, and include vomiting, profuse sweating, piloerection ('gooseflesh'), intermittent brady- or tachyarrhythmias, abdominal colic, diarrhea, loss of sphincter control, and priapism. Subsequently adrenergic symptoms develop, such as hypertension, shock, tachyarrhythmias, ECG changes, pulmonary edema and myocardial dysfunction (Gueron *et al.*, 1992). Convulsions are commoner in infants and young children (Waterman, 1938). Acute pancreatitis and pancreatic cysts have also been described (Waterman, 1938). Although the duration of symptoms is usually 24–48 h, neurological features may last up to one week. Rapid progression of symptoms in the first 2–4 h after the sting indicates a poor outcome. Survival after 48 h is usually followed by recovery, although deaths have been recorded up to four days after the sting.

Mortality is greatest in young children. In the cane fields and the cocoa plantations of Trinidad, stings by *Tityus trinitatis* are an occupational hazard; there was an overall mortality of 4.7% following 698 bites during 1929–1933, with a mortality rate of 25% in children less than five years old compared to 0.25% in adults over 21 years (Waterman, 1938). In Brazil mortality is 15–25% in children less than six years compared to 1% in adults. In the Colima state of Mexico there are 1000–2000 deaths per year (incidence of 84 deaths/100 000/year), with a mortality rate of 50% in children less than four years old. Mortality rates are declining with increasing availability of anti-venoms, but remain high in many regions.

The venoms of scorpions are complex, and few samples of venom have been systematically analyzed. There is little doubt that most venoms contain a number of distinct neurotoxic polypeptides targeting specific ion channels as well as other toxins that are responsible for hematological disturbances, cardiac myotoxicity, edema, etc. These complexities give rise to a number of associated symptoms that contribute to the overall syndrome. Some general points can be made with respect to particular genera.

Buthus

This genus occurs throughout Southern Europe, Africa, and the Middle East. The best known species is *B. occitanus*, which is divided into two races. The northern race (southern France, Spain, and Portugal) possesses a mild venom which is not of major clinical significance, whereas the southern race (North Africa, Middle East) has a highly toxic venom. Stings by this southern race are extremely painful and give rise to cardiovascular complications. Other features of the syndrome include thirst, urinary retention, pupillary dilatation, and aphonia.

Leiurus

This genus is very common in the Middle East and north Africa, the most notable species being *L. quinquestriatus*. This species produces a very painful sting. Cardiac and respiratory failure is commonly seen in addition to muscle spasms and twitching, excessive sweating, lacrimation, priapism, and irritability.

Centruroides

This genus is found in the New World, and two species have been imported into west Africa. All species are nocturnal, and often inhabit human dwellings. The most important species is *C. sculpturatus*, which produces a painful but almost invisible sting. The venom has neurotoxic effects, producing fasciculation, spasms, respiratory paralysis, and convulsions (Curry *et al.*, 1983); death may occur from cardiovascular collapse due to myocarditis. Although hematological disturbances from scorpion bites are uncommon, venom from *C. sculpturatus* can prolong platelet aggregation in children (Longnecker and Longnecker, 1981). Other features seen include nervousness, hyper-salivation, gastric distension, and temporary visual impairment (blurring, temporary blindness).

Androctonus

This genus is found widely over North Africa and the Middle East. The most notable species for causing human envenomation is *A. australis*, causing 80% of all stings on humans in north Africa. Symptoms are similar to envenomation by *B. occitanus* (vide supra).

Tityus

This genus occurs throughout most of South America and the Caribbean. Important species include *T. serrulatus*, *T. bahiensis*, *T. trivittatus*, and *T. trinitatis*.

The sting causes local burning pain which characteristically spreads to involve the whole limb. The pain may last several hours but resolves, in most cases, within 24 h. In more severe cases the patient may experience numbness, tightness around the throat, speech difficulties, and involuntary muscle twitching. Death may result from respiratory paralysis. Stings by the Trinidadian species causes severe abdominal pain, pancreatitis, hematemesis, hyperglycemia, and cardiac irregularity.

Heterometrus

This genus includes many species of large jungle scorpions, which are often kept as pets. The effects of stings are milder than those from the Buthidae. Local pain and a burning sensation occur at the sting site. Nose itching, salivation, and labored breathing may occur in milder cases. More severe stings cause local swelling, hemorrhage, and muscle paralysis in the affected limb; cardiovascular symptoms are prevalent. Symptoms generally disappear within 24 h, although fatalities have been recorded.

Treatment of scorpion stings

Treatment is generally supportive. Pain at the sting site can be relieved by local infiltration or ring lock. Although a local injection of emetine or dehydroemetine has been advocated, it can also cause soft tissue necrosis. Parenteral opioids may be considered, but their use can be dangerous in victims of neurotoxic envenoming. Treatment may also be required to control any cardiac arrhythmias. Atropine should be avoided except in cases of life-threatening sinus bradycardia. The use of cardiac glycosides and β-blockers is controversial. Anticonvulsants (for example phenobarbitone) have been recommended for central 'neurotoxic' effects.

If specific anti-venom is available it should be administered as soon as possible to young children stung by dangerous species or to patients with systemic involvement, although the efficacy of such treatment is debatable if delayed for more than 2 h after the sting. If given early (i.e. within 30 min) to patients with systemic manifestations of envenomation, complete recovery may occur within 2–3 h and overall mortality is reduced (Dehesa-Davila, 1989).

BITES BY SPIDERS

Spiders bite prey or potential predators with fangs mounted on the chelicerae. With the exception of one small family, the Uloboridae, the fangs are attached to venom glands that are located within the basal segments of the chelicerae and may extend back into the head.

When the spider bites, the fangs are raised and then stabbed into the prey. Simultaneously the muscles surrounding the venom glands contract and venom is inoculated.

Most spiders are not medically important; their fangs are too small and fragile to penetrate human skin and their venom's are of no significance to humans. The diagnosis of spider bites is notoriously difficult, but there is little doubt that only three genera are of significant interest to the neurologist or neurotoxicologist.

Latrodectus

The genus *Latrodectus* comprises the redback spiders, known throughout the warm-temperate sub-tropical and tropical world. Many species of *Latrodectus* are known to be dangerous; possibly all are. Bites usually occur when the spiders are disturbed. It is not an aggressive animal.

Bites by this spider have been responsible for many fatalities in southern Europe, North America and Australia, especially before the availability of anti-venom. Bites are still common – for example more than 200 bites per year are recorded in Australia, although fatalities are now very rare.

The species most frequently associated with medically important bites are *Latrodectus mactans* (the Americas), *Latrodectus hasselti* (Australasia and New Zealand (Figure 8.5 above and in color plate section), and *Latrodectus tredecimguttatus* (southern Europe).

Bites by Latrodectus are usually very painful and needle-like, but local signs may be minimal (*L. mactans*) or moderate (*L. hasselti*). About 30 min later there is a painful enlargement of local lymph nodes, followed by headache, nausea, vomiting, sweating, and piloerection. Painful muscle spasms and cramps spread throughout the body, leading to rigidity of abdominal, chest, and back muscles; respiration may be impaired if involvement is severe. Other features include constipation, tachycardia, hypotension, restlessness, irritability, psychosis, priapism, and rhabdomyolysis. The 'facies latrodectismica' refers to the painful grimace caused by facial spasm and trismus associated with swollen eyelids, conjunctival congestion, flushing, and sweating following envenomation by *L. tredecimguttatus*. The duration of illness in untreated cases is usually one week, although convalescence may last a month or more. The mortality in untreated cases is said to be 5% (Ori, 1982), most fatal cases involving children weighing less than 15 kg.

Phoneutria

This aggressive South American genus includes the two well known species *P. fera* and *P. nigriventer*. Their common name (wandering or banana spiders) reflects their habits. These spiders hunt actively for prey and do not construct a web. This method of hunting can often lead them into human dwellings, especially during winter months when the warmth is an added attraction. Bites can occur when they get into clothing and bedding. Their alternative name of banana spider reflects their occurrence on bunches of bananas, resulting in a high incidence of bites from such spiders in plantation workers. Such spiders may also be inadvertently exported with shipments of bananas, and bites have been recorded by this means in various destinations of such shipments (Trestrail, 1983).

The bite is extremely painful, producing a local burning sensation. The pain then spreads proximally in the limb to the trunk. Other features of envenomation include tachycardia, hypertension, fever, nausea, vomiting, vertigo, sweating, temporary blindness, respiratory distress, and paralysis. Hypothermia and priapism have also been recorded (Trestrail, 1983). Death is most likely to occur within the first 6 h of envenomation, and is due to respiratory failure. After this time the chances of survival are good, and a healthy adult will usually recover within 48 h.

Atrax

The genus *Atrax* was once used to include all known Australasian funnel web spiders, but they are now included in two genera: *Atrax* and *Hadronyche*.

Atrax includes the most notorious of the funnel web spider, *Atrax robustus*.

Atrax robustus is a large spider with a restricted range enclosed within a 160 km radius of Sydney. The male spider is the dangerous animal, typically encountered when it is searching for a receptive female (Sutherland, 1984).

The bite is extremely painful due to the long fangs and the acidic venom. The pain can last for a few days but there is no necrosis.

The venom is potently neurotoxic, initiating the release of transmitters from the autonomic and somatic nervous systems. Symptoms appear within 10 min of the bite with perioral anesthesia and fasciculation, and spasm of the tongue. This is followed by nausea, vomiting, abdominal pain, diarrhea, sweating, salivation, lacrimation, fasciculation and spasm of skeletal muscles, respiratory difficulties, and visual disturbances. There may also be rapid changes from hypo- to hypertension. Fatalities are rare because of the availability of anti-venom, but untreated victims can die as late as six days after the bite, usually of an insidious progressive hypotension that leads to heart failure.

The toxins of spider venoms

The toxins of spider venoms are typically small polypeptides, evolved for the subduing, killing or partial digestion of invertebrate prey. The venoms contain very rich supplies of proteases. Some of the neurotoxins – particularly those elaborated by *Latrodectus* – are extremely large toxins that precipitate the accelerated release of neurotransmitters. Because few of the toxins of spider venoms are of direct relevance to human toxicology, they are not discussed further.

Treatment of spider bites

Immediate first-aid measures for the seriously envenomed patient include maintenance of the airway and respiration. First aid should consist of reassurance, and splinting or immobilization of the bitten limb. This aspect is particularly important in cases involving rapidly acting and potent venoms from spiders such as *Atrax robustus*. Minor analgesics can be used to control pain. Calcium gluconate relieves the pain of muscle spasms caused by *Latrodectus* venom rapidly and more effectively than muscle relaxants (for example diazepam, methocarbamol). Atropine and diazepam are effective for funnel-web spider bites. Corticosteroids relieve symptoms, but have no effect on overall mortality. Specific anti-venoms for *Latrodectus* (made in Australia, USA, Russian Federation, Italy, Yugoslavia, South Africa, and South America), *Phoneutria* (Brazil) and *Atrax* (Australia) are available for seriously envenomed patients. They should be used with usual precautions to minimize adverse reactions.

ACARI

Approximately 25 000 species of ticks and mites collectively form the order Acari of the class Arachnida. Adult females of about 34 out of approximately 650 species of hard ticks (family *Ixodidae*) and immature specimens of nine out of approximately 170 species of soft ticks (family *Argasidae*) have been implicated in human tick paralysis.

Human tick paralysis occurs most commonly in eastern Australia from north Queensland to Victoria, and western and eastern North America. In Australia, where the disorder is often referred to as bush or scrub paralysis, most human cases are due to *Ixodes holocyclus*; there has been one case of a three-year-old boy requiring ventilation after envenomation by *I. cornuatus* (Tibballs and Cooper, 1986). In North America different species of tick are involved in cases of tick paralysis in western and eastern areas (*Dermacentor andersoni* and *D. variabilis*, respectively).

Tick paralysis is caused by neurotoxins in the tick's saliva. The toxins are introduced by the prominent barbed hypostome and two hooked chelicerae which are inserted into the host's tissues when the tick embeds itself into the skin and engorges itself with blood. Paralysis in the host usually develops as the tick becomes fully engorged. The primary neurotoxin of *Ixodes* is a protein with a molecular weight of 40 000–80 000 (Stone, 1988), and causes a presynaptic neuromuscular block, possibly by reducing calcium availability and thereby impairing the excitation–secretion coupling at the neuromuscular junction (Cooper and Spence, 1976). There is also evidence for autonomic and central involvement but the signs and symptoms are not well defined.

Ticks can be picked up from the countryside or from domestic animals, particularly dogs; in Australia *I. holocyclus* is therefore also known as the dog tick. The majority of patients, and almost all fatal cases, are children. Initial symptoms include anorexia, lethargy, and irritability. Vomiting is a feature of the more acute course associated with *Ixodes holocyclus*. Five to six days after the tick bite the victim may develop a progressive ascending lower motor neurone paralysis with paraesthesiae. Ticks embedded behind the ear or in the external auditory meatus are a well-recognized cause of unilateral facial weakness (Hamilton, 1940; Pearn, 1977). The diagnosis depends on finding the tick, which may prove difficult as it is likely to be concealed in a crevice, orifice or hairy area of the body. The scalp is a common site. Fatal tick paralysis has been caused by a single tick attached to the tympanic membrane.

Tick-bite paralysis caused by the North American ticks is similar to that seen in Australia, but there is no information on the toxins involved.

In the absence of definitive features, a fretful, irritable child exhibiting progressive neuromuscular weakness should be considered as possibly carrying a tick.

Diagnosis can be confused with Guillain–Barré syndrome, snakebite, tetrodotoxic poisoning, myasthenia gravis, Lambert–Eaton syndrome, poliomyelitis, paralytic rabies, and infantile botulism. A good guide to differential diagnosis is provided by Grattan-Smith *et al.*, 1997.

Treatment consists of carefully detaching the tick whilst keeping the tick intact and causing as little trauma as possible. Killing the tick with pyrethrin-based insecticides prior to removal may help. Older techniques – applying heat, lighted matches, alcohol, etc. – should be avoided.

Following tick removal there is usually a rapid and complete recovery in cases involving *D. andersoni* and *D. variabilis* (Garrettson, 1984), but in cases involving *I. holocyclus*, maximal weakness may not be reached until 48 h after the tick has been removed, and recovery may take several weeks. A hyperimmune serum prepared from dogs, available since 1935, is the standard treatment for paralyzed animals. More recently rabbits have been used to produce an antitoxin against *I. holocyclus* saliva. Antitoxin use is not very effective and is associated with a high incidence of acute allergy and serum sickness. It is therefore only recommended for those at exceptionally high risk, such as severely affected, very young patients. Fatalities are rare.

POISONOUS AMPHIBIANS

The moist skin of amphibians is an accessory respiratory organ, and is protected by highly toxic secretions. The skin of the 'poison dart frogs' (*Dendrobatidae*) of Central and South America contains steroidal toxins known as batrachotoxins. These toxins cause the activation of sodium channels, resulting in muscular paralyis. The skin secretions are used by some Colombian Indians to coat the tips of their hunting darts (Myers *et al.*, 1978). The skin of three species of newts (genus *Taricha*) from the western United States contain 'tarichatoxins', identical to the tetrodotoxins found in marine fish (vide infra-tetrodotoxin poisoning). Tetrodotoxins can be absorbed through the gastric mucosa. A man who swallowed a 20 cm long Oregon rough-skinned newt (*Taricha granulosa*) developed perioral paresthesia, which progressed to more generalized numbness and weakness, and a fatal cardiopulmonary arrest 2 h after ingestion (Bradley and Klika, 1981).

POISONOUS BIRDS

The feathers and breast muscles of three species of pitohui or thickhead (genus *Pitohui*) passerine birds from New Guinea contain homobatrachotoxin, a steroidal alkaloid that activates sodium channels (Dumbacher *et al.*, 1992). Contact with feathers from these birds causes numbness and burning of tongue, lips or skin wounds, in addition to sneezing.

VENOMOUS MARINE INVERTEBRATES

Mollusca

The most important marine molluscs are the cone snails and octopuses. There are around 500 species of cone snails (genus *Conus*). Most are algal grazers but many are carnivores, feeding on other gastropods, polychaete worms, nematodes, and fish. The carnivores all possess modified grazing teeth that have evolved into barbed arrows. When ejected, the arrows are filled with a venom elaborated in a venom bulb. The venom toxins are used to paralyze the prey, thus allowing the prey to be swallowed by the cone snail without difficulty.

The fish-eating cones can cause a fatal sting to a human. Stinging usually occurs when the snails are handled. The venom of the cones contains many small polypeptides – the conotoxins. Three classes of these toxins are dangerous: α-conotoxins, which bind to the α-subunit of the ACh receptor thus blocking neuromuscular transmission; μ-conotoxins which block the fast, voltage-gated sodium channel, thus blocking action potential generation; and ω-conotoxins, which block voltage-gated calcium channels, thus blocking transmitter release from motor nerve terminals.

The symptoms of envenoming are paraesthesia, perioral numbness, neuromuscular weakness, and, ultimately, respiratory paralysis.

Deaths usually involve shell-collecting children paddling in shallow tropical waters but fatality rates are highly variable, ranging from <10% to approximately 70% for *Conus geographus*.

The only octopuses involved in neurotoxic envenoming are the two species of blue-ringed octopus (*Octopus maculosus* (Figure 8.6, above and in color plate section) and *O. lunulatus*) found in the shallow coastal waters of the Australian and west Pacific regions. They are small animals, often found under rocks at low tide, and may, therefore, be disturbed by holidaymakers. They inject a salivary tetrodotoxin (vide infra-tetrodotoxin poisoning) when they bite. The bites are extremely painful and cause local bleeding, swelling, and inflammation; severe neurotoxicity and even fatal generalized paralysis may develop within 15 min of the bite.

No specific anti-venoms are available. Treatment is therefore generally supportive.

Cardiopulmonary resuscitation and mechanical ventilation may be needed.

Echinodermata

The hard exoskeletons of the Echinodermata (for example starfish and sea urchins) contain numerous long, sharp projecting spines which can release venom when embedded into the skin. Severe pain and local swelling may result. Systemic effects include respiratory distress, cardiac arrhythmias, syncope, numbness, aphonia, generalized paralysis, and even death. There are no specific antivenoms. Skin penetrated by the spines (usually the soles of the feet) should first be softened with 2% salicylic acid ointment or acetone. The spines can then be squeezed out or surgically removed.

Coelenterates

Coelenterates (for example jellyfish, cubomedusoids, sea wasps, Portuguese man-of-war or bluebottles, hydroids, sea anemones) produce venoms that contain or release vasoactive substances (for example histamine and kinins). The sea nettle (*Chrysaora quinquecirrha*) contains a neurotoxin that causes a reversible but non-specific membrane depolarization in muscles and nerves. Intense pain and shock are the dominant features of coelenterate stings (Burnett and Calton, 1987). Severe systemic effects include convulsions.

Ichthyosarcotoxism

Ichthyosarcotoxism – poisoning as the result of the consumption of poisonous fish – is a growing problem. It is almost certainly under-reported. There are numerous causes of poisoning, but there are certain common features in terms of symptomology: acute nausea, vomiting, abdominal colic, tenesmus, and watery diarrhea. Associated features include paraesthesia of the lips, buccal cavity and extremities, painful reversal of hot–cold temperature sensation (for example cold objects impart a burning sensation, like dry ice), myalgia, progressive flaccid paralysis, ataxia, cardiovascular disturbances (for example bradycardia, profound hypotension), and rashes. The main differential diagnoses to consider include bacterial and viral food poisoning, and allergic reactions (Hughes and Merson, 1976). Diagnosis may be facilitated by a history of ingestion of a species of fish associated with this type of poisoning. Preventive measures are limited. Cooking does not prevent poisoning as most marine toxins involved in seafood poisoning are heat stable. Water in which fish have been cooked should be avoided, as some toxins are water soluble and may be partially leached out by soaking. In regions where poisoning occurs the flesh of the fish should be separated as soon as possible from parts where the toxins are concentrated, such as the head, skin, intestines, gonads, and other viscera. The risks of ciguatera poisoning can be minimized by avoiding the consumption of very large fish (vide infra); moray eels also carry a high risk of an unusually rapid and severe type of ciguatera poisoning. All scaleless fish should be considered as potentially tetrodotoxic. Scombroid poisoning can be prevented by eating very fresh fish or fish frozen immediately after being caught. Shellfish should not be eaten during the recognized dangerous seasons and during 'red tides' (vide infra).

Ciguatera fish poisoning

Occasional references to disorders suggestive of ciguatera poisoning exist in the world literature dating back to the sixteenth century, with clearer descriptions originating from the West Indies since the eighteenth century. The term ciguatera is derived from the American–Spanish word cigua, the name for a poisonous sea snail (*Livona pica*), which produces a similar illness in the Spanish Antilles.

Most cases of poisoning are seen in the Caribbean, Pacific Islands, and the United States. Estimates for the annual incidence of ciguatera poisoning in such regions varies from five per 100 000 (Lawrence *et al.*, 1980) to 100–300 per 100 000 (Bagnis *et al.*, 1979; Morris, 1980; Centers for Disease Control 1982). In the United States the disease is the most commonly reported illness associated with eating fish, occurring mostly in Hawaii and south eastern Florida (Hughes and Merson, 1976; Lawrence *et al.*, 1980; Morris, 1980), with illness in other states associated with travel in the Caribbean (Halstead, 1978; Gelb and Mildvan, 1979) or with eating fish from Florida (Centers for Disease Control, 1980). The incidence of poisoning is growing rapidly and serious outbreaks in areas previously considered free of ciguatera are regularly reported. The increasing importation of exotic fish from the Caribbean has led to cases of such poisoning in other parts of the world, including Europe. The global incidence of such poisoning is estimated at between 50 000 and 500 000 cases per year.

Ciguatera is commonly associated with the ingestion of either small reef grazers, such as parrot fish and surgeon fish, or the larger pelagic fish that enter reef areas to feed on the grazers. Typical pelagic fish are red snapper (*Lutjanus bohar*), amberjack (*Seriola dumerili*), barracuda (*Sphyraeniadae*), Spanish mackerel (*Scomberomorus* sp.) and moray eel (*Gymnothorax*). To date over 400 species of fish have been reported as potentially ciguatoxic, and most are prized food items. The toxins responsible for the clinical features include ciguatoxin (which can exist in several forms), maitotoxin and scaritoxin, and are thought to be initially formed by the dinoflagellate *Gambierdiscus toxicus* (Adachi and Fukuyo, 1979; Bagnis *et al.*, 1980). The toxins are first accumulated by grazing fish and then concentrated along the food chain in the liver, viscera, and gonads (Helfrich and Banner, 1963; Halstead, 1978). The toxins are present in fish when they are caught, and are unaffected by handling procedures or cooking. The toxins are lipid soluble, relatively heat stable and resistant to gastric acid.

Features of poisoning usually develop within 1–6 h (range of few minutes up to 30 h) of ingestion (Halstead, 1964). Ciguatera is characterized by the onset of gastrointestinal (abdominal cramps, nausea, vomiting, and watery diarrhea) or neurological symptoms (most commonly circumoral or limb numbness and paraesthesiae, or painful reversal of hot–cold sensation). Other symptoms include malaise, dry mouth, a metallic taste, dental pain or a sense of looseness of teeth, pruritus, arthralgia, myalgia, blurred vision, photophobia, transient blindness, vertigo, and ataxia. The average duration of illness is 8.5 days, with a median hospital stay of six days (Hughes and Merson, 1976), although symptoms of malaise and depression may persist for weeks or months. Bagnis *et al.* (1979) reported that diarrhea and abdominal pains may be commoner in males, with arthralgia and myalgia commoner in females. They also reported a possible ethnic difference in presenting symptoms, with Melanesian patients experiencing pruritus, ataxia, abdominal pains, and ataxia more frequently than Polynesians (Bagnis *et al.*, 1979); indeed, in New Caledonia, ciguatoxin poisoning has the common name la gratte which means 'the itch'. In the more severe cases reversal of hot–cold sensation, sinus bradycardia, hypotension, cranial nerve palsies, respiratory paralysis, and coma have been reported early in the course of the illness. A clinically more severe illness may develop during the second or more episode of poisoning (Bagnis *et al.*, 1979); the Florida Division of Health have therefore advised persons affected by ciguatoxin to avoid potentially toxic fish for several months. There is no reliable immunodiagnostic procedure available.

Therapy is essentially supportive. Further absorption of toxin may be reduced by inducing emesis or by gastric lavage, and by the administration of activated charcoal. Drugs used to treat ciguatera have included atropine, vitamin B complex, ascorbic acid, calcium gluconate, and steroids (Russell, 1975; Gelb and Mildvan, 1979), but their routine use cannot be recommended. Initial reports of the toxin inhibiting human red-cell cholinesterase *in vitro* have led to the use of pralidoxime (an acetylcholinesterase reactivator) as a potential treatment for cases of poisoning. However, more recent studies have not confirmed any effects of toxin on cholinesterase activity. The intravenous use of mannitol has been reported as producing a positive response within 10 min in all of 24 patients treated, with a mean time to complete resolution of neurological symptoms of 10 h and complete recovery in 17 patients within 48 h; this included a full recovery from coma in two patients (Palafox *et al.*, 1988). Gastrointestinal symptoms took longer to resolve. The mechanism of action may be by competitive inhibition of the toxin's effect on sodium channels, or by neutralization of the toxin. Overall mortality of ciguatera was recorded as 0.1% in a series of 3009 poisonings during 1964–1977 in the French Polynesia and New Caledonia Pacific Islands groups (Bagnis *et al.*, 1979), and zero in a series of 33 patients during a 14-week period on St Thomas in the US Virgin Islands (Morris *et al.*, 1982).

Various public health regulations have been enacted in an attempt to prevent cases of ciguatera poisoning. However, this has proved to be difficult as affected fish have a normal appearance and taste. As barracuda has often been implicated in ciguatera poisoning in the Caribbean and Miami, the Miami City Code has prohibited the sale of barracuda. Other measures have included attempts at increasing general awareness on the features of ciguatera poisoning; the Florida State Division of Health has circulated an information sheet about the disorder amongst physicians in Florida, and have also alerted the public through press releases. A radioimmunoassay (RIA) for the toxin (Hokama *et al.*, 1977) has been used to screen all amberjack sold in commercial fish markets on Oahu (in Hawaii) in an effort to identify affected fish before marketing, but it is neither sufficiently sensitive nor specific and is no longer used. Since the toxin is concentrated along the food chain, large fish are likely to be more toxic than small. In a study of red snapper caught in the Pacific Ocean, 69% of fish weighing more than 2.8 kg were toxic compared to only 18% of smaller fish (Hessel *et al.*, 1960). It has therefore been suggested that ingestion of fish larger than 2.3 kg, or of fish caught during red tides, should be avoided (Lewis, 1986).

Tetrodotoxin poisoning

Puffer fish ('fugu') is considered a gourmet dish in Japan and in Japanese communities settled elsewhere. Despite stringent regulations their consumption results in 250 cases of tetrodotoxin poisonings each year, with an associated 60% mortality. This is reflected by the Japanese saying 'Great is the temptation to eat fugu but greater is the dread of losing life.'

Fish belonging to the order Tetraodonitiformes (for example scaleless porcupine, sun, puffer, and toad fish) may become highly poisonous during the spawning season.

The poison tetrodotoxin is concentrated in the ovaries, gonads, live, bile, and skin of such fish; it has also been isolated from the skin of newts (genus *Taricha*), frogs (genus *Atelopus*) and salamanders, the saliva of the blue-ringed octopus, and the digestive glands of several species of gastropod mollusc, flatworms (*Planorbis*) and nemertine worms in Japan, and in some bacteria. Tetrodotoxin is a non-protein (an aminoperhydroquinazoline) and heat-stable, having both neurotoxic and cardiotoxic effects. It blocks the fast voltage-gated sodium channels, causing a loss of action potential generation in peripheral nerves and skeletal muscle. The toxin can also produce vomiting and respiratory depression by a direct action on the medulla.

Neurotoxic symptoms develop within 3 h of ingestion (usually within 1–45 min). If death occurs (from respiratory paralysis) it is usually within 2–6 h of ingestion. There may be no gastrointestinal symptoms. General features include lethargy, vomiting, hypersalivation, dysphagia, erythema, petechiae, skin blistering, and desquamation. Neurological features including paraesthesia, numbness, a floating sensation, weakness, and ataxia. Hypotension, bradycardia, and fixed dilated pupils indicate severe poisoning. In a report of a severe case of poisoning the patient became apnoeic and deeply comatosed with brainstem arreflexia, and developed features of cranial diabetes insipidus – the latter was attributed to a direct central action of tetrodotoxin on the neurohypophysis (Tambyah et al., 1994). Despite being in a coma without any brainstem reflexes for 36 h, the patient showed signs of improvement and had recovered by 50 h. Diagnosis is usually suggested by an appropriate history of ingestion, although it may be assisted by demonstrating the presence of tetrodotoxin using gas chromotography where that is available (Ohtsuka, 1984). Treatment is essentially supportive (Torda et al., 1973). Gastric lavage and activated charcoal may limit toxin absorption. Symptoms resolve over a period of days, with a good prognosis if the patient survives 18–24 h (Bower et al., 1981).

Shellfish poisoning

Poisoning as a result of the consumption of shellfish (for example clams, mussels, oysters, etc.) is a common problem. Animals most likely to be involved are filter feeders or grazers feeding on detritus (for example mud crabs and horseshoe crabs). All forms of poisoning result from the ingestion of toxic algae. It should be noted that both wild and cultured stocks of shellfish can be poisonous, and that the incidence of poisoning is increasing. This is probably because the combination of rising temperatures and the dumping of organic matter at sea is creating enriched environments that stimulate algal growth. The definitive study of the relationship between algal growth and human health is a UNESCO report (1996).

There are four medically important forms of shellfish poisoning: paralytic shellfish poisoning (PSP), neurotoxic shellfish poisoning (NSP), amnesic shellfish poisoning (AS) and diarrhetic shellfish poisoning (DSP). Only the first three are considered here.

PARALYTIC SHELLFISH POISONING

Paralytic shellfish poisoning is the most common form of shellfish poisoning. It is a world-wide problem, most common in temperate and warm temperate areas.

The causative agents are dinoflagellates. It is not known how many species of dinoflagellates are involved, but four genera are known to be very important: *Alexandrium*, *Gyomnodinium*, *Pyrodinium*, and *Gonyaulax*.

Most incidents of poisoning occur when shellfish are collected during blooms of the dinoflagellates, but a bloom is not an essential requirement because all of the responsible dinoflagellates form resting cysts. The cysts

can be accumulated by detritus grazers or, at early stages of activation before a bloom, by filter feeders.

The toxins involved

The toxins are members of a specific class of toxins known as gonyautoxins. The best known toxin is saxitoxin. The gonyautoxins block the fast, voltage-gated sodium channel. The result is paraesthesiae, neuromuscular weakness as well as nausea, vomiting, and diarrhea. Death is uncommon, but is typically the result of neuromuscular paralysis and respiratory failure.

Treatment

Supportive treatment is all that is necessary. There is no specific treatment. The symptoms resolve after a few days. Gastric lavage and artificial ventilation may be required in seriously ill patients. Fatalities are rare, and always occur within 12 h. Early treatment is required.

Avoidance

It is important to obey strictly warnings against collecting and eating shellfish during algal blooms or from sheltered waters where blooms have been recorded in previous years.

NEUROTOXIC SHELLFISH POISONING

This is a much rarer problem, with outbreaks of poisoning recorded off the Florida coast, South America, and, possibly, South Africa. It is caused by major blooms of the dinoflagellate *Ptychodiscus brevis*.

Major outbreaks are always associated with massive kills of fish and sea birds. Victims can be poisoned either by eating filter feeding shellfish or as a result of aerosols blown off the sea during violent storms (Pierce, 1986).

The toxins involved

The toxins are complex lipid soluble toxins known as brevetoxins. These toxins activate fast voltage-gated sodium channels. The symptoms of poisoning are very similar to those of paralytic shellfish poisoning, but lacrimation, salivation, headache, palpitations and fasciculation, and asthma-like conditions are common (Asai et al., 1982).

Treatment

There is no specific treatment. Human fatalities are rare.

Avoidance

Avoid the consumption of shellfish when there is a bloom and/or when there is evidence of unusually high deaths of marine fauna.

AMNESIC SHELLFISH POISONING

This is a rare and poorly documented form of poisoning confined, to date, to the west coast of

America, the Baltic, eastern Canada and North Island, New Zealand.

The responsible alga appears to be *Pseudonitzschia* and the toxin is domoic acid. The symptoms are gastrointestinal, associated with memory loss and ataxia.

There is no specific treatment.

REFERENCES

Adachi, R. and Fukuyo, Y. 1979: The thecal structure of a marine toxic dinoflagellate *Gambierdiscus toxicus gen. et sp. Nov.* collected in a ciguatera-endemic area. *Bulletin of the Japanese Society of Science of Fish*, **45**, 67–71.

Amaral, C.R.S., Campolina, D., Dias, M.B., Bueno, C.M. and Rezende, N.A. 1998: Tourniquet ineffectiveness to reduce the severity of envenoming after *Crotalus durissus* snake bite in Belo Horizonte, Minas Gerais, Brazil. *Toxicon*, **36**, 805–8.

Asai, S., Krzanowski, J., Anderson, W. *et al.* 1982: Effects of the toxin of red tide, *Ptychodiscus brevis*, on canine tracheal smooth muscle: a possible new asthmas-triggering mechanisms. *Journal of Allergy and Clinical Immunology*, **69**, 418–28.

Bagnis, R., Chanteau, S., Chungue, E. *et al.* 1980: Origins of ciguatera fish poisoning: a new dinoflagellate, *Gambierdiscus toxicus* Adachi and Fukuyo, definitely involved as a causal agent. *Toxicon*, **18**, 199–208.

Bagnis, R., Kuberski, T. and Laugier, S. 1979: Clinical observations on 3009 cases of ciguatera (fish poisoning) in the South Pacific. *American Journal of Tropical and Medical Hygiene*, **28**, 1067–73.

Bower, D., Hart, R., Matthews, P. *et al.* 1981: Non-protein neurotoxins. *Clinical Toxicology*, **18**, 813–63.

Bradley, S.C. and Klika, L.J. 1981: A fatal poisoning from the Oregon rough skinned newt (*Taricha granulosa*). *Journal of the American Medical Association*, **246**, 257.

Burnett, J.W. and Calton, G.J. 1987: Venomous pelagic coelenterates: chemistry, toxicology, immunology and treatment of their stings. *Toxicon*, **25**, 581–602.

Centers for Disease Control 1980: Ciguatera fish poisoning: Maryland. *MMWR* **29**, 610.

Centers for Disease Control 1982: Ciguatera fish poisoning: Bahamas, Miami. *MMWR* **31**, 391–2.

Cooper, B.J. and Spence, I. 1976: Temperature-dependent inhibition of evoked acetylcholine release in tick paralysis. *Nature*, **263**, 693–5.

Curry, S.C., Vance, M.V., Ryan, P.J. *et al.* 1983: Envenomation by the scorpion *Centruroides sculpturatus*. *Journal of Toxicology and Clinical Toxicology*, **21**, 417–49.

Dehesa-Davila, M. 1989: Epidemiological characteristics of scorpion sting in Leon, Guanajuato, Mexico. *Toxicon*, **27**, 281–6.

Dixon, R. and Harris, J.B. 1999: Nerve terminal damage by β-bungarotoxin: its clinical significance. *American Journal of Pathology*, **154**, 447–55.

Dumbacher, J.P., Beehler, B.M., Spande, T.F. *et al.* 1992: Homobatrachotoxin in the genus *Pitohui*: chemical defense in birds? *Science*, **258**, 1867.

Fritts, T.H., McCoid, M.J. and Haddock, R.L. 1990: Risk to infants on Guam from bites of the brown tree snake (*Boiga irregularis*). *American Journal of Tropical and Medical Hygiene*, **42**, 607–11.

Garrettson, L.K. 1984: Poisoning. In *Neurological Emergencies in Infancy and Childhood*, Pellock, J.M. and Myer, E.C. (eds), p 187. Philadelphia, PA: Harper & Row.

Gelb, A.M. and Mildvan, D. 1979: Ciguatera fish poisoning. *New York State Journal of Medicine*, **79**, 1080–1.

Gratton-Smith, P.J., Morris, J.G., Johnston, H.M. *et al.* 1997: Clinical and neurophysiological features of tick paralysis. *Brain*, **120**, 1975–87.

Gueron, M., Ilia, R. and Sofer, S. 1992: The cardiovascular system after scorpion envenomation. A review. *Clinical Toxicology*, **30**, 245–8.

Halstead, B.W. 1964: Fish poisonings – their diagnosis, pharmacology and treatment. *Clinical Pharmacology and Therapeutics*, **5**, 615–27.

Halstead, B.W. 1978: *Poisonous and Venomous Marine Animals of the World*. Princeton, NJ: Darwin Press.

Hamilton, D.G. 1940: Tick paralysis, a dangerous disease in children. *Medical Journal of Australia*, **1**, 759–65.

Harris, J.B. 1997: Toxic phospholipases in snake venom: an introductory review. In *Venomous Snakes*, Thorpe, R.S., Wüster, W. and Malhotra, A. (eds) pp 235–50. Oxford: Oxford University Press.

Helfrich, P. and Banner, A.H. 1963: Experimental induction of ciguatera toxicity in fish through the diet. *Nature*, **197**, 1025–6.

Hessell, D.W., Halstead, B.W. and Peckham, N.H. 1960: Marine biotoxins. I. Ciguatera poison: some biological and chemical aspects. *Annals of the New York Academy of Science*, **90**, 788–97.

Hokama, Y., Banner, A.H. and Boylan, D.B. 1977: A radioimmunoassay for the detection of ciguatoxin. *Toxicon*, **15**, 317–25.

Hughes, J.M. and Merson, M.H. 1976: Fish and shellfish poisoning. *New England Journal of Medicine*, **295**, 1117–20.

Lawrence, D., Enriquez, M. and Lumish, R. *et al.* 1980: Ciguatera fish poisoning in Miami. *Journal of the American Medical Association*, **244**, 254–8.

Lewis, N. 1986: Disease and development: ciguatera fish poisoning. *Social Science and Medicine*, **23**, 983–93.

Longnecker, G.L. and Longnecker, H.E. 1981: Centruroides sculpturatus venom and platelet reactivity: possible role in scorpion venom-induced defibrillation syndrome. *Toxicon*, **19**, 153–7.

Malasit, P., Warrell, D.A., Chanthavanich, R. *et al.* 1986: Prediction, prevention and mechanism of early (anaphylactic) anti-venom reactions in victims of snake bites. *British Medical Journal of Clinical Research*, **292**, 17–20.

Morris, J.G. 1980: Ciguatera fish poisoning. *Journal of the American Medical Association*, **244**, 273–4.

Morris, J.G., Lewin, P., Hargrett, N.T. *et al.* 1982: Clinical features of ciguatera fish poisoning – a study of the disease in the US Virgin Islands. *Archives of International Medicine*, **142**, 1090–2.

Myers, C.W., Daly, J.W. and Malkin, B. 1978: A dangerously toxic new frog (*Phyllobates*) used by the Embera Indians of Western Columbia with discussion of blowgun fabrication and dart poisons. *Bulletin of the American Museum of Natural History*, **161**, 307–66.

Ohtsuka, Y. 1984: Determination of globefish poison by mass fragmentography. In *Proceedings of the 21st International Meeting of Forensic Toxicologists (Brighton, UK)*, pp 355–40.

Ori, M. 1982: In *Handbook of Natural Toxins*, Ju (ed.).

Palafox, N.A., Jain, L.G., Pinano, A.Z. *et al.* 1988: Successful treatment of ciguatera fish poisoning with intravenous mannitol. *Journal of the American Medical Association*, **259**, 2740–2.

Pearn, J. 1977: The clinical features of tick bite. *Medical Journal of Australia*, **2**, 313–18.

Pierce, R. 1986: Red tide (*Ptychodiscus brevis*) toxin aerosols: a review. *Toxicon*, **24**, 955–65.

Reid, H.A. 1979: Symptomatology, pathology and treatment of the bites of sea snakes. In *Snake Venoms. Handbook of Experimental Pharmacology*, Lee, C-Y. (ed.), Vol. 52, p 922. Berlin: Springer.

Russell, F.E. 1975: Ciguatera poisoning: a report of 35 cases. *Toxicon*, **13**, 383–5.

Stone, B.F. 1988: Tick paralysis, particularly involving *Ixodex holocyclus* and other Ixodes species. In *Advances in Disease Vector Research*, Harris, K.F. (ed.), Vol. 5, pp 61–85. New York: Springer.

Sutherland, S.K. 1984: Management of venomous bites and stings. *Medicine International*.

Tambyah, P.A., Hui, K.P., Gopalakrishnakone, *et al.* 1994: Central nervous system effects of tetrodotoxin poisoning. *Lancet*, **343**, 538–9.

Tibballs, J. and Cooper, S.J. 1986: Paralysis with *Ixodes cornualus* envenomation. *Medical Journal of Australia*, **145**, 37–8.

Torda, T.A., Sinclair, E., Ulyatt, D.B. 1973: Puffer fish (tetrodotoxin) poisoning: clinical record and suggested management. *Medical Journal of Australia*, **i**, 599–602.

Testrail, J.H. 1983: *Bites and Stings of Poisonous Insects*. National Poisons Information.

Warrell, D.A. 1991: Tropical snake bite: clinical studies in south-east Asia. In *Natural Toxins*, Harris, J.B. (ed.), Vol. 25, p 45. Oxford: Oxford University Press.

Waterman, J.A. 1938: Some notes on scorpion poisoning in Trinidad. *Transactions of the Royal Society of Tropical Medicine and Hygiene*, **31**, 607–24.

9

Parasitic disorders of neurological significance

PETER K NEWMAN

INTRODUCTION

Human infection with protozoa and helminths comprises an enormous global problem. Recent figures suggest that worldwide there are 2400 million people at risk of malaria, with 300–500 million infected with the parasite. For schistosomiasis the estimate of current infection is 200 million, lymphatic filariasis infects 117 million, trypanosomiasis more than 18 million, leishmaniasis 12 million, and onchocerciasis 17.5 million. Cysticercosis is present in between 1–4% of the population in some endemic regions. Transmitted by insect vector, in impure water sources and via the feco-oral route, these zoonotic infections are traditionally associated with poor hygiene, inadequate living conditions, malnourishment, and deficient or absent health facilities. Commonly, but not exclusively, such factors are found in poor developing countries in tropical areas where resources are not available for prevention and treatment, which could theoretically eradicate many of these conditions. However, with ever expanding movements of individuals, families, and groups in and out of endemic zones, dissemination of these disorders is increasingly seen. Thus, for example, there are 2000 cases of malaria imported each year into the UK. Furthermore, immunosuppression, whether it be iatrogenic or due to human immunodeficiency virus (HIV) infection, increases the possibility of parasitic infection in millions of people worldwide. Finally, predictions on global warming suggest that vast new habitats may become available for the vectors which spread infections such as malaria (Sharp, 1996).

The protozoa, which are pathogens in humans, are divided into four phyla or subphyla: Sarcodina, Mastigophora, Ciliospora, and Saporozoa. Helminths are the most complex of infectious agents causing disease and are classified into nematodes (roundworms), trematodes (flatworms) and cestodes (segmented worms).

Many of the human parasitoses have a predilection for neurological involvement. The following short account of these conditions is intended only as a summary of a huge topic (Table 9.1). Greater detail will be found in the references given with each section and also in the Further reading section at the end of the chapter.

PROTOZOAL INFECTIONS

Trypanosomiasis

American trypanosomiasis (Chagas' disease; *Trypanosoma cruzi*) and African trypanosomiasis (sleeping sickness; *Trypanosoma brucei gambiense* and *Trypanosoma brucei rhodesiense*) are clinically distinct entities but there are some similarities in the organisms, each of which has epimastigote, trypomastigote, and mastigote forms. Reservoirs of infection are found in domestic and wild animals in the locality. Transmission of the protozoal parasite is by the tsetse fly (*Glossinia* species) in Africa (see Figure 9.1, overleaf and in color plate section) and the assassin bug (*Triatomina* species) in Latin America (see Figure 9.2, overleaf and in color plate section).

American trypanosomiasis is endemic in most Latin American countries and has spread with migrants into North America (Kirchhoff, 1993). It is said to affect 20 million people, generally in low socio-economic circumstances, when the human host, usually a child,

Table 9.1 *Parasites and neurological disease*

Group	Organism	Neurological features	Main geographical regions
Protozoa	Plasmodium falciparum	Cerebral malaria	Throughout the tropics and subtropics
	Trypanosoma cruzi	Peripheral neuropathy, myositis and stroke	Central and South America
	Trypanosoma brucei (gambiense and rhodesiense)	Sleeping sickness	Equatorial, west and east Africa
	Entamoeba histolytica	Meningoencephalitis, cerebral abscess	Throughout the tropics and subtropics
	Free living amoebae (Naegleria fowleri and Acanthamoeba)	Meningitis, granulomatous meningoencephalitis	Worldwide (rare)
	Toxoplasma gondii	Encephalitis, cerebral abscess	Worldwide
	Sarcocystis	Muscle pain and swelling	Worldwide (rare)
	Microsporidiosa	Encephalitis	Japan (case report)
Helminths			
Nematodes	Angiostrongylus cantonensis	Eosinophilic meningoencephalitis	Widespread in tropics, esp. SE Asia, Pacific Islands
	Gnathostoma spinigerum	Eosinophilic meningoencephalitis	Widespread in tropics, esp. Thailand and Japan
	Trichinella spiralis	Muscle pains, meningoencephalitis	Temperate and tropical areas
	Strongyloides stercoralis	Meningitis, encephalopathy	Patchy in tropics and subtropics
	Toxocara canis	Eosinophilic meningitis, myelitis, encephalitis	Worldwide
	Loa loa	Meningoencephalitis	Central and west Africa
	Dracunculus medinensis	Spinal cord compression	Africa and Asia
	Onchocerca volvulus	Optic atrophy, epilepsy	Mainly west Africa, also South America and Middle East
	Wuchereria bancrofti	Filariae in CNS	India, widely in tropics and subtropics
	Dipetalonema perstans	Meningoencephalitis	Tropical Africa and America
	Micronema deletrix	Meningoencephalitis	North America (case reports)
Trematodes	Schistosoma mansoni	Spinal cord (esp. S. mansoni) and cerebral lesions (esp. S. japonicum)	Africa, Brazil, Arabia
	Schistosoma japonicum		China, Indonesia, Philippines
	Schistosoma hematobium		Africa, Arabia, SW Asia
	Paragonimus	Epilepsy, cerebral mass lesion, encephalopathy, cord compression	Widespread in tropics, esp. Far East
Cestodes	Echinococcus granulosus and multilocularis	Cerebral or spinal hydatid cysts	Worldwide
	Taenia solium	Fits, cerebral cysts, rarely spinal	Widespread, esp. Latin America and India
	Spirometra	Cerebral and spinal sparganosis (mass lesions)	SE Asia, E Africa and N America
	Taenia (Multiceps)	Similar to T. solium	Temperate and tropical areas (rare)
	Diphyllobothrium latum	B12 deficiency	Northern temperate areas and worldwide

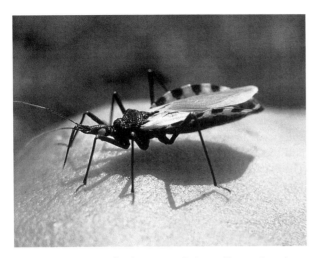

Figure 9.1 *A tsetse fly. (Courtesy of The Wellcome Trust.)*

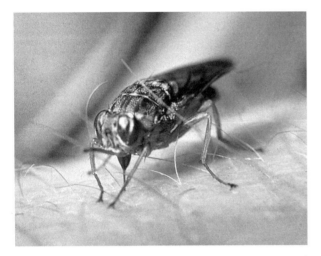

Figure 9.2 *The assassin bug. (Courtesy of The Wellcome Trust.)*

is bitten at night by the insect vector. Transplacental injection and injection via blood transfusion is also well recognized (Leiguarda *et al.*, 1990). A local reaction takes place at the site of inoculation from which there is hematogenous spread with parasitization of distant cells. Further cycles of hematogenous dissemination occur and variably effective immune mechanisms are activated. In most cases the clinical manifestations are not serious but in some, and especially in hosts who are immunosuppressed, for example those with the HIV infection, the condition may eventually prove fatal (Rocha *et al.*, 1992).

Acute Chagas' disease is usually a trivial illness but there may occur fever, local oedema, lymphadenopathy, hepatoslenomegaly, myocarditis, and rarely meningoencephalitis. Low-grade parasitaemia persists and years later the unfortunate patient may present with the classical features of Chagas' cardiomyopathy, megaoesophagus or megacolon. In this chronic stage of Chagas' disease there may be seen an encephalopathy, often subtle and suspected only as a result of cognitive

disturbance, a slowly progressing peripheral neuropathy or embolic cerebral infarction, the latter complicating the associated cardiomyopathy.

Diagnosis in the acute stage is confirmed by identification of the trypanosome in blood or cerebrospinal fluid (CSF), either by direct examination or after culture. The chronic stages are characterized by an antibody response which can be identified by a variety of serological tests, of which the enzyme-linked immunosorbent assay (ELISA), compliment fixation, and indirect immunofluorescence reactions are all in use.

Treatment with nifurtimox or benznidazole may abolish parasitaemia and be helpful in the acute phase of Chagas' disease. However, the response in the chronic illness is less certain and side effects are common. More effective, less toxic, trypanocidal drugs are desperately needed but, until available, public health measures are essential.

African trypanosomiasis, the sleeping sickness, is an equally devastating scourge affecting sub-Saharan populations in the east of the continent (*T.b. rhodesiense*) and the west (*T.b. gambiense*). A century ago the population around Lake Victoria was decimated by this disease and, although prevention measures later proved very successful, there has been a resurgence in recent decades. This has resulted in an estimated 50 million people being exposed in the endemic zones, including the many tourists who visit the east African game parks.

When the African trypanosome has been inoculated into its human host, there arises a local inflammatory reaction and a papule may be noticed. A few days later there is hematogenous dissemination with lymphoid involvement and this stage may persist for months or years, with periods of remission and sometimes without symptoms. A variable immunological response is degraded by the ability of the parasite to alter its surface antigenicity, and pathological changes are seen in the lymph nodes, spleen, heart, and central nervous system. The latter take the form of a meningoencephalitis with marked perivascular proliferation, the presence of characteristic modified plasma cells (Mott cells), and later gliosis. Clinically, in the later stages as nervous system invasion occurs, months or even years after the primary inoculation, insidious and progressive neurological dysfunction develops (Boa *et al.*, 1988). Early neuropsychiatric features are soon joined by the typical characteristics of lassitude and somnolence. As the encephalitis proceeds, any combination of pyramidal, extrapyramidal, cerebellar, sensory, and involuntary movement disorder is seen. Progressive dementia, stupor, and coma, accompanied by profound wasting, leads eventually to death due to malnutrition and intercurrent infection. There are many diseases which may cause a similar pattern of progressive encephalitis, although the particular pattern of sleep disturbance is rather characteristic. The diagnosis is confirmed by the identification of the trypanosome in the CSF or, in an earlier stage, in the lymph node and, rarely, in the initial skin lesion. Brain imaging, the electroencephalogram (EEG) and the CSF cellular reaction are non-specific. Serological tests are not foolproof but there is an IgM response in the CSF. Inoculation of mice with infected blood or CSF leads to demonstrable parasitaemia in *T.b. rhodesiense* but is not reliable in *T.b. gambiense* infection.

Pentamidine or suramin are used in early disease before CNS manifestations have occurred, but these drugs do not cross the blood–brain barrier and hence neurological reservoirs of infection remain. If neurological features develop, or if sequential CSF examinations indicate activity, then the arsenical drug, melarsoprol, is used. This drug has serious local and generalized toxicity including a reactive encephalopathy, but treatment can lead to a good outcome; other drugs may show promise (Dumas *et al.*, 1985), but less toxic alternatives must be found. Untreated sleeping sickness is invariably fatal. As with American trypanosomiasis, and so many other parasitic diseases, prevention is well within the bounds of possibility, but the lack of local resources and the frequent fractures of society in endemic regions does not inspire hope.

Cerebral malaria

Approximately half of the world's population live in malarial endemic regions. About 250 million people are affected by malaria and at least 2 million fatalities each year are attributed to the disease, usually in young children living in poverty. On a smaller but significant scale, some 2000 cases are imported into the UK each year, and increasingly these are due to the dangerous *Plasmodium falciparum*, the cause of cerebral malaria. The other human malarial parasites (*P. vivax, ovale*, and *malariae*) do not cause cerebral disease. Drug resistance is increasingly common in sub-Saharan Africa, southeast Asia and South America, and there is comparatively little investment in new drugs. Anti-malarial vaccines have not, as yet, shown the effectiveness in field trials that had been promised from the laboratory. Prevention by draining or spraying stagnant water is successful, as recommended a century ago in the pioneering work of Ronald Ross, but such simple measures are only taken where good public health systems flourish. Trials have also shown the effectiveness in prevention of excluding the insect vector by sleeping under impregnated bed-nets, if only these could be widely available to poor people in the endemic regions. Thus, all the evidence points to a continuous resurgence of all forms of malaria, including cerebral malaria.

The life cycle of the malarial parasite is shown in Figure 9.3 opposite (and see color plate section).

Cerebral malaria is associated with a high level of erythrocyte parasitization. In fatal cases at autopsy the brain is oedematous, congested, shows multiple petechie, and the small vessels are seen to be packed with infected red cells. Various theories have been advanced to explain the pathogenesis of cerebral malaria and none are entirely satisfactory. Disseminated intravascular coagulation is unlikely to be the causative event, and there is little evidence of immune complex disease. The mechanical theory postulates a progressive obstruction of the cerebral microcirculation by the dysfunctional parasitized erythrocytes, which exhibit a pathological degree of adherence to the blood vessel endothelium. An alternative and plausible theory implicates tissue necrosis factor and other cytokines. Perhaps the answer lies in a combination of interlinked pathogenetic mechanisms (Warrell, 1987; White and Ho, 1992).

A clinical diagnosis of cerebral malaria is made when the infection is associated with progressive drowsiness leading to coma. The term should not be applied to cases of high fever with 'toxic' confusion, irritability, and lesser degrees of obtundation. In adults the fever is usually present for several days but children have a much more rapid deterioration into coma (Molyneux *et al.*, 1989). Convulsions are common in children and adults, as are signs of meningeal irritation, and it is vitally important to differentiate cerebral malaria from meningitis. Clinical discrimination between these two conditions only achieved an accuracy of 77% in a Liberian study which emphasized the importance of CSF analysis (Wright *et al.*, 1993). Gaze disturbances, jaw clenching, and retinal hemorrhages are frequent; extensor posturing and pyramidal tract signs are seen at all ages. Hypoglycemia frequently complicates severe falciparum malaria in children and was present in 15 of 47 Gambian children in a prospective study (White *et al.*, 1987). It is of obvious importance to recognize and treat this consequence of disordered hepatic gluconeogenesis. Despite the desperately ill condition of patients with cerebral malaria, those that are appropriately treated and survive have a relatively low risk of significant neurological sequelæ, although epilepsy and other chronic disabilities, both physical and mental, may follow.

The diagnosis is supported by microscopy of thick and thin blood films which will show a high degree of parasitemia in proportion to the clinical severity. Of course, children and adults becoming ill in a malarial zone with a febrile encephalopathy may have conditions other than cerebral malaria, and the presence of parasites on a blood film may be coincidental to another underlying disease.

The treatment of severe *P. falciparum* malaria is usually with quinine or quinidine given by intravenous infusion. A bolus injection should be avoided as this can cause dangerous hypotension. Chloroquine resist-

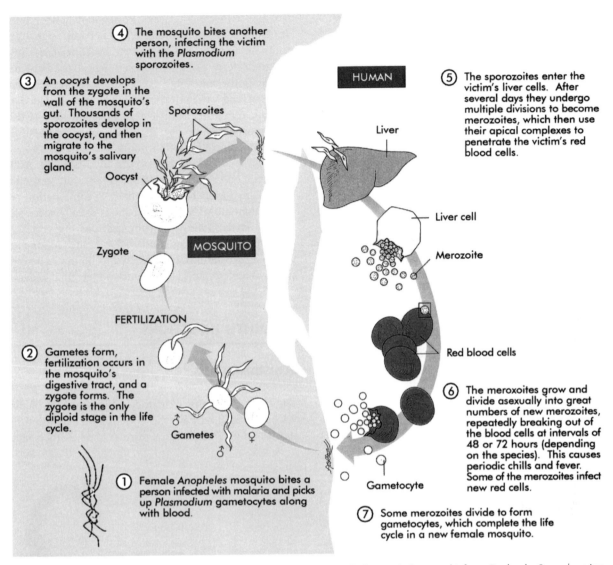

Figure 9.3 *The life cycle of the malarial parasite. Amended from Campbell. Permission sought from Benjamin Cummings Inc.*

ance is now so widespread that this drug is best avoided in treatment. The artemisin derivatives artesunate and artemether are becoming increasingly used for the treatment of severe infections (Boele van Hensbroek *et al.*, 1996; Hien *et al.*, 1996). The whole subject of the treatment of malaria, doses, resistances, and choice of drugs has been recently reviewed by White (1996). Fits can be treated with phenobarbitone or other appropriate anticonvulsant. Hypoglycemia, anemia, renal failure or shock have to be considered and treated as indicated. A high standard of nursing care is desirable to avoid complications such as aspiration pneumonia. Raised intracranial pressure may require mannitol, but it is now accepted that steroids are to be avoided (Warrell *et al.*, 1982). Exchange transfusion has been used successfully in desperately ill cases, but this has not been subjected to a controlled evaluation (Looareesuwan *et al.*, 1990).

It is worth mentioning briefly that falciparum malaria without coma may be followed by the onset of a cerebellar syndrome with ataxia, dysarthria, tremor, and nystagmus. This has been reported from India and Sri-Lanka and, like other postinfectious cerebellar disorders, may have an immunological cause (de Silva, 1993).

Cerebral amoebiasis

Entamoeba histolytica is the organism responsible for amoebic dysentery, sometimes also causing liver abscess or pleuropulmonary complications. It is not common for cerebral involvement to occur, but one Mexican study found this in 8.1% of cases (Lombardo *et al.*, 1964), and in all instances there was associated hepatic disease. A patient with amoebiasis who deteriorates neurologically showing a meningoencephalitic picture or focal features should be suspected of having cerebral spread of the infection. Blood amoebic serology should be positive and a computerized tomography (CT) brain scan will reveal diffuse low-density or ring-enhancing lesions. CSF examination is not helpful but aspiration biopsy and direct microscopy may reveal trophozoites. Treatment with surgical aspiration and debridement combined with intravenous metronidazole has been successful (Shah *et al.*, 1994). However, the condition is more commonly fatal and often found only at autopsy in patients who succumbed to an overwhelming infection.

Primary amoebic meningoencephalitis

This relatively recently recognized zoonosis was first described in 1965 from Australia (Fowler and Carter, 1965). It is caused by infection of the brain by the free living amoebae *Naeglaria fowleri* and *Acanthamoeba* species. As a result of swimming in infected freshwater lakes or pools, or from inhaling dustborn cysts, ingress is effected through the nose. *Naegleria* then finds a route to the brain via the olfactory bulbs. The patient presents with a suppurative meningitis. *Acanthamoeba* infects immunosuppressed individuals and causes multiple granulomatous lesions in the brain. The mortality of *Naegleria* meningitis is high and in granulomatous meningoencephalitis the outlook is even grimmer. This topic is fully reviewed by Duma (1991).

Toxoplasmosis

Toxoplasma gondii is a ubiquitous obligate intracellular sporozoan found throughout the world but with a vastly increased significance in this era of the acquired immune deficiency syndrome (AIDS) epidemic. Infection can occur congenitally, with resultant intracerebral calcification, mental retardation, ocular abnormalities or hydrocephalus. Congenital infection may reactivate in later life. Intrauterine infection is usually asymptomatic but can cause stillbirths and neonatal deaths (Eichenwald, 1960).

Acquired toxoplasmosis may present at the time of primary infection or later by reactivation of latent disease in immunocompromised individuals. Infection may follow ingestion of tainted meat (tissue cysts) or by feco-oral spread from infected pets, especially the cat. The primary infection is usually silent but sometimes causes an acute systemic illness with fever, myalgia, lymphadenopathy, rash, and occasionally a meningoencephalitis. The AIDS patient is more likely to show a florrid reaction. Following a latent period a relapse may be triggered by immunoincompetence and here the most common presentation is with a sub-acute encephalitis. Cancer or iatrogenic immunosuppression may underlie the relapse but usually it is the AIDS

patient in whom it is seen (Porter and Sande, 1992; Harrison and McArthur, 1995). Focal signs are common and the patients often have headache and low-grade fever. Toxoplasma serological tests are not helpful as the raised IgG level only indicates previous infection and an IgM response has usually failed to develop. CT and magnetic resonance imaging (MRI) appearances are of characteristic enhancing lesions, sometimes single but often multiple.

Cerebral toxoplasmosis occurs in 5–20% of AIDS patients (Luft and Remington, 1988) but responds remarkably well to treatment. A combination of pyrimethamine with sulphadiazine is usually successful (Leport *et al.*, 1988) but complications are common and alternatives such as clindamycin or atovaquone are used. Corticosteroids are indicated to inhibit hypersensitivity manifestations and insignificant cerebral oedema.

HELMINTH INFECTIONS

Schistosomiasis

The life cycle of this trematode is illustrated in Figure 9.4 below (and see color plate section). There are three species whose distribution mirrors that of their snail

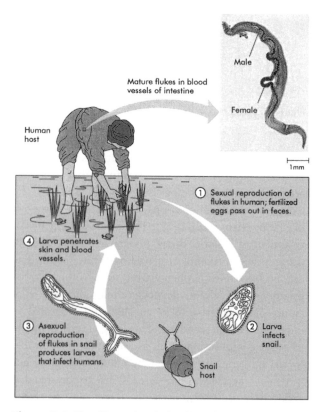

Figure 9.4 *The life cycle of the blood fluke Schistosome. Amended from Campbell. Permission sought from Benjamin Cummings Inc.*

hosts. *Schistosoma mansoni* is widespread in Africa but is also found in South America, the Caribbean, and the Middle East. *Schistosoma hematobium* is predominantly an African scourge, whereas *Schistosoma japonicum* is prevalent in south-east Asia, China, and Japan.

Human infestation with these freshwater parasites has a predilection for the young. Fever and itching may occur when the cercariae first penetrate the skin. At about six weeks the characteristic Katayama fever is seen, accompanied by sysemic symptoms and eosinophilia. Later as a chronic phase develops, there is a granulomatous response to ova deposited in various tissues, and this produces the characteristic hepatosplenic picture with *S. mansoni* and *japonicum* and obstructive uropathy with *S. hematobium*. Varices and ascites are the end result of hepatosplenic disease and bladder cancer is a common sequela of the chronic bladder irritation caused by *S. hematobium*. Allergic responses and reactions to eggs in the lungs may lead to pneumonitis or cor pulmonale, and immune complex glomerulonephritis is common but usually asymptomatic.

Central nervous system schistosomiasis is rare. Ova embolize through the cerebral or spinal cord vasculature and induce a granulomatous response or infarction. Access probably occurs when increased intra-abdominal pressure allows reverse flow in the venous system, from the mesenteric veins to the spine, and into the brain via the internal jugular veins. Most cases of cerebral schistosomiasis are due to *S. japonicum*, in which 2–5% of infections may have brain involvement; *S. mansoni* is the more usual cause of spinal disease.

In cerebral schistosomiasis there may be acute or chronic reactions and in some cases the infestation may be clinically silent (Blankfein and Chirico, 1965; Liu, 1993). The acute form presents as an encephalitis or encephalomyelitis with fever, headache, neck stiffness, seizures, speech disturbance or behavioral changes; less commonly stupor or coma, long tract signs or cranial nerve palsies are seen. Leucocytosis and eosinophilia are to be expected. The chronic form presents as a space-occupying lesion with raised intracranial pressure, focal signs and, commonly, focal seizures.

Many other conditions may manifest similar clinical features, but the correct diagnosis would usually be suspected in its appropriate setting, with ova identified in the feces and often in the context of systemic disease. The CSF and EEG (if available) will show non-specific features and a CT scan may reveal focal contrast enhancing lesions which at biopsy will show ova surrounded by inflammatory or granulomatous reactions. In recent years praziquantel has replaced other drugs as a safe and very effective treatment in all forms of CNS schistosomiasis; cerebral disease responds rapidly with clinical and CT resolution of the lesions, but seizures may persist longer term.

Spinal schistosomiasis is caused predominantly by *S. hematobium* in Africa and by *S. mansoni* worldwide (Scrimgeour and Gajdusek, 1985; Haribhai *et al.*, 1991). It is more common than cerebral involvement and it is almost certainly underreported. As well as the common cases in endemic regions, imported cases are seen, for example, in the returned traveler who has unwisely swum in an African lake (Cetron *et al.*, 1996). Deposition of schistosomal ova in veins which connect with the spinal canal may lead, after an incubation interval, to an acute or sub-acute transverse myelitis usually localized in the lower thoracic cord. Alternatively, it may lead to a granulomatous intramedullary lesion at the conus level, often with involvement of the cauda equina (bilharzial radiculitis).

Clinically, spinal schistosomiasis presents as a painful and rapidly progressing paraplegia with sphincter involvement and a clear sensory level; a more leisurely progression is seen in smaller numbers of cases. In an endemic area where the patient has a history of exposure, hematuria (*S. hematobium*) or diarrhea, there may be a high index of suspicion supported by identification of ova in urine, feces or rectal biopsy. Eosinophilia is probably present but blood serology is often unhelpful. The CSF contains a pleocytosis with an elevated protein level, sometimes with features of a spinal block, and the ELISA test may be positive. Imaging is not always available, but myelography, CT myelography or MR scanning will usually identify the site of a granulomatous lesion and often, but not always, confirm transverse myelitis; MR imaging is of course the superior investigation. The differential diagnosis may test the clinician as the young African in an endemic area may not have bilharzia but tuberculous arachnoiditis, paraplegia due to human T-cell lymphocytotrophic virus (HTLV)-1 infection or malignant cord compression. In cases of transverse myelitis the diagnosis may be particularly difficult, whereas in granulomatous presentations with a spinal block, biopsy of the lesion may confirm the expected pathology.

In most cases the triad of schistosomal infection, an appropriate clinical presentation and radiological support will be considered evidence enough to begin treatment. Praziquantel is lethal to the adult worm and, when given with corticosteroids, leads to a rapid improvement in those cases in which spinal cord function is recoverable. This treatment may be combined with surgical decompression where indicated, but medical therapy alone can be monitored by repeat imaging to show a rapid reduction in the bulk of the lesion. One-third to one-half of cases can be expected to recover fully, and one-third partly, but these figures can be improved further with early diagnosis and prompt treatment (Blansjaar, 1988).

In all forms of schistosomiasis, prevention is the primary aim of health workers.

Neurocysticercosis

After malaria, neurocysticercosis is the parasitic infection most commonly affecting the nervous system. Infestation with this cestode can range from the clinically trivial to severe disability and death. *Tenia solium*, the pork tapeworm, is spread by poor hygiene. Intestinal tapeworm infection can develop in pork eaters who have consumed 'measly meat' but it is often not appreciated that pork avoiders can also be infected by the feco-oral route if they should ingest food that has been contaminated by an unhygienic food handler. Thus, in India where the condition is widespread, the Muslim may be infected in the same way as the Hindu. The point is well illustrated by a recent outbreak in an orthodox Jewish community in New York (Schantz *et al.*, 1992).

The life cycle of the worm is illustrated in Figure 9.5 opposite (and see color plate section), but in essence *T. solium* has a two-host cycle. Humans as the definitive host harbor the mature worm in the intestine, excreting ova which may be consumed by the intermediate host, the pig, transforming into cysticercal larvae which then lodge in muscle or other organs. When humans become the intermediate host, by cross- or autoinfection, human cysticercosis is the outcome.

High infestation rates are found in parts of South and Central America and in India, but there is a worldwide prevalence of the parasite. Where cysticercosis is found in Western countries the source of infection is usually traced to migrants from endemic regions; in the USA the condition is commonly seen in Mexican immigrants. Although stringent public health controls will avoid locally acquired infection, for example only three of 83 million pigs inspected after slaughter in the USA had cysticerci (Schantz and McAuley, 1991), targeting control measures in particular risk groups is a problem.

All authors emphasize the varied pathologic and clinical manifestations of neurocysticercosis. These depend on the parasite load, site of involvement and the immune response of the host, and can range from a single intracerebral cyst acting as an epileptic focus to a massively disseminated infection peppering the brain with multiple lesions and giving the characteristic appearance seen on brain scanning or at autopsy. An evaluation of a large Mexican series is summarized in Table 9.2.

Reviews from other parts of the world, especially India, do not suggest any major regional variations (Wadia, 1996). Although the classical presentation with multiple active cerebral cysts may be ominous, it has been increasingly recognized that a benign presentation is common where a single parenchymal brain cysticercus is detected on scanning patients from an endemic area who have presented with epilepsy. The seizures may be focal or generalized and an EEG is often normal.

Table 9.2 *Classification of neurocysticercosis (Sotelo et al., 1985)*

Active forms	Occurrence in 753 cases (%)
Arachnoiditis	48.2
Hydrocephalus (meningeal inflammation)	25.7
Parenchymal cysts	13.2
Brain infarction	2.3
Mass effect	1.0
Intraventricular cysts	0.7
Spinal cysts	0.7
Inactive forms	
Parenchymal calcifications	57.6
Hydrocephalus (meningeal fibrosis)	3.8

If CT or MR scanning is available then the characteristic lesion is revealed and this should lead to anticysticercal therapy, for these cases are readily treatable. Several large series have now been published which illustrate this manifestation of cysticercosis (Rajshekher *et al.*, 1993; Del Brutto, 1995). Cerebral cysticercosis may be the underlying cause of epilepsy in greater than 50% of cases in highly endemic zones.

It is evident from Table 9.2 that neurocysticercosis may present as a case of focal or generalized epilepsy, with features of raised intracranial pressure, as dementia or other neuropsychiatric disorder, with focal neurological signs, or rarely as a spinal disorder. The clinician should not forget the non-neurological manifestations, which may give confirmatory support to the diagnosis, especially muscle involvement (including tongue nodules) seen in about 5% of cases. Ocular disease, where the larvae may be seen in the aqueous and vitreous chambers of the eye or cause retinal inflammatory changes is seen in 3%.

Cysticercosis should be suspected in patients who are resident in or have traveled from an endemic area in whom appropriate clinical features are demonstrated. Stool examination may reveal ova of *T. solium*. Blood and CSF may contain non-specific reactions of eosinophilia and leucocytosis. Serological tests have been available for many years and are more likely to be positive in the CSF than in the blood. Complement fixation tests have been gradually superceded by ELISA and immunoblot techniques which have good specificity but are more likely to be positive with a full parasite load than in the presence of a single cerebral cyst. It would be unwise to rely too heavily on serological tests alone in a suspect patient from a prevalent region. In some cases there may be changes evident on plain X-rays of the skull or limb muscles, due to calcified cysts in these organs. More usually, however, the diagnosis is supported by CT or MR images of the brain which will show single or multiple

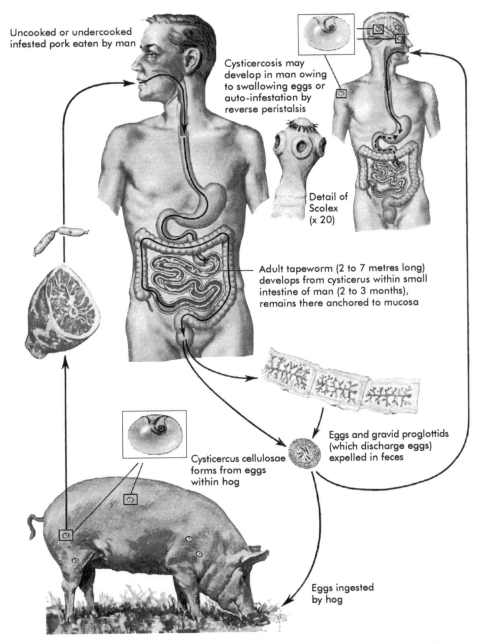

Uncooked or undercooked infested pork eaten by man

Cysticercosis may develop in man owing to swallowing eggs or auto-infestation by reverse peristalsis

Detail of Scolex (x 20)

Adult tapeworm (2 to 7 metres long) develops from cysticerus within small intestine of man (2 to 3 months), remains there anchored to mucosa

Eggs and gravid proglottids (which discharge eggs) expelled in feces

Cysticercus cellulosae forms from eggs within hog

Eggs ingested by hog

Figure 9.5 *The life cycle of the pork tapeworm. Reproduced from* The CIBA Collection of Medical Illustrations, Volume 3. *Permission sought from Novartis Pharmaceuticals Corp.*

parenchymal lesions, calcified in later stages, and with varying degrees of local reaction in the surrounding brain, ranging from the entirely inert to massive amounts of oedema. Careful evaluation of CT or MR images can indicate the stage of development of the cysts and whether the enclosed larvae are still living. Biopsy of a sub-cuticular lesion or of a brain cyst, aided by stereotactic localization, is usually unnecessary but is perhaps more likely to be performed in cases seen in non-endemic areas.

Calcified and dead cysts will of course be unaffected by cysticidal drugs, but both praziquantel and albendazole have been shown to kill parenchymal and

meningeal cysts and the results of treatment are excellent. The choice of drug has given rise to some debate but there is now a consensus to give albendazole in the first instance and then a further treatment course with praziquantel if a suitable response is not evident after a reasonable interval (Takayanagui and Jardim, 1992). In a heavy infestation the death of a large number of parasites may lead to an aggressive immunological reaction, in turn creating a potentially dangerous level of intracranial hypertension. Thus, dexamethasone and sometimes mannitol may be needed in these cases. Pretreatment with corticosteroids has been suggested to avoid this complication in patients with a heavy infestation.

Hydrocephalus may require ventricular shunting; intraventricular cysts, which cannot be reached by drug therapy, should be excised. Spinal cord compression probably needs combined medical and surgical treatment. Anticonvulsants are effective in controlling the epileptic seizures which so commonly mark cerebral cysticercosis and, in many cases where the cysts are inactive, constitutes the only treatment necessary.

Cysticercosis could be eradicated in endemic zones if food handlers practiced thorough personal hygiene, pigs were effectively inspected, and human and animal living environments were separated.

Echinococcosis

Two species of *Echinococcus* commonly cause hydatid disease in humans. *E. granulosus* is widespread and infection occurs when close proximity exists between humans, their dogs and domestic animals. The dog is the definitive host, sheep and cattle are intermediate hosts, and humans are infected when ova excreted in canine feces are present in the living environment. Ingestion of the eggs allows the oncosphere to traverse the gut mucosa and develop into a hydatid cyst in a target organ, usually the liver and/or the lungs. CNS involvement arises in up to 2% of cases, either as a single cerebral cyst or much less commonly with multiple cerebral lesions (Carcassonne *et al.*, 1973). Spread to the spinal cord is a very rare complication in hydatid disease, and develops when vertebral involvement broaches directly into the extradural space (Pamir *et al.*, 1984). *E. multilocularis* finds its definitive host in the cat, rodents are the intermediate hosts, and this is a much less common cause of human, including CNS, disease (Aydin *et al.*, 1986).

Older children and young adults are those usually infected, and typically the cerebral hydatid cysts present with features of raised intracranial pressure, with or without focal signs or seizures. The uncommon spinal form may cause root pain followed by paraplegia and sphincter dysfunction. Orbital hydatid cysts have occasionally been reported (Lerner *et al.*, 1991). Embolization from cardiac hydatid disease has caused acute stroke (Benomar *et al.*, 1994). Cerebral hydatid disease should be suspected when a child or young adult in an endemic area presents with the appropriate clinical scenario; blood eosinophilia, serology, and skin testing are often unhelpful but CT scanning demonstrates characteristic findings.

The treatment of cerebral and spinal hydatid disease is often unsatisfactory. Albendazole is active in extra-cerebral disease (Liu and Weller, 1996) and has a role in CNS disease but treatment is essentially surgical. Superficial cysts may be delivered intact at craniotomy but only aspiration or partial excision is likely to be possible in large or deep-seated lesions. In all cases a delicate avoidance of cyst spillage will prevent iatrogenic dissemination of infective protoscolices. A recent review of a large surgical series is rather more optimistic than previous reports (Cataltepe *et al.*, 1992), giving a recurrence rate of just over one-quarter. Radical and sometimes repeated surgery is required for spinal hydatid disease, in which widespread bone resection is necessary, and the prognosis is usually guarded although sometimes surprisingly good (Karray *et al.*, 1990).

Paragonimiasis

This relatively common trematode infestation is seen predominantly in Japan, Korea, Taiwan, and China, where seven species of the genus *Paragonimus* are known to infect humans. The final (definitive) host, humans or other animals, becomes infected by ingesting raw crabs or crayfish (the second intermediate hosts), from which metacercariae migrate from the gut to the lungs, develop into adults and produce the familiar condition of pulmonary paragonimiasis. The life cycle completes when eggs produced in the lungs are expectorated or swallowed, eventually being passed in the feces into freshwater. These form miracidia which in turn are taken up by freshwater snails (first intermediate host) and hence to the crustacean. It is obvious from knowledge of the life cycle that paragonimiasis could be eradicated by improving hygiene and avoiding ingestion of uncooked crustacea in endemic areas.

Pulmonary paragonimiasis is a chronic condition which is often mild, causing a persistent cough productive of rusty sputum and with typical radiological features. If the lung fluke migrates, it may find its way to the brain and, much less commonly, to the spinal extradural and intradural compartments. A meningoencephalitic phase is followed by parenchymal granuloma or abscess formation, triggered by the host reaction to the adult worm and its eggs, which manifests clinically with raised intracranial pressure, seizures, and focal features. Meningitis may be associated with cranial nerve palsies. Blood eosinophilia, raised sedimentation rate, hypochromic anemia, and hypergammaglobulinemia are non-specific features in pulmonary and extrapulmonary disease. Eggs may be found in the sputum or the feces. An ELISA test has good specificity and sensitivity. Plain skull X-rays may show typical 'soap bubble' calcified lesions; CT and MR scanning reveal more definitive findings.

Bithionol, niclofolan, and praziquantel have all been used successfully in paragonimiasis and, in some CNS cases, surgery is unnecessary. The aim of surgery is to remove the worm as well as the surrounding tissue and it should not be performed without concomitant chemotherapy. There is a significant mortality attached to cerebral paragonimiasis, with or without surgical intervention.

CNS paragonimiasis has been thoroughly and authoritatively reviewed by Hung and Chen (1996).

Eosinophilic meningitis

Distinctive clinical syndromes are seen with CNS infection by the rat lungworm *Angiostrongylus cantonensis* and by *Gnathostoma spinigerum*. The former is widespread but seen most frequently in south-east Asia, Papua New Guinea, Pacific Islands, and in Australia; the latter is found also throughout south-east Asia but especially in Thailand and Japan. Each produces an eosinophilic meningitis and will be readily diagnosed by the local physician in an endemic region. Widespread travel by tourists to Thailand and other south-east Asian destinations should foster a wider awareness of these conditions. A variety of other disorders may also cause CSF eosinophilia, including alternative parasitic infections, fungal or lymphoproliferative diseases, and drug allergies.

A cantonensis is a roundworm that lays its eggs in the lungs of the rat. Larvae then migrate into the gastrointestinal tract and are excreted in rat feces, finding their way to snails or slugs which are the intermediate hosts. Humans are infected as incidental hosts, either by ingesting raw snails (Vejjajiva, 1978) or from eating contaminated unwashed vegetables (Fuller *et al.*, 1993). The larva makes its way to the brain where in humans it dies and fails to complete the life cycle. In the rat it matures into the adult worm which migrates to the lung to produce its eggs. While moving through the brain the worm causes extensive damage characterized by lymphocytic and eosinophilic infiltration, hemorrhage, and granuloma formation around dead worms. An afebrile meningitis is the rule in angiostrongyliasis, sometimes with radiculitis, cranial nerve palsies, paraplegia or an encephalitis. The CSF is turbid with a high white count which may comprise 75% or more eosinophils. Blood eosinophilia is usually present and an ELISA test is sometimes positive. Often the diagnosis cannot be confirmed but is suspected from a history of having recently consumed Pila snails in Thailand (Schmutzhard *et al.*, 1988). The treatment is symptomatic and the disease usually runs its course over about a month, leading to recovery in most cases but sometimes to persisting neurological disability or death. Antihelminth drugs are ineffective.

Gnathostoma spinigerum lives in the adult form in the stomach of cats and dogs from which eggs are excreted in the feces and, if freshwater is found, develop into larvae and infect *Cyclops*. Fish or frogs may then ingest the *Cyclops* and, if this second intermediate host is eaten by humans, or if infected water is drunk, then the migrating worm will produce cutaneous swellings and eosinophilia as well as a variety of other systemic features. The less common CNS involvement is typified by intense nerve root pain followed by sudden paraplegia or cerebral hemorrhage as the worm creates havoc in its neurological wanderings. The CSF reaction is less cellular than in angiostrongyliasis, eosinophils are still plentiful, but the hallmark is the presence of xanthochromia and red blood cells produced by the hemorrhagic tendencies of the migrating parasite. In Thailand gnathostomiasis is a common cause of hemorrhagic stroke (Punyagupta *et al.*, 1990). Serological tests are not usually helpful but the condition may be fatal and the worm identified at autopsy. There are claims of successful treatment of human gnathostomiasis with albendazole (Kraivichian *et al.*, 1992) but attempts at treating the CNS infections may be less impressive.

Toxocariasis

Children with pica may eat dirt contaminated by eggs of *Toxocara canis* or other roundworms, passed in the feces of dogs. This is the setting in which visceral larva migrans or ocular larva migrans may develop, although most such cases of ingestion are asymptomatic. Ocular involvement can produce an inflammatory mass which can be mistaken for retinoblastoma. Visceral larva migrans rarely causes neurological symptoms but cases have been reported of encephalitis, myelitis, and meningitis (Sommer *et al.*, 1994).

Trichinosis

The nematode *Trichinella spiralis* is an important worldwide parasitosis. Consumption of infected undercooked meat is followed by maturation of larvae to mature adults in the host gut, and then production of further larvae which migrate usually to striated muscle. The migration may be clinically silent or produce systemic symptoms. If invasion of the CNS occurs then meningoencephalitis, seizures, cerebral thrombosis or hemorrhage may all be seen, and fatal cases have been reported. An ELISA test is useful and muscle biopsy may be diagnostic. The protean neurological and cardiac features have been recently ascribed to the associated hypereosinophilia syndrome (Fourestie *et al.*, 1993). Mild cases of trichinosis require only symptomatic treatment but for more severe manifestations, steroids and mebendazole are recommended.

Filariasis

Filarial infection only rarely leads to neurological involvement but the microfilarie of *Loa loa* may cause a meningoencephalitis. *Dracunculus medinensis*, the guinea worm, has been known to cause a spinal block due to extradural infiltration by the adult filarie. *Onchocerca volvulus* has been associated with a higher than expected epilepsy prevalence, the significance of which is disputed. *Dipetalonema perstans* is reported to have caused encephalitis. *Wuchereria bancrofti* is also occasionally implicated in neurological disturbance due to microfilarial activity (Dumas and Avode, 1988).

Stongyloidiasis

Strongyloides stercoralis is a widespread but uncommon gut parasite. In the presence of immunosuppression, a disseminated hyperinfection develops, and larvae invade capillaries in the brain leading to stupor and coma. A further complication may be a bacterial meningitis, possibly caused by gut flora adhering to the migrating larvae, or by hematogenous spread during bacteremia (Cook, 1987). This may be seen in AIDS and also in HTLV-1 infection.

Sparganosis

The *Spirometra* species of tapeworm contaminates drinking water. It may cause cerebral or spinal disease in south-east Asia and cases are not unknown in the southern USA. Usually infecting subcutaneous tissues and muscle, the larva may create a granulomatous reaction in the brain which mimics a tumor. CT and MR scanning will define the lesion but it is commonly not until histological examination that the diagnosis is made. The results of surgery can be good (Tsai *et al.*, 1993). Spinal sparganosis is exceptionally rare and presents with paraparesis caused by a granulomatous spinal block which may be successfully treated with decompressive surgery (Cho *et al.*, 1992).

Coenuriasis

Sheep and dogs are the usual hosts of *Taenia* (*Multiceps*) species. Eggs may, however, be ingested by humans and develop into coenuri in the muscle and the CNS, rather like in neurocysticercosis, although, in the case of coenuriasis, the cyst in the brain or spinal cord is usually single. Surgical excision combined with praziquantel or albendazole is the treatment. In sheep, this condition causes a common condition known as the staggers (McGreevy and Nelson, 1991).

Diphyllobothriasis

Eating raw or undercooked fish in areas where *Diphyllobothrium latum* flourishes may lead to the harboring of this large tapeworm in the gut. Although often asymptomatic and not associated with changes in the intestinal mucosa, in some cases there are abdominal pains, bloating, and anorexia. Rarely, the appetite of the worm for vitamin B_{12} leads to deficiency in the host with resulting megaloblastic anemia. Neurological manifestations are comparable to those seen in subacute combined degeneration of the cord complicating pernicious anemia, and may develop without associated anemia. Once the worm has been expelled using niclosamide or praziquantel, and the B_{12} deficiency is treated, there should be no long-term deficit, providing that treatment was started before irreversible changes had developed (Tanowitz and Wittner, 1991).

REFERENCES

Aydin, Y., Barlas, O., Yolas, C. *et al.* 1986: Alveolar hydatid disease of the brain. *Journal of Neurosurgery*, **65**, 115–19.

Benomar, A., Yahyaoui, M., Birouk, N. *et al.* 1994: Cerebral artery occlusion due to hydatid cysts of myocardial and intraventricular cavity cardiac origin. *Stroke*, **25**, 886–8.

Blankfein, R. J. and Chirico, A-M. 1965: Cerebral schistosomiasis. *Neurology*, **15**, 957–67.

Blansjaar, B.A. 1988: Schistosomiasis. In *Handbook of Clinical Neurology*, Vinken, P.J., Bruyn, G.W. and Klawans, H.L. (eds), Vol. 52, pp 533–43. Amsterdam: Elsevier Science.

Boa, Y.F., Traore, M.A., Doua, F. *et al.* 1988: Les différents tableaux cliniques actuels de la trypanosomiase humaine africaine à *T.b. gambiense*. Analyse de 300 dossiers du foyer de Daloa, Côte d'Ivoire. *Bulletin de la Societe de Pathologie Exotique et de ses Filiales*, **81**, 427–44.

Boele van Hensbroek, M., Onviorah, E., Jaffar, S. *et al.* 1996: A trial of artemether or quinine in children with cerebral malaria. *New England Journal of Medicine*, **335**, 69–75.

Carcassonne, M., Aubrespy, P. and Dor, V. 1973: Hydatid cysts in childhood. *Progress in Pediatric Surgery*, **5**, 1–35.

Cataltepe, O., Colak, A., Özcan, O. *et al.* 1992: Intracranial hydatid cysts: experience with surgical treatment in 120 cases. *Neurochirurgia*, **35**, 108–11.

Cetron, M.S., Chitsulo, L., Sullivan, J.J. *et al.* 1996: Schistosomiasis in Lake Malawi. *Lancet*, **348**, 1274–8.

Cho, Y.D., Huh, J.D., Hwang, Y.S. and Kim, H.K. 1992: Sparganosis in the spinal cord with partial block: an uncommon infection. *Neuroradiology*, **34**, 241–4.

Cook, G.C. 1987: *Strongyloides stercoralis* hyperinfection syndrome: how often is it missed? *Quarterly Journal of Medicine*, **64**, 625–9.

Del Brutto, O.H. 1995: Single parenchymal brain cysticercus in the acute encephalitic phase: definition of a distinct form of neurocysticercosis with a benign prognosis. *Journal of Neurology, Neurosurgery and Psychiatry*, **38**, 247–9.

de Silva, H.J. 1993: Cerebellar involvement in falciparum malaria: investigation of an epidemic. *Journal of the Ceylon College of Physicians*, **26**, 12–23.

Duma, R.J. 1991: Primary amoebic meningoencephalitis: infection by free living amoebae. In *Infections of the Central Nervous System*, Lambert, H.J. (ed.), pp 253–63. London: Edward Arnold.

Dumas, M. and Avode, G. 1988: Filariasis. In *Handbook of Clinical Neurology*, Vinken, P.J., Bruyn, G.W. and Klawans, H.L. (eds), Vol. 52, pp 513–21. Amsterdam: Elsevier Science.

Dumas, M., Breton, J.C., Alexandre, M.P. *et al.* 1985: Etat actuel de la thérapeutique de la trypanosomiase humaine africaine. *Presse Médecin*, **14**, 253–6.

Eichenwald, H.F. 1960: A study of congenital toxoplasmosis with particular emphasis on clinical manifestations, sequelæ and therapy. In *Human Toxoplasmosis*, Siim, J. (ed.), pp 41–9. Copenhagen: Munksgaard.

Fourestie, V., Douceron, H., Brugieres, P. *et al.* 1993: Neurotrichinosis. *Brain*, **116**, 603–16.

Fowler, M. and Carter, R.F. 1965: Acute pyogenic meningitis due to *Acanthamoeba* species. *British Medical Journal*, **2**, 740–2.

Fuller, A.J., Munckhoff, W., Kiers, L. *et al.* 1993: Eosinophilic meningitis due to *Angiostrongylus cantonensis*. *Western Journal of Medicine*, **159**, 78–80.

Haribhai, H.C., Bhigjee, A.I., Bill, P.L. *et al.* 1991: Spinal cord schistosomiasis. *Brain*, **114**, 709–26.

Harrison, M.J. and McArthur, J.C. 1995: Opportunistic infections – parasites. In *AIDS and the Nervous System*, pp 171–81. Edinburgh: Churchill Livingstone.

Hien, T.T., Day, N.P., Phu, N.J. *et al.* 1996: A controlled trial of artemether or quinine in Vietnamese adults with severe falciparum malaria. *New England Journal of Medicine*, **335**, 76–83.

Hung, T. and Chen, E-R. 1996: Paragonimiasis of the central nervous system. *Neurological Infections and Epidemiology*, **1**, 11–29.

Karray, S., Zlitric, M., Fowles, J.V. *et al.* 1990: Vertebral hydatosis and paraplegia. *Journal of Bone and Joint Surgery*, **72**, 884–8.

Kirchhoff, L.V. 1993: American trypanosomiasis (Chagas' disease): a tropical disease now in the United States. *New England Journal of Medicine*, **329**, 639–44.

Kraivichian, P., Kulkumthorn, M., Yingourd, P. *et al.* 1992: Albendazole for the treatment of human gnathostomiasis. *Transactions of the Royal Society of Tropical Medicine and Hygiene*, **86**, 418–21.

Leiguarda, R., Roncoroni, A., Taratuto, A.L. *et al.* 1990: Acute CNS infections by *Trypanosoma cruzi* (Chagas' disease) in immunosuppressed patients. *Neurology*, **40**, 850–1.

Leport, C., Raffi, F., Matheron, S. *et al.* 1988: Treatment of central nervous system toxoplasmosis with pyrimethamine/sulphadiazine combination in 35 patients with acquired immune deficiency syndrome. *American Journal of Medicine*, **84**, 94–100.

Lerner, S.F., Morales, A.G. and Croxatto, J.O. 1991: Hydatid cyst of the orbit. *Archives of Ophthalmology*, **109**, 285.

Liu, L.X. 1993: Spinal and cerebral schistosomiasis. *Seminars in Neurology*, **13**, 189–200.

Liu, L.X. and Weller, P.F. 1996: Drug therapy. Antiparasitic drugs. *New England Journal of Medicine*, **334**, 1178–84.

Lombardo, L., Alonso, P., Arroyo, L.S. *et al.* 1964: Cerebral amoebiasis. Report of 17 cases. *Journal of Neurosurgery*, **21**, 704–9.

Looareesuwan, S., Phillips, R.E., Karbwang, J. *et al.* 1990: *Plasmodium falciparum* hyperparasitemia: use of exchange transfusion in seven patients and a review of the literature. *Quarterly Journal of Medicine*, **75**, 471–81.

Luft, B.J. and Remington, J.S. 1988: Toxoplasmic encephalitis. *Journal of Infectious Disease*, **157**, 1–6.

McGreevy, P.B. and Nelson, G.S. 1991: Coenuriasis. In *Hunter's Tropical Medicine*, Strickland, G.T. (ed.), 7th edn, pp 858–9. Philadelphia, PA: W.B. Saunders.

Molyneux, M.E., Taylor, T.E., Wirima, J.J. and Borgstein, A. 1989: Clinical features and prognostic indicators in pediatric cerebral malaria: a study of 131 comatose Malawian children. *Quarterly Journal of Medicine*, **265**, 441–59.

Pamir, M.N., Akalan, N., Özgen, T. *et al.* 1984: Spinal hydatid cysts. *Surgical Neurology*, **21**, 53–7.

Porter, S.B. and Sande, M.A. 1992: Toxoplasmosis of the central nervous system in the acquired immune deficiency syndrome. *New England Journal of Medicine*, **327**, 1643–8.

Punyagupta, S., Bunnag, T. and Juttijudata, P. 1990: Eosinophilic meningitis in Thailand. *Journal of the Neurological Sciences*, **96**, 241–56.

Rajshekher, V., Haran, R.P., Prakash, S.G. and Chandy, M.J. 1993: Differentiating small cysticercus granulomas and tuberculomas in patients with epilepsy. *Journal of Neurosurgery*, **78**, 402–7.

Rocha, A., Meneses, A.C., Silva, A.M. *et al.* 1992: Pathology of patients with Chagas' disease and acquired immune deficiency syndrome. *American Journal of Tropical Medicine and Hygiene*, **50**, 261–8.

Schantz, P.J.M., Moore, A.C., Munoz, J.L. *et al.* 1992: Neurocysticercosis in an orthodox Jewish community in New York City. *New England Journal of Medicine*, **327**, 692–5.

Schantz, P.M. and McAuley, J. 1991: Current status of foodborne zoonoses in the United States. *South-east Asian Journal of Tropical Medicine and Public Health*, **22**, 65–71.

Schmutzhard, E., Boongird, P. and Vejjajiva, A. 1988: Eosinophilic meningitis and radiculomyelitis in Thailand, caused by *Gnathostoma spinigerum* and *Angiostrongylus cantonensis*. *Journal of Neurology, Neurosurgery and Psychiatry*, **51**, 80–7.

Scrimgeour, E.M. and Gajdusek, D.C. 1985: Involvement of the central nervous system in *Schistosoma mansoni* and *Schistosoma hematobium* infection. *Brain*, **108**, 1023–38.

Shah, A.A., Shaikh, H. and Karim, M. 1994: Amoebic brain abscess: a rare but serious complication of *Entamoeba histolytica* infection. *Journal of Neurology, Neurosurgery and Psychiatry*, **57**, 240–1.

Sharp, D. 1996: Malarial range set to spread in a warmer world. *Lancet*, **347**, 1612

Sommer, C., Ringelstein, E.B., Biniek, R. and Glockner, W.M. 1994: Adult *Toxocara canis* encephalitis. *Journal of Neurology, Neurosurgery and Psychiatry*, **57**, 229–31.

Sotelo, J., Guerrero, V. and Rubio, F. 1985: Neurocysticercosis: a new classification based on active and inactive forms – a study of 753 cases. *Archives of Internal Medicine*, **145**, 442–5.

Takayanagui, O.M. and Jardim, E. 1992: Therapy of neurocysticercosis. Comparison between albendazole and praziquantel. *Archives of Neurology*, **49**, 290–4.

Tanowitz, H.B. and Wittner, M. 1991: Diphyllobothriasis. In *Hunter's Tropical Medicine*, Strickland, G.T. (ed.), 7th edn, pp 834–6. Philadelphia, PA: W.B. Saunders.

Tsai, M.D., Chang, C.N., Ho, Y.S. and Wang, A.D. 1993: Cerebral sparganosis diagnosed and treated with stereotactic techniques. *Journal of Neurosurgery*, **78**, 129–32.

Vejjajiva, A. 1978: Parasitic diseases of the nervous system in Thailand. *Clinical and Experimental Neurology. Proceedings of the Australian Association of Neurology*, **15**, 92–7.

Wadia, N.H. 1996: Neurocysticercosis. In *Tropical Neurology*, Shakir, R.A., Newman, P.K. and Poser, C.M. (eds), pp 247–73. London: W.B. Saunders.

Warrell, D.A. 1987: Pathophysiology of severe falciparum malaria in man. *Parasitology*, **94**, 553–76.

Warrell, D.A., Looareesuwan, S., Warrell, M.J. *et al.* l982: Dexamethasone proves deleterious in cerebral malaria. A double-blind trial in 100 comatose patients. *New England Journal of Medicine*, **306**, 313–19.

White, N.J. 1996: The treatment of malaria. *New England Journal of Medicine*, **335**, 800–6.

White, N.J. and Ho, M. 1992: The pathophysiology of malaria. *Advances in Parasitology*, **31**, 83–173.

White, N.J., Miller, K.D. and Marsh, K. 1987: Hypoglycemia in African children with severe malaria. *Lancet*, **i**, 708–11.

Wright, P.W., Avery, W.G., Ardill, W.D. and McLarty, J.W. 1993: Initial clinical assessment of the comatose patient: cerebral malaria vs meningitis. *Pediatric Infectious Diseases Journal*, **12**, 37–41.

FURTHER READING

Cook, G.C. (ed.) 1996: *Manson's Tropical Diseases*, 20th edn. London: W.B. Saunders.

Harris, A.A. 1988: In *Handbook of Clinical Neurology*, Vinken, P.J., Bruyn, G.W. and Klawans, H.L. (eds), Vol. 52. Amsterdam: Elsevier Science.

Shakir, R.A., Newman, P.K. and Poser, C.M. 1996: *Tropical Neurology*. London: W.B. Saunders.

Spillane, J.D. (ed.) 1973: *Tropical Neurology*. London: Oxford University Press.

Strickland, G.T. (ed.) 1991: *Hunter's Tropical Medicine*, 7th edn. Philadelphia, PA: W.B. Saunders.

10

Genetically determined susceptibility to environmental toxins

HARUO KOBAYASHI AND TADAHIKO SUZUKI

INTRODUCTION: NEUROGENETIC INVOLVEMENT IN ENVIRONMENTAL HAZARDS

In the past decade, great advances have been made in our understanding of the molecular basis of brain functioning. A large number of phenotypically distinct cell types, genes, that appear to be expressed solely in the central nervous system (CNS) and the vast numbers of synaptic connections that can be made by most neurons have exemplified the complexities of the brain. Input from hundreds of different synapses are translated, integrated, and modified in single neurons, resulting in the production or control of some aspect of behavior.

Environmentally induced neurological disorders are well documented. A few examples are mercury poisoning in consumers of fish or wheat bread tainted with methyl mercury, extrapyramidal disorders in manganese miners, lathyrism from excessive consumption of the chickling pea, lead poisoning in children, amnestic shellfish poisoning associated with domoic acid contamination, and sequelae of poisoning by organophosphorus nerve agents such as sarin and soman (Dawson et al., 1995). While there is no question that focal populations exposed to unusual environmental chemicals or to high levels of neurotoxicants in the workplace may manifest overt symptoms of neurological disease, the broader questions, such as neurogenotoxicity, teratogenicity, apoptogenicity and psychodysleptogenicity, and of the long-term effects of sporadic or chronic low-dose exposure remain largely unanswered (Johannessen, 1995).

GENETICS AND NEURODEGENERATIVE DISORDERS

There are two classes of nucleic acids, deoxyribonucleic acid (DNA), and ribonucleic acid (RNA). DNA is found in the nucleus and in mitochondria of cells and carries all hereditary information. Parts of the DNA called genes are transcribed into RNA. One of the several classes of RNA that gives rise to proteins is called messenger RNA (mRNA). Receptors, neurotransmitter-synthesizing enzymes, neurotransmitter-degrading enzymes, re-uptake transporters, and ion channels are the typical proteins in the nervous system (Eberwine, 1994).

It has long been suspected that genetic predisposition plays an important role in the etiology of neurodegenerative disorders. Recent advances in genetics have made substantial progress in identifying the genetic basis of many human diseases, at least those with conspicuous determinants. These successes in neurogenetic involvement include Huntington's disease and Alzheimer's disease. Families with a high incidence of Parkinson's disease and amyotrophic lateral sclerosis are also well documented. However, the detection of genetic factors for complex neurodegenerative diseases, such as schizophrenia and double personality disorder, has been far more complicated. Although there have been numerous reports of genes or loci that might give rise to these disorders, few of these findings have been replicated. Under such circumstances, it may be premature to refer to neurogenotoxicity of causative substances, such as drugs and environmental agents, inducing neurodegenerative alteration. Attempts to identify a specific exposure or causative environmental agents have been unsuccessful. Table 10.1 represents environmental neurotoxicants which are suspected to have neurogenetic effects.

TYPES OF NEUROGENETIC DISORDERS

Neurogenetic disorders are divided into four classes: genetically heritable diseases as formalized by Mendel's law, including non-mendelian inheritance (Price, 1994); cellular phenotypic alterations induced by expression of immediate early genes (IEGs), such as the proto-oncogenes c-fos and c-jun within the neuron (Hughes and Dragunow, 1995); neuro-oncogenesis or brain tumors (Kleihues *et al.*, 1995); and apoptosis of neuron (Eastman, 1993) (Figures 10.1 and 10.2).

The first disorders, such as Huntington's disease and Parkinson's disease, are transmitted by autosomal dominant inheritance and mutation. Some environmental toxins, infectious agents, and environmental stresses have been proposed to transform autosomal recessive inheritance to an autosomal dominant one, or cause mutation. For example, genetic factors can influence the susceptibility of certain alcoholics to neurological complications.

The IEGs act as transcription factors and couple cell-surface stimulation to gene transcription. The changes in IEG expression underlie physiological processes, such as learning and memory, and excessive changes in IEG expression may lead to abnormal or pathological processes, such as drug abuse/tolerance/sensitization and neurotoxicosis by methyl mercury and trimethyltin (LoPachin and Aschner, 1993; Zawia and Harry, 1993, 1996). For example, chronic administration of an opiate-like morphine induces behavioral changes, such as tolerance and dependence, and biochemical changes such as an up regulation of several components of the cyclic adenosine-3′,5′-monophosphate (cAMP) signal transduction cascade. The cAMP-responsive element-binding protein (CREB) has been proposed to be one of

Table 10.1 *Environmental agents suspected to have neurogenetic toxicity directly or indirectly*

A Heavy metals and metals
  Organomercury: methyl mercury, ethyl mercury
  Lead: inorganic lead; organolead
  Organotin: trimethyltin, triethyltin
  Aluminum
  Arsenic
  Manganese
  Copper
B Insecticides, nerve gases
  Organophosphate (antiChE): parathion, DFP, DDVP (dichlorvos), sarin, soman, chlorpyrifos
  Carbamate: carbaryl (denapon), propoxur, eserine, neostigmine
  Organophosphate (organophosphorus-induced delayed neuropathy, OPIDN): TOCP
  Organochlorine: DDT, BHC, polychlorinated biphenyl, chloropicrin
C Abuse and addiction drugs
  Opiates and opiate analogs: morphine, diacetylmorphine (heroin), codeine, thebaine, fentanyl, meperidine
  Cannabinoid: tetrahydrocannabinol
  Hallucinogen: methanphetamine, amphetamine, methylphenidate, phencyclidine, cocaine, 4-methylaminorex (U4Euh), lysergic acid diethylamide (LSD)
  Alcohol (alcoholism): ethanol
  Nicotine
D Organic solvent
  1,1,1-Trichloroethane, toluene, carbon tetrachloride, acetone, xylene
E Uncoupler-like agents
  Cyanide: KCN, NaCN
F Miniencephalotics
  Methylazoxymethanol, N-methyl-N-nitrosourea, cytosine arabinoside
G Therapeutics
  Reserpine
  Muscarinic antagonists: atropine, scopolamine
  Muscarinic agonists: pilocarpine, alecoline, carbachol
  Dopamine
H Natural toxins
  Marine toxin: domoic acid
  Plant toxin: 3-nitropropionic acid
  Mycotoxin: 3-nitropropionic acid
  Phenylketoneuria: inability to metabolize the amino acid phenylalanine
I Epileptics
  Pentylentetrazol, kainic acid, glutamate
J Free radicals
  Hydrogen peroxide (H_2O_2), peroxynitrite ($ONOO^-$)
K CNS trauma
  1,3-Dinitrobenzene
  Triethyltin (see also A)

the components. In this case, CREB-dependent gene transcription is a factor in the onset of behavioral manifestation of opiate dependence.

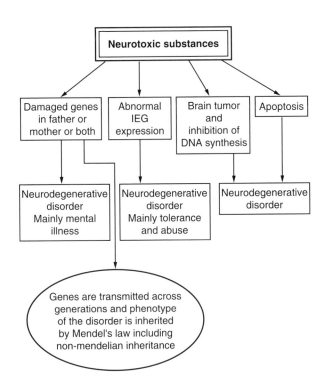

Figure 10.1 *Various neurogenetic mechanisms suspected to be involved in neurotoxicity caused by environmental agents.*

Although the incidence of brain tumors is estimated to be less than 2% of all malignant neoplasms, a significant proportion of central nervous system (CNS) neoplasms affect children. Tumors of the nervous system, including retinoblastomas and peripheral neuroblastomas, rank second in incidence after leukemias in children. In recent years, experimental studies have shown chemical carcinogens and viral oncogenes to be highly susceptible to malignant transformation.

While free radicals such as superoxide (O_2^-) and hydroxyl (OH) are normal products of cellular aerobic metabolism, reactive oxygen species (ROS), such as hydrogen peroxide (H_2O_2) and peroxynitrite ($ONOO^-$), contribute importantly to the cellular redox state. ROS can damage lipids, proteins and DNA, and induce necrosis and apoptosis.

Genetic approaches in inheritance

Genetic approaches in inheritance include examinations of phenotype definition, familial aggregation, genetic involvement, mode of inheritance, heterogeneity, and specific mechanisms (Price, 1994).

NEUROGENETIC DISORDERS

It has long been suspected that genetic predisposition plays an important role in the etiology of neurodegen-

erative disorders. The typical example is believed to be Huntington's disease, which is transmitted by autosomal dominant inheritance. Various neurogenetical disorders suspected to be genetic, in part, probably include Alzheimer's disease, Parkinson's disease, amyotrophic lateral sclerosis, prion diseases, transmissible sponge-form encephalopathies, such as scrapie in sheep, Creutzfelt–Jakob disease in humans, and most recently bovine spongiform encephalopathy (BSE) or 'mad cow disease' in cattle. They are primarily disorders of later life, developing in individuals who are neurologically normal, although childhood-onset forms of each of the disorders are recognized (Cordell, 1994; Joyce and Hurtig, 1994; Albin and Tagle, 1995; Higgins and Cordell, 1995; Risch and Merikangas, 1996; Standaert and Young, 1996).

NEUROLOGICAL COMPLICATION OF CHEMOTHERAPY AND INSECTICIDE EXPOSURE

Some experimental studies suggest that exposure to apparently subtoxic doses of organophosphorus insecticides, such as chlorpyrifos, can cause specific inhibition of DNA and protein synthesis in the immature brain (Whitney *et al.*, 1995). These insecticides are widely applicable to domestic and agricultural use, and are believed to be much safer compared to parathion.

Certain antineoplastic agents are commonly associated with particular neurological syndromes apparent as a central nervous system or peripheral nervous system disease. A recent new approach, using both potent antineoplastic agents and radiation, will produce a higher risk for developing long-term and irreversible toxicity. High doses of this kind of chemotherapy will also expose the nervous system to very high doses of chemotherapeutic agents that do not normally have any neurotoxicity (Fan and Howd, 1995).

Intracellular pools of reduced folate are necessary for thymidylate and purine metabolism; these are necessary for the synthesis of DNA. Since methotrexate is a folic acid analogue that inhibits dihydrofolate reductase, it depletes the pools of reduced folate and inhibits the synthesis of DNA. Although low-dose oral or parenteral methotrexate results in little or no neurotoxicity, intrathecal methotrexate may develop neurotoxicity in patients by up to 30%. Leucovorin, a reduced folate, can prevent methotrexate toxicity to the bone marrow and gastrointestinal tract, but cannot prevent the neurotoxicity (Cascino, 1995).

Fludarabine phosphate, which has been used for hematological malignancies and solid tumors, is a purine nucleoside antineoplastic agent that will inhibit the synthesis of DNA.

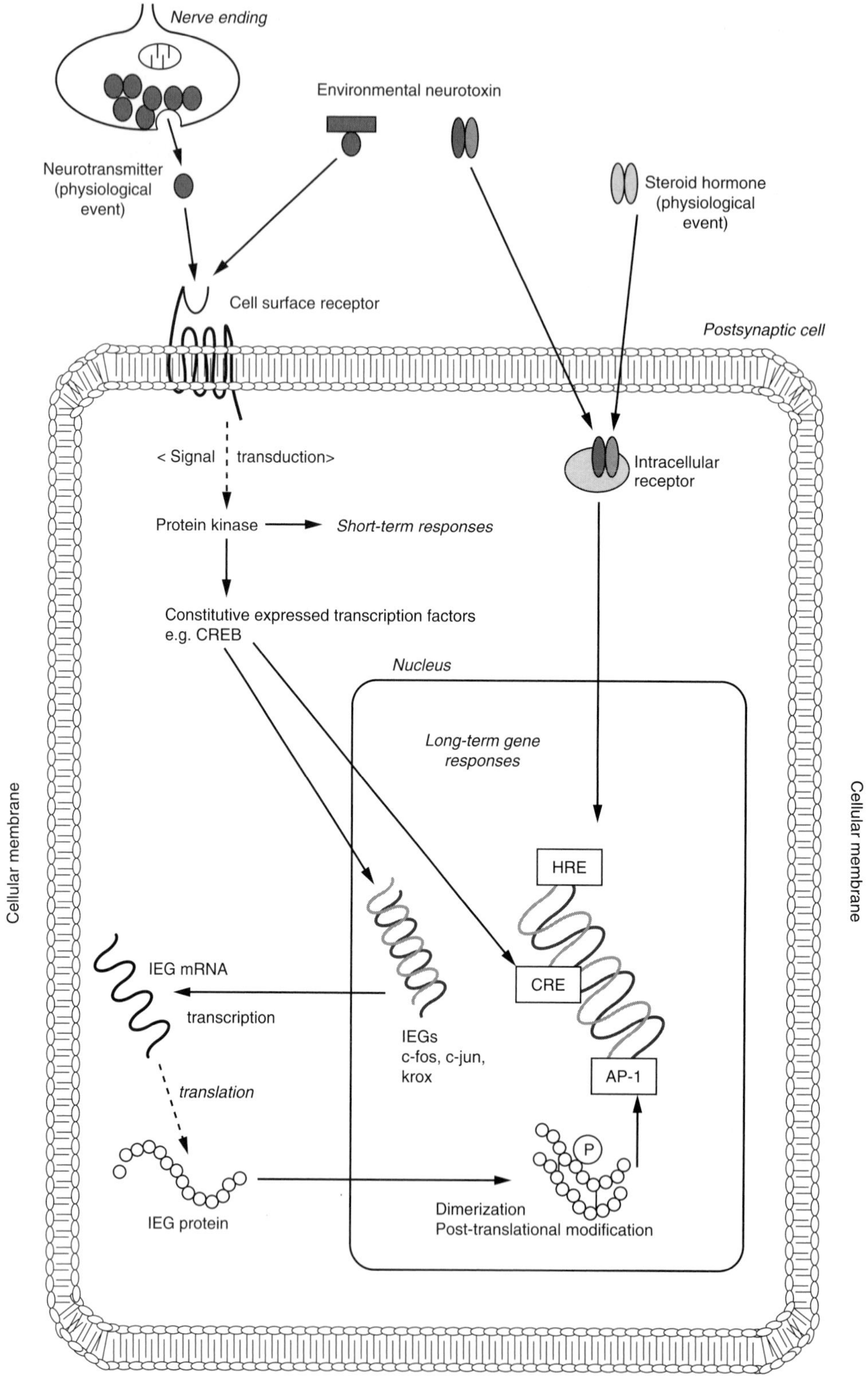

Figure 10.2 *Cell signaling pathways from the cell surface to the nucleus to activate the immediate early genes (IEGs). The responses of the neuron to its environment including physiological first messengers (neurotransmitter, growth factor or steroid hormone) and environmental neurotoxins may be divided into short- and long-term responses. Short-term responses are produced by activated protein kinases and last within the limits of the persistence of protein phosphorylation. Long-term responses involve changes in neuronal gene expression. These changes in gene expression are controlled by signal-regulated transcription factors (TFs; DNA binding effector molecules). Three families of signal regulated TFs exist: ligand-activated TFs (intracellular receptor) of the steroid hormone family; post-translationally activated TFs (e.g. CREB family); IEGs family (e.g. c-fos, c-jun). This figure was prepared from the illustrations in Figure 1 in the review by Hughes and Dragunow (1995).*

5-Fluorouracil, an antiprimidine, inhibits the synthesis of DNA by inhibiting thymikylate synthetase and can cross the blood–brain barrier. This drug is used for the treatment of breast cancer, colorectal cancer and other solid tumors, and has neurotoxicity as characterized mainly by cerebellar ataxia.

L-asparaginase is an enzyme which catalyzes the hydrolysis of L-asparagine to L-aspartic acid and ammonia. This drug is useful for therapy in patients with acute lymphoblastic leukemia who do not have the ability to synthesize their own asparagine.

Other antineoplastic agents that are found in the central nervous system are procarbazine, isosfamide, etoposide, cytosine arabinoside, and nitrosoureas like N,N-bis (2-chloroethyl)-N-nitrosourea. On the other hand, cisplatin, carboplatin, vinca alkaloids, such as vincristine, vindesine and vinblastine, taxol, and suramin, which are useful for tumors and cancers, are reported to cause neurotoxicity especially in the peripheral nervous system.

CREB-DEPENDENT GENE EXPRESSION

Adaptations in the cAMP signal transduction pathway underlie the mechanisms of tolerance to and dependence on opiates. Up-regulation of the cAMP signal transduction pathway plays an important role in the onset of the withdrawal syndrome. The CREB genes involved in a hypomorphic allele are CREB α, β, and δ.

MENDELIAN INHERITANCE AND NON-MENDELIAN INHERITANCE

Hereditary diseases in humans can result from chromosome alterations, either structural or numerical, a variety of changes within structural or regulatory genes, or polygenic mutations. Since cellular, organic, and environmental factors affect the mechanisms of inheritance, some environmental toxins may have genetic effects on the structure and function of the nervous system.

In spite of more complicated forms of single gene expression, multigene traits have also been reported, Mendel's laws still hold for many human genetic diseases, such as phenylketonuria, neurofibromatosis, Duchenne's muscular dystrophy, and cystic fibrosis (Price, 1994).

A gene is a sequence of nucleotides (constituting a small part of a DNA molecule) which provide codes for the production of a single polypeptide chain. Genes provide codes for protein structure and function. They occur in chromosomes in precise sequences, and their location on a chromosome is termed their 'loci.'

Homologous genes on homologous chromosomes occur at corresponding loci. Any given change in some part of the DNA is called a mutation and results in an alteration in the code of instructions for protein. Mutations are usually lethal since they can result in the production of defective protein or the cessation of protein synthesis. On rare occasions, however, mutations can manifest changes in some measurable attributes, termed traits or characters, which are inheritable. Any given gene may have two or more alternative forms that may coexist on homologous chromosomes as alleles. A gene pair or allelic pair are alleles occurring at the same locus on homologous chromosomes, and may be constituted by identical or different alleles. In the case of alleles which are identical, the organism is said to be homozygous for that trait; in the case of different alleles, the organism is said to be heterozygous for the trait. The genetic makeup of an organism for a single allelic pair and for the total complement of genes is termed the genotype. Phenotype is the structural and functional manifestations of an organisms's genotype.

Genotype and phenotype in mendelian inheritance

In sexually reproducing organisms, during gametogenesis, each member of a pair of alleles segregates to a different gamete. When fertilization occurs, each parent contributes an allele resulting in a zygote that is heterozygous (for example the stem length of pea plants). The offspring (the F1 generation) are termed hybrids, and monohybrids when organisms are heterozygous for only one trait.

As illustrated in standard genetic text books, the phenotype of all F1 offspring is dominant and the genotype of all F1 offspring is heterozygous dominant (Aa). The phenotypes in F2 offspring of matings between hybrid F1 offspring is formalized into the 3 (dominant) : 1 (recessive) ratio. There are three different genotypes: one homozygous dominant (AA), two heterozygous dominants (Aa) and one homozygous recessive (aa).

Non-mendelian inheritance

Most genes interact with others to produce some phenotypic effect. Epistatic genes interfere with or prevent the expression of other genes. M modifier genes alter the phenotypic expression of other genes.

INCOMPLETE DOMINANCE

Incomplete dominance is the incomplete masking of a recessive allele by a dominant allele in the heterozygous condition. The resultant phenotype is unlike that of either homozygous state. For example, a cross between one red allele and one white allele results in hetero-zygous offspring with a pink phenotype.

CODOMINANCE

Codominance is the phenotypic expression of both alleles of a gene locus. AB-type blood in humans is an example: A-allele provides the codes for the production of A-type antigens on the surface of red blood cells and B-allele provides the codes for the production of B-type antigens on the same red blood cells.

MULTIPLE ALLELES

Multiple alleles are the condition in which plural alleles exist for a given gene locus. The typical example is ABO blood groups in humans in which six possible genotypes result.

GENETIC FACTORS IN NEUROTOXICITY

Genetic factors may also be involved in the suscepti-bility of individuals to certain neurological compli-cations such as in alcoholism (Finnegan, 1995).

It is well known that excessive ethanol consumption is capable of producing deleterious effects on virtually any organ, and the CNS appears particularly suscep-tible. Although the reasons why manifestations of ethanol toxicity in the CNS are so common or why given neurological complications develop in some alcoholics and not in others remains poorly under-stood; a complex interplay among nutritional de-ficiencies, a direct toxic effect of ethanol, and genetic factors is presumed to be responsible. Wernicke's encephalopathy and Korsakoff's psychosis, neurological complications associated with chronic alcoholism, are thought to be mainly due to a deficiency in thiamin.

Wernicke's encephalopathy is a preventable disorder associated with a deficiency in thiamin. The activity of several enzyme systems, including transketolase, pyr-uvate dehydrogenase, and α-ketoglutarate dehydrogen-ase, depends on the availability of the cofactor thiamin. Variants of transketolase that differ in their binding affinity for thiamin have been known. It is possible that genetically determined alterations in thiamin-depen-dent enzymes develop into Wernicke's syndrome in only a relatively small proportion of thiamin-deficient alcoholics.

Korsakoff's psychosis is a syndrome showing ante-rograde amnesia (impairment of learning) most commonly and retrograde amnesia (disturbance of past memory) as well. Treatment involves thiamin replacement, but once established the memory deficit recovers in only a small proportion of patients. As well as Wernicke's encephalopathy, genetic factors are also important.

Induction of immediate early genes (IEGs) within the central nervous system

Numerous recent studies have shown that various treatments to the nervous system result in an increased expression of IEG mRNA and protein in both neurons and non-neuronal cells. Long-term, high-dose and repeated effects on the central nervous system and peripheral nervous system functions, which result from exposure to neurotoxicant(s), are mediated at a multitude of cellular levels (Hughes and Dragunow, 1995). However, changes in differential gene expression may greatly contribute to the neuropathological effects of the toxicant(s). For example, seizure activity induced toxicologically or pharmacologically and electrically; kindling, brain injury caused mechanically, by hypoxia ischemia and by spreading-depression; sensory stimu-lation, noxious, visual, olfactory, and somatosensory; stress; and long-term potentiation all result in increased expression of IEGs within the nervous system.

Immediate early genes and drug-induced seizure

Chemically and electrically induced seizures rapidly increase the expression of IEGs in mouse and rat brain. c-Jun, jun-B, zif268, and jun-D mRNA are induced in rat brain neurons when animals are given convulsant drugs or electric shock-induced seizure (Costa, 1994; Hughes and Dragunow, 1995). For example, pentyle-netetrazole, an epileptic convulsant, is known to induce c-fos mRNA and protein in various brain areas. Kainic acid, bicuculline, pilocarpine, lithium with pilocarpine, and MK801 with pilocarpine also result in increased expression of IEGs.

Immediate early gene proteins in drug dependence

A recent review has suggested that sensitization to psychosocial stressors may be encoded at the level of gene expression and that immediate early gene proteins (IEGPs) may play a role in this process (Hughes and Dragunow, 1995). Eventually, these genetically encoded stressful events may manifest themselves in the form of a major affective disorder.

IEGPs are very important molecules in the action of drugs of abuse (Hughes and Dragunow, 1995; Beno-witz, 1996). A number of drugs of abuse, such as morphine, cocaine, amphetamine, phencyclidine, and MK801, induce IEGPs principally in neurons of the striatum, but also in the cortical regions. IEGPs may also be involved in the chronic effects of opiates like morphine in the locus coeruleus. Opiate withdrawal after chronic treatment induces c-fos in this area.

Immediate early genes in brain injury and nerve cell death

Glutamate receptors, particularly the N-methyl-D-asparate (NMDA) receptors, play important roles in neuronal injury and brain plasticity. c-Jun expression is closely coupled to glutamate receptor activation. Low-level glutamate receptor activation at physiological events may produce a transient induction of c-jun, whereas activation of glutamate receptors producing neurotoxicity leads to prolonged c-jun and perhaps c-fos expression. Thus, a prolonged expression of c-jun may be necessary for nerve cell death in the brain.

Axotomy of nigrostriatal neurons with 6-hydroxy-dopamine (6-OHDA) produces a strong but short (two weeks) expression of c-jun in nigral dopamine neurons (Hughes and Dragunow, 1995).

The production of c-jun in axotomized peripheral nervous system and CNS neurons may be initiated by the absence of retrogradedly transported growth-, survival- or maintenance factors. The nerve growth factor (NGF) reduces c-jun expression in axotomized peripheral neurons. Antisence DNA studies are required to determine the role of neuronal c-jun expression in neuronal injury/repair/regeneration mechanisms.

NEUROTOXIN-INDUCED APOPTOSIS

Apoptosis in the nervous system

Cell death in the nervous system can occur through one of several mechanisms. Two distinct morphological cell deaths, apoptosis or necrosis, involve either active or passive cellular mechanisms, respectively. Up to 50% of many types of neurons normally die during maturation of the vertebrate nervous system. This elimination of neurons is essential for the appropriate structural and functional maturation of the nervous system (Charriaut-Marlangue et al., 1996).

Apoptosis is a form of cell death defined by morphological and biochemical features, the participation of specific genetic programs, and no inflammation. By contrast, necrotic cell death is characterized by a severe and sudden injury associated with an inflammatory response. The process of apoptosis is usually considered an active death that requires participation of cellular processes, unlike necrosis which appears to be a passive death. This active nature of apoptosis requires new protein synthesis. Within a dying cell, chromatin is condensed at the nuclear membrane concurrently with internucleosomal fragmentation of the chromatin. Cells undergoing apoptosis, and in general the nucleus, shrink remarkably and electron micrographs show a condensed cytoplasm with organelles that appear normal. Finally, it breaks into several dense spheres known as apoptotic bodies. This DNA digestion is a direct cause of the morphological changes. Early in the process of apoptosis, DNA is cleaved into fragments by Ca^{2+}/Mg^{2+}-dependent endonuclei. Apoptosis requires lethal proteins to be synthesized. Necrosis is a product of random DNA fragmentation only as a late consequence of release of lysosomal enzymes.

Unfortunately, most cytotoxic agents can induce apoptosis, and some may also induce necrosis in an appropriate system, even though they interact with many different primary targets. However, necrosis will occur only at higher concentrations, whereas apoptosis will be induced at only marginally toxic concentrations. Cytotoxin-induced apoptosis is expected to be prevented or inhibited by modulation of damage at the primary target, such as by drug export or enhanced DNA repair.

Apoptotic effects of neurotoxins

Oxidative stress refers to the cytologic consequences of a mismatch between the production of free radicals and the ability of the cell to defend itself against them. Oxidative stress induces both necrosis and apoptosis (Simonian and Coyle, 1996). In necrosis, a selective loss of membrane permeability occurs, which results in swelling of organelles, loss of membrane depolarization, and rupture of the plasma membrane. In apoptosis, a death-promoting signal activates a program of cell death through either new protein and RNA synthesis or depression of existing pathways. Cells undergoing apoptosis show shrinkage of the nucleus, condensation and fragmentation of chromatin, and usually DNA degradation by endonuclei into fragments in multiples of 180–200 base pairs. Although oxidative stress is not essential for all apoptotic cell death, oxidative DNA damage is believed to be a trigger for apoptosis.

Epileptogenic compound, such as kinate and glutamate, anticarcinogens, such as actinomycin D, herbicides, such as paraquat, and cycloheximide can also induce apoptosis in the central nervous system.

GENETIC AND ENVIRONMENTAL FACTORS INVOLVED IN BRAIN TUMORS

Epidemiology on brain tumors induced by chemical carcinogens

Brain tumors amount to less than two percent of all malignant neoplasms. About five to nine cases of primary brain tumors occur per 100 000 inhabitants in Western Europe and North America every year.

Approximately half of them are of glial origin and the remainder are of neuronal origin or are metastatic tumors from peripheral origin (Kleihues, *et al.*, 1995). Epidemiological statistic shows that the morbidity is higher in Caucasians than in people of African or Asian descent. Males are affected approximately 1.4 times more often than females. In children, tumors of the nervous system, including retinoblastomas and neuro-blastoma, rank second in incidence after leukemias. A significant proportion of brain tumors affect children.

Although epidemiological attempts to identify causative environmental agents have been unsuccessful, they have revealed an increased risk of brain tumor development in association with some occupations, for example farmers, dentists, fire fighters, metal workers, and the rubber industry. Multicenter studies have not proved the hypothesis of an increased incidence of brain tumors in certain occupational exposures, such as formaldehyde in anatomists and embalmers, vinyl chloride in plastic industry employees and electromagnetic fields in industrial workers.

Brain tumors induced by chemical carcinogens in experimental animals

Simple alkylating agents can induce tumors selectively in the rodent central nervous system. The typical carcinogens demonstrated are nitrosourea derivatives, dialkyl-aryltriazenes, azo compounds, azoxi compounds, and hydrazo compounds (Kleihues *et al.*, 1995). The probability of brain tumorgenesis with ethylnitrosourea and related ethylating agents is particularly high when a single or pulse dose of the carcinogen is administered transplacentally at a day after the 10th prenatal day or shortly after birth. The susceptibility of the rat brain with a single dose of the compound reaches its maximum at birth when a single dose is about 50 times more effective than in adult rats. There exists a species difference in the oncogenicity of ethylnitrosourea such that the brains of mice and gerbils do not express a significant tumor.

Experimental brain neoplasms induced by alkylating agents are classified into three categories. They are oligodendrogliomas, which originate from the white matter, astrocytomas, which originate from the sub-ependymal plate, and mixed gliomas.

As illustrated in Figure 10.3, the mechanism of carcinogenesity by alkylating agents is thought to result from the interaction of the ultimate carcinogen, a methyl cation or an ethyl cation, with cellular DNA. In this interaction, transition mutations from G : C to A : T are caused by O^6-alkylguanine, the major promutagenic base. Repair by the O^6-alkylguanine-DNA alkyltransferase responds much less efficiently in the central nervous system than in other peripheral organs, like the liver.

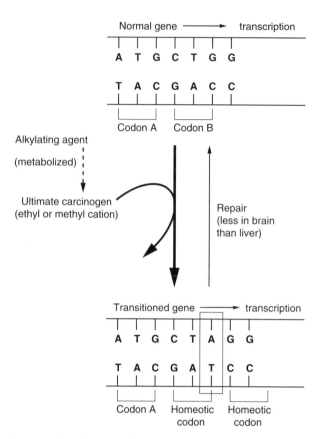

Figure 10.3 *Brain oncogenesis by alkylating agents. Interaction of the ultimate carcinogen from the alkylating agent with DNA causes transition of G : C to A : T mutation. A: adenine, C: cytosine, G: guanine, T: thymine.*

p53 mutations and human brain tumors

GLIOMAS

Gliomas amount to 30–40% of brain tumors. They are classified as: neurogliomas – astrocytomas, oligoden-drogliomas, ependymomas, and glioblastomas; neuro-cytomas – medulloblastoma, medullo-epithelioma, neuroblastoma, ganglioneuroma, and ganglioglioma; and pyneoparenchymas – pyneocytoma and pyneoblastoma. The rank order of incidence of gliomas are astrocytomas, glioblastomas, ependymomas, medullo-blastoma, and oligodendrogliomas. These five tumors amount to 80–90% of all gliomas.

p53 MUTATIONS

Carcinogenesis is a multistage process involving activation of protooncogenes, for example ras, and inactivation of tumor suppresser genes, for example p53 and p16^{INK4} (Kleihues, *et al.*, 1995). Mutation of the p53 tumor gene is the most frequent single genetic legion detected in human tumors. The mutation is found more frequently in the more malignant late stages of tumor development than in early stages, suggesting that loss of function of p53 is important in malignant progression. p53 is a prototype tumor suppresser gene and is useful for analysis of the mutational spectrum in human cancers. The p53 mutational spectrum differs among cancers of the brain, colon, lymphoid, liver, lung breast, esophagus, reticuloendothelial tissues, and hemopoietic tissues. Transitions predominate in malignant tumors of brain, colon, and lymphoid. Mutational hotspots at CpG dinucleotides in codon 175, 245, 248, 273, and 282 are thought to reflect endogenous mutagenic mechanisms, for example deamination of 5-methylcytosine to thymidine.

Since p53 mutations are observed during glioma progression, analyzing p53 mutations is useful in assessing a possible potential source of information on the etiology of human brain tumors. p53 mutations in sporadic astrocytic brain tumors are mainly located in the highly conserved region of the gene, with clusters at codons 175, 248, and 273. These codes are located among the six hot spots and are found in various human tumors. Transitions from G : C to A : T are most frequent (52%) and are predominantly located at CpG sites among p53 mutations in astrocytic brain tumors. However, since the transition mutations at CpG sites can best be explained as being endogenous events, the deamination of 5-methylcytosine residues but not exogenous events caused by genotoxic environmental carcinogens. Until now, any specific mutations or mutational hot spots, which could demonstrate or suggest environmental carcinogens operative in the etiology, have not been found in human brain tumors.

GLIOMA PROGRESSION AND p53 MUTATIONS

Astrocytoma progression is supposed to reflect the sequential accumulation of genetic alterations. Astrocytomas, benign brain tumors, have an intrinsic tendency to progress towards a more malignant tumor, a glioblastoma, phenotypically, histopathologically, and clinically. For example, diffusely infiltrating low-grade astrocytomas (WHO Grade II) tend to progress to anaplastic astrocytoma (WHO Grade III) and glioblastoma (WHO Grade IV) (Kleihues, et al., 1995). p53 mutations, with or without loss of heterozygosity on chromosome 17p, are the principal detectable changes in low-grade astrocytomas. Anaplastic astrocytomas show p53 mutations at an overall incidence of 34%, with loss of heterozygosity on chromosome 19q and frequently with homozygous deletion of the p16 tumor suppresser (MTS-1) gene is observed. Glioblastoma, the most malignant astrocytoma, shows loss of chromosome 10 and amplification of the epidermal growth factor receptor (EGF-R) gene at overall incidences of 66 and 34%, respectively.

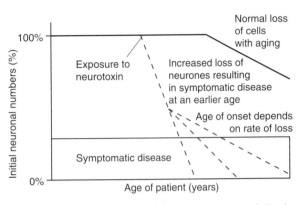

Figure 10.4 *Increase rate of loss of neurones following exposure to a neurotoxin producing symptomatic neurological disease at an earlier stage.*

BIOCHEMICAL MECHANISMS

There is a natural decrement in both neuronal numbers and functional efficiency with age. Increasing evidence suggests that the effects of some neurotoxic chemicals and drugs may not become apparent unless neuronal numbers and function are below a critical threshold, which then produce deficits that are apparent to both the individual and the clinician. In some cases of parkinsonism a genetic variation in the response of cells in the nigrostriatal tracts to neurotoxic oxidative stress may exist. The adverse effects of exposure to a neurotoxic chemical may not be apparent unless the functional activity and number of dopaminergic cells in these tracts has fallen below a critical threshold (Figure 10.4).

Genetic polymorphisms

Genetic polymorphisms in metabolism are increasingly being seen to also play a significant role in an individual's susceptibility to neurotoxicity. The clinical consequences of slow acetylator phenotype include increased susceptibility to peripheral neuropathies produced by isoniazid, hydrallazine, and dapsone. Similarly, following the administration of methoin, poor metabolizers of this drug have increased somnolence and intellectual impairment (Relling, 1989). Phenotypic variation in plasma esterases, especially cholinesterases, may contribute to the toxicity of some anticholinesterases affecting both the toxicity of these compounds directly, but also influencing their metabolism and elimination.

Genetic differences in the activity of a specific enzyme may be associated, in an individual, with an increased risk of developing certain neurological disorders. It is not yet clear how important these differences are for many drug-related adverse neurological effects since experience to date has been principally with non-drug chemicals. Nevertheless, useful risk indicators can be derived and these will now be described.

ACETYLATOR STATUS

Acetylation is a conjugation reaction, usually for aromatic amines or hydrazines, where an acetyl group is transferred from acetyl co-enzyme A, by acetyltransferases, to receptor amines resulting in the formation of an amide. Many drugs and other chemicals are metabolized by this pathway and the slow gene frequency in a population varies from 20 to 90%, showing marked racial differences. Inheritance is as an autosomal recessive trait. Isoniazid is a potent irritant of the central nervous system but an isoniazid-induced polyneuropathy was the first neurological adverse reaction to be recognized as associated with slow acetylation (Weber et al., 1983). The neurotoxic effect has been shown to be a consequence of isoniazid-induced vitamin B6 (pyridoxime) deficiency. A modest excess of slow acetylators in motor neurone disease and faster acetylators in Parkinson's disease has been reported (Heathfield et al., 1990).

DEBRISOQUINE-4-HYDROXYLASE DEFICIENCY

Debrisoquine is metabolized by ring hydroxylation, and polymorphic differences in metabolism have been established. The phenotype is determined from the ratio of the percentage of a dose excreted as unchanged debrisoquine to that excreted as the metabolite, 4-hydroxydebrisoquine (metabolic ratio) (Ohta et al., 1990). Family studies on the phenotype have indicated that it is an autosomal recessive trait with the enzyme deficiency present in approximately 6–8% of the UK population. Mutations in regulatory genes seem to be involved and at least four P450 proteins are involved (Gonzalez et al., 1987, 1988; Gonzalez, 1988). Cloning and sequencing of cDNAs from the livers of poor metetabolizers have identified at least three variant RNAs, but these have been the products of intron mutants producing an incorrectly spliced P450 pre-RNA.

Several studies of this phenotype have found no differences in the frequency of Parkinson's disease, amyotrophic lateral sclerosis or dementia from the general population. However, some studies do suggest a shift in the metabolic ratio in favor of poor metabolism in these patients, although the percentage of poor metabolizers is not significantly different from controls (Barbeau et al., 1985; Steventon et al., 1989a). Phenotype studies may not be the best predictors of abnormal genotypes since recent molecular studies suggest a modest but significant increase in poor

metabolizer mutations in Parkinson's disease (Smith et al., 1992).

SULFUR METABOLISM

The phenotype for this oxidation polymorphism is determined by measuring sulfur oxides in urine following the administration of S-carboxymethyl-cysteine. The enzyme involved, cysteine dioxygenase, is the rate-limiting step in the conversion of cysteine to sulfate. Patients with Parkinson's disease, amyotrophic lateral sclerosis, and presumed Alzheimer's disease are, as a group, very poor metabolizers. Cysteine dioxygenase has also been found to be deficient in Hallervorden–Spatz disease. The results suggest that individuals born with underactivity of this metabolic pathway are less capable of dealing with sulfur compounds used as drugs or found in the environment and food. Brassica vegetables (cabbages, etc.) have a high sulfur load and Parkinson's disease has been related to a high intake of raw vegetables. Sulfur availability may reduce the capacity to detoxify drugs and compounds, such as cyanide and heavy metals, and may also be responsible for excess production of free radicals.

MONOAMINE OXIDASE B

MPTP (1-methyl-4-phenyl-1,2,3,6-tetrahydropyridine), a contaminant of illicit designer drugs, causes selective neuronal death resulting in a neurological disorder similar to Parkinson's disease (Davis et al., 1979; Adams and Odunze, 1991). The neurotoxic metabolite is the N-methyl-4-phenyl pyridinium ion (MPP+). Conversion, via the enzyme monoamine oxidase B (MAO-B), is an intoxication step when it occurs in the brain, but could be considered a detoxification if it occurs outside the brain, such as in the liver or gut, since MPP+ cannot cross the blood–brain barrier. MAO-B is found in platelets and there is evidence that the activity of this enzyme is closely related to that in the liver and brain (Steventon et al., 1989b). MPTP is a relatively simple chemical and similar compounds could be derived from tryptamine metabolism, endogenously or exogenously, or possibly from plants in food (Ramsden and Williams, 1985). There is also the possibility that beta-carbolines, tetrahydroisoquinolones, and trichlorethylene share the same pathway for metabolism, mechanism, and site of toxicity with MPP+.

A study using phenylethylamine as a substrate found an increased MAO-B activity in untreated patients with Parkinson's disease, although there was overlap with the normal range. When dopamine was used as a substrate there was a much reduced activity. There may be several isoenzymes of MAO-B which could function as risk markers for screening, since inefficient enzymes may allow MPTP, or similar compounds, to reach the brain before conversion to MPP+. Alternatively, the reduced metabolism of dopamine in Parkinson's disease may produce a rise in dopamine levels resulting in shunting down other metabolic pathways with the production of toxic metabolites, such as an orthohydroxylated derivative of dopamine, which has neuroexcitotoxic properties.

METHYLATION

The enzyme, thiolmethyltransferase (TMT), carries out *S*-methylation, which masks functional chemical groups and reduces water solubility impairing further conjugation (Waring *et al.*, 1989). TMT is involved in the detoxification of substances such as hydrogen sulfide and other free sulfydryl compounds including the thioesters of glutathione conjugates (a final common pathway for many toxic xenobiotics).

Hydrogen sulfide has a similar toxic mechanism to cyanide, acting as a mitochondrial poison, and may cause an acquired defect in mitochondrial function similar to that described in Parkinson's disease. Patients with amyotrophic lateral sclerosis have high activity of TMT, when assessed by *in vitro* test systems, but in Parkinson's disease and patients with Alzheimer's disease, low activity is found. The low enzyme activity has a high heritability, but it is possible for some individuals to have reduced activity of the normal enzyme or an isoenzyme. Heavy metals, such as mercury, form toxic derivatives with the enzyme and increased enzyme activity, such as that reported in the motor neurone diseases, might predispose to heavy metal poisoning.

N-methylation is carried out by *N*-methyltransferases, which can act on a number of different substrates, including substituted 4-phenyl pyridines to form MPTP (Ansher *et al.*, 1986). The level of enzyme activity can be determined by measurement of *N*-methylnicotinamide excretion in urine following administration of nicotinamide. In one study, patients with amyotrophic lateral sclerosis had normal excretion but those with Parkinson's disease excreted considerably increased amounts of this *N*-methyl derivative (Green *et al.*, 1991).

SUMMARY

Neurological adverse reactions are determined by the rates of absorption, distribution, biotransformation, and excretion as well as the toxicodynamics of a chemical. The body's defenses against toxic effects are complex and there are considerable interindividual, genetic, inter-racial, and interspecies variations in both toxicokinetics and toxicodynamics. Many of these variations will be dependent on genetic polymorphisms in the specific enzymes involved in the toxic mechanisms. Perhaps uniquely, in the nervous system early damage to neuronal function may not become clinically

important until the natural decrease in neuronal numbers and function with age passes a critical threshold. This concept can explain why some neurodegenerative disorders may appear at an unusually early age in certain patients.

REFERENCES

Adams, J.D. Jr. and Odunze, I.N. 1991: Biochemical mechanisms of 1-methyl-4-phenyl-1,2,3,6-tetrahydropyridine toxicity: could oxidative stress be involved in the brain? *Biochemical Pharmacology*, **8**, 1099–105.

Albin, R.L. and Tagle, D.A. 1995: Genetic and molecular biology of Huntington's disease. *Trends in Neurosciences*, **18**, 11–4.

Ansher, S.S., Cadet, J.L., Jakoby, W.B. and Baker, J.K. 1986: Role of *N*-methyl-transferases in the neurotoxicity associated with the metabolites of 1-methyl-4-phenyl-1,2,3,6-tetrahydropyridine (MPTP) and other 4-substituted pyridines in the environment. *Biochemical Pharmacology*, **35**, 3359–62.

Barbeau, A., Cloutier, Y. and Roy, M. 1985: Ecogenetics of Parkinson's disease: 4 hydroxylation of debrisoquine. *Lancet*, **2**, 1213–15.

Benowitz, N.L. 1996: Pharmacology of nicotine: addiction and therapeutics. *Annual Review of Pharmacology and Toxicology*, **36**, 597–613.

Cascino, T. 1995: Clinical neurotoxic concerns on antineoplastic agents. In *Neurotoxicology Approaches and Methods*, Chang, L.W. (ed.), pp 657–70. San Diego, CA: Academic Press.

Charriaut-Marlangue, C., Aggoun-Zouaoui, D., Represa, A. and Ben-Ari, Y. 1996: Apoptotic features of selective neuronal death in ischemia, epilepsy and gp 120 toxicity. *Trends in Neurosciences*, **19**, 109–14.

Cordell, B. 1994: β-Amyloid formation as a potential therapeutic target for Alzheimer's disease. *Annual Review of Pharmacology and Toxicology*, **35**, 69–89.

Costa, L.G. 1994: Signal transduction mechanisms in developmental neurotoxicity: the phosphoinositide pathway. *Neurotoxicology*, **15**, 19–28.

Davis, G.C., Williams, A.C., Markey, S.P. *et al.* 1979: Chronic parkinsonism secondary to intravenous injection of meperidine analogs. *Psychiatry Research*, **1**, 249.

Dawson, R., Beal, M.F., Bondy, S.C., Di Monte, D.A. and Isom, G.A. 1995: Contemporary issues in toxicology. Excitotoxins, aging, and environmental neurotoxins: implications for understanding human neurodegenerative diseases. *Toxicology and Applied Pharmacology*, **134**, 1–17.

Eastman, A. 1993: Highlights. Apoptosis: a product of programmed and unprogrammed cell death. *Toxicology and Applied Pharmacology*, **121**, 160–4.

Eberwine, J.H. 1994: Molecular biological techniques applied to the study of the central nervous system. In *Biological Bases of Brain Function and Disease*, Frazer, A., Molinoff, P. and Winokur, A. (eds), pp 61–83. New York: Raven Press.

Fan, A. and Howd, R. 1995: Risk assessment of environmental chemicals. *Annual Review of Pharmacology and Toxicology*, **35**, 341–68.

Finnegan, K.T. 1995: Clinical neurotoxicological concerns on drugs of abuse. In *Neurotoxicology Approaches and Methods*, Chang, L.W. (ed.), pp 641–55. San Diego, CA: Academic Press.

Gonzalez, F.J. 1988: The molecular biology of cytochrome P450s. *Pharmacological Reviews*, **40**, 243–88.

Gonzalez, F.J., Matsunaga, T., Nagata, K. *et al.* 1987: Debrisoquine-4-hydroxylase: characterization of a new P450 gene subfamily regulation, chromosomal mapping and molecular analysis of the DNA rate polymorphism. *DNA*, **6**, 149–61.

Gonzalez, F.J., Skoda, R.C., Kimura, S. *et al.* 1988: Characterization of the common genetic defect in humans deficient in debrisoquine metabolism. *Nature*, **331**, 442–6.

Green, S., Buttrum, S., Molloy, H. *et al.* 1991: *N*-methylation of pyridines in Parkonson's disease (letter). *Lancet*, **338**, 120–1.

Heafield, M.T.E., Waring, R.H., Sturman, S.G. *et al.* 1990: *N*-acetylatic status in neurodegenerative disease. *Medicine and Science Research*, **18**, 963–6.

Higgins, L.S. and Cordell, B. 1995: Review article. Genetically engineered animal models of human neurodegenerative diseases. *Neurodegeneration*, **4**, 117–29.

Hughes, P. and Dragunow, M. 1995: Induction of immediate early genes and the control of neurotransmitter-regulated gene expression within the nervous system. *Pharmacological Reviews*, **47**, 133–78.

Johannessen, J.J. 1995: Biomolecular approaches to neurotoxic hazard assessment. In *Neurotoxicology: Approaches and Methods*, Chang, L.W. and Sukker, W. (eds), pp 399–421. San Diego, CA: Academic Press.

Joyce, J.N. and Hurgig, H.I. 1994: Neurodegenerative disorders. In *Biological Bases of Brain Function and Disease*, Frazer, A., Molinoff, P. and Winokur, A. (eds), pp 427–48. New York: Raven Press.

Kleihues, P., Aguzzi, A. and Ohgaki, H. 1995: Genetic and environmental factors in the etiology of human brain tumors. *Toxicology Letters*, **82/83**, 601–5.

LoPachin, R.M. and Aschner, M. 1993: Contemporary issues in toxicology. Glial-neuronal interactions: relevance to neurotoxic mechanisms. *Toxicology and Applied Pharmacology*, **118**, 141–58.

Ohta, S., Tachikawa, O., Makino, Y. *et al*. 1990: Metabolism and brain accumulation of tetrahydro-isoquinoline (TIQ), a possible parkinsonism-inducing substance, in an animal model of a poor debrisoquine metabolizer. *Life Sciences*, **46**, 599–605.

Price, R.A. 1994: Genetic approaches to mental illness. In *Biological Bases of Brain Function and Disease*, Frazer, A., Molinoff, P. and Winokur, A. (eds), pp 281–99. New York: Raven Press.

Ramsden, D.B. and Williams, A.C. 1985: Production in nature of compound resembling methylphenyltetrahydropyridine, a possible cause of Parkinson's disease. *Lancet*, **1**, 215–16.

Relling, M.V. 1989: Polymorphic drug metabolism. *Clinical Pharmacy*, **8**, 852–63.

Risch, N. and Merikangas, K. 1996: The future of genetic studies of complex human diseases. *Science*, **273**, 1516–17.

Simonian, N.A. and Coyle, J.T. 1996: Oxidative stress in neurodegenerative diseases. *Annual Review of Pharmacology and Toxicology*, **36**, 83–106.

Smith, C.A.D., Gough, A.C., Leigh, P.N. *et al*. 1992: Debrisoquine hydroxylase gene polymorphism and susceptibility to Parkinson's disease. *Lancet*, **339**, 1375–7.

Standaert, D.G. and Young, A.B. 1996: Treatment of central nervous system degenerative disorders. In *Goodman and Gilman's The Pharmacological Basis of Therapeutics*, Hardman, J.G., Limbrid, L.E., Molinoff, P.B. and Ruddon, R.W. (eds), 9th edn, pp 503–19. New York: McGraw-Hill.

Steventon, G.B., Heafield, M.T.E., Sturman, S.G. *et al*. 1989a: Degenerative neurological disease and debrisoquine-4-hydroxylation capacity. *Medicine and Science Research*, **17**, 163–4.

Steventon, G.B., Sturman, S.G., Heafield, M.T.E. *et al*. 1989b: Platelet monoamine oxidase-B activity in Parkinson's disease. *Journal of Neurological Transmission*, **1**, 255–61.

Waring, R.H., Steventon, G., Heafield, M.T.E. *et al*. 1989: *S*-Methylation in Parkinson's disease and motor neurone disease. *Lancet*, **2**, 356–7.

Weber, W.W., Hein, D.W., Litwin, A. and Lower, G.M. 1983: Relationship of acetylator status to isoniazid toxicity, lupus erythematosus and bladder cancer. *Federation Proceedings*, **42**, 3086–97.

Whitney, K.D., Seidler, F.J. and Slotkin, T.A. 1995: Developmental neurotoxicity of chlorpyrifos: cellular mechanisms. *Toxicology and Applied Pharmacology*, **134**, 53–62.

Zawia, N.H. and Harry, G.J. 1993: Trimethyltin-induced c-fos expression: adolescent vs neonatal rat hippocampus. *Toxicology and Applied Pharmacology*, **121**, 99–102.

Zawia, N.H. and Harry, G.J. 1996: Developmental exposure to lead interferes with glial and neuronal differential gene expression in the rat cerebellum. *Toxicology and Applied Pharmacology*, **138**, 43–7.

Prion disease

MARTIN ZEIDLER

INTRODUCTION

The prion diseases are a group of fatal human and animal neurodegenerative conditions (Table 11.1) associated with an infectious agent whose nature is currently unknown. The history of prion disease starts over 250 years ago with the recognition of a disorder of sheep called scrapie. In the early 1920s the first descriptions of the most common human prion disease, Creutzfeldt–Jakob disease (CJD), were published and 15 years later the infectious nature of scrapie was first demonstrated. Kuru, a condition largely confined to a single region in Papua New Guinea, was brought to the world's attention in the late 1950s. The alarming conclusion that this human prion disease was passed via ritualistic cannibalism raised much interest at the time. In 1965 kuru was reported to be transmissible by intracerebral inoculation to the chimpanzee, prompting similar transmission studies of a number of other human neurodegenerative conditions. These were unsuccessful for all but one condition: CJD, which shares many histological features with kuru, including spongiform change. Hence the term transmissible spongiform encephalopathy (TSE). Although it was generally assumed at this time that the TSEs were due to infection with a 'slow virus', such an agent could not be identified and in 1967 a mathematician, Griffiths, wrote to *Nature* to suggest the infective particle might be a protein. His theory was largely ignored for the next 15 years. In 1974 the first iatrogenic case of CJD was reported in a patient who developed CJD 18 months after receiving a corneal transplant from a donor with CJD. Tragically, over 170 iatrogenic cases have now occurred, mainly following the use of contaminated human cadaveric-derived growth hormone or dura mater homografts, but also as the result of contaminated neurosurgical instruments and human cadaveric-derived gonadotropin.

About 10–15% of human prion diseases are hereditary and include, in addition to familial CJD, the disorders fatal familial insomnia (FFI) and Gerstmann–Sträussler–Scheinker syndrome (GSS). In 1986 the gene associated with these autosomal dominant disorders was mapped to the short arm of chromosome 20. In the same year as this important genetic discovery was made the first case of a novel prion disease of cattle was reported in England. The subsequent epidemic of bovine spongiform encephalopathy (BSE) raised much concern for public health. However, this was tempered by the reassurance that the most likely cause of this new disease was sheep scrapie, a disorder to which humans were not known to be susceptible. Measures to protect humans from exposure to the BSE agent were quickly put in place but there still remained a window between 1986 and 1989 when a potentially large proportion of the UK population could have been exposed to the BSE agent in their diet.

In March 1996, the occurrence of 10 cases of a new variant of CJD (nvCJD) was announced by the UK government. These patients exhibited an apparently novel and distinct clinicopathological phenotype and, although unproven, an etiological link with the BSE agent, given the temporo-spatial association, was considered likely (Will *et al.*, 1996). There was

Table 11.1 *Human and animal prion diseases*

Human	First reported
Creutzfeldt–Jakob disease	
Sporadic	1921
Familial	1924
Iatrogenic	1974
New variant	1996
Gerstmann–Sträussler–Scheinker syndrome	1928
Kuru	1955
Fatal familial insomnia	1986

Animal	First reported
Scrapie	
Sheep	1730
Goat	1872
Moufflon	1992
Transmissible mink encephalopathy	1965
Chronic wasting disease of mule and elk deer	1967
Bovine spongiform encephalopathy	1986
Feline spongiform encephalopathy	
Domestic cat	1990
Puma	1992
Cheetah	1992
Ocelot	1994
Tiger	1996
Spongiform encephalopathy of captive wild ruminants	
Nyala	1987
Gemsbok	1988
Arabian oryx	1989
Eland	1989
Kudu	1989
Scimitar-horn oryx	1993
Ankole	1995

the tongue more easily). It was first coined in 1982 by the American neuroscientist Stanley Pruisiner (Prusiner, 1982). The prion theory postulates that the infectious TSE agent (the prion) is composed largely, if not entirely, of an abnormal isoform of a normal membrane protein. Although this hypothesis appears to fly in the face of conventional microbiological wisdom, with the passage of time, and an impressive array of supportive evidence, initial scepticism has largely dwindled. The prion hypothesis is now the convention. However, it may not be the whole answer. A characteristic of many TSEs is the presence of different strains of agent, a concept that, as explained in more detail later, fits much easier with a viral-like rather than protein-only agent.

Whatever the nature of the TSE agent, it clearly possesses unusual and fascinating properties. For example, it is unique in causing a disease that is both hereditary and infectious. Furthermore, its remarkable resistance to sterilization is noteworthy and raises many concerns, including the possibility of as yet unrecognized modes of iatrogenic transmission. This chapter will review the present state of knowledge on human and animal prion diseases, including a further discussion on the nature of the infectious agent, safety issues, and the possible link between CJD and BSE.

HUMAN TRANSMISSIBLE SPONGIFORM ENCEPHALOPATHIES

Sporadic Creutzfeldt–Jakob disease

BACKGROUND AND EPIDEMIOLOGY

In 1920 Hans Gerhard Creutzfeldt, a German neuroscientist, reported the case of a 22-year-old women with a six-year history of progressive cerebral dysfunction. A year later another German neuroscientist, Alfons Jakob, described further cases and in 1922 the term Creutzfeldt–Jakob disease was first introduced. Although some of these first cases would not have met modern neuropathological criteria, a retrospective analysis suggests at least half were the condition we now know as CJD. However, CJD remained an obscure and poorly understood condition over the ensuing four decades, a situation not helped by the use of the multiple synonyms (listed below):

- disseminated encephalopathy;
- spastic pseudosclerosis;
- cortico-pallido-spinal degeneration;
- cortico-striato-spinal degeneration;
- Jakob's syndrome;
- presenile dementia with cortical blindness;
- Heidenhain's syndrome;

subsequently heightened public concern in Britain, Europe and the rest of the world, and an immediate global ban on beef exports from the UK was imposed. In April 1996 a case of nvCJD was reported in France and by August 1997 a total of 21 cases had been confirmed in the UK. At present too little information is available to accurately predict the future number of cases of this new disease, which has potentially far-reaching implications for public health in both the UK and further afield.

Although it is claimed that more is known about the molecular biology of the TSEs than any other group of neurodegenerative diseases, the search for diagnostic tools and potential treatments is currently hampered by the elusive nature of the infectious agent. However, increasing evidence is accumulating in support of the radical 'infectious protein' theory first proposed by Griffiths 30 years ago. The term prion (pronounced pree-on) stands for PROteinaceous INfectious particle (with the o and i switched to allow the word to role off

- subacute vascular encephalopathy with mental disorder;
- subacute presenile spongiosus atrophy;
- Nevin–Jones disease;
- Brownell–Oppenheimer syndrome.

Following the identification of the transmissibility of CJD to primates in 1968, epidemiological surveys, including case-control studies, have been undertaken in France, the USA, Israel, Japan, the UK, and more recently collaboratively in the European Union. Our current understanding of CJD epidemiology is indebted to these studies which have led to a greater insight of the clinical and pathological features of CJD in addition to addressing the difficult question, given the rarity of disease, of etiological risk factors.

The incidence of CJD is approximately 0.5–1.0 cases per million persons per year. The female to male ratio is representative of the general population and no distinct pattern of socio-economic incidence prevails. The majority of cases occur sporadically, and in this group there is no evidence of geographical clustering or case-to-case transmission (Will *et al.*, 1986). The mean age at onset of disease is approximately 65 years but is known to range from 14–92 years of age. Case-control studies have yielded controversial results, suggesting an association of CJD with various factors including surgery to the head, surgery requiring sutures, herpes zoster infection, trauma to the head or body, tonometry, consumption of various meats, farming, and exposure to a range of animals including fish and squirrels. However, none of these associations have consistently been found and therefore they may simply reflect the difficulty of obtaining reliable associations from small studies. A recent meta-analysis, comprising 178 cases and 333 control patients, found no statistical evidence for an association between the development of sporadic CJD and diet (including consumption of brain), previous surgery, blood transfusion, occupation or animal exposure (Wientjens *et al.*, 1996). However, even this relatively large analysis may lack the statistical power to detect minor, but relevant, risk factors. In the near future data from over 400 case-control pairs identified as part of the recent European Union Collaborative Study Group of CJD will be available, with a greater power to detect potentially relevant risk factors than the previous smaller national studies.

CLINICAL FEATURES

The classical diagnostic triad of CJD is a rapidly progressive dementia, myoclonus, and a characteristic electroencephalogram (EEG). The median and mean duration of illness are 4.5 and 8 months, respectively, and only 4% of cases survive longer than two years (Brown *et al.*, 1994). Patients usually present (in order of decreasing frequency) with cognitive decline, ataxia or visual disturbance, either alone or in combination.

Less common presenting features include behavioral disturbance or a rapid evolution resembling a stroke. There is sometimes a history obtained of non-specific symptoms, such as headache, fatigue, sleeping difficulties, weight loss, malaise or anxiety, in the illness prodrome. Dementia is invariably present during the course of the illness and myoclonus, although a rare presenting feature, is observed at some stage in 80% of cases. Visual abnormalities are also common and include non-specific blurring, visual field defects, perceptual abnormalities, and occasionally hallucinations. Seizures virtually never occur at presentation and are only observed later in the clinical course in 10% of patients. As the disease progresses multi-focal central nervous system failure occurs with increasing global cognitive dysfunction, urinary incontinence, ataxia and dependency, culminating in the patient becoming bedbound, mute, and unresponsive. Physical pain is an uncommon feature at any stage of the illness and, due to the rapid progression of cognitive impairment, any retained insight is usually soon lost. Terminally, the patients are usually rigid, frequently cortical blind, dysphagic (predisposing to aspiration and pneumonia, the commonest cause of death), and may develop Cheyne–Stokes respiration.

Physical signs correspond with the global central nervous system involvement and may include a combination of cerebellar, pyramidal, and extrapyramidal signs. Primitive reflexes, paratonic (gegenhalten) rigidity, cortical blindness, and akinetic mutism are also common, whereas lower motor neuron signs are rarely observed. Myoclonus is probably the most important clinical sign. It usually shows some asymmetry; is typically arrhythmic, asynchronous, and stimulus sensitive; and noted most frequently in the limbs, but also commonly affects the body and/or face. Stimulus sensitive myoclonus or a startle reaction can occur in response to sudden noise, visual threat, touch, noise, or muscle stretch, but usually myoclonus can also be noted at rest. Attempted movement may induce the jerks as may a maintained posture such as holding the arms outstretched.

DIFFERENTIAL DIAGNOSIS

The characteristic clinical features of CJD – rapidly progressive dementia and myoclonus – can rarely occur in patients with Alzheimer's disease, the most common condition mimicking CJD. Reports exist of the characteristic EEG appearances of CJD occurring in Alzheimer's disease but these are exceptional. Other conditions that are important in the differential diagnosis are listed below:

- multi-infarct dementia/cerebrovascular disease;
- diffuse Lewy body disease;
- brain tumors (both primary and secondary);
- motor neuron disease;

- cerebellar degeneration;
- Pick's disease;
- progressive supranuclear palsy;
- multiple system atrophy;
- corticobasal degeneration;
- metabolic encephalopathies;
- drug-induced encephalopathies, e.g. bismuth, amitriptyline, mianserin, lithium, baclofen;
- viral encephalitis.

PATHOLOGY

As with animal TSEs, no specific macroscopic abnormalities are detected outside the central nervous system (CNS) at autopsy in CJD. Although macroscopic examination of the brain may be unremarkable, cortical atrophy is often found, although this may vary greatly from case to case and within the various regions of the cortex in each individual. Sometimes the pattern of atrophy may correspond with the clinical syndrome, such as involvement of the occipital lobes in cases with relevant visual symptoms, or may occasionally extend to involve the basal ganglia, thalamus, and hypothalamus.

The microscopic hallmarks of sporadic CJD are spongiform change, neuronal loss, and astrocytosis. Amyloid plaques, similar to those of Alzheimer's disease but composed of prion protein (PrP) rather than β-amyloid, are seen in about 10% of sporadic CJD cases, but are much more common in kuru, iatrogenic CJD, and the familial forms of disease. Spongiform change consists of a fine vacuolation of the gray matter neuropil in which vacuoles vary from 2 to 20 μm in size, with larger vacuoles becoming confluent to form irregular cavities. In long-standing cases severe spongiform change, neuronal loss, and astrocytosis may occur, leading to status spongiosus with collapse of the cytoarchitecture. Neuronal loss and reactive astrocytosis generally tend to be most apparent in the gray matter areas with spongiform change (Ironside, 1996).

An adjunct to the neuropathological investigation of CJD and related disorders has come from advances in PrP immunocytochemistry. In this technique tissue sections are stained using monoclonal or polyclonal antibodies directed against PrP. Because tissues may normally express PrP^C (the normal cellular PrP isoform), pre-treatment is required to ensure that only the pathological PrP^{Sc} (the abnormal isoform, sc = scrapie form) is detected. Although the pattern of PrP positivity may be as variable as standard pathology, certain generalities can be made. PrP immunostaining patterns appear to be of two main types: perivacuolar deposits and discrete plaques. In the presence of severe spongiform change in the neocortical gray, irregular strongly positive PrP deposits are present within coalescing vacuoles and around the periphery of these lesions. The second type of distinctive abnormality, PrP positive plaques, may be more conspicuous with immunocytochemistry compared to routine hematoxylin and eosin staining. The most frequent sites of plaque formation include the granular layer and, to a lesser extent, the central white matter and molecular layers of the cerebellum. Well-defined plaques may also be seen in the basal ganglia, thalamus, brain stem, and cerebral cortex. More subtle staining patterns are often seen, in particular some neurons may be outlined by granular PrP depositions, and in addition to this perineuronal pattern, sometimes intraneuronal staining may be detected (Bell, 1996).

FAMILIAL DISEASE

The entire open reading frame of all known mammalian and avian PrP genes resides within a single exon. In humans this encodes a product of 253 amino acids, which includes four octapeptides contiguous with a preceding nonapeptide of similar sequence. To date 12 point mutations and eight different length octorepeat insertions have been associated with genetic prion disease. Familial disease, inherited as an autosomal dominant trait, accounts for approximately 10–15% (Laplanche et al., 1994) of all cases of CJD and is associated with greater clinicopathological diversity than sporadic disease. The most common disease-associated mutations are codon 102 (Pro → Leu) and codon 200 (Gln → Lys). Tables 11.2 and 11.3 list the clinical and pathological features of the conditions that result from the various known point mutations (Table 11.2) and octarepeat inserts (Table 11.3). Also listed are the country of origin of the known cases and a general description of the condition, such as 'spastic paraparetic GSS' or 'familial CJD'. The condition is described as 'sporadic' when none of the cases with the particular genetic defect are known to have a relevant family history. Such cases could arise, for instance, if other relatives had been asymptomatic carriers or were unrecognized as having the condition; the genetic abnormality had occurred de novo in the affected individual; or if the mutation was an incidental finding, not related to the development of disease. To date, no instance of a case with a genetic defect shown to have arisen de novo has been identified. However, detecting such a case requires the exclusion of the genetic abnormality in both parents, information which is frequently difficult to obtain. Deletions have been identified in the PrP gene of asymptomatic controls as well as patients with CJD (and are therefore probably only an incidental finding). An octarepeat insert has been identified in only a single control patient, who had no relevant personal or family history to suggest CJD. The failure to identify insert or point mutations in a large number of further control subjects implies that a PrP genetic mutation in a case of CJD is likely to be causative.

Table 11.2 *Characteristics of genetic prion disease*

Codon/ mutation	Condition	Epidemiology	Clinical findings	Neuropathology
102 (Pro → Leu)	Usually ataxic GSS	Most common GSS mutation. France, USA, Germany, Italy, UK, Israel, Austria and Japan.	Early cerebellar ataxia, myoclonus, nystagmus, aphasia, pyramidal tract and lower motor neuron signs. Later: dementia.	PrP plaques +++, kuru and multilobular type, slight spongiform change, system atrophies of the spinocerebellar tracts, posterior columns, atrophy of brain stem, subcortical nuclei and fiber systems.
105 (Pro → Leu)	Spastic paraparetic GSS	Japan	Spastic gait disturbance and progressive dementia without either cerebellar signs, myoclonus, or periodic complexes (PCs) on the EEG. Onset in the fourth or fifth decades and long duration.	Numerous amyloid plaques in the cerebral cortex, severe gliosis but no spongiform changes. Cerebellum histologically preserved except for scant PrP plaques.
117 (Ala → Val)	Dementing GSS	Alsatian family; American family of German descent; and a British family.	The clinical picture became more severe over the generations, and consisted of dementia, pyramidal and extrapyramidal signs, pseudobulbar features, and cerebellar signs in some family members.	PrP positive uni- and multi-centric plaques, neuronal degeneration, moderate spongiform change.
145 (Tyr → Stop)	Familial CJD	Japan	Single case reported. Twenty-one year duration of a progressive dementia starting at age 38.	Many PrP positive amyloid plaques and neurofibrillary tangles.
178 (Asp → Asn) Codon 129 Met	Fatal familial insomnia	Italian, Italian-American, German, French, Australian and British families.	Average age at onset is ~50. Onset is with progressive insomnia, autonomic failure, endocrine and memory disturbances. Later dementia, cerebellar ataxia and myoclonus. Duration 7–36 months.	Atrophy of the anterior ventral and mediodorsal thalamic nuclei, olivary atrophy, varying degree of cerebral and cerebellar cortical gliosis. No plaques. Spongiform change rare.
178 (Asp → Asn) Codon 129 Val	Familial CJD	Finnish, French, Hungarian, Dutch, Canadian and British families	Average age at onset is ~47, and relatively long average duration of ~15 months. Patients usual present with memory impairment, behavior and mood changes, and although myoclonus was usual Pcs were reported in only one of over 40 cases.	Considerable diversity, cerebral cortex and basal ganglia most severely involved, prominent spongiform change and gliosis, less prominent neuronal loss, no plaques
180 (Val → Ile)	'Sporadic' CJD	Japan	66- and 79-year-old women. Older case had an extrapyramidal syndrome, dementia, myoclonus, and akinetic mutism. Duration 1–2 years. No PCs seen in either case.	Cortical spongiform change. No plaques. Weak synaptic PrP staining.
180 (Val → Ile) on one allele and 232 (Met → Arg) on other allele	'Sporadic' CJD	Japan	85-year-old man. No PCs	'Sporadic-type'
198 (Phe → Ser)	GSS with neurofibrillary tangles	Indiana kindred	Characteristically the disease leads to dementia, ataxia and an extrapyramidl syndrome with an average duration of illness around 6 years.	PrP positive amyloid plaques widespread; neurofibrillary tangles numerous in the cerebral cortex, hippocampus, and substantia innominata, spongiform change is occasional and mild.
200 (Gln → Lys)	Familial CJD	Commonest mutation causing familial CJD. Slovakia, Chile, Japan, USA, Sephardic Jews, and families of Greek, British, French, Tunisian, and Polish origin.	Very similar to sporadic CJD, but with slightly earlier average age at onset (56 vs 65 years)	As in sporadic CJD with spongiform change, gliosis, neuronal loss, very rarely amyloid plaques
208 (Arg → His)	Sporadic CJD	USA	Single case, aged 62, progressive dementia, hallucinations, ataxia myoclonus, and a characteristic EEG. Died 7 months after the onset of dementia.	Astrocytosis, extensive spongiform change without plaques or neurofibrillary tangles.
210 (Val → Ile)	Familial CJD	Italian, French, Japanese, and Chinese families.	Phenotype similar to sporadic CJD. Asymptomatic 81 and 82-year-old relatives carried mutation.	'Sporadic-type'
217 (Gln → Arg)	GSS with neurofibrillary tangles	Swedish family	Patients present with dementia and later developed gait ataxia and dysphagia.	Numerous neurofibrillary tangles in the neo-cortex, PrP positive plaques in cerebral and cerebellar cortex.
232 (Met → Arg)	'Sporadic' CJD	Japan	Patients presented with rapidly progressive dementia, myoclonus, became akinetic mute and had PCs. Illness duration 4–24 months.	Spongiform changes, neuronal loss and severe astrocytosis. No plaques.

Table 11.3 *Characteristics of genetic prion disease with insert mutations*

Insert size	Condition	Epidemiology	Clinical findings	Neuropathology
24 base pairs (one extra repeat)	Familial CJD	French. Single case	Age 73, dizziness, visual agnosia, ataxia, dementia, cortical blindness and akinetic mutism. Death occurred 4 months from onset.	Nil available
48 base pairs (two extra repeats)	Familial CJD	North America. Single family.	Patient aged 58 with typical CJD-like phenotype including PCs. Patient's mother had a slowly progressive dementia over many years and also carried the insert mutation.	Typical of CJD
72 base pairs (three extra repeats)	No case reported			
96 base pairs (four extra repeats)	Sporadic CJD	Single French, Japanese and British cases.	Ranges from classical CJD to a slower dementia with myoclonus. Ages 56, 62, 82.	One case had cerebellar plaques, another had classical pathological and PrP staining of molecular layer of the cerebellum.
120 base pairs (five extra repeats)	Familial CJD	North America	Age onset between 31 and 45. Duration 5–15 years. Progressive dementia, extrapyramidal, pyramidal cerebellar signs, and myoclonus	Classical with no plaques. One case had minimal pathological abnormalities.
144 base pair (six extra repeats)	Familial CJD	British and Japanese families.	Age of onset 22–53. Duration 2–18 years. Progressive dementia ± cerebellar, extrapyramidal and pyramidal signs; myoclonus, chorea, seizures. A long psychiatric prodrome is sometimes noted. EEG may show PCs.	Very variable from classical changes ± plaques to cases without any specific features to suggest CJD.
168 base pairs (seven extra repeats)	Familial CJD	Single Japanese case and North American family.	Age at onset 23–35. Duration 7 to >13 years. Slowly progressive dementia, rigidity and cerebellar signs ± myoclonus	Varying degree of spongiform change, neuronal loss, gliosis ± plaques.
192 base pairs (eight extra repeats)	Familial GSS	French and Dutch families.	Age at onset 21–55. Duration 3 months–13 years. Intellectual slowing, behavioral change extrapyramidal and cerebellar signs, myoclonus.	Neuronal loss, spongiform change, gliosis and multicentric plaques.
216 base pairs (nine extra repeats)	Familial GSS	British and German	Reported cases aged 54 and 32 at onset. FH of dementia in both cases. Slowly progressive dementia in one case >6 years. No PCs. One case had myoclonus.	Available in one case. Marked PrP positive amyloid plaques in cerebellum and basal ganglia. No spongiform change. A few neurofibrillary tangles.

Gerstmann–Sträussler–Scheinker syndrome and fatal familial insomnia (FFI) can be considered as variants of familial CJD as they are all transmissible neurodegenerative conditions associated with mutations of the PrP gene. Gerstmann–Sträussler–Scheinker syndrome has traditionally been described as an autosomal dominant disorder that presents with a progressive cerebellar ataxia and leads characteristically to multicentric amyloid plaques seen on neuropathology. However, the illness phenotype in a single kindred of GSS can vary considerably, with some affected individuals having a disease characterized by a rapidly progressive

myoclonic dementia indistinguishable from classical CJD. Gerstmann–Sträussler–Scheinker syndrome can more simply be used to refer to the forms of hereditary disease in which a characteristic pathological phenotype predominates, in particular the presence of numerous cerebellar multicentric PrP positive amyloid plaques.

The first report of FFI was made in 1986 and relates to an Italian kindred. The disease is characterized clinically by severe insomnia and autonomic failure, and pathologically by marked thalamic gliosis and little or no spongiform change. The genetics of FFI are particularly interesting: although a mutation at codon

178 is necessary for the development of disease, it is the presence of a polymorphism coding for methionine 'downstream' at codon 129 on the abnormal allele that appears to determine the FFI phenotype. The same 178 mutation but coding for valine at codon 129 of the affected allele is associated with a clinicopathological phenotype clearly distinct from FFI, thus illustrating the dramatic effect on disease that can result from a subtle change in prion protein structure.

Approximately 50% of hereditary cases lack a clear family history of a similar disorder. This is probably due largely to incomplete penetrance and the mis-diagnosis of other affected family members (for example with conditions such as Huntington's chorea, Alzheimer's disease or multiple sclerosis). Genetic penetrance appears to vary somewhat between the various genetic forms. For example, individuals carry-ing the codon 102 mutation almost invariably develop disease, unless they succumb to another condition, whereas carriers of the codon 200 mutation are relatively more likely to remain disease-free (Palmer and Collinge, 1997).

Approximately 2% of apparently sporadic cases of CJD, with no relevant family history, are found to carry a mutation. This percentage increases further if there is a family history of dementia or other neurological or psychiatric disorder. Prion protein gene analysis should only be performed after a full explanation of the possible implications of the test and obtaining informed consent from the patient or, more usually, their relatives. Genetic material is commonly extracted from a small sample of ethylenediaminetetraacetic acid (EDTA)-preserved blood (10–20 ml) but can also be obtained from other tissues, for example brain obtained at autopsy.

The human PrP gene plays a central role in conferring susceptibility to disease by means of a methionine/valine polymorphism at codon 129; iatro-genic cases of CJD have a high frequency of homo-zygosity (either methionine or valine), whilst in sporadic CJD 80% of cases are methionine homo-zygotes (compared with 37% of controls) (see Figure 11.1). Furthermore, it has been observed that the codon 129 polymorphism influences the age of onset and clinical presentation in some cases of hereditary CJD by interaction with pathogenic mutations in other parts of the PrP gene. It also influences the nature and distribution of neuropathological lesions in sporadic CJD, in particular PrP plaques are more common in valine homozygotes (VV) or heterozygotes (MV) than in methionine homozygotes (MM). Evidence also suggests that the EEG of cases with valine homozygosity are much less likely to show the classical periodic complexes compared with other genotypes. The duration of illness is slightly prolonged in those carrying at least one valine allele.

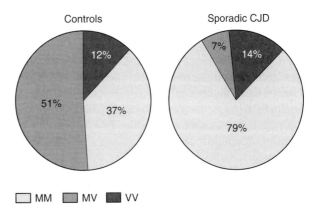

Figure 11.1 *Codon 129: controls and sporadic CJD.*

It is noteworthy that the association with codon 129 status and susceptibility to sporadic CJD has not been seen in Japan where the population has a different distribution of codon 129 genotype (MM = 92%, MV = 8%, and no VV). However, there appears to be no difference in the incidence between sporadic CJD in Japanese and Caucasians. Similarly the distribution or PrP genotypes in cases of kuru (MM = 30%, MV = 50%, and VV = 20%) does not differ significantly from a group of controls of the same ethnic background (MM = 30%, MV = 48%, and VV = 22%).

Iatrogenic Creutzfeldt–Jakob disease

In 1974 a CJD case suspected to have arisen from an environmental source was reported in the USA. The patient had received a corneal transplant when aged 55 because of a corneal dystrophy. Eighteen months later she developed lethargy and ataxia, followed by myo-clonus, spasticity, and akinetic mutism. She died eight months after the onset of her symptoms. The donor of the graft had died after a two-month history that included ataxia, memory loss, and myoclonus. Both the recipient and donor had typical neuropathological features of CJD at autopsy. Studies have subsequently demonstrated infectivity in corneas of animals inocu-lated with the CJD agent. Corneal donation from patients dying with dementia is now prohibited.

Further cases of iatrogenic CJD were reported in 1977. Two young patients from North America had undergone electrocorticography in 1974 for intractable epilepsy. During the procedure the same two previously used and sterilized silver electrodes had been inserted into their cerebral cortices for several hours. The patients developed progressive neurological disease, after a delay of 16 and 20 months, and subsequently died from histologically confirmed, and transmitted, CJD. The electrode probes used in both cases had previously been implanted for two days into the brain of a 70-year-old women with a four month history of mood disturbance, ataxia, mental deterioration, and involuntary movements. She died three months later of histologically confirmed CJD. The electrodes had been cleaned with benzene, disinfected with 70% ethanol, and sterilized in formaldehyde between each use. Twenty-eight months after their implantation in the original CJD case, the electrodes were inserted into the frontal lobes of a chimpanzee, who, after a period of 18 months, developed an encephalopathy histologically confirmed as CJD.

Although the above were the first iatrogenic cases reported, it seems likely that four other instances of contaminated neurosurgical instruments transmitting CJD had occurred in the UK and France in the 1950s and 1960s. It is presumed that in these cases routine sterilization procedures were insufficient to abolish infectivity and it is now strongly recommended that instruments used for neurosurgical and invasive ophthalmological procedures on patients with CJD (or at risk of developing CJD, such as individuals with a family history of CJD, human dural homograft recipients, and human cadaveric-derived pituitary hormone recipients) should be discarded (WHO, 1997).

In 1987 the first case of CJD linked with the use of a cadaveric-derived dural homograft during a neurosurgical procedure was reported. Subsequently a further 68 similar cases have been identified, including cases from the UK, Canada, the USA, Italy, Spain, Germany, Australia, New Zealand, and Japan. The majority of the implicated grafts were Lyodura, produced by a single manufacture between 1982 and 1986 (when Lyodura was often pooled), and most, if not all, of the patients received dura produced prior to the introduction of a decontamination procedure involving treatment with 1 N sodium hydroxide for 1 h and rigorous donor selection. However, experimental evidence suggests that sodium hydroxide is not always a reliable disinfectant for TSE agents. Furthermore, even the most stringent donor screening may not detect presymptomatic, but potentially infective, carriers of the TSE agent. The use of commercial cadaveric-derived dural homografts has therefore been largely discontinued in New Zealand, Australia and the UK, and the use of dura mater

replaced with suitable synthetic or autologous alternatives.

Cadaveric-derived human growth hormone (hGH) has been used since 1958, mainly for the medical treatment of children with growth hormone deficiency. The hormone had been manufactured in batches, each produced from a large number of pituitary glands (up to 2000), and was administered by intramuscular or subcutaneous injection. In 1985, the first case of CJD in a patient who had received hGH occurred; and subsequently a further 93 cases have been reported, mainly in France, the UK, and the USA. However, cases have also been identified in Brazil and New Zealand in patients who received hGH manufactured in the USA, and in Australia in patients who had received locally produced hGH. Four cases of CJD were also recorded in Australian women treated with cadaveric-derived pituitary gonadotropin. It is thought that the incriminating batches used to treat these hGH- and gonadatropin-related CJD cases had been contaminated by donors with CJD, and that sterilization methods employed were not sufficient to inactivate the infectious agent. It is of note that a sample of one such batch transmitted CJD to primates and that experiments have shown that the infectious agent can survive methods of 'inactivation' used in commercial production. The use of cadaveric-derived growth hormone has now been replaced by recombinant growth hormone, but due to the long incubation period of CJD, it is likely that more cases will appear in years to come.

The clinical phenotype of iatrogenic CJD is largely dependent on the route of agent inoculation: patients inoculated peripherally (for example hGH recipients) usually develop a progressive cerebellar syndrome reminiscent of kuru; whilst those inoculated centrally (for example through the use of stereotactic EEG probes or neurosurgical instruments) typically develop a rapidly progressive dementia similar to sporadic CJD. The illness resulting from the use of contaminated dural homografts can resemble either of these phenotypes. The incubation period is also largely determined by the route of infection, with central inoculation leading to the onset of disease more rapidly than peripheral inoculation (Table 11.4, modified from Brown, 1996).

Table 11.4 *Summary of all proven or highly probable cases of iatrogenic Creutzfeldt–Jakob disease*

Mode of infection	Number of patients	Agent entry into brain	Mean incubation period, range	Clinical presentation
Stereotactic EEG	2	Intracerebral	18 months (16,20)	Dementia/cerebellar
Neurosurgery	4	Intracerebral	20 months (15–28)	Visual/dementia/cerebellar
Corneal transplant	3	Optic nerve	17 months (16, 18)[a]	Dementia/cerebellar[a]
Dura mater graft	69	Cerebral surface	5.5 years (1.5–12)[a]	Cerebellar (visual/dementia)[a]
Gonadotropin	4	Haematogenous	13 years[b] (12–16)	Cerebellar
Growth hormone	94	Haematogenous	12 years[b] (5–30)[a]	Cerebellar[a]

[a]Although clinical information not available for all cases.
[b]Calculated from the midpoint of hormone therapy to the onset of CJD symptoms.

The main neuropathological characteristics of sporadic CJD, spongiform change, neuronal loss and astrocytosis, occur in iatrogenic disease, although the distribution of lesions varies from case to case. However, the neuropathology of hGH-related cases is noteworthy as there is usually pronounced cerebellar atrophy associated with neuronal loss, widespread spongiform change, and PrP amyloid plaque formation. Immunocytochemistry also shows a more widespread distribution of PrP in a diffuse pattern within the cerebellar granular layer in many of these cases (Ironside and Bell, 1997). Furthermore, neuropathological changes in the spinal cord, particularly the presence of PrP amyloid plaques, are more frequent in hGH-related iatrogenic cases than in sporadic CJD.

Possible occupational risks from prion disease

Although CJD has been documented in a neurosurgeon, two neuropathology technicians, an orthopedic surgeon, and a pathologist, it is reassuring to note that in none of these individuals was there a history of a definite infective event. The orthopedic surgeon had however worked with human and ovine dura mater 20 years prior to his illness. Case-control studies do not suggest that individuals potentially exposed to the TSE agent in the health care setting are at an increased risk of developing CJD. However, the possibility that cases of CJD have rarely occurred in such circumstances cannot be confidently dismissed. It is noteworthy, and of some further reassurance, that no case of CJD has been documented in any person working in a research laboratory studying human or animal prion disease (Brown, 1996).

A statistically significant excess of cases of CJD in cattle farmers has been reported in the UK since 1990. Of concern, four of these six cases were known to have had BSE-affected animals in their herds. However, analysis of the clinical and pathological features of these cases shows that none had the nvCJD phenotype. This observation has been strengthened by recent molecular biological data that demonstrate that the PrP glycosylation pattern characteristic of both BSE and nvCJD was not present in any of these cases. Furthermore, analysis of the incidence of CJD in dairy farmers from other European countries, in which BSE is rare or absent, reveals a similar excess of cases. This observation suggests that dairy farmers may be at increased risk of CJD for reasons other than exposure to the BSE agent. One possible explanation for the apparent excess of cases in dairy farmers, particularly in the UK, is that case ascertainment in this group has been better than in other groups because of concern of a possible link between the bovine and human diseases.

Possible risk of CJD from blood products

Although there is no proven or even probable instance of transmission of CJD by blood, blood components or plasma derivatives, increased awareness has recently raised concern about such a possibility. Numerous attempts have been made to detect the infective agent in the blood of experimentally infected animals. Although some results have been negative, several laboratories have reported the irregular presence of small amounts of infectivity in blood and particularly in buffy coat during both the preclinical incubation period and clinical phase of the disease. A recent experiment has demonstrated a low level of infectivity in the plasma and cryoprecipitate fraction from mice experimentally infected with CJD. A few attempts have also been made to detect the infectious agent in the blood of humans with CJD, four of which were successful (one from serum and three from buffy coat). It is important to emphasize that the presence of the infectious agent in the blood of either experimentally infected animals or naturally infected humans has been determined by transmission of disease to laboratory rodents only by intracerebral inoculation, and that the single experiment using an intravenous route of inoculation failed to transmit disease (units of blood from three CJD patients transfused into three chimpanzees). Taken together, these data suggest that blood components from patients with CJD may contain low levels of infectivity. However, it is considered difficult to extrapolate from experimental data to the situation in a medical setting. Furthermore, epidemiological studies have yet to identify a single instance in which disease was actually transmitted by blood. It is reassuring that in a population highly exposed to specific blood products, as is the case of hemophiliacs, there are no reports of CJD to date (WHO, 1997).

The appearance of a nvCJD raises new concerns. Because of a possible oral route of infection and a novel strain of infectious agent, the distribution of tissue infectivity in nvCJD may differ from that of other forms of CJD. This is supported by evidence that suggests that at least one part of the lymphoreticular system, the palatal tonsil, may harbor the abnormal PrP isoform in nvCJD but not sporadic disease. However, the weight of evidence suggests that the risk of parenteral transmission of any TSE by blood is remote, if not nil, and there is currently little evidence to consider that nvCJD will necessarily be any different in this respect. Transmission studies using blood from cases of nvCJD are currently ongoing.

In view of the theoretical possibility that blood from patients incubating prion disease may harbor the infective TSE agent the World Health Organization recommends that the following groups should be excluded as blood donors:

1 recipients of extracts derived from human pituitary glands (growth hormone and gonadotropin);
2 those with a family history of CJD, GSS or FFI;
3 those who have received a human dura mater graft.

Kuru

Kuru is a prion disease confined to the people originating from a number of adjacent valleys in the mountainous interior of Papua New Guinea. It was first described in 1955, although cases had probably been occurring for several decades before this. The term 'kuru' means shivering or trembling in the language of the Fore, the cultural and linguistic group in which more than 80% of cases occurred. The point prevalence of the disease in this population was about 1%, which was also the yearly incidence. Women and children were much more commonly affected than adult males, leading to a male/female ratio of more than 3 : 1 in some villages, and suggesting (incorrectly) that sex-linked genetic factors were important in disease etiology. Although the cause of kuru was initially unclear, intensive study concluded that the disease resulted from the practice of ritualistic cannibalism, a rite of mourning and respect for dead kinsmen, with resulting conjunctival, nasal, skin, mucosal, and gastrointestinal contamination with highly infectious brain tissue. For cultural reasons men were only infrequently exposed to infectious tissues during these funeral rituals, thus explaining the relative scarcity of the disease in adult males. The recognition that other tribes remained free of kuru despite cannibalistic practices similar to the Fore led to the suggestion that kuru may have initially arisen following the ritualistic cannibalism of a sporadic or familial CJD victim in the Fore region, and it is of note that CJD has been reported in Papua New Guinea. Kuru has gradually been disappearing since cannibalistic rituals ceased toward the end of the 1950s, and with the passage of time progressively older age groups have become free of kuru (Gajdusek, 1977). Between four to eight cases still occur annually, thus demonstrating that the incubation period can range from ≤4.5 years (the age of the youngest victim) to >35 years. It is noteworthy that no child born after the cessation of cannibalism, from a mother affected with kuru, is known to have developed the disease, suggesting that direct maternal transmission rarely, if ever, occurs.

In 1959 an American veterinary pathologist, Dr William Hadlow, drew attention to the similarity between the neuropathology of kuru and scrapie. It was known at this time that scrapie was transmissible and subsequently Drs Clarence Gibbs Jr and Carlton Gajdusek demonstrated transmission of kuru to a chimpanzee in 1965.

The clinical course of kuru is remarkably uniform, with cerebellar symptoms progressing to total incapacitation and death, usually within three to nine months. The disease has been divided into three clinical phases. The first, or ambulant, stage starts with unsteadiness of stance or gait and often of the hands. This is preceded in some cases by symptoms of headache and limb pains. Dysarthria starts early, and speech progressively deteriorates as the disease advances. Convergent strabismus often appears early too, and persists. Shivering tremors are also noted during this phase. The second, or sedentary stage, is reached when the sufferer can no longer walk without complete support. Tremors and ataxia become more severe, rigidity of the limbs often develops, associated with widespread involuntary movements, particularly myoclonus ± choreoathetosis, and a startle reaction may be seen. Emotional lability, leading to outbursts of pathological laughter, frequently occurs and although most patients show a resignation to, and a light-hearted attitude toward their illness, some patients become depressed. Mental slowing is apparent, but severe dementia is conspicuously absent. The third, or terminal, stage is reached when the patient is unable to sit up without support; ataxia, tremor, and dysarthria become progressively more severe and incapacitating. Pyramidal, extrapyramidal and frontal release signs may be seen at this stage, and in time plasticity, inanition, and signs of bulbar involvement develop. The patient becomes mute and unresponsive, deep decubitus ulceration and hypostatic pneumonia often occur, and the patient finally succumbs, usually, but not always, in a state of emaciation.

In keeping with the prominent cerebellar clinical features of kuru, neuropathology demonstrates macroscopic atrophy of the cerebellar vermis in most cases. Microscopically, changes are more widespread in the CNS and are characterized by marked astrocytosis throughout the brain; mild spongiform change of the gray matter; diffuse neuronal degeneration that is most severe in the cerebellum and its afferent and efferent connections; and minimal demyelination. Typical intracytoplasmic vacuolation is usually observed in the large neurons of the striatum. The most striking histological abnormality however is the presence of PrP-positive amyloid plaques, most conspicuous in the cerebellum, and occurring in about 70% of cases.

New variant Creutzfeldt–Jakob disease

BACKGROUND TO THE IDENTIFICATION OF NEW VARIANT CJD

In 1990 surveillance of CJD was reinstituted in the UK because of concern that the agent responsible for the epidemic of BSE in British cattle might transmit to humans. The rare occurrence of two teenage patients with CJD in the second half of 1995 was followed over the next few months by the identification of eight further young cases. All 10 patients shared a distinct and previously unseen clinicopathological phenotype (Will *et al.*, 1996). A review of the literature and consultation with experts in CJD pathology and epidemiology from Europe and the rest of the world failed to reveal any further cases. It was therefore concluded, in light of the temporo-spatial association with the occurrence of BSE, that this apparently new variant of CJD was most likely causally linked with exposure to the BSE agent. A further 12 cases were diagnosed between March 1996 and July 1997, 11 in the UK and a single case in France. During this period further scientific evidence in support of a link with the BSE agent has become available: the identification of pathological features similar to nvCJD in macaque monkeys inoculated with BSE, and the demonstration that nvCJD is associated with a pattern of PrP glycosylation that distinguishes it from other forms of CJD and which resembles that seen in BSE, and BSE transmitted to a number of other species. Furthermore, no additional cases of nvCJD were identified in other countries over this time period or retrospectively. However, proof of an association between nvCJD and BSE has not been established, and is likely to depend on the results of experiments to determine if the diseases share the same 'strain type' and continued epidemiological vigilance in the UK, Europe, and the rest of the world (Figure 11.2).

EPIDEMIOLOGY OF nvCJD

With reference to the cases mentioned above, 12 of the 22 cases were female and 10 male. Their age at onset of symptoms ranged from 16 to 48 years (mean 27 years). All the patients lived in the UK, apart from the single French case (who had never traveled to Great Britain).

Some of the patients had been long-standing residents in Wales, Scotland or Northern Ireland, and spatial analysis fails to show clustering of cases to any particular part of the UK. Information on potential risk factors has been published for 10 cases. Four had no history of any operation, four had undergone minor surgery (two tonsillectomy in 1975 and 1991, one a foot operation in 1984, one a dilatation and curettage in 1989), one had had surgery for congenital glaucoma twice around 1970, and another had had a cesarean section (1974), colonoscopy (1992, 1994), and laparoscopy (1986). One patient had worked as a butcher from 1985 to 1987 and another had visited an abattoir for two days in 1987, but was not known to have had contact with animals or animal products. None had ever worked on farms with livestock, although one patient had spent one week's holiday a year on a dairy farm between 1976 and 1986. There was no record of BSE in this herd. Dietary histories are available for nine cases, all were reported to have eaten beef or beef products since 1986, but none were reported to have eaten brain. One of the cases had been a strict vegetarian since 1991.

nvCJD – CLINICAL FEATURES

In this next section a detailed description of the features of the first 14 histologically confirmed cases of nvCJD identified in the UK will be given.

Early features
The two striking early features of nvCJD are sensory disturbance and behavioral change (see Table 11.6), both of which are unusual in sporadic CJD. Four of the 14 cases initially complained of sensory symptoms. One case developed foot pain severe enough to warrant referral to a rheumatologist; another presented with foot pain followed within a fortnight by hand and face

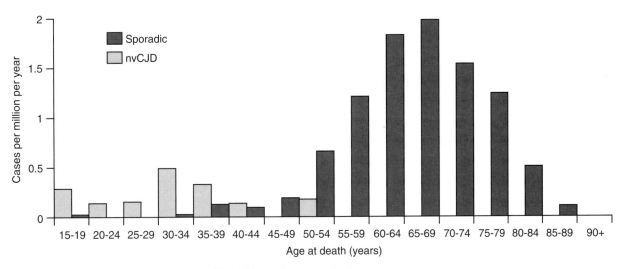

Figure 11.2 *Sporadic and nvCJD: age-specific incidence for age at death.*

dysesthesia; two further patients initially complained of sensory changes (dysesthesia ± paresthesia) in the legs. Four of the other 10 patients, although not initially complaining of sensory symptoms, developed these during an early stage of their illness – two had persistently cold feet, one hemi-dysesthesia, and another pain below both knees. The sensory symptoms were continuous and persistent throughout most of the illness in all these cases. Another patient, without overt sensory symptoms, was noted to have hyperesthesia. Five patients underwent electromyography and/or nerve conduction studies. These were normal in four cases and abnormal in one, which showed minor changes of uncertain significance.

All but one patient saw a psychiatrist during their illness, six as the initial referral. Most cases were depressed, apathetic, and withdrawn early in the clinical course, often accompanied by weight loss and mild insomnia. Fleeting delusions were common, for example microscopic people living in the body, a new-born baby was dead, and two patients developed a schizophrenia-like psychosis. One of these, following treatment with neuroleptic medication, made an almost complete recovery for about a month before becoming withdrawn, developing sensory symptoms, and a progressive dementia.

Clinical course

Although a minority of cases suffered from forgetfulness or mild unsteadiness of gait from an early stage, frank neurological signs were not apparent for many months (median 6.25, range 4–24.5 months) after

disease onset (see Table 11.5). During this period the most prominent clinical features were psychiatric disturbance and/or sensory symptoms. After the onset of frank neurological dysfunction, mainly in the form of ataxia, the illness rapidly progressed with global cognitive impairment, involuntary movements, incontinence of urine, and progressive immobility leading to increasing dependency, unresponsiveness, and mutism. Preterminally, the patients were usually akinetic mute and at least three developed cortical blindness. Dysphagia usually developed, predisposing to aspiration and pneumonia, the most frequent terminal event. The mean delay from developing unsteadiness to becoming bed-bound was six months (range 2.5 to 12.5 months), and from bed-bound to death 1.5 months (range one week to six months), although two patients remained alive 6.5 and 18 months after becoming bed-bound. Most patients had minor fluctuations in their clinical course with cognitive or neurological dysfunction varying over a few hours or days, often related to a change of medication or infective episode.

Clinical signs (Table 11.7)

The neurological signs were cerebellar: limb or gait ataxia, in nine cases. These occurred in isolation in three, or in combination with either involuntary movements, pyramidal signs, primitive reflexes, or sensory signs, in the others. The remaining cases first developed either pyramidal signs (± dysphasia), dysarthria or involuntary movements, although unsteadiness of gait was noted within weeks even in these

Table 11.5 *Clinical features and months to clinical milestones of the first 14 cases of nvCJD in the UK*

Presenting features	Sensory symptoms	Forgetful	Unsteady	Neurological signs	Involuntary movements[a]	Mute	Bed-bound	Abnormal EEG	Normal EEG	Duration
Withdrawn	No	5	6	6.5	8[M]	10	11	6	–	11
Dysaesthesia	Yes	5.5	4.5	5.5	5.5[C]	13	17	–	5.5 and 8.5	>35[b]
Foot pain	Yes	4	4	6	8.5[M]	9.5	8.5	6	–	10
Psychosis	Yes	6.5	6.5	8.5	9[C]	15	16	9.5	8.5	18
Forgetful	No	0	2.5	4.5	7[M]	6	5	1.5	–	11
Aggression and apathy	No	1	5	9	9[M]	10.5	10	10	–	11
Paraesthesia	Yes	9	10	3.5	11[C]	20	20	–	11.5 and 14.5	22.5
Dysaesthesia	Yes	5	11	11	16.5[M]	17	17	16	–	17.5
Personality change	Yes	1	4.5	5.5	5.5[C]	8	9	5	–	9.5
Depression	No	3.5	3.5	4	5[C]	7.5	11	12.5	4.5 and 6.5	13
Withdrawn	Yes	0	23.5	24.5	23[M]	28.5	28.5	25	–	28.5
Withdrawn	Yes	10.5	12	14	14[C]	17	16.5	14	–	17
Emotional lability	No	5.5	9.5	11	13.5[M]	13.5	13	12	–	14
Agitation, weight loss, and insomnia	No	1	0	4	4[C]	7.5	7	6.5	–	>15.5[b]
Median		4.5	5.5	6.25	8.75	11.75	12	9.75		14

[a]First involuntary movements either chorea (C) or myoclonus (M); [b]alive.

Table 11.6 *Psychiatric features of the first 14 cases of nvCJD in the UK*

Initial psychiatric diagnosis	Anxiety	Aggression	Emotional lability	Apathic/ withdrawn	Depression	Delusions	Auditory hallucinations	Visual hallucinations
Major depressive illness	+	+	−	+	+	+	−	+
Nil	+	−	+	+	−	+	−	−
Organic rather than functional[a]	+	+	+	+	−	+	−	−
Paranoid illness with possible first rank symptoms	+	+	+	+	+	+	+	−
Thought that amnesia may well be hysterical rather than organic[a]	+	+	+	+	−	+	+	+
Severe agitated depression	+	+	−	+	+	+	+	+
Neurodegenerative disorder[a]	+	−	+	+	+	−	−	−
Depressive illness with significant anxiety symptoms[a]	+	+	−	+	+	+	+	+
Both organic and functional symptoms – thought to be developing a psychosis[a]	+	+	+	+	−	+	−	+
Major depressive illness	+	−	+	+	+	+	−	+
No evidence of depression or any other psychiatric disorder	−	+	−	+	+	+	−	−
Schizophreniform psychosis[a]	−	+	−	+	−	+	+	+
Anxiety, hyperventilation – possible underlying depression	+	+	+	−	+	+	−	+
Severe depression without psychotic features. Marked agitation	+	+	+	+	+	−	−	−
Total	12	11	9	13	9	12	5	8

[a]Possibility of an organic cause raised.

cases. Those with the longest delay to the development of neurological signs had a long prodrome with mild personality change or forgetfulness followed by sensory disturbance. The majority of cases developed primitive reflexes, cerebellar, and pyramidal signs. All patients developed persistent involuntary movements, initially chorea (seven cases) or myoclonus (seven cases), and five of the seven patients who initially had chorea were later noted to also have myoclonus. Although seven cases were not formally noted to have chorea four of these were described as 'fidgety'. Seven cases were noted to have upgaze paresis, an uncommon feature of sporadic CJD, after the development of other focal neurological signs.

Formal neuropsychometry was performed in six cases after their routine clinical examination had suggested cognitive impairment. All assessments revealed evidence of global cognitive dysfunction.

nvCJD – INVESTIGATIONS

Below is a summary of the neurophysiological, biochemical, neuroradiological, and other investigations performed on the cases described above. There is further discussion of the laboratory investigation of CJD later in this chapter.

EEG

Each case underwent electroencephalography on multiple occasions (two to five times). The characteristic EEG pattern of CJD was not seen, even though four patients had recordings in the final month of illness (in one case two days predeath). Initial tracings were normal in four cases and in three of these the subsequent recording was also unremarkable. These three patients had a normal EEG even though they had documented cognitive impairment, cerebellar signs, and involuntary movements prior to the recording. Abnormal recordings were noted in 12 patients and all

Table 11.7 *Neurological signs noted during the clinical of the first 14 cases of nvCJD in the UK*

Myoclonus	Chorea	Pyramidal signs	Cerebellar signs	Rigidity	Primitive reflexes	Upgaze paresis	Akinetic mutism	Cortical blindness
+	−	+	+	+	−	+	+	−
+	+	+	+	+	+	−	+	−
+	−	+	+	+	+	−	+	−
−	+	+	+	+	−	−	−	+
+	−	+	−	+	+	+	+	+
+	−	+	+	+	+	−	+	−
+	+	+	+	+	+	−	+	−
+	−	+	+	+	+	+	+	−
+	+	+	+	−	+	+	+	−
−	+	+	+	−	+	+	+	−
+	−	−	+	+	−	−	+	−
+	+	+	−	+	+	+	−	−
+	−	+	+	+	+	−	+	−
+	+	+	−	+	+	+	−	+
Total 12	7	13	11	12	11	7	11	3

showed pathological slow wave activity. This tended to deteriorate as the illness progressed. The majority of cases thought to have a functional psychiatric illness developed an abnormal EEG within three months of their psychiatric diagnosis. However, one patient had a normal recording 7.5 months after the diagnosis of a schizophreniform psychosis.

Cerebrospinal fluid analysis

All patients had cerebrospinal fluid (CSF) analysis. A leucocyte response was not seen in any case. Four patients had a slightly raised CSF protein (0.5–0.9 g/l) but in nine the level was normal. The results of CSF electrophoresis are available for 11 cases and in none were oligoclonal bands detected. The analysis of 14-3-3 protein is discussed later in this chapter.

Neuroimaging

Ten cases underwent brain computerized tomography (CT), eight patients were reported to have normal scans and two non-specific abnormalities: dural calcification in one case and a slightly enlarged lateral ventricle and cerebellar interhemispheric cistern in another. Cranial magnetic resonance imaging (MRI) was reported to show no significant abnormalities in eight cases, three of whom had normal repeat studies. Four patients were reported to have mild generalized atrophy; one case as having slightly prominent ventricles with one or two small areas of high signal in the left frontal white matter; and two others had posterior thalamic high signal on T2-weighted (and one case also proton density-weighted) images. A retrospective analysis of MRI from these cases is ongoing, and provisional information (without comparison with controls) suggests that most, if not all, cases show abnormal high signal from the posterior thalamus on T2-weighted or proton density-weighted images or both.

Abnormal areas of cerebral perfusion were detected in both cases that had single photon emission computed tomography (SPECT) studies. A single patient underwent positron emission tomography (PET) which was normal.

Genetic analysis

Sequencing of the open reading frame of the PrP gene identified no mutations in the cases screened so far. All 21 cases tested to date have the methionine–methionine genotype (MM) at codon 129 which differs significantly from Caucasian controls (37%, $p < 0.0001$) and sporadic CJD (79%, $p = 0.02$). It is interesting to postulate why this might be. It is thought that the ability to transmit a prion disease between species is determined by the homology of the central residues of their prion protein structures (which includes residue 129). Recent evidence suggests that, unlike humans, bovines only code for methionine at the equivalent site to the human codon 129 polymorphism. Therefore, if nvCJD is due to infection with the BSE agent, and bovine PrP is usually, if not always, homozygous for methionine at codon 129, the MM genotype in humans may confer an increased susceptibility to bovine prions.

Differential diagnosis

A number of cases of suspect nvCJD have subsequently been shown to have an alternative diagnosis. The commonest condition that may closely resemble nvCJD appears to be sporadic CJD in young persons. Even in retrospect the clinical features of one case of sporadic CJD in a 46-year-old man were not readily distinguishable from those of nvCJD, and illustrate the importance of neuropathological examination. Furthermore genetic/familial CJD tends to occur at a younger age than sporadic CJD, may present with a prolonged psychiatric prodrome, and run a relatively protracted clinical course. Approximately half of genetic cases have no clear family history of CJD emphasizing the importance of analysis of the PrP gene in all suspect cases of nvCJD. Other conditions that were referred to the UK National CJD Surveillance Unit initially as suspect nvCJD are listed below:

- transient encephalopathy of unknown cause with recovery (three cases);
- encephalitis with inflammatory CSF but no definite diagnosis (three cases);
- Hashimoto's encephalitis (one case);
- multiple system atrophy (one case);
- vascular encephalopathy (one case).

Pathology

Neuropathological examination in nvCJD shows spongiform change and PrP plaques confirming the diagnosis of CJD. Spongiform change, neuronal loss, and astrocytosis is most evident in the basal ganglia and thalamus, and is present focally in the cerebrum and cerebellum, most evidently in areas with confluent spongiform change.

The most striking and consistent neuropathological abnormality is PrP plaques. These are extensively distributed throughout the cerebrum and cerebellum, with smaller numbers in the basal ganglia, thalamus, and hypothalamus. Many of these resemble kuru-type plaques with a dense eosinophilic center and pale periphery and, unusually for this type of lesion, were surrounded by a zone of spongiform change. Although extremely rare in other forms of CJD, similar lesions have been described in scrapie, where they have been referred to as 'florid' plaques. Immunocytochemistry for PrP shows strong staining of these plaque-like lesions, but also shows many other smaller plaques, which appeared both as single and multicentric deposits. Prion protein deposition is also seen in a pericellular distribution in the cerebral cortex and in the molecular layer of the cerebellum, the pattern of which suggests deposition around small neurons. Plaque and pericellular PrP deposits occur throughout the cerebrum and cerebellum, and are clearly visible in the absence of confluent spongiform change in the surrounding neuropil. In the basal ganglia and thalamus, a perivacuolar pattern of PrP staining is also seen, with linear tract-like deposits within the gray matter. Prion protein plaques are also noted in these regions although there are fewer than in the cerebrum and cerebellum (Will et al., 1996).

Predicting the future number of cases of nvCJD

Statistical modeling of the size of a potential nvCJD epidemic has been performed. This was based on the dates of onset of the first 14 cases identified in the UK and the assumption of a causal link between nvCJD and BSE. The estimate for the total number of infections occurring in the UK ranged from less than 100 to greater than 80 000 cases. This large variability reflects the difficulty of modeling based on a relatively small number of cases and uncertainties relating to incubation period. It was concluded that even though only 14 cases had been identified at that time it would be premature to assume that any subsequent epidemic would be small. Furthermore, it was noted that although the number of cases over the next few years might provide a better indication of how large any potential epidemic might eventually be, much uncertainty could remain even after four years (Cousens et al., 1997).

ANIMAL TRANSMISSIBLE SPONGIFORM ENCEPHALOPATHIES

Scrapie

Scrapie, the prototype TSE, is an insidious degenerative disease affecting the CNS of sheep and goats. Natural scrapie has also been reported in moufflon, a primitive relative of sheep, but only in Great Britain. The term 'scrapie' describes the tendency for affected sheep to scrape themselves against trees or bushes and the disease was known as la tremblante (trembling disease) in France, as Gnubberkrankheit (itching disease) or Traberkrankheit (trotting disease) in Germany, rida in Iceland, súrlókór (brushing disease) in Hungary. As a clinical entity it was recognized in sheep in England as early as 1730 and has subsequently been reported in many other countries throughout the world. Although scrapie occurred due to importation of sheep to Australia and New Zealand, the disease was successfully eradicated through stringent and immediate efforts to depopulate the imported sheep as well as their animal contacts (Bradley, 1997).

Scrapie was experimentally transmitted by inoculation of a ewe in the 1930s. Demonstration of transmission of mice in the early 1960s permitted the disease to be intensively studied but in spite of this the exact mechanism(s) of scrapie spread in nature remains obscure. It is commonly accepted that the disease is infectious and contagious but that genetic factors are also important. Infection is most commonly transmitted from ewe to lamb, both up to the time of parturition and afterwards when the ewe and lamb run together. There is also horizontal spread of infection between unrelated adults and this may account for some of the scrapie cases in older sheep. Placental tissue is known to be infectious and this is commonly postulated as a possible source of transmission both to the lamb and unrelated animals sharing the same pasture. The exact routes of infection are unresolved but possibilities include transplacental, oral, nasal, optic or cutaneous. Complex genetic factors are known to affect incubation period and susceptibility of sheep to scrapie, and the possibility of engineering animals resistant to disease has been raised.

In natural scrapie the onset of disease is often insidious. Early signs are apprehension, restlessness, hyperexcitability and aggressiveness, and some animals even manifest apparent dementia. Fine tremors of the head and neck are observed, and as the disease progresses these become more generalized, involving the whole body and producing a shivering effect. Fasciculations of superficial skeletal muscles may occur, and signs of coetaneous irritation, self-induced by rubbing and scratching, constitute one of the most characteristic clinical features. As the disease evolves the gait becomes ataxic with severely affected animals unable to stand or walk without falling. In the advanced stages of the disease, animals become stuporous and manifest visual impairment, excessive salivation, and incontinence. The duration of natural disease is usually less than four months.

In keeping with other TSEs the neuropathological triad of spongiform change, neuronal loss, and astroglial proliferation occur in scrapie. Vacuolation of the neuronal cytoplasm is a marked and pathognomonic feature, being particularly evident in the brain stem and the ventral and lateral horns of the spinal cord. Another characteristic feature of scrapie and other TSEs is the presence of rod-shaped structures seen on electron microscopy and known as scrapie-associated fibrils. The nature of these bodies is a matter of some debate, with some scientists claiming they are a viral-like agent and others that they are composed of chains of prion protein. Although there is no currently available clinical diagnosis test for the disease, a recent study has identified the presence of abnormal prion protein in tonsillar tissue from sheep with naturally occurring scrapie, long before the occurrence of clinical signs. This raises the possibility of tonsillar biopsy as a clinical diagnostic, and possibly presymptomatic, test.

Bovine spongiform encephalopathy

Bovine spongiform encephalopathy was first reported in British cattle in November 1986. Most cases were infected as calves; the modal age of disease occurrence is five years (range 29 months to 18 years) and the average incubation period four to five years. Current evidence suggests that the disease originated from the use of feed supplements containing meat and bone meal (MBM) contaminated by a TSE agent. The stringency of the rendering procedure, by which animal materials were processed to produce MBM, changed during the early 1980s and decreased use of hydrocarbon solvents and the adoption of lower temperatures may have resulted in increased survival of the infective agent. These changes were adopted in response to a fall in the value

of tallow (the fat-rich fraction of the process whose yield is increased by using solvent), a rise in the cost of energy, and a need to replace old plant with safer systems not using potentially carcinogenic solvents. Epidemiological evidence suggests that sheep scrapie, endemic in Great Britain, was the likely source of the infective agent that initiated the BSE epidemic. However, experiments indicate that BSE is associated with a single strain of infective agent and, although over 20 different scrapie strains are recognized, to date, none appear to match that seen in BSE. This has led to the further hypothesis that BSE may have been an uncommon sporadic and/or hereditary disease of cattle that was dramatically amplified as a result of infected bovine material entering the modified rendering process. Whatever the origin of the agent responsible for BSE it is likely that the recycling of infected cattle through the rendering process in the 1980s was largely responsible for fuelling the large and explosive epidemic. It is of note that BSE has been experimentally transmitted via the oral route to cattle by as little as 1 g of BSE-infected bovine brain.

The British government made BSE notifiable in June 1988 and shortly afterwards a statutory ban on the feeding of ruminant-derived protein to ruminants was introduced. In November 1989 a ban was enforced on the use of certain specified 'high risk' bovine offals (SBO) for human consumption (brain, spinal cord, tonsils, spleen, and intestines from animals >30 months old). The selection of which offals should be included in the SBO ban was based on the evidence of infectivity of tissues from scrapie-infected sheep. BSE infectivity has now been demonstrated in the brain, spinal cord, and retina of naturally affected cattle and the distal ileum of those infected experimentally. However, a wide range of tissues from clinically affected cases of BSE have shown no detectable infectivity using the mouse bioassay (which has potential limitations, in particular the 'species barrier' – see later), and these include muscle, milk, and a range of lymphoreticular tissues. In September 1990 the use of SBO was further restricted, being prohibited for use in feed for all animals and birds. At the end of 1992 BSE reached its peak incidence (see Figure 11.3) in the UK but thereafter declined rapidly, almost certainly in response to the statutory measures. However, new cases of BSE were being observed in cattle that were born after the implementation of the feed ban. It has been suggested that most of these cases occurred because of the continued use of feed rations produced before the ban; cross-contamination of cattle feed by feed containing MBM intended for pigs or poultry; and an incomplete adherence by some manufactures to the SBO ban. Further measures were instituted to address these particular issues and following the announcement of a possible link between BSE and a nvCJD in March 1996, cattle >30 months old and heads from all bovines over six months old were excluded from all food or feed chains.

Although the pattern of the epidemic remains consistent with the hypothesis that the vast majority of cases arose through infection with contaminated feed, it remains possible that other routes of transmission may occur infrequently, in particular maternal transmission from dam to calf. A study to assess maternal transmission suggests that this may occur at a low rate (estimated to be responsible for only about 1% of cattle expressing disease) but also tentatively suggests that genetic factors may also influence susceptibility.

The appearance of a number of novel TSEs, causally linked with BSE, in domestic and captive animals raises the question of whether BSE occurs, or will occur, in further animal species. Particular concern has been expressed regarding the possibility of BSE in sheep, pigs, and poultry. BSE has been experimentally transmitted to sheep by feeding as little as 0.5 g of infected bovine brain and it is known that some sheep were fed MBM until this practice was banned in 1988. In this regard the lack of evidence of a BSE-related epidemic of sheep scrapie is reassuring, but concern was sufficient to lead to the ban of ovine brain from sheep over six months of age for human consumption in the UK. Pigs, but not chickens, have been shown to be susceptible to BSE by parenteral inoculation of infected bovine brain homogenate. However, challenging pigs with a very large oral dose of BSE-infected brain failed to produce disease, at least up to 6.5 years post challenge.

By the end of 1996, over 168 000 confirmed cases of BSE had been reported in the UK. Relatively small numbers of cases have also been reported in native-born cattle in Switzerland, the Republic of Ireland, France, Portugal, and the Netherlands. Small numbers of cases have also been reported in Germany, Italy, Oman, Canada, Denmark, and the Falkland Islands, but solely in animals imported from the UK.

The duration of the clinical course of BSE is typically one or two months, but ranges from seven days to 14 months. The most commonly observed signs are apprehension, hyperesthesia, and ataxia, but affected animals may also show a decreased milk yield and loss of condition. There is no effective treatment and the disease always progresses to death in the affected animal. A number of other bovine conditions can mimic the illness phenotype of BSE, for example magnesium deficiency ('staggers'), and currently no reliable laboratory diagnostic disease marker has been reported, emphasizing the importance of pathological diagnosis.

Pathological changes are similar to scrapie in many respects with vacuolar lesions largely confined to the brain stem and accompanied by neuronal degeneration and an astrocytic reaction. Sparse cerebral amyloid plaques are seen in a small proportion of cases. In contrast to scrapie, greater diagnostic importance is attributed to the neuropil vacuolation than neuronal vacuolation.

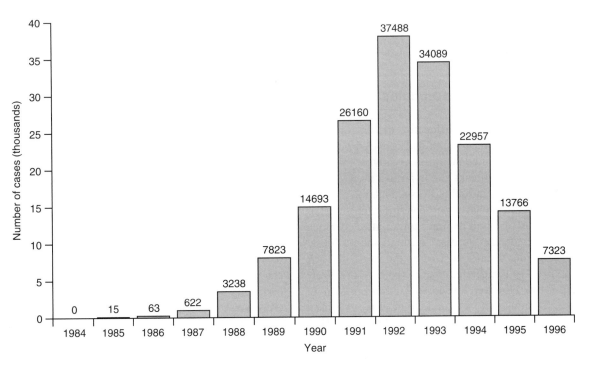

Figure 11.3 *Number of cases of BSE per year.*

Chronic wasting disease of mule and elk deer

Chronic wasting disease (CWD) is a TSE of deer and elk that has only occurred in limited areas in the western United States. It was first recognized as a clinical syndrome in 1967 and is typified by chronic weight loss leading to death. There is no known or suspected relationship between CWD and any other animal TSE.

CWD has occurred in four captive wildlife research facilities in northern Colorado and one in south-eastern Wyoming. Although cases of CWD have been seen in two zoological parks, the affected animals all originated from the above-mentioned research facilities. Soon after recognition of the disease, animal movement from these facilities was stopped. CWD has also been confirmed in fewer than 70 free-ranging deer and elk in a limited number of counties in northern Colorado and south-eastern Wyoming.

Species that have been affected with CWD are Rocky Mountain elk, mule deer, white-tailed deer, and black-tailed deer. Other ruminant species, including wildlife and domestic cattle, sheep and goats, have been housed in wildlife facilities in direct and indirect contact with CWD-affected deer and elk, but no cases of CWD in these ruminant species have been detected. The origin and mode of transmission of disease is unknown. Animals born in captivity and those born in the wild have been affected with the disease. Based on the epidemiology of CWD, transmission is thought to be lateral, and possibly maternal. Transmission via feed is not believed to occur as affected animals have been fed a variety of foodstuffs. It is of note that painstaking attempts to eradicate CWD from captive facilities, including thorough decontamination and a 12-month period free of elk or deer, failed to prevent disease recurrence (Bradley, 1997).

Transmissible mink encephalopathy

Transmissible mink encephalopathy (TME) was first described in the mid 1960s but had occurred on mink farms in Minnesota and Wisconsin as early as 1947. The disease occurs as outbreaks and in farmed mink only. It has been recognized in Idaho, Russia, Finland, Canada, and Germany. Although a rare condition, mortality is high, with nearly all adult mink on an affected ranch succumbing to the disease during an outbreak. Evidence points to infected feed as the cause of TME and it has been suggested that scrapie is the likely contaminant. However, experimental transmission of scrapie to mink via the oral route has not been successful to date, although this may be because TME is caused by a different scrapie strain than those used experimentally. The possibility of a bovine origin of TME has also been raised. Products from fallen or sick cattle ('downer cows') were said to have been fed to a colony of affected mink in the USA and that these animals had been fed a diet free of any ovine material. However, surveillance of cattle in the USA has not revealed a single case of BSE, thus arguing against a bovine origin of TME infection. Furthermore, although BSE has been experimentally transmitted to mink, the incubation period, clinical signs, and neuropathology showed significant differences from natural TME. No convincing evidence for maternal or horizontal transmission of natural disease exists.

Feline spongiform encephalopathy

In 1990 the first case of feline spongiform encephalopathy (FSE) in a domestic cat was reported. The six-year-old animal had been referred to the Bristol Veterinary School, in England, with a progressive neurological condition. He failed to respond to treatment and subsequent neuropathological examination revealed a scrapie-like spongiform encephalopathy. Although no previous naturally occurring TSE had been documented in a feline, CJD had been experimentally transmitted to a cat in 1972. Since 1990 cats with FSE have been reported from most regions of the UK (total 78 up to May 1997) and single cases have been documented in an indigenous cats from Norway and Liechtenstein. Feline spongiform encephalopathy has also been documented in captive large cats: three pumas, five cheetahs (including one in Australia and one in the Republic of Ireland), a tiger, and two ocelots. Experimental evidence supports the hypothesis that these novel feline diseases are causally related to BSE (see end of section on animal encephalopathies). It is suggested that the domestic cats may have been infected through the consumption of commercially produced cat food, and it is of note that no case has been reported in a cat born after the potentially infective bovine offals were banned from use in cat food in September 1990. It is assumed that disease in the captive large cats arose though the consumption of infected bovine materials, and it is likely that some were fed carcasses from BSE-affected cattle before the offals ban was instituted.

Based on an analysis of FSE in 11 domestic cats the average age of an affected animal is just over six years (range 2–10 years). The onset of disease usually develops slowly, over weeks or months. Behavioral changes are frequently the first noted, with the animal becoming increasingly aggressive or timid. Altered grooming, polyphagia, and polydipsia are also common signs. Cases often develop hyperesthesia, a startle reaction, and tremor and ataxia invariably occurs. The typical clinical duration is between two and three months.

Spongiform encephalopathies of captive wild ruminants

In a British zoo in 1986 a nyala (which belongs, like cattle, to the family 'Bovidae') died of a spongiform encephalopathy, alerting the British veterinary community to the possibility that a TSE of cattle could exist. Subsequently, additional cases of spongiform encephalopathy occurred in other captive wild Bovidae in Britain: gemsbok, Arabian oryx, greater kudu, eland, and scimitar-horned oryx. As with FSE, the temporospatial clustering of these novel spongiform encephalopathies would be consistent with a causative link to BSE. Although it would seem likely that dietary exposure was of most importance, it is noteworthy that one of the kudu was the offspring from an affected mother, at least raising the additional possibility of maternal transmission in this species.

Strain typing studies of the TSE agents in animals

The 'strain' of a TSE can be defined by characteristic features when transmitted to mice. For example, when inoculated into genetically similar mice a particular scrapie strain leads to a consistent incubation period and pattern of neuropathology. Using a range of genetically distinct mice allows a strain profile based on incubation period and neuropathological distribution to be produced (see Figure 11.4). Such experiments have suggested that scrapie exists as over 20 separate strains, whereas BSE is due only to a single strain of agent, which is distinct from those of scrapie (Bruce et al., 1994). Furthermore, the transmission characteristics of FSE and the novel spongiform encephalopathies of kudu and nyala resemble those of BSE, and thus provide supportive evidence for a causative association. Similar strain typing experiments for nvCJD are currently in progress.

DIAGNOSTIC TESTS FOR CREUTZFELDT–JAKOB DISEASE

Routine blood tests

Routine hematological and biochemical investigations, including inflammatory markers, are usually normal in CJD. In about one-third of cases the liver function tests are deranged, usually in the form of mildly

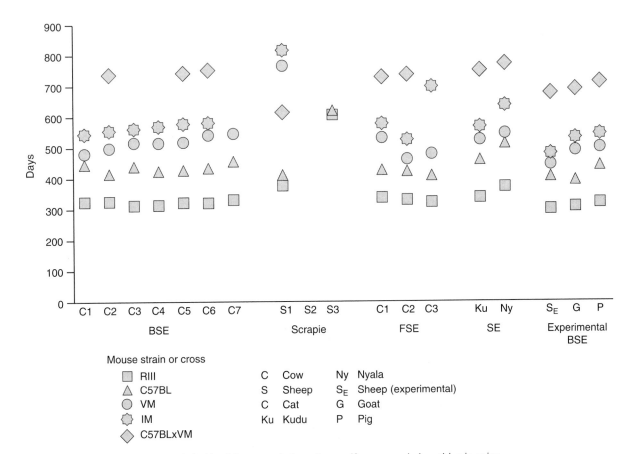

Figure 11.4 *Mean incubation periods (days) in transmission of spongiform encephalopathies in mice.*

elevated transaminases – the reason for this is not known.

Electroencephalography

The EEG was first recognized as an important aid to the diagnosis of CJD in 1954 and was included as a component of the first published diagnostic criteria in 1979 (Masters *et al.*, 1979). The EEG has traditionally been considered the most reliable non-invasive diagnostic of CJD. Approximately 60–70% of cases are reported to develop the diagnostic 'classical' appearance of 1–2 Hz generalized bi/triphasic periodic complexes (see Figure 11.5), the remainder usually show non-specific slow wave abnormalities only. As the possibility of a characteristic tracing increases with time, it is recommended that following a non-diagnostic recording further tracings should be repeated at regular intervals (days or weeks). The response to diazepam is unpredictable with the classical appearances being either abolished or unaltered by its administration. The typical EEG appearance has not been reported in kuru, nvCJD or 'classical' GSS, and has only rarely been described in growth hormone related iatrogenic disease. A normal EEG does not exclude the diagnosis of CJD, indeed, there are exceptional reports of such records, even in the late stages of the disease. Although the

Table 11.8 *Differential diagnosis of CJD-like EEG*

Alzheimer's disease
Lewy body disease
MELAS syndrome
Hyperparathyroidism
Anoxic encephalopathy
Binswanger's disease
Baclofen, mianserin, metrizamide, and lithium toxicity
Hyperammonemia
Hypo- and hypernatremia
Hypoglycemia
Hepatic encephalopathy
AIDS dementia

characteristic EEG is virtually diagnostic of CJD in the correct clinical context, similar appearances have very rarely been described in other conditions, such as Alzheimer's disease or metabolic encephalopathies (Table 11.8).

Brain biopsy

This procedure is unlikely to significantly benefit the patient unless a potentially treatable condition is also considered a possibility. Therefore, although diagnostic

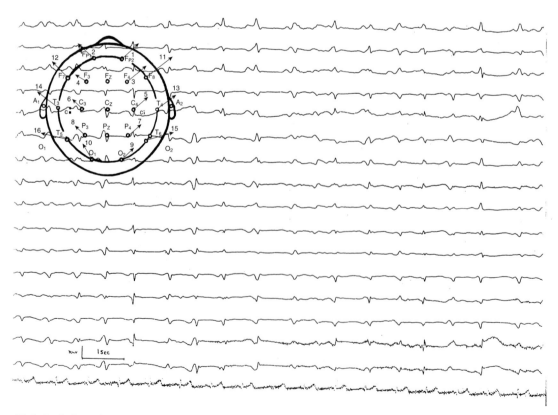

Figure 11.5 *Typical ECG in CJD.*

in most cases, brain biopsy cannot be recommended as a procedure to confirm the clinical suspicion of CJD. It is potentially hazardous, not only to the patient (who may develop a surgical complication such as infection or hemorrhage) but also to hospital staff. It is mandatory that the neurosurgical instruments are stored and destroyed if the diagnosis of CJD is confirmed, as adequate sterilization cannot be guaranteed. Approximately 5% of biopsies from definite cases are non-diagnostic, reflecting the potentially uneven distribution of pathology in CJD.

Neuroimaging

The main role of neuroimaging is to exclude other conditions. Computerized tomography is usually normal in CJD (80% of cases), but sometimes atrophy is found, especially in patients with a protracted illness (de Silva, 1996). Magnetic resonance imaging abnormalities have been reported, particularly an abnormal high signal from the basal ganglia on T2-weighted images (noted in only 4% of MRI reports in one series but 79% of retrospectively reviewed scans in another). However, most MRI scans are reported as being normal or showing generalized atrophy only. High T2-weighted signal abnormalities largely confined to the posterior thalami have been reported in two cases of nvCJD, a pattern not previously reported in other forms of CJD and therefore possibly specific for the new variant.

Magnetic resonance spectroscopy (for N-acetylaspartate) has been disappointing as an early diagnostic tool in CJD.

Positron emission tomography has been reported in only a few cases and the clinical usefulness of this technique remains to be established. Using [^{18}F]2-fluoro-2-deoxy-D-glucose, regional hypometabolism of glucose has been shown to correlate in general with neuropathological lesions in familial and sporadic cases. The hypometabolism is thought to reflect loss of neuronal function.

Single photon emission computed tomography (SPECT) scanning has also been reported in only a few cases of CJD, and frequently showed abnormal perfusion when contemporaneous imaging by MRI or CT was unremarkable. However, the specificity of SPECT abnormalities, and hence its use as a diagnostic tool, also remains to be established.

Cerebrospinal fluid

The CSF usually contains no inflammatory cells but a slightly elevated protein (0.5–1 g/l) is detected in about one-third of cases. The presence of oligoclonal bands confined to the CSF has only rarely been described.

Recent reports have suggested that the detection of a 'marker of neuronal death' in the CSF, the 14-3-3 protein, is both a highly sensitive and specific test for CJD (this immunoassay is derived from on an older and more complex technique using 2D-gel electrophoresis to detect two proteins designated p130 and 131) (Hsich et al., 1996). The results of a small number of blinded samples from the UK has been promising, including positive results from two confirmed cases of nvCJD. However, three further nvCJD samples were falsely negative. The detection of another CSF marker, neuron-specific enolase, is said to be a more rapid and simple, although less accurate, test than the detection of p130/131.

As the diagnosis of CJD is usually straightforward the clinical usefulness of these or other diagnostic tests is likely to depend on their ability to correctly detect those cases in which diagnostic difficulty occurs. This group largely consists of those in which the typical EEG appearance is not seen: the minority of sporadic cases, nvCJD, and most iatrogenic cases. Although results to date have been promising, too little information is currently available to reliably predict how clinically useful these CSF tests will be. At present the above-mentioned CSF assays are only available in a few centers in Europe and the USA.

Future diagnostic tests

Recent studies have demonstrated that the abnormal form of human PrP may exist as at least four distinct 'strains' determined, in part, by sites of glycosylation within the protein structure (Collinge et al., 1996). The strain appears to be associated with the clinical phenotype and may reflect disease etiology; for example, the 'type 4' strain pattern is associated with nvCJD. Another report describes the presence of abnormal PrP in palatal tonsillar tissue obtained at autopsy from a patient with nvCJD. Furthermore, it was possible to demonstrate the 'strain type' from this tissue. This raises the possibility that palatal tonsillar biopsy may be a useful test for nvCJD. However, it is not known when in the clinical course tonsillar biopsy would be diagnostic, whether tonsillar tissue is always affected in nvCJD, and if similar changes would be detectable in other forms of CJD. Indeed, a recent study from Japan failed to identify abnormal PrP in tonsillar tissue from a group of 11 sporadic CJD or GSS patients.

Prion protein is normally expressed on white blood cells and platelets but there is currently no convincing evidence that they carry the abnormal PrP isoform. However, the possibility that small amounts may be detectable, leading in a blood test for CJD, cannot be dismissed.

THE NATURE OF THE INFECTIOUS AGENT

The infectious nature of scrapie was discovered in 1935 when a previously healthy ewe developed the disease following inoculation with spinal cord from an affected sheep. Transmissibility of the human diseases kuru (1966), CJD (1968), GSS (1981), and FFI (1995) followed but the exact nature of the infectious agent remained elusive. In 1954 the concept of 'slow-virus disease' was first mooted. Certainly the long incubation period and predilection for the CNS of kuru is very much in keeping with known human slow-viral infections, such as subacute sclerosing panencephalitis. However, exhaustive, but unfruitful, efforts to find the 'TSE virus', and a conspicuous lack of inflammatory response, argued against a viral etiology. Furthermore the infectious pathogen shows a remarkable resistance to treatments that would normally be expected to inactivate viruses, such as ultraviolet and ionizing radiation. In 1967 a radical theory was put forward suggesting that the infectious agent could be a self-replicating protein. Subsequent experiments showed that scrapie infectivity was associated with a protease resistant protein, and in 1982 the term 'prion' was introduced for this hypothetical proteinaceous infectious particle. Advances in molecular biology have subsequently contributed greatly to our knowledge of the TSE agent, often supporting the protein-only hypothesis. Prion protein is now known to be a normal outer cellular membrane glycoprotein, expressed on most cell types, but predominantly in the CNS. This normal protease sensitive cellular form is transformed into the abnormal protease resistant isoform in the disease state. The difference between the normal and pathological isoforms appears to be solely conformational. The prion hypothesis states that, once produced, the abnormal isoform, PrP^{Sc}, acts as a template for the conversion of more PrP^{C} to PrP^{Sc}, thus, a chain reaction is set in motion with more and more PrP^{C} being transformed into the pathological PrP^{Sc} isoform. The prion theory may help explain the central paradox of the TSEs: how a disease can develop as an inherited, sporadic, and infective disorder. It is suggested that the mutations associated with these hereditary disorders renders the mutant PrP^{C} inherently unstable, with a high tendency to fold into the disease-causing PrP^{Sc} isoform. In sporadic disease the initial pathogenic prion protein needed to seed the production of PrP^{Sc} occurs as a rare spontaneous event, perhaps due to a somatic mutation of PrP gene in one or more cells. Finally in infective disease the inoculated PrP^{Sc} initiates the chain reaction of host PrP^{C} conversion to PrP^{Sc}.

Although the prion theory has gained increasing popularity over the past 15 years, many scientists still believe the transmissible agent is viral-like, containing DNA. Some have argued that perhaps the infectious DNA is associated with, and protected by, host protein – the 'virino hypothesis'. In support of these 'viral' hypotheses is the demonstration that different 'strains' of agent can be detected in hosts with identical PrP genotypes, thus suggesting the presence of a strain-specific informational molecule independent of the prion protein. The obvious candidate for such a particle would be nucleic acid, and it is difficult to explain strain variation in the context of the prion hypothesis. Although recent evidence suggests that PrP may be able to retain strain information by adopting different three-dimensional structures, the large number of scrapie strains would require ovine PrP to form an extraordinary range of different conformations.

Properties of the infectious agent

The efficiency of TSE transmission from donor to host is dependent on several factors, including route of infection. Experimental evidence suggests that ease of transmissibility decreases in the following order:

- intracerebral — most efficient
- intravenous
- intraperitoneal
- subcutaneous
- intragastric — least efficient.

It is of note that the intragastric route has the lowest efficiency requiring about 10^5 times more LD_{50} than the highly efficient intracerebral route. Animal studies show that when peripheral routes of infection are used replication of the TSE agent occurs early in the spleen and lymph nodes. The agent reaches the brain from the spleen probably via the visceral sympathetic fibers of the splanchnic nerves which facilitate the agent entering the mid-thoracic spinal cord, from where it appears to pass caudally at a maximum rate of about 1 mm/day. It is interesting to note that splenectomy in the early stages of the disease delays neuroinvasion. Once infection has passed to the brain and spinal cord it can pass centrifugally to the peripheral tissues, and this may account for the low and inconsistent infectivity at these sites.

Another important factor determining the transmissibility of the TSE agent is this 'species barrier'. This refers to the greater difficulty that exists when trying to transfer infection across species compared to within the same species. This was discovered in the 1960s when it was found to be difficult to transmit scrapie from sheep to rodents. Evidence suggests that PrP structure may play an important role in the determination of the species barrier: the greater the homology between the PrP structure of the donor and the host, the more likely the host will acquire prion disease. This may have particular relevance when considering the susceptibility of humans and other animals to the BSE agent. The bovine/human species barrier is not known but it is reassuring to note that transgenic mice expressing human rather than murine PrP have not developed disease over 500 days postinoculation with BSE. However, the human gene inserted into these mice is homozygous for valine at residue 129, in contrast with all the cases of nvCJD screened to date who are homozygous for methionine. Furthermore, recent *in vitro* studies of the efficiency of human PrP conversion by bovine prions has suggested a more efficient reaction if the human PrP has methionine rather than valine at polymorphic residue 129. The results of further studies with transgenic mice homozygous for methionine at codon 129 of their human transgene are awaited.

TREATMENT

Good nursing care to prevent the complications of immobility, such as pressure sores, is likely to be the most important treatment for a patient with CJD. Therapies aimed at palliation of any distressing symptoms, such as clonazepam or sodium valproate for myoclonus, are frequently successfully administered. Sedatives may be required for agitation, but such symptoms, if present, often abate at the illness progresses.

No treatment has been proven to halt the course of CJD, although a number of specific therapies have been tried including magnesium, amantidine, interferon, and other antiviral agents. Patients are frequently administered steroids, acyclovir or thiamin in the hope that they may have an occult, treatable condition such as a cerebral vasculitis, viral infection or Wernicke's encephalopathy. None of these therapies have an appreciable effect in CJD. Amphoteracin and doxorubicin have been found to delay death in hamsters infected with scrapie. However, both these drugs are toxic and needed to be injected directly into the brain. Amphoteracin has been tried in human CJD without success. Prophylactic administration of Congo red, a sulfonated amyloid-binding dye commonly used as a diagnostic stain for amyloids, before or shortly after experimental scrapie infection, may significantly delay the onset of clinical disease.

It has been shown that transgenic mice in whom the gene for PrP has been removed (and therefore who do not produce PrP naturally or following inoculation with prions) appear clinically well. This has led to the suggestion that ablative gene therapy, or the use of antisense oligonucleotides to 'turn off' the production of PrP, may be a useful treatment strategy. It is possible that through an increased understanding of the three-dimensional structure of PrP other therapies might evolve. Evidence suggests that PrP^C contains four

central α-helices whereas the pathological form, PrP^{Sc}, has a greater β-sheeted structure. If a molecule could be found that was able to bind and stabilize the central α-helices, this may in turn prevent the conversion of PrP^C to the putative disease-causing moiety. However, such therapies are purely theoretical at present (Table 11.9).

TISSUE HANDLING AND SAFETY PRECAUTIONS

Although the TSE agent is known to be infectious it is not contagious in the usual sense. Individuals exposed to patients with CJD: their spouses, nurses, and doctors, do not appear to have an increased risk of developing the disease. Furthermore, professionals who might be considered 'high risk' in relation to exposure to TSE agents, for example neuropathologists, veterinarians, butchers, etc., also do not appear to be at an increased risk of developing CJD. No proven instance of CJD contracted occupationally has been identified. However, the over 170 cases for iatrogenic CJD contracted through inoculation of contaminated CNS tissue or corneal transplantation serve to remind those of us involved in the management of CJD patients of the importance of safety procedures in relation to the TSE agents.

Table 11.10 shows the comparative frequency of infectivity in organs of human or animals with TSEs, and it is apparent that although the greatest infectivity is found in the CNS lower levels may be found in other tissues (Brown, 1996). However, it is of note that there is no proven instance of iatrogenic CJD arising from any tissues other than brain, dura mater, and cornea.

The resistance of the TSE agent to standard medical sterilization procedures is of concern. Experimental evidence demonstrates that the agent shows resistance to the following: exposure to boiling, freezing, ethanol, H_2O_2, permanganate, iodine, ethylene oxide vapor, detergents, organic solvents, formaldehyde, UV and gamma irradiation, and standard autoclaving.

Which decontamination measures should be followed for surfaces, instruments, gloves, and other devices that come in contact with tissues or body fluids from patients with TSEs? Since conventional methods of sterilization and disinfection do not decontaminate CJD infectious agents, specific measures must be used. Below is a section from guidelines produced for the European Union Biomed-1 Concerted Action 'The human prion diseases: from neuropathology to pathology and molecular genetics' (Budka *et al.*, 1995). Detailed recommendations on the performance of an autopsy of a suspect case of CJD are also included in these guidelines but are beyond the scope of this chapter.

Table 11.9

1. Sporadic CJD
Definite:
  Neuropathologically confirmed *and/or*
  Immunocytochemically confirmed PrP positive (Western blot) *and/or*
  Presence of scrapie associated fibrils
Probable:
  Progressive dementia and
  Typical EEG and
  At least two out of the following four clinical features: myoclonus; visual or cerebellar, pyramidal/extrapyramidal, akinetic mutism
Possible:
  Progressive dementia and
  No EEG or atypical EEG and
  Duration < 2 years and
  At least two out of the following four clinical features: myoclonus; visual or cerebellar, pyramidal/extrapyramidal, akinetic mutism

2. Iatrogenic CJD
  Progressive cerebellar syndrome in a recipient of human cadaveric-derived pituitary hormone or
  Sporadic CJD with a recognized exposure risk

3. Familial CJD
  Note: for the purpose of surveillance this includes GSS and FFI
  Definite or probable CJD plus definite or probable CJD in a first degree relative and/or
  Neuropsychiatric disorder plus disease-specific PrP mutation

4. New variant CJD
  Neuropathology is mandatory for the diagnosis of a definite nvCJD which is based on the following features:
  Abundant kuru-like amyloid plaques surrounded by vacuoles (clearly visible on H&E and PAS stains)
  Abundant PrP deposits on immunocytochemistry, including prominent 'pericellular' deposition in cerebral and cerebellar cortex (especially in the molecular layer)
  Spongiform change most prominent in the basal ganglia
  Marked thalamic astrocytosis

The following features are characteristic of nvCJD, although not sufficient for a definite diagnosis. Other forms of CJD may share some of these features and not every case of nvCJD cases demonstrates all these characteristics. Validated diagnostic criteria for a clinically 'probable' or 'possible' case are not yet available.

- A psychiatric presentation with depression and/or psychosis lasting weeks or months
- Onset of progressive unsteadiness within weeks or months of presentation
- Early and persistent paraesthesia/dysaesthesia
- Chorea and/or myoclonus
- Late illness progression similar to classical CJD, with dementia and multifocal neurological signs
- EEG does not show 'typical' appearance and may be normal
- MRI scan showing posterior thalamic high signal on T2- and/or proton density-weighted images
- Prolonged illness duration
- Young age
- Genetic analysis to exclude familial CJD is important and patients should have no history of exposure to a known risk factor for iatrogenic disease.

1. Steam autoclaving (glassware, instruments, safety gloves, etc.) 134°C recommended for 1 h. Comment: porous load is considered more effective than gravity displacement autoclaves (Advisory Committee on Dangerous Pathogens, 1994), the required time periods have been debated. For porous load autoclaving, only 18 min at 30 psi, or six separate cycles for 3 min each at 30 psi have been recommended. However, some laboratories recommend two cycles of autoclaving for at least 1 h during, or subsequent to, soaking in NaOH (see below).

2. Chemical decontamination of non-autoclavable materials and surfaces:
(a) 2NaOH (80 g/liter) for 1 h is recommended; alternately, 1 N NaOH may be used for 2 h. Comment: some laboratories consider mere wiping off as sufficient for surfaces, but others require more extensive washes. Do not use NaOH for aluminum material.

Table 11.10 *Distribution of comparative frequency of infectivity in organs of human or animals with spongiform encephalopathy*

Host tissue	Human/ kuru[a]	Sheep/goat scrapie	Cattle BSE
Brain	+++	+++	+++
Spinal cord	++	+++	(++)
Cerebrospinal fluid	++	+++	(0)
Eyeball	+++	+++	(0)
Peripheral nerve	(0)	+++	(0)
Pituitary gland	NT[b]	+++	NT
Spleen	+	+++	(0)
Lymph nodes	+	+++	(0)
Leucoctyes	+	NT	(0)
Serum	(0)	0	(0)
Whole or clotted blood	0	±	(0)
Bone marrow	(0)	0	(0)
Lung	+	±	(0)
Liver	+	+	(0)
Kidney	+	0	(0)
Pancreas	NT	0	(0)
Thymus	NT	±	NT
Intestine	(0)	+++	(0)
Heart	0	0	(0)
Skeletal muscle	0	0	0
Fat	(0)	NT	(0)
Testis	(0)	0	(0)
Semen	(0)	0	0
Ovary	NT	+	(0)
Uterus	NT	+	(0)
Placenta	(+)	(++)	0
Amniotic fluid	(0)	(±)	(0)
Cord blood	(+)	NT	(0)
Colostrum	(+)	0	NT
Milk	(0)	(0)	0

Based on isolations of the infectious agent from the natural hosts of each disease.

[a]Dem, Infectivity: +++ almost always present, ++ frequent, + irregular, ± rare, 0 undetectable. Parentheses indicate very few tested specimens.

[b]NT: not tested.

(b) Alternatively 5% NaOCl (at least 20 000 ppm free chloride, fresh solution) for 2 h. Comment: very irritating and corrosive for steel. Some laboratories use boiling of instruments or material in 3% SDS for at least 3 min as another option, either alone or in combination with autoclaving at 121°C for 1 h.

CONCLUSIONS

The past decade has seen a dramatic rise in the scientific understanding of the group of conditions that constitute the prion diseases. This explosion of knowledge is particularly timely given the tragic occurrence of the two novel prion diseases, BSE and nvCJD. What will the next decade hold? An accurate prediction of the numbers of nvCJD is currently beyond our grasp and we can only hope that the bovine/human species barrier is sufficiently large to prevent many further cases. We can perhaps be less guarded in predicting the demise of BSE in cattle, which many observers think will become virtually extinct shortly after the year 2000. But what of the prion 'Holy Grail': the nature of the infectious particle? This single discovery would be of enormous benefit, hopefully opening up numerous possibilities of diagnostic tests and therapeutic interventions. We must hope it comes soon.

Acknowledgements

I would like to thank Dr Gillian Stewart for helpful comments on this manuscript and Dr Robert Will, Dr Richard Knight, Dr Paul Brown, and Dr Clarence Gibbs for kindly providing information and illustrations.

REFERENCES

Advisory Committee on Dangerous Pathogens 1994: *Precautions for Work with Human and Animal Transmissible Spongiform Encephalopathies*, pp 1–35. London: HMSO.

Bell, J.E. 1996: Neuropathological diagnosis of human prion disease: PrP immunocytochemistry. In *Prion Diseases*, Baker, H.F. and Ridley, R.M. (eds), pp 59–83. Totowa, NJ: Humana Press.

Bradley, R. 1997: Animal prion diseases. In *Prion Diseases*, Collinge, J. and Palmer, M.S. (eds), pp 89–129. Oxford: Oxford University Press.

Brown, P. 1996: Environmental causes of human spongiform encephalopathy. In *Prion Diseases*, Baker, H.F. and Ridley, R.M. (eds), pp 139–54. Totowa, NJ: Humana Press.

Brown, P., Gibbs, C.J. Jr, Rodgers-Johnson, P. *et al.* 1994: Human spongiform encephalopathy: the National Institutes of Health series of 300 cases of experimentally transmitted disease. *Annals of Neurology*, **35**, 513–29.

Bruce, M., Chree, A., McConnell, I., Foster, J., Pearson, G. and Fraser, H. 1994: Transmission of bovine spongiform encephalopathy and scrapie to mice: strain variation and the species barrier. *Philosophical Transactions of the Royal Society of London – Series B: Biological Sciences*, **343**, 405–11.

Budka, H., Aguzzi, A., Brown, P. *et al.* 1995: Tissue handling in suspected Creutzfeldt–Jakob disease (CJD) and other human spongiform encephalopathies (prion diseases). *Brain Pathology*, **5**, 319–22.

Collinge, J., Sidle, K.C.L., Meads, J., Ironside, J. and Hill, A.F. 1996: Molecular analysis of prion strain variation and the etiology of 'new variant' CJD. *Nature*, **383**, 685–90.

Cousens, S.N., Vynnycky, E., Zeidler, M., Will, R.G. and Smith, P.G. 1997: Predicting the CJD epidemic in humans. *Nature*, **385**, 197–8.

de Silva, R. 1996: Human spongiform encephalopathy: clinical presentation and diagnostic tests. In *Prion Diseases*, Baker, H.F. and Ridley, R.M. (eds), pp 15–33. Totowa, NJ: Humana Press.

Gajdusek, D.C. 1977: Unconventional viruses and the origin and the disappearance of kuru. *Science*, **197**, 943–60.

Hsich, G., Kenney, K., Gibbs, C.J. Jr, Lee, K.H. and Harrington, M.G. 1996: The 14-3-3 brain protein in cerebrospinal fluid as a marker for transmissible spongiform encephalopathies. *New England Journal of Medicine*, **335**, 924–30.

Ironside, J.W. 1996: Neuropathological diagnosis of human prion disease: morphological studies. In *Prion Diseases*, Baker, H.F. and Ridley, R.M. (eds), pp 35–57. Totowa, NJ: Humana press.

Ironside, J.W. and Bell, J.E. 1997: Pathology of prion diseases. In *Prion Diseases*, Collinge, J. and Palmer, M.S. (eds), pp 57–88. Oxford: Oxford University Press.

Laplanche, J.L., Delasnerie-Laupretre, N., Brandel, J.P. *et al.* 1994: Molecular genetics of prion diseases in France. French Research Group on Epidemiology of Human Spongiform Encephalopathies. *Neurology,* **44**, 2347–51.

Masters, C.L., Harris, J.O., Gajdusek, D.C., Gibbs, C.J. Jr, Bernoulli, C. and Asher, D.M. 1979: Creutzfeldt–Jakob disease: patterns of worldwide occurrence and the significance of familial and sporadic clustering. *Annals of Neurology,* **5**, 177–88.

Palmer, M.S. and Collinge, J. 1997: Human prion diseases. In *Prion Diseases*, Collinge, J. and Palmer, M.S. (eds), pp 1–17. Oxford: Oxford University Press.

Prusiner, S.B. 1982: Novel proteinaceous infectious particles cause scrapie. *Science,* **216**, 136–44.

Wientjens, D.P., Davanipour, Z., Hofman, A. *et al.* 1996: Risk factors for Creutzfeldt–Jakob disease: a reanalysis of case-control studies. *Neurology,* **46**, 1287–91.

Will, R.G., Ironside, J.W., Zeidler, M. *et al.* 1996: A new variant of Creutzfeldt–Jakob disease in the UK. *Lancet,* **347**, 921–5.

Will, R.G., Matthews, W.B., Smith, P.G. and Hudson, C. 1986: A retrospective study of Creutzfeldt–Jakob disease in England and Wales 1970–1979. II: Epidemiology. *Journal of Neurology, Neurosurgery and Psychiatry,* **49**, 749–55.

World Health Organization 1997: *Report of WHO Consultation on Medicinal and Other Products in Relation to Human and Animal Transmissible Spongiform Encephalopathies.* Geneva: World Health Organization.

Specific environmental hazards

12

Metals and neurotoxicology

CHRISTOPHER G GOETZ AND KURT R WASHBURN

INTRODUCTION

Exposure to toxic metals is a continuing hazard of modern society. Although the danger of intoxication is greatest among workers directly exposed to metallic products or fumes, the ubiquity and widespread metal dissemination of many metals exposes large segments of the population to potentially damaging influences. The growing trend to set safety limits of exposure in the workplace may help curtail several toxic syndromes, but many metals are likely to remain problems for many decades. The most significant intoxicant metals are reviewed in this chapter.

LEAD

Lead poisoning has long been and continues to be a major environmental health problem in industrialized societies. Despite some recent animal research indicating a possible nutritional requirement for lead, there is no information to indicate that it is essential to humans (Mahaffey, 1984). The toxic effects of lead have been well documented and efforts to reduce exposure to lead and lower blood lead levels remain the primary goals of most health organizations worldwide. For example, in 1991, the Centers for Disease Control and Prevention, Atlanta, US (CDC) established new guidelines for the screening of lead and intervention due to increased awareness of neurobehavioral deficits found in children with low-level lead exposure (Centers for Disease Control, 1991). Based upon their recommendations, pediatricians were advised to intervene at blood lead levels $\geq 10\,\mu$g/dl as opposed to previous guidelines of $\geq 25\ \mu$g/dl.

The source of exposure most often linked to pediatric lead toxicity has been leaded paint, found in most houses built in the United States (and Europe) before the 1960s (Binns et al., 1994). In urban environments the deterioration of these houses and lack of adequate or complete restoration has provided a chronic lead burden to the pediatric population. Ingestion of non-food products, whether it be leaded paint, soil, or dust, and even consumption of lead contaminated food items remain the primary methods for elevated blood lead levels in children (Mahaffey, 1983). Inorganic lead found in paints, alloys, and plastics is generally either inhaled as a vapor or ingested. There have even been cases of lead intoxication from gunshot wounds (Manton, 1994).

Combustion of leaded gasoline raises air lead levels and is considered the major contributor to contamination of soil, dust, or food. Tetraethyl and tetramethyl lead (TEL and TML) are the most important alkyl lead derivatives used in petrol and reach the bloodstream via inhalation, or less frequently, by means of penetration of the skin (Marconi and Catenacci, 1994). Introduction of the catalytic converter in US automobiles in 1973 and the conversion to unleaded gasoline have helped in the reduction of blood lead levels in the United States (United States Environmental Protection Agency, 1991) and such measures are being introduced across the developed world.

There are numerous occupations which place workers at risk of lead exposure, including such fields as battery making/recycling, painting, printing, welding, firearm manufacturing, and smelting. Safety limits have been established for inorganic lead (dust or fumes) and lead arsenate exposure in the workplace. The current threshold limit value–time weighted average or TLV–TWA representing the concentration limit for chronic exposure in the workplace is 0.15 mg/m^3. The threshold limit value–short-term exposure limit or TLV–STEL representing the concentration limit for 15 minutes of exposure is 0.45 mg/m^3. For TEL and TML the TLV–TWAs are 0.10 and 0.15, respectively (Marconi and Catenacci , 1994).

Pathogenesis and pathophysiology

In the adult between 30% and 50% of lead that penetrates the lowest airways reaches the bloodstream, whereas only 5–10% of ingested lead is absorbed by the gastrointestinal tract. Lead absorption does, however, vary with age. In children, gastrointestinal absorption of lead can reach 40–50%, resulting in higher blood levels and consequently greater toxicity to the maturing brain.

There is evidence that nutritional factors influence the amount of lead absorption. Total food intake, calcium intake, and iron intake are three major factors which can influence absorption of lead, and may be areas of intervention in regards to treatment and prevention of lead poisoning. Lead is more readily absorbed if ingested without food compared to with food. This factor may play a role in the increased risk of lead poisoning among the urban poor who lack adequate availability of food or fail to attain the proper nutritional requirements. Either a low-calcium or a low-iron diet will result in increased lead absorption and toxicity as well. Lead may compete with calcium and accumulate not only in bone but also non-osseous sites. Although iron deficiency alone can cause behavioral and cognitive dysfunction in children, there is also evidence that iron deficiency enhances the retention and subsequent toxicity of lead (Mahaffey, 1990).

Once absorbed, inorganic lead is generally distributed into three major pools: blood and soft tissues (rapidly exchangeable pool); skin, muscles and trabeculated bone (exchangeable at an intermediate rate); and dense bone and teeth (slowly exchangeable) (Marconi and Catenacci, 1994). In the adult the majority of lead is found in bone. The total blood lead concentration reflects the plasma lead level and only comprises 0.2% of total lead burden. Once in plasma, inorganic lead is primarily cleared via renal excretion.

Organic lead differs from inorganic lead in that it easily penetrates the skin and is highly lipid soluble. It is metabolized in the liver and its byproducts, most notably triethyl lead, readily cross the blood–brain barrier to induce central nervous system (CNS) toxicity. Renal clearance is again the main route of excretion.

Many of the biochemical effects of lead are well known and can be predicted on the basis of its divalent, cationic structure. Lead interferes with several enzymes and compounds containing sulfhydryl groups. It acts on enzymes in glycolysis, the tricarboxylic acid cycle and even the electron transport system (Goetz, 1985).

An important pathway affected by lead poisoning is heme biosynthesis (see Figure 12.1). Lead interferes with conversion of delta aminolevulenic acid (ALA) to porphobilinogen by binding to the dithiol groups of delta aminolevulenic acid dehydrase (ALAD). In addition to inhibition of ALAD in the cytosol, lead can also act indirectly on membrane-bound proteins such as ALA synthetase (the rate limiting step in heme biosynthesis), coproporphyrinogenase, and heme synthetase (the final enzymatic pathway in the synthesis of heme). In the latter pathway, lead prevents incorporation of the ferrous ion into the protoporphyrin tetrapyrrole ring, thereby inhibiting the formation of heme, and concomitantly disrupting hemoglobin production.

Lead has been found to bind to high affinity proteins, similar to metallothionenes, which may facilitate translocation of lead into mitochondria. It is unclear, however, whether these binding proteins actually worsen lead toxicity through this mechanism, or whether they act to prevent lead binding to ALAD, and therefore, lessen toxicity (Goering, 1993).

There are other mechanisms by which lead acts to affect cell function. Lead has been found to influence the role of calcium as a second messenger via binding of calmodulin and activation of calmodulin-dependent phosphodiesterase, calmodulin inhibitor sensitive potassium channels, and calmodulin independent protein kinase C (Goldstein, 1993). It is theorized that by disrupting the normal functioning of these enzymes lead may interfere with neurotransmitter function, ion transport, and cell differentiation and proliferation.

Lead affects neurotransmitter release either by competing with calcium entry into the cell or by increasing the availability of intracellular calcium. Lead is a potent blocker of voltage-sensitive calcium channels and interferes with normal synaptic transmission. At low concentrations, lead enhances the spontaneous release of neurotransmitters, yet blocks the normal evoked neurotransmitter release produced by depolarization of the nerve (Bressler and Goldstein, 1991). Minnema and colleagues found that micromolar concentrations of lead increased the spontaneous

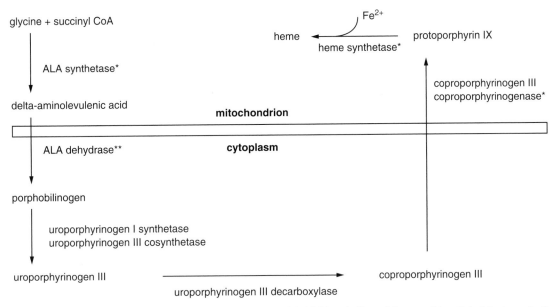

Figure 12.1 *The heme biosynthetic pathway with sites of head inhibition indicated by asterisks. ALA dehydrase is the most sensitive to lead poisoning.*

release of dopamine, acetylcholine, and gammaamino-butyric acid in rat hippocampal synaptosomes (Minnema *et al.*, 1986, 1988; Minnema and Michaelson, 1986). In addition, there is evidence that lead may act as a dopamine receptor agonist and even alter opioid peptides (Cory-Slechta *et al.*, 1993; Kitchen, 1993).

The neurotransmitter effects of lead may have significant influences on the neural network of a maturing brain, and supports the belief that lead is particularly toxic to the very young, and at low levels. It is known that as the brain develops the density of synapses is low at birth and much higher as a toddler before undergoing pruning and neural selection into adulthood. Bressler and Goldstein (1991) speculate that throughout these early stages of development lead may interfere with normal synaptic pruning leading to the learning and behavioral disabilities found in late childhood and early adulthood in those with chronic exposure to lead.

Clinical features

The syndrome associated with lead poisoning in children differs significantly from that seen in adulthood. Whereas peripheral neuropathy is the primary manifestation of lead neurotoxicity in adults, in the pediatric population encephalopathy is the hallmark of acute lead poisoning. Blood lead levels of 45 μg/dl or more are usually considered neurotoxic to children and warrant chelation therapy. However, there has been an abundance of recent research which has shown neurologic sequelae at lower lead levels than previously realized. The CDC's recommendations for intervention at lower blood lead levels stemmed from numerous studies suggesting an inverse ratio between body lead burden and neuropsychological and cognitive performance of children. The Port Pirie Cohort Study documented this inverse association between blood lead concentrations and developmental indices, including performance on the Bayley Mental Developmental Index and IQ measurement, measured longitudinally at the ages of 2, 4, and 7 within their cohort (Baghurst *et al.*, 1992). Other prospective studies have shown similar trends (Landsdown *et al.*, 1986; Fulton *et al.*, 1987; Hatsakis *et al.*, 1987; Ferguson *et al.*, 1988; Bergomi *et al.*, 1989; Hansen *et al.*, 1989; Binns *et al.*, 1994). Despite these reproducible results, there remains concern that confounding variables such as genetic and environmental factors were not adequately controlled in many of these studies.

The clinical manifestations of acute lead intoxication in children have been well described and typically develop over several weeks. Initial signs are often subtle and consist of alterations in behavior, such as irritability and listlessness. The child who continues to ingest lead will often develop clumsiness and ataxia, and gastrointestinal symptoms such as abdominal pain and vomiting. If not recognized at this time, signs of lead poisoning can rapidly progress causing seizures, coma or respiratory arrest. Although there is no precise correlation, lead levels greater than 70 μg/dl warrant immediate chelation therapy due to risk of sudden deterioration. However, children with blood lead levels less than 70 μg/dl may have signs and symptoms of lead toxicity and should also be treated.

On a pathologic basis the most common finding in a child with lead induced encephalopathy that leads to death is cerebral edema. At high lead levels, the blood–brain barrier is disrupted and there is a loss of interendothelial tight junctions and an influx of plasma constituents leading to increased intracranial pressure, diminished cerebral perfusion, and eventually, ischemia, necrosis, and hemorrhage. There is deposition of a proteinaceous material which can be found in the perivascular regions. Both gray and white matter undergo degeneration, although white matter is typically more damaged. The cerebellum seems preferentially affected and in those children who have died with acute lead encephalopathy there is often herniation of the cerebellum and temporal lobes on autopsy.

In the adult, lead poisoning can also cause encephalopathy but is rare and usually secondary to either ingestion of illicit liquor contaminated by lead or inhalation of TEL or TML from gasoline fumes. The latter method of exposure is often via the intentional 'sniffing' of gasoline. Initial manifestations range from confusion and irritability to frank psychosis. In addition to the neurobehavioral symptoms, adults with lead intoxication may demonstrate myoclonus (Hansen and Sharp, 1978). Occasionally, seizures and other extrapyramidal effects, such as ataxia, chorea and tremor, may be present. Chronic exposure in adults can lead to dementia.

Classically, adults with chronic lead intoxication will present with colic, anemia, blue lead lines along the gingiva, and peripheral neuropathy. Peripheral neuropathy is generally indicative of chronic lead exposure with blood lead levels over 70 μg/dl. The neuropathy is predominantly a motor neuropathy, although pain and paresthesias can occur. The characteristic nerve affected is the radial nerve with resultant wrist drop. Typically the finger extensors are involved first with progression to the wrist extensors. There will often be signs of lower motor neuron injury including atrophy, fasiculations, and hyporeflexia without significant sensory loss.

In addition to the radial nerve there may be nerve root involvement with, not only wrist drop, but weakness of the thenar muscle and interossei as well.

There may also be a loss of strength in the muscles of the shoulder girdle but this is rare (Windebank, 1984).

Foot drop is the most common manifestation of lead-induced peripheral neuropathy in the lower extremity and is more apt to be found in children rather than adults (Seto and Freeman, 1964).

Although both segmental demyelination and axonal degeneration have been found in nerves of lead-exposed animals, axonal degeneration is the prominent lesion in humans with lead neuropathy. Electrophysiologic studies generally confirm these findings by demonstrating active denervation and fibrillations, with relatively normal nerve conduction velocities in intact axons. Pathologically, there is controversy as to the direct effects of lead on the peripheral nerve. However, there is some evidence that lead accumulates in both the endoneurium and Schwann cells with resultant perineural edema. How this leads to axonal degeneration is not clear.

Evaluation

To make a diagnosis of lead poisoning there must be confirmation of exposure and an appropriate clinical presentation. Numerous laboratory tests exist which can be used to confirm clinical suspicion of lead toxicity.

Venous blood sampling for whole blood lead is the primary method for confirmation of lead poisoning. In the pediatric population there are new recommendations for intervention based upon whole blood lead levels (see Table 12.1). In adults with peripheral neuropathy levels are generally >70 μg/dl.

Routine blood testing can often demonstrate an anemia which is usually microcytic and hypochromic, with basophilic stippling of erythrocytes. Additionally, free erythrocyte protoporphyrin, urine coproporphyrins, and urine ALA are usually elevated. All of these findings can be attributed to lead's inhibition of the enzymes in heme synthesis.

The lead mobilization test (LMT) utilizes the urine lead excreted in response to a single dose of $CaNa_2$

Table 12.1 *Class of child and recommended action according to blood lead measurement*

Class	Blood lead (μg/dl)	Recommended action
I	≤9	Rescreen in 6 months
IIa	10–14	Rescreen in 3–4 months. If many children in this range begin communitywide prevention activities.
IIb	15–19	Rescreen in 3–4 months. Begin nutritional and educational intervention. Test for iron deficiency. Investigate environment.
III	20–44	Complete medical evaluation. Identify and eliminate lead source. Consider chelation with PCA or DMSA.
IV	45–69	Begin chelation with $CaNa_2$EDTA or DMSA. Environmental assessment within 48 hours.
V	≥70	Emergent chelation with BAL and $CaNa_2$EDTA. Environmental assessment immediately.

PCA = D-penicillamine; DMSA = 2,3 dimercaptosuccinic acid; BAL = dimercaprol. Adapted from Centers for Disease Control 1991: Preventing Lead Poisoning in Young Children. Atlanta, GA: US Department of Health and Human Services.

ethylenediaminetetraacetic acid (EDTA) as an index of chelatable body burden (Angle, 1993). This provocative test can determine more subtle lead exposure and can also be used to predict the response to chelation.

In patients with lead-induced encephalopathy a lumbar puncture is often performed and typically reveals non-specific findings such as increased cerebral spinal fluid (CSF) pressure, mild lymphocytosis, elevation of protein, and normal glucose. Caution should always be used however with this test due to possible high intracranial pressure (ICP) secondary to edema. In peripheral neuropathy from lead poisoning the CSF is usually normal but may show elevation of protein.

Other studies can be used to confirm chronic lead exposure. In children, roentograms of the long bones will often reveal lead lines at the metaphyses. X-ray fluorescence is a newer radiographic technique which may offer a better index of lead burden in children (Rosen and Markowitz, 1993). Analysis of lead in hair and teeth is generally not very practical or necessary in the determination of total body lead burden.

Management

The key to treatment of lead poisoning is identification of the source of lead and removal from exposure. Without taking these measures chelation therapy often fails or potentially worsens toxicity secondary to increased lead absorption (Goldstein, 1992). Therefore, the CDC's strategy for investigation and treatment of lead intoxication stresses early detection with screening of children via questionnaires for the determination of risk and the analysis of blood lead levels on those suspected of lead exposure. Initial steps involve investigation into the child's household and search for potential lead contamination in such items as paint, glasses, pottery, dishes or even cosmetics. In adults, the workplace is the usual source of lead poisoning and questions regarding occupational exposure are paramount.

Once measures are taken to eliminate or at least limit lead exposure, chelation therapy is often begun in those who are symptomatic or with elevated blood lead levels. The most commonly used agents are calcium disodium EDTA, dimercaprol (BAL), D-penicillamine (PCA), and dimeso-2,3-dimercaptosuccinic acid (DMSA).

In children with symptoms of acute lead encephalopathy or with significant elevation in blood lead levels ($>70\,\mu g/dl$), therapy generally consists of hospital admission, hydration to ensure adequate renal function and urine output, frequent neurological monitoring, and chelation with $CaNa_2EDTA$ and BAL. The beneficial effects of $CaNa_2EDTA$ and BAL on mortality in acute lead encephalopathy have been well described over the past 50 years (Chisolm, 1968). Administration

of intravenous $CaNa_2EDTA$ at a dose of 1000–1500 mg/m^2/day for five days is indicated in this setting as it results in the greatest urinary excretion of lead when compared to other chelating agents (Selander, 1967). However, drawbacks of this medication are its lack of oral dosing, potential nephrotoxicity, primary effect on bone lead rather than blood or soft tissue lead, and significant depletion of zinc as it is non-selective in its metal chelation. Zinc monitoring, and often supplementation, is therefore recommended. Chisolm has favored the use of BAL in conjunction with $CaNa_2EDTA$ because of the presumption that BAL reaches the spinal fluid and chelates brain lead (Chisolm, 1971). BAL is generally administered at a dose of 450 mg/m^2/day in divided doses every 4 h by deep intramuscular injection. However, it too has potential toxicity and can cause rapid elevation in blood pressure, headaches, nausea, and vomiting.

PCA has long been used for treatment of heavy metal intoxication, including lead, and has the advantage of oral administration. It has been used satisfactorily for the treatment of blood lead levels of 20–40 $\mu g/dl$ (Shannon et al., 1988, 1989). The usual dosage is 25–35 mg/kg/day in two to three doses for weeks or even months. Glotzer et al. (1995) determined that chelation with $CaNa_2EDTA$ or PCA could alleviate, partially, the reading disability of those who had elevated lead levels, and was cost effective when compared to the treatment of the learning disability. Therefore, PCA has a role in the asymptomatic child with mild to moderate elevations in blood lead levels. It also has been used effectively in adults with lead-induced peripheral neuropathy. However, due to frequent side effects, including penicillin-like sensitivity reactions and occasionally nephrotoxicity, PCA has limitations as well.

DMSA is a newer chelating agent that is structurally related to BAL but has the advantage of oral administration. Unlike other agents DMSA has been found to reduce the gastrointestinal absorption and retention of lead in addition to decreasing brain lead levels (Aposhian and Aposhian, 1990). It is currently recommended for moderate elevations in blood lead levels (20–69 $\mu g/dl$) and is well suited for out-patient administration. The initial dose of DMSA in children is 30 mg/kg/day in three divided doses for five days, followed by 20 mg/kg/day in two divided doses for two weeks. Although it seems to have a better side-effect profile when compared to other chelating drugs, DMSA can cause elevation of liver transaminases and occasionally thrombocytopenia. This warrants monitoring of liver function and complete blood counts during administration.

Despite the recent addition of DMSA to the armament of chelating agents used in treating lead toxicity, the most important aspect in managing lead toxicity remains prevention. Investigations into the households of children, or workplaces of adults, with lead toxicity remains vital to the determination, and eventual elimination, of the source of lead. Should more evidence build linking low blood lead levels in children to neurobehavioral sequelae, the issue of lead toxicity will gain even more attention.

MERCURY

Inorganic mercury

Historically, inorganic mercury compounds have been used as antiseptics, disinfectants, purgatives, and in industrial use of processing felt. Mercury is also found in the form of cinnabar, a red pigment used for painting and coloring (Bates, 1912). By current National Institute for Occupational Safety and Health (NIOSH) estimates, 65 000 workers have potential exposure to mercury. The occupations significantly at risk for mercury intoxication include alcohol distillation and brewing, chlorine production for antiseptics, dental preparations and pharmaceuticals, agricultural pesticides, and paper and pulp production. Other sources of exposure include disinfectants, cosmetics, dyes, furs, leather tanning goods, paints, photographic equipment, and storage batteries. There appears to be a wide range of individual susceptibility to the toxic effects of mercury; these may depend on the form of mercury, hygiene such as the frequency of hand washing, diet, specifically vitamin deficiency, and some intrinsic differences in mercury metabolism. Metallic mercury volatilizes at room temperature and thus generally enters the body through the inhalation of mercury vapors (Hunter, 1978). Whereas dental amalgams release small amounts of mercury, available data do not indicate that this exposure represents a significant clinical risk of intoxication (Levy, 1995), but dentists may be exposed to mercuric fumes on a chronic basis (Mantyla and Wright, 1979).

Elemental mercury is transported in blood plasma, proteins, and hemoglobin. Once incorporated into the body, mercury can be found in the urine as long as six years after cessation of exposure. Inorganic mercury has the greatest affinity for the kidney. Although concentrations are lower in the central nervous system, under the appropriate conditions it may be incorporated rapidly into the brain. Animal studies demonstrate that the highest concentrations of mercury occur in the brain stem followed by the cerebellum, cerebral cortex, and hippocampus (Kark, 1979). Although it is generally accepted that inorganic mercury exerts its neurotoxic effects by 'altering membranes', there is a paucity of information on specific pathological mechanisms and so such terms are almost meaningless. Very few postmortem studies have been published, and results vary from normal to slight neuronal damage with evidence of intracellular mercury (Battigelli, 1960).

Acute mercury poisoning usually results from the accidental ingestion of an antiseptic in the medicine cabinet. Patients presenting to the emergency room with bloody diarrhea, brownish lesions in the mouth, and massive vomiting may be experiencing a case of inorganic mercury toxicity. Erosive colitis with renal failure follow. The breath has a metallic odor, and a brownish mercurial linear streak may be visible along the margin of the teeth. Symptoms of mental irritability, rapid onset of weakness in the lower limbs, psychotic behavior with delirium, and hallucinations develop. The major threat to these patients is gastrointestinal hemorrhage, but after 24 h renal failure becomes the predominant cause of morbidity (Bates, 1912; Levy, 1995).

Chronic mercury toxicity can result in tremor and weakness of the limbs or progressive personality change. Mercury-induced tremor, also known as 'Hatters shakes' or 'Danbury shakes' consists of fine and regular tremor interrupted by much coarser myoclonic jerks. This can be seen at rest and often diminishes with activity. In later stages, gait and balance can be altered because of the continuous trembling. At times, these patients present a typical picture of parkinsonism, but with mercurial intoxication, tremor is usually both resting and postural or action-induced, having also a coarser quality than that found with Parkinson's disease. Mercury can also cause peripheral polyneuropathy (sensorimotor axonopathy), which affects the lower more than the upper extremities. In these cases, signs of sensory dysfunction in the form of paresthesia and sometimes extreme pain develop along with distal weakness with occasional muscle atrophy. A pure motor syndrome resembling amyotrophic lateral sclerosis can also develop (Kantarjiam, 1961). Cortical and subcortical signs include cognitive decline, personality changes, and seizures. Brain stem and cranial nerve signs include vertigo, nystagmus, blurred vision, narrowing of the visual fields, optic neuritis, and late optic atrophy. Ataxia is due to both the sensory loss and cerebellar dysfunction (Kark, 1979).

Of particular note, personality changes can develop before the appearance of neurological signs. Mercurial neurasthenia may insidiously occur over weeks or months before the patient seeks treatment. This syndrome consists of extreme fatigue, hyperirritability, insomnia, pathological shyness, and depression. The hyperirritability may become so severe that extreme violent behavior develops, possibly including homicidal acts.

Acrodynia, a chronic mercury toxicity syndrome in children, consists of painful neuropathy and significant autonomic changes. This syndrome includes hands and feet that are red and cold, painful limbs, profuse sweating of the trunk, severe constipation, and weakness. Tremors, similar to those found in adults, and personality change may also occur (Hamilton, 1925).

Serum mercury concentrations are unreliable indicators of inorganic and organic mercury toxicity since blood levels show large inter- and intra-individual variability. The threshold (BEI) for blood is 15 μg/l and for urine 35 μg/g creatine. However, urinary excretion is not a good measure of toxicity since there seems to be little correlation between symptomatology and the amount of mercury excreted in the urine. Because mercury intoxication may mimic some common neurological syndromes, the correct diagnosis is dependent on a good occupational history, clinical symptomatology, and the documentation of mercury in the patient's blood, urine or hair.

Organic mercury

Sources of organic mercury include contaminated seafood, ingestion of livestock feed grain that has either been treated with mercurial fungicides or the direct exposure to alkyl mercury used in the antifungal treatment of seed grains. There have been reports of massive intoxications resulting from ingestion of fish containing methyl mercury or from eating homemade bread prepared from seed treated with methyl mercury fungicide (Gotelli et al., 1985; Franchi et al., 1994).

Absorption routes of organic mercury are primarily dermal and gastrointestinal. Organic mercury is slowly excreted through the kidneys, its half-life varying between 40 and 105 days. It readily crosses the placenta resulting in blood concentrations in the fetus that are equal to or greater than in the maternal blood. There are several reports of fetal methyl mercury poisoning in asymptomatic mothers. Methyl mercury is also secreted in breast milk, although whether it induces toxicity by this route is unclear. In a community based study in the Faroe Islands where mothers consume large quantities of contaminated whale meat and blubber, breast-fed infants were compared to non-breast fed infants over their first year. The breast-fed babies developed their motor milestones earlier than the babies who were not breast-fed, in spite of higher mercury levels. The authors concluded that mercury was not toxic in these cases or the benefits of breast-feeding outweighed toxic signs (Grandjean et al., 1995).

Organic mercury readily crosses the blood–brain barrier, and its turnover in the brain is slow. In chronic exposure, approximately 10% of the body burden localizes in the brain. With acute intoxication, less than 3% is degraded into inorganic mercury localized to the brain, but this rate may change with time. Specifically, inorganic mercury levels may account for 82–100% of brain mercury after organic mercury exposure, if the autopsy is done several years after exposure (Davis et al., 1994). Once biotransformation to inorganic mercury occurs, excretion rates are extremely low since inorganic mercury crosses the blood–brain barrier very poorly. Excretion is primarily through the gastrointestinal tract, mostly through biliary secretion, and with almost immediate gastrointestinal reabsorption into the blood stream. Neuropathologic changes based on 10 cases found damage to the myelin sheath of peripheral neurons accompanied by glial proliferation and mobilization of phagocytes (Shiraki, 1979). Anatomically, the most severe damage was found in the primary visual cortex followed by the cerebellar cortex, pre- and postcentral gyri, the transverse gyrus, and the putamen. In a single case study, histological cases and high mercurial content were noted in the corpus callosum.

CLINICAL FEATURES

There are several typical clinical syndromes associated with organic mercury intoxication, the syndrome varying with age and exposure. The classical clinical triad of organic mercury toxicity is peripheral neuropathy, ataxia, and cortical blindness. There may be a delay of two weeks to several months before the appearance of symptoms after mercury exposure. The earliest symptoms may be paresthesia of the extremities beginning distally and extending to a glove-stocking distribution. Touch and pain are most impaired. Constriction of visual fields is generally seen (Chang and Dyer, 1995). In infants born of intoxicated mothers, severe brain damage including retardation and cerebral palsy develops.

Motor neuron disease resembling amyotrophic lateral sclerosis (ALS) is another notable and prominent clinical pattern. In these patients, gradual weakness develops with features of both upper neuron disease (increased reflexes and prominent jaw jerk) and lower motor neuron disease (fasciculations and atrophy) (Franchi et al., 1994).

A family that had ingested contaminated pork over a three-month period in 1969 was examined at the time of intoxication and followed for 22 years thereafter. Four children developed severe acute methyl mercury poisoning and the most profound signs occurred in the youngest, a neonate exposed in utero. Siblings exhibited poor balance, co-ordination, pyramidal function, and cortical blindness. The adults, although exposed, had no acute symptoms of intoxication. At 22-year follow-up, the two oldest children had cortical blindness, and the two younger ones had died during early adulthood, each demented, mute, quadraparetic with choreoathetosis and seizures. One adult had developed poor tandem gait. In the autopsy specimen, regional mercury levels correlated with the extent of brain damage which was most marked in the paracentral and parietal-occipital cortex. Since most mercury was inorganic, the authors suggested that methyl mercury had entered the brain, but was endogenously biotransformed, and thereafter remained in high concentrations in the inorganic form because this chemical does not easily cross the blood–brain barrier (Davis *et al.*, 1994).

It is difficult to diagnose mercury toxicity from laboratory data because of variability of blood and urine measurements. While measurements in blood and hair are less variable than those in urine, these do not necessarily reflect the degree of mercury toxicity. In urine, levels higher than 35 μg/g creatinine are elevated. Hair samples must be collected according to specific protocols. For example, samples must be taken close to the scalp and then washed to remove contaminants such as hair dyes or hair treatments. The advantage of hair samples is that they provide exposure information for the past year. Hair sample levels are usually 300–500 times those seen in blood (Takeuchi *et al.*, 1968).

MANAGEMENT

The management of mercury toxicity first depends on eliminating the exposure. Other remedies include the use of mercury-binding chelators such as D-penicillamine, BAL or DMSA which may accelerate the excretion of mercury (Marsh, 1979). However, chelation mobilizes mercury from bones and thus may worsen clinical symptoms and cause greater deposits of mercury into the brain (especially BAL). Penicillamine may be a most effective treatment in improving the effects of mercury on the nervous system. However, side effects of penicillamine treatment include hematopoietic suppression, alterations in cognitive and renal functioning, symptoms of myasthenia gravis, occasional hepatitis, and allergic reactions such as pruritus and swelling. With chelation, blood concentrations usually begin to decline after approximately three days (Tokuomi *et al.*, 1961). In asymptomatic individuals with increased blood concentrations of mercury, the administration of selenium and vitamin E may prevent the development of symptoms. In patients with mild contractures, physical therapy can be helpful.

Most of the patients with severe mercury poisoning die within a few weeks of the onset of symptoms. Some may survive with major neurological disability. In those with mild or moderate neurological symptoms, improvement may occur within the first six months. This occurs mostly in children and young adults. Examples have also been reported of ataxic, bedridden individuals who regained the ability to walk and some children who were totally blind regained vision. The family reported by Davis *et al.* (1994), however, demonstrated that generally the age at time of exposure is important to long-term outcome, and that young children have far greater residual neurological damage than adults (Davis *et al.*, 1994).

ARSENIC

Epidemiology

Arsenic has been used for centuries as both a medicinal treatment and a poison. In the past, it was recommended for a number of disorders ranging from arthritis to tuberculosis (Sollman, 1957). However, arsenic became more widely used in the treatment of syphilis in the early twentieth century before the advent of penicillin. Although no longer utilized in western medicine, arsenic continues to be used in some areas as a treatment for trypanosomiasis and is found in various traditional remedies such as Fowler's solution (potassium arsenite) (Windebank, 1984).

Despite its known toxicity and carcinogenic effect, arsenic can still be found in many households and work environments. Many pesticides and herbicide preparations contain arsenic and are potential sources of accidental ingestion in the pediatric population. Arsenic is also used in a number of industries, including taxidermy and welding, and the manufacture of paints, glass, enamels, and dyes. The smelting of copper and lead is still a means of producing arsenical compounds. Feldman *et al.* (1979) correlated increased arsenic levels with both subclinical and clinical evidence of peripheral neuropathy in smelter workers exposed to arsenic trioxide. Although modern smelting practices have improved, the use of arsenic-containing antiques, such as copper kettles, may still produce cases of arsenic poisoning (Jones, 1981).

Arsenic compounds can be divided into three major groups: inorganic compounds, organic compounds, and arsine gas. Most arsenic insecticides and weed killers contain inorganic arsenic and are therefore more frequently associated with accidental ingestion than organic compounds. Organic arsenic was more commonly used in medicinals but can be ingested by consuming fish and crustaceans (in the form of arsenobetaine), and by exposure to herbicide. Arsine gas was an agent used in chemical warfare in World War I but can be generated as a byproduct of tin refining. The TLV-TWA for arsenic is 0.01 mg/m^3 for elemental arsenic and its inorganic compounds and 0.16 mg/m^3 for arsine (Marconi and Catenacci, 1994). These standards reflect not only the knowledge of arsenic's neurotoxic effects but also its role as a carcinogen and have helped reduce the incidence of arsenic intoxication in the workplace.

Pathogenesis and pathophysiology

Although arsenic can be absorbed from the skin and mucous membranes, arsenic poisoning generally occurs through ingestion or inhalation of arsenic-containing products. Once absorbed into the bloodstream, arsenic is widely distributed throughout the body. The primary route of elimination is urinary.

The biochemical effects of arsenic depend on the particular form of the arsenic. Arsenates or pentavalent (+5) arsenic, the primary forms of arsenic in shellfish, are considered less toxic as they are readily methylated and excreted in the urine and do not directly bind thiol groups. Since arsenates do not directly bind to keratin-SH groups, the measurement of arsenic levels in hair or nails is not an appropriate assessment of arsenate exposure. Pentavalent arsenic produces its toxic effects at a cellular level by substituting for inorganic phosphate and uncoupling oxidative phosphorylation, preventing formation of ATP.

Arsenites or trivalent (+3) arsenic compounds are considered more toxic because they can directly bind to sulfhydryl groups of proteins. Similar to lead toxicity, many enzyme systems are affected; the pyruvate dehydrogenase complex, the bridge between glycolysis, and the citric acid cycle being particularly sensitive. By binding to dihydrolipoate dehydrogenase, arsenite compounds may prevent formation of acetyl coenzyme A and succinyl coenzyme A, thereby interrupting oxidative phosphorylation. As these are thiamine-dependent reactions, arsenic poisoning may mimic thiamine deficiency not only in its clinical signs (peripheral neuropathy) but in its biochemical effect as well. This observation may explain, in part, an increased susceptibility to arsenic toxicity in subjects who consume large amounts of alcohol (Massey, 1981). Trivalent arsenic, like pentavalent arsenic, may also disrupt phosphorylation and ATP production by substituting for inorganic phosphate. Both pentavalent and trivalent arsenic are eventually methylated to less toxic compounds, notably monomethylarsenic acid (MMA) and dimethylarsenic acid (DMA), which have lower affinity for tissues and are readily excreted in the urine.

Clinical features

Acute arsenic intoxication is more common than chronic arsenic poisoning and generally presents as a systemic illness. Gastrointestinal symptoms are pronounced, with nausea, vomiting, abdominal pain, and diarrhea being early manifestations. There can be profound fluid loss leading to circulatory collapse, renal failure, shock, and death. Initial neuropsychiatric symptoms may include nervousness, psychosis, paranoia, delirium, stupor or even coma and death with severe intoxications. As with other metals, the organic compounds tend to produce these CNS symptoms more rapidly than the inorganic compounds. Other manifestations may include fever, convulsions, and cardiac arrhythmias. Neurological examination may reveal nystagmus, exaggerated reflexes or even nuchal

rigidity (Goetz, 1985). A prolonged encephalopathy with features of a Korsakoff psychosis has been reported with arsenic poisoning, but is relatively uncommon (Freeman and Couch, 1978).

Reports of CNS pathology attributed to acute arsenic intoxication comes predominantly from those treated with organic arsenicals in the early 1900s. Autopsy cases generally revealed pericapillary hemorrhages, most notably in the midbrain and pons with perivascular demyelination, small vessel thrombosis and areas of necrosis (Hurst, 1959). 'Hemorrhagic purpura' have been described in these fatal cases.

Symptoms or signs of a peripheral neuropathy can occur with chronic arsenic exposure or, more commonly, following a single ingestion of arsenic. Neuropathic symptoms generally begin one to three weeks following exposure. Initial manifestations are predominantly sensory, often with significant pain, hyperalgesia, and paresthesias. Most typically, the neuropathy develops thereafter into a mixed sensorimotor type with some weakness. Guillan–Barré syndrome and diabetic neuropathy may be considered in the differential diagnosis. Arsenical neuropathy is usually symmetrical involving both lower extremities, but in more severe cases can involve upper extremities as well. Occasionally, a pure sensory neuropathy has been reported with arsenic intoxication.

Pathological studies of affected nerves generally reveal axonal degeneration (LeQuesne and McLeod, 1977). There may be segmental demyelination as well and degenerative changes with a fragmented appearance to the nerve (Chhutani and Chopra, 1979). There may even be a loss of anterior horn cells in the spinal cord. However, the hallmark finding remains axonal degeneration.

Although subacute or chronic exposure to arsenic has been associated with a prolonged encephalopathy, peripheral neuropathy is the most common neurological finding. Chronic systemic signs of arsenic poisoning, either from chronic exposure or from a single large exposure, help in making the diagnosis. Of all the systemic abnormalities, dermatological changes are the most pronounced. Hyperkeratosis and skin desquamation are commonly found over the palms and soles. Hyperpigmentation in a 'raindrop' or 'teardrop' configuration may form on the trunk or neck region. Brittle nails with transverse bands (Mees lines) above the lanulae may be present, although not specific for arsenic intoxication. There may be various hematological abnormalities as well, ranging from hemolysis and hemoglobinuria to aplastic anemia.

Evaluation

As with any other poisoning, a diagnosis of arsenic intoxication needs to be considered in the appropriate clinical setting and when exposure can be documented. There are numerous tests which may be helpful in confirming clinical suspicion of arsenic poisoning. Blood arsenic levels are not very helpful due to the rapid distribution of arsenic in body tissues. Urine arsenic concentration is considered the best index of recent exposure. Although laboratory values may vary among institutions, a 24-h urinary arsenic excretion $>100 \mu g$ may be considered elevated. A mobilization test may even be performed using penicillamine to monitor urinary clearance of arsenic. However, both blood and urine arsenic concentrations may be influenced by diet, specifically seafood ingestion. Other laboratory abnormalities may include elevated liver function tests or pancytopenia.

Hair and nails have been studied in cases of chronic arsenic intoxication due to their slow turnover and increased binding affinity for arsenic. Although hair may be influenced by external contamination with arsenic, neither hair nor nail arsenic concentrations are rapidly affected by diet. Arsenic concentrations in slow-growing hair such as pubic hair may be elevated ($>1 \mu g/g$) as long as eight months following exposure (Choucair and Ajax, 1988).

Since arsenic is radiopaque, plain radiographs may demonstrate recent ingestion. Other neurological studies such as CSF analysis or electroencephalograms usually reveal non-specific findings, but can be helpful in differentiating arsenic poisoning from other neurological disorders. Nerve conduction velocities show absent or reduced amplitudes of sensory potentials and compound muscle action potentials. Motor conduction velocities are relatively preserved suggesting an axonal rather than demyelinating process.

Management

Although removal from exposure is important in chronic arsenic intoxication, most presentations are in the acute setting following arsenic ingestion. In these situations, initial management involves evaluation of the airway and breathing, circulatory support and pain management. Gastric lavage should be initiated with 2–3 l of water followed by a glass of 1% thiosulfate or milk. Chelation therapy is generally indicated for severe cases of arsenic poisoning. However, there is no consensus on which agent is optimal. BAL given intramuscular (IM) at an initial dose of 3 mg/kg every 4 h with a slow taper is recommended by some authors, but is difficult to administer and has serious side effects (Greenhouse, 1982). Duration of therapy is also unclear, ranging from five to 10 days, or even longer depending on urinary excretion of arsenic and clinical course. Penicillamine has also been advocated at a dose of 250 mg four times daily for five days or until urinary arsenic has significantly dropped. Although it may be

considered an ideal medication for arsenical neuropathy due to few side effects and oral dosing, there still is a lack of convincing evidence for efficacy. DMSA is a newer chelating agent and like penicillamine has the advantage of oral dosing. Fornier et al. (1988) reported success with the use of 30 mg/kg/day for five days in the treatment of arsenic poisoning. Treatment with thiamin supplementation may be warranted especially in those suspected of alcohol abuse. Physical therapy may also be of benefit in those with arsenic neuropathy, as these patients tend to improve very slowly over months or even years.

MANGANESE

Mining dust and industry are the primary sources of manganese, although, like organic lead, manganese is also an antiknock additive in gasoline. In industry, it is used in the manufacture of chlorine gas, storage batteries, paints, varnish, enamel, and linoleum. Inhalation is the primary source of exposure (Mena et al., 1967). Also, patients with chronic liver failure cannot eliminate manganese well and therefore accumulate the metal (Hauser et al., 1994). Exposure levels reported to lead to neurological effects in humans range from $0.14–30 \, mg \, Mn/m^3$. Although most studies are not able to define a dose–response curve or a minimal neurotoxic threshold, Iregren (1990) and Roels et al. (1987) identify early effects at 0.14 and $1 \, mg \, Mn/m^3$.

In humans exposed to high levels of manganese, cells of the pallidum show histological changes at autopsy. Damage to the reticular portion of the substantia nigra as well as nerve cell alterations in the subcortical basal nuclei, frontal and parietal cortex, cerebellum, and hypothalamus occur. On magnetic resonance (MR) T1-weighted images, signal hyperintensity is seen in the globus pallidus (Hauser et al., 1994). Positron emission tomography (PET) scans, using 6-fluorodopa as a measure of dopamine activity, demonstrate normal findings in patients with clinical parkinsonism and manganese intoxication, even when they show clinical signs of parkinsonism (see below), suggesting that the presynaptic nigrostriatal system remains intact (Wolters et al., 1989). These data support the idea that the prominent target is in the striatum or globus pallidus. In experimental animals intoxicated with manganese, likewise, damage is directed towards the globus pallidum and reticular portion of the substantia nigra, sparing the nigrostriatal pathway typically lesioned in Parkinson's disease (Shinotoh et al., 1995; Olanow et al., 1996).

The onset of neurotoxic symptoms is extremely variable from individual to individual. Symptoms may appear as early as one or two months after exposure or as late as 20 years with chronic exposure. The earliest signs of manganism include anorexia, asthenia, apathy, somnolence, headaches, and social withdrawal. Personality changes are common and consist of irritability, emotional lability, and periods of hyperexcitability (manganese psychosis) (Cotzias et al., 1968). Facial expression becomes fixed and masked, resembling parkinsonism. Speech is affected, becoming faint with a monotone quality and occasionally becomes unintelligible or even mute. Most motor symptoms are confined to the extrapyramidal system, and include dystonia, bradykinesia, gait difficulties like retropulsion on rising and propulsion on walking. Awkwardness of extremity control and fine or gross rhythmic tremors of the extremities, trunk, and head may also occur. Motor deficits may develop without behavioral changes (Huang et al., 1989). Although it may be difficult to differentiate manganese toxicity from idiopathic Parkinson's disease, the tremor is less frequent and typically larger in amplitude (flapping) with manganese intoxication (Huang et al., 1993). Retropulsive gait is particularly prominent in manganese intoxication, and response to dopaminergic agents is generally less marked than in Parkinson's disease (Calne et al., 1994). Although frank weakness from upper or low motor neuron dysfunction is unusual, patients complain of slowness, weakness and fatigue, and signs like micrographia can be seen. Autonomic dysfunction can include impotence.

Meta-analysis techniques have been applied to case reports and worker cohort studies in order to clarify toxic ranges for extrapyramidal signs in different occupational settings (Feldman, 1992). Data from 18 references on 60 individual cases reports and population studies in 325 workers and control subjects formed the basis of this analysis. Of 117 workers, 6% with an exposure greater than $5 \, mg/m^3$ had acute extrapyramidal features, and in follow-up studies, 14% exposed to manganese dust had parkinsonism 11–20 years after cessation of exposure. The median latency period between exposure and development of parkinsonism ranged from six months to two years (Meco et al., 1994; Rodier, 1955).

Outside of the occupational setting, hospitalized patients receiving total parenteral nutrition (TPN) therapy, that includes manganese, can develop distinctive T1-weighted hyperintense patterns in the region of the globus pallidus (Mirowitz et al., 1991). These seeming lesions disappear after cessation of the TPN and in some patients their presence correlates with clinical parkinsonism and high manganese blood levels (Ejima et al., 1992; Mirowitz et al., 1992).

Evaluation

The diagnosis of manganism requires a history of manganese exposure in combination with physical findings. About 43% of the body burden of manganese is in the bone. Excretion is biphasic with a rapid phase having a half-life of four days and a second slower phase having a half-life of 39 days. Methods of biological monitoring are poor and individual manganese levels in blood and urine do not correlate with either present or past exposure.

Management

Management involves removal from exposure. The chronic movement disorder may respond modestly to the use of levodopa and sometimes 5-hydroxytryptophan. Patients studied by Mena responded well to doses greater than 3 g levodopa per day with a marked reduction in rigidity and all other symptoms except speech (Mena et al., 1970). Those treated by Huang and colleagues improved by 50% in objective assessments (Huang et al., 1993). Traditional chelation therapy has not proven to be helpful (Cook et al., 1974).

Once a syndrome develops, full recovery is rare. Signs and symptoms remain for many months after cessation of exposure. However, some symptomatic improvement may occur. This improvement is not felt to correlate well with reductions in the body concentrations of manganese (Mena et al., 1970).

ALUMINUM

Aluminum is the most abundant metal in the earth's crust. Due to its lightweight and corrosion resistant properties, aluminum alloys are of vital importance in the construction of modern aircraft and rockets. Aluminum compounds can also be found in the cosmetics field, food packaging, glassmaking, and water purification. Aluminum is used in the medical arena as well, in the form of antacids and antidiarrheal agents. Although aluminum continues to be used in many industries, toxicity from occupational exposure occurs only rarely. Intoxication, in recent years, has been most frequently identified in patients with renal failure through ingestion of aluminum-containing phosphate binders or through aluminum-contaminated dialysate.

The average amount of aluminum ingested by humans is 3–5 mg/day, mainly through food products. Only a small fraction of this is generally absorbed from the gastrointestinal tract. Once in plasma, aluminum may be distributed to a number of tissue stores, including the brain. The absorbed aluminum is cleared predominantly through renal filtration, with urinary aluminum concentrations averaging $10–15 \, \mu g/day$ (Kaehny et al., 1977).

The biochemical and toxic effects of aluminum are not well understood. Aluminum may affect a number of enzyme systems. It has been shown to inhibit hexokinase, an important step in glycolysis (Trapp, 1980). It has also been linked to inhibition of dihydro-pteridine reductase (DHPR) in both the brain (Cowburn and Blair, 1987) and erythrocytes (Altmann et al., 1987). This enzyme is vital to aromatic amino acid metabolism and may lead to toxic accumulation of tyrosine in nerve cells (Murray et al., 1991). Even with a mild aluminum overload, assays of erythrocyte DHPR have been reduced, suggesting some degree of aluminum toxicity to the human brain (Altmann et al., 1989). By interfering with calmodulin, aluminum may also cause an abundance of intracellular calcium. In addition, aluminum has been associated with alterations in cyclic adenosine-3,5-monophosphate (cAMP) levels (Johnson and Jope, 1987) and inhibition of acetylcholinesterase (Patocka, 1971).

The neurologic condition most commonly linked to aluminum intoxication is the dialysis encephalopathy syndrome (DES). Although once occurring in epidemics in the 1970s, DES is now infrequently encountered due to improved water purification methods and effective removal of aluminum from dialysate. The classic description of DES is a subacute progressive syndrome seen in chronic hemodialysis patients, presenting initially with a hesitant dysarthria, myoclonus, and behavioral changes. Patients generally progress over months developing focal or generalized seizures, psychotic features, and eventually, dementia and death. Other features of aluminum poisoning may include osteomalacia and anemia. Typically, the electroencephalogram (EEG) will reveal frontally predominant high voltage delta waves with multifocal spike activity. Treatment with deferoxamine, used mainly for iron chelation in the USA, may be of benefit, but has been associated with transient worsening or precipitation of the encephalopathy as well (Sherrard et al., 1988).

Pathologic features seen in the brains of DES patients are non-specific, but often include shrunken neurons with accumulation of aluminum in neuronal cytoplasm. However, in animal studies, pathological investigations have revealed neurofibrillary changes resembling, but not identical to, the helical filaments seen in the neurofibrillary tangles of Alzheimer's disease. In fact, raised aluminum levels have not only been found in the neurofibrillary degeneration of Alzheimer's disease, but also in the neurofibrillary degeneration of the amyotrophic lateral sclerosis–parkinsonism–dementia complex, another progressive neurologic disorder affecting some inhabitants of Guam. Although aluminum levels in drinking water have been elevated in Guam and some believe a correlation exists between aluminum in drinking water and Alzheimer's disease (Martyn et al., 1989), conclusive evidence linking aluminum ingestion with these neurologic disorders is still lacking. Mere presence of aluminum in the brains of demented patients may reflect secondary injury to the neuron

from a yet unidentified cause, rather than a direct causal relationship.

ANTIMONY

Antimony is a crystalline powder with a metallic taste. In action, it resembles arsenic, but is absorbed more slowly. Intoxication has resulted from the use of tartar emetic to provoke vomiting or with homicidal or suicidal intent. Poisoning has also resulted during the use of antimony in the treatment of bilharziasis, filariasis, and trypanosomiasis (Renes, 1953).

The acute intoxication manifests itself in abdominal pain, profuse vomiting, and diarrhea. The patient soon becomes weak, drowsy, and finally comatose. Occasionally, fainting spells or spasmodic contractions of the limbs may be present (Taylor, 1966). After a period of apparent improvement, there may be suppression of urine, the temperature drops to subnormal, and delirium, convulsions, and coma may be present for hours or days before death. In less severe cases, drowsiness and weakness persist for days, often accompanied by tetanic spasms of the limbs. The symptoms gradually subside, leaving only a persistent enteritis and loss of hair (Goetz and Cohen, 1989).

BARIUM

Barium is an abundant metal used extensively by people in a number of industries. Barium is utilized in the manufacture of alloys, valves, and flares, in the ceramic, paint and glass industries, in insecticides and rodenticides, and in the field of diagnostic radiology. Barium sulfate is the poorly soluble barium compound used as a contrast material for roentgenographic studies of the gastrointestinal tract and has been associated with toxicity. Occupational exposure can occur as well, particularly in welders who may inhale fumes containing barium compounds. A case of life-threatening barium poisoning has even been reported in a man exposed to barium carbonate used for cleaning chrome tanks (Shankle and Keane, 1988). However, the most important route of exposure is through ingestion of contaminated food or drinking water.

Soluble barium salts tend to be rapidly absorbed from the gastrointestinal (GI) tract and even the insoluble barium salts used in radiological studies have been shown to be taken up by intestinal absorption (Clavel et al., 1987). Once absorbed barium, like calcium, is preferentially deposited in bone, specifically at the sites of active bone growth and turnover. Barium is also distributed to a variety of soft tissues. Once ingested, barium is primarily eliminated via the fecal route with urinary excretion playing a minor role.

At a cellular level, barium's cationic, divalent structure allows it to mimic calcium in its physiologic effect. It can impede both calcium and potassium efflux from cells, and thereby interfere with depolarization of nerves and subsequent neurotransmitter release. Similar to familial periodic paralysis, chronic potassium deficiency, and thyrotoxicosis, barium poisoning results in an excess of intracellular potassium, leading to improper depolarization and resultant muscle weakness or paralysis (Layzer, 1982).

Clinically, patients with acute barium intoxication will present with nervousness, abdominal pain, nausea, and vomiting. These initial GI manifestations generally give way to progressive muscle weakness and loss of reflexes. These three features of gastroenteritis, progressive weakness, and hyporeflexia are most characteristic of barium poisoning. Although most cases of barium intoxication tend to recover without the need for medical intervention, occasionally treatment with intravenous or oral potassium is warranted to correct the hypokalemia (Smith and Gosselin, 1976). Only in the most severe cases is respiratory failure present requiring ventilatory support.

BROMIDES

Medicinal bromides, available as inorganic salts or organic compounds, have been used historically in the treatment of epilepsy and various psychoneuroses. The mechanism of action of bromides remains unknown, but may well relate to a general effect on neuronal membranes rather than a selective alteration of enzyme systems. Abuse or inadvertent intoxication has become less common in the USA since proprietary bromide was removed from the market in 1971 (Josse et al., 1965). Currently, triple bromide, containing potassium, sodium, and chloride salts, is available in the USA by prescription. In Europe, bromide-containing 'nerve tonics' remain available and are the major source of cases of intoxication (Siebner and Berndt, 1995).

Following ingestion, bromides are rapidly absorbed into the bloodstream and are distributed to all body organs with only minimal amounts reaching the brain. Bromides appear in all secretions and are present in breast milk in sufficient amounts to affect a nursing infant. Acute poisoning is distinctly uncommon, since doses sufficient to cause acute toxicity induce nausea and vomiting with expulsion of the irritant. Chronic intoxication with bromides, however, is observed and the clinical manifestations of poisoning may be divided into: excessive sedation, 30%; delirium, 65%; and hallucinosis, 5%. Excessive sedation begins at blood bromide levels above 150 mg/dl, and is an accentuation

of the medicinal effect. A mild drowsiness develops, associated with loss of concentration and occasional insomnia. In bromide delirium, the patient becomes disoriented, with mood disturbances, delusions, and possibly hallucinations. The hallucinatory type of toxicity differs from the delirium in that the hallucinations are experienced in an otherwise lucid setting (Moses and Klawans, 1979).

Neurologic findings are present in approximately 60% of chronically intoxicated patients and are commonly fluctuating. Tremor, ataxia, autonomic disturbances, and eye abnormalities appear as the most frequent abnormalities. The tremor is a fine postural one and is frequently most pronounced in the tongue on extension. As intoxication progresses, speech becomes slurred and gait ataxic, although unlike barbiturate intoxication, limb and truncal co-ordination are less compromised. Autonomic disturbances with unexplained fever and cardiac arrhythmias are also common, and eye signs have been a frequent source of diagnostic error. Anisocoria, extraocular palsies, and dilated pupils with light/near association are reported and, on occasion, small irregular pupils suggesting neurosyphilis. Furred tongue, headache, constipation, digestive disturbances, palpitations, fatigue, masked facies, and insomnia have also been attributed to bromide toxicity, although they cannot be reproduced by experimental intoxication (Moses and Klawans, 1979).

Two non-neurologic characteristics are common in patients with bromide toxicity and may help to suggest the diagnosis in confusing cases. The first is a state of general cachexia suggesting some form of chronic disease, neoplasm or vitamin deficiency. The physiologic basis of this picture is unclear, but when evaluation does not reveal an explainable cause for the cachexia, bromide toxicity should be considered. Second, skin involvement is present in approximately one-third of cases, usually manifested as an acneiform eruption over the face, arms, and upper trunk. Folliculitis or pemphigoid blisters may also appear.

Treatment involves the removal of all bromide substances, and the institution of hydration to promote diuresis. One liter of sodium chloride solution may need to be given intravenously every 4 h. Diuretics like furosemide (1 mg/kg) will also enhance the excretion of bromide. For chronic intoxication, 2–3 g of sodium chloride three or four times daily may be given by mouth with at least 4 l of fluids daily. Ammonium chloride in a dose of 2–3 g four times daily may be substituted for the sodium chloride if high sodium concentrations are felt undesirable in the patient. Severe psychosis has been managed with 300–500 mg of chlorpromazine daily. Patients with chronic exposure to bromide should be observed for three weeks.

CADMIUM

Cadmium is a relatively rare element which is generated as a byproduct of zinc production, but may be liberated with volcanic activity or from waste disposal as well. Cadmium is used as a component of various alloys, and can be found in pigments, fertilizers, and stabilizing compounds. The production of cadmium and nickel batteries continues to rise, particularly in Japan where the vast majority of cadmium is used for this purpose (Wilson, 1988). This rise represents not only an increased risk for occupational exposure but also a threat to the environment in regards to waste disposal. Inhalation of cadmium-containing compounds is also the major source of exposure in the workplace. Due to a growing demand for cadmium in a variety of industries, increased production has resulted in greater environmental contamination, particularly in food and drinking water. These are the main routes of human exposure to cadmium. Tobacco has also been implicated as a cause of increased body burden of cadmium in cigarette smokers (Webb, 1975).

Whereas only 5% of ingested cadmium is absorbed, 50% of inhaled cadmium will reach the bloodstream. Once absorbed from the lower airways or gastrointestinal tract, cadmium generally is distributed in the soft tissues, predominantly the kidney and brain. It is in these regions that cadmium toxicity is usually manifest. Binding to metallothionenes intracellularly is thought to be a protective measure against direct tissue toxicity. However, speculation still exists as to the role of this binding protein. Once in the body cadmium has a very long half-life, lasting for up to 30 years. Urinary excretion is difficult to assess with cadmium poisoning and varies depending on the degree of exposure and renal function. Measuring cadmium in feces will usually provide evidence of any recent ingestion.

Acute cadmium intoxication occurs most frequently in workers who inhale fumes or dust containing cadmium. A common presenting sign is respiratory distress. Acute pneumonitis and pulmonary edema are often diagnosed in these occupational exposures. With significant intoxication or prolonged exposure, workers may develop symptoms of chronic obstructive pulmonary disease. Renal tubular dysfunction is also characteristic of cadmium poisoning. Those exposed to cadmium may demonstrate proteinuria, glucosuria, aminoaciduria, or even hypercalciuria with formation of renal stones (Scott et al., 1976). Other manifestations of poisoning include osteomalacia and multiple fractures.

Neurologic toxicity from cadmium is not well documented in humans. However, in animal studies, both the central and peripheral nervous system are affected. In neonatal mice, subcutaneously administered cadmium chloride resulted in hemorrhagic changes, and subsequent neuronal destruction, in both the cerebrum and cerebellum (Webster and Valois, 1981). The predominant abnormalities were in capillaries, with disruption of the endothelium and secondary neuronal damage. The same mechanisms of injury have been reported in the peripheral nervous system. Most pathology in the peripheral nervous system is found in the sensory and autonomic ganglia (Arvidson and Tjalve, 1986). Sato et al. (1978) reported demyelination of peripheral nerves in rats with long-term exposure to cadmium.

Current therapy for cadmium intoxication is similar to all other poisonings, in that removal from exposure and supportive measures are usually indicated. Due to cadmium's strong affinity for metallothionein and the unproven efficacy of most chelating agents, specific therapy is often lacking. However, newer chelating agents are being investigated which may be helpful not only in treating cadmium poisoning but also in assessing body burden of cadmium (Jones and Cherian, 1990).

GOLD

Gold compounds, such as aurothioglucose, gold sodium thiomalate, and auranofin, are used in the treatment of rheumatoid arthritis (RA) and represent the principal mode of gold intoxication in humans. However, due to increased awareness of the serious side effects of gold and the availability of more efficacious medications, gold preparations are no longer frequently prescribed, even as second line arthritic therapy (Cash and Klippel, 1994). Although the mechanism by which gold compounds arrest the progression of RA is unknown, many hypothesize that its efficacy is related to inhibition or suppression of macrophage activity and T-cell response. The main route of administration is generally intramuscular injection, except for auranofin, which is given orally. Gold is absorbed rapidly into the bloodstream when taken intramuscularly and has a half-life of approximately seven days with a 50 mg dose (Insel, 1996). Once in plasma, gold compounds are distributed to a number of sites, including the synovium, kidney, and liver. Elimination is predominantly via renal clearance, except in the case of auranofin which is excreted mainly in the feces.

The exact mechanism of gold neurotoxicity is poorly understood, but there is some evidence that gold acts directly on peripheral nerves. However, speculation also exists regarding an immunologic basis for toxicity.

The most common clinical manifestations of gold toxicity involve lesions of the skin and mucous membranes. Cutaneous effects ranging from pruritis to exfoliative dermatitis are frequently seen, and may not be dose related. Ulcerations of the mucous membranes are often encountered as well. Hypersensitivity reactions with anaphylaxis have been reported. Blood dyscrasias, ranging from thrombocytopenia to aplastic anemia, have also been observed. Toxicity to the proximal renal tubules may lead to proteinuria and hematuria.

Peripheral neuropathy is the most common neurologic complication of gold intoxication. The classic description is that of an acute, symmetrically progressive polyneuropathy, with focal or generalized myokymia, and findings of axonal degeneration and segmental remyelination that improves with cessation of gold therapy (Katrak et al., 1980). Distal limb parasthesias are usually the first symptoms of gold neuropathy. They are generally followed by distal symmetric muscle weakness and atrophy (Windebank, 1984). The myokymia may resemble fasiculations but are slower and more undulating. Electrophysiologic studies typically reveal reduced amplitude of sensory nerve and compound muscle action potentials with slowing of conduction velocity. There may be repetitive discharges of muscle in those patients with myokymia. Since RA itself may cause a mononeuritis multiplex syndrome, differentiating gold neurotoxicity from symptoms of RA may be difficult. Increased joint inflammation or pain, asymmetry of the neuropathy, the presence of vasculitis, and the absence of myokymia may be factors which favor a diagnosis of rheumatoid rather than gold neuropathy.

Peripheral neuropathy is not the only neurologic complication of gold therapy. Meningitis has been reported (Myerson, 1950). Encephalopathy, cranial neuropathies, and psychiatric symptoms have also been described with gold intoxication (Fam et al., 1984).

Discontinuation of gold therapy is the primary means of treating gold toxicity. The neuropathy will generally improve following cessation of the medication, providing further evidence of a correct diagnosis. Chelating agents do not play a major role in the treatment of gold intoxication, as many patients will recover spontaneously.

IRON

Poisoning from iron preparations affects approximately 2000 individuals annually in the USA, with a mortality of up to 45% (Anderson, 1994). With iron toxicity, the onset of symptoms occurs as early as 30 min after ingestion; vomiting, which is frequently bloody, is an initial manifestation. Many patients have accompanying diarrhea, which may also be bloody. In severe cases, coma or convulsions may occur. The diagnosis is confirmed by demonstrating elevated concentrations of serum iron.

Induction of vomiting, gastric lavage, maintenance of adequate ventilation, correction of acidosis, and control of shock are the essential therapeutic measures (Chan et al., 1992). Chelation with deferoxamine is the specific treatment for iron toxicity. Using nasogastric tube, 5–10 g is administered following lavage (Cheney et al., 1995). With milder intoxication, 1–2 g is administered intramuscularly every 3–12 h, depending upon the degree of intoxication. For more severely ill patients, 1 g of the chelating agent is administered intravenously at a rate not exceeding 15 mg/kg/h. The dose may be repeated in 4–12 h for periods up to three days. BAL should not be administered, since it may form a toxic compound with iron (Kontoghiorghes, 1995).

SELENIUM

Selenium, ubiquitous in nature, is an essential trace element at low concentrations in humans. It is felt to be important in several enzyme systems, including glutathione peroxidase, and may have carcinostatic properties (Spallholz, 1994). Selenium has also demonstrated protective effects against intoxication from other metals, notably mercury and cadmium. The main route of human exposure to selenium is through food. However, the dietary intake of selenium is quite variable, dependent upon selenium concentrations in soil and plants, and the degree to which it is incorporated into the food chain in a particular geographic region. Many farmers have supplemented selenium into animal feeds due to concern over selenium deficiency diseases of livestock (Anonymous, 1971).

Exposure to selenium may also occur in the workplace through dermal contact or inhalation of selenium compounds in fumes or dust. Selenium may be found in the smelting and refining industries, and in the production of glass and electronic equipment.

Selenium is readily absorbed from the gastrointestinal tract and distributed to all major body tissues, but preferentially to the kidney and liver. Excretion is both through urine and feces, although respiratory excretion has been noted with high selenium exposures in animals (Olson et al., 1963).

Selenium toxicity in animals has been well described. The 'blind stagger' and 'alkali' diseases of livestock were commonly encountered by ranchers in the USA, and typically presented as stumbling and impaired vision in the former, and liver cirrhosis, hoof malformations, loss of hair, and lameness in the latter disease.

Although human toxicity from selenium exposure is usually more difficult to recognize, symptoms are often similar to those experienced in animals (Neve and Favier, 1989). In human populations exposed to excessive selenium, the most common clinical manifestations have been alopecia and nail pathology. Gastrointestinal disturbances, dermal eruptions, and dental caries have also been documented. Neurologic findings are rarely encountered. Selenium toxicity has been described in a man who ingested selenious acid in the form of gun blueing and developed a garlicky odor to his breath, hypotension, and a myopathy leading to respiratory failure and death (Pentel et al., 1985). A ranching family with chronic exposure demonstrated neuropsychiatric symptoms characterized as a clouding of the sensorium and emotional instability (Lemley and Merryman, 1941). Kilness and Hichgerg (1977) reported four cases of amyotrophic lateral sclerosis in male farmers living in a seleniferous area, and suggested that elevated environmental selenium may be a risk factor for this motor neuron disease. However, this interpretation has been disputed and no definite correlation has been established.

THALLIUM

Poisoning due to thallium is now uncommon. Thallotoxicosis has resulted from industrial use, clinical use, from homicidal and suicidal attempts, and through inadvertent use in foods. Industrially, thallium occurs as a waste product in manufacture of sulfuric acid. Thallium acetate has been used clinically in the treatment of dysentery and ringworm, and as a depilatory. Thallium acetate creams have accounted for many cases of thallotoxicosis, since thallium is readily absorbed through the skin. The chief source of thallium in cases of homicide or suicide has been Zelipaste, or 'Zello,' a rodent and ant poison containing 2.5% thallium sulfate. A few cases have been reported in which thallium sulfate had been accidentally mixed with food and eaten. The lethal dose of thallium in adults is approximately 1.7 g (Papp et al., 1969).

Recently, thallium poisoning has been implicated as the cause of numerous political poisonings. A 1980 news release by Amnesty International reported political suspects in Iraq poisoned while in custody. Some of these patients, examined and treated in the UK later, had varied thallium poisoning. It was suspected that thallium was added to the prisoners' food (Thompson, 1981).

Like other heavy metals and metalloids, thallium ions have a particular affinity for SH groups, and are capable of binding these groups in many sulfhydryl enzymes and certain proteins. Additionally thallium ions have the capacity to replace potassium ions and may affect systems such as the Na^+/K^+ ATP-ase. Porphyrin metabolism is also affected as evidenced by the appearance of porphyrins in the urine (DeBacker et al., 1982).

Characteristically, thallium toxicity focuses on combined neurologic, gastrointestinal, and hair abnormalities (Herrero et al., 1995). Severe abdominal cramps are often the earliest sign. Alopecia usually is not seen for two to four weeks after the acute exposure. This triad of system involvement should suggest thallium poisoning, although additional hepatic and renal disorders can also be seen (Thompson, 1981).

Neurologically, the onset of symptoms may be explosive or gradual, depending on the amount of thallium ingested. The earliest symptoms consist of neuritic pains in the extremities, followed by progressive, widespread flaccid paresis or paralysis, and even generalized convulsive seizures. The patient may become restless, irritable, mildly confused, and sometimes severely depressed. Often, as the illness progresses, the restlessness is replaced by lethargy and coma. In many cases of chronic or subacute thallotoxicosis, the patients will manifest choreiform movements, tremors or myoclonic jerks of the extremities and head. A secondary neuropathy similar to that seen with arsenic toxicity may occur, or an ascending weakness that resembles Guillain–Barré syndrome or even polio. In acute intoxication, faster conducting fibers are affected preferentially, and slower conducting fibers are not specifically affected (Yokoyama et al., 1990).

Cranial nerve involvement includes facial palsies and vocal cord involvement. Several ophthalmic lesions can develop including optic neuritis, optic atrophy, blindness, as well as ptosis, strabismus, dilated pupils, and lens opacification. Prior to frank optic atrophy, diminished contrast sensitivity and scotomas can predominate the clinical picture (Tabandeh et al., 1994).

Although most cases are isolated, in 1988, five of seven members of a US family were intoxicated. Two remained asymptomatic whereas three developed a severe acute peripheral neuropathy that led to respiratory compromise, and one of these people died. Medico-detective work led to identification of putatively fatal levels of thallium in glass soft drink bottles; a neighbor was later arrested and convicted of poisoning and murder (Desenclos et al., 1992).

Recovery is uncommon, and prolonged when it does occur. Patients continue to be weak and tired, and seem unable to return to a normal state. Striking residuals persist in the form of scattered pareses, visual disturbances, or severe emotional instability.

Prick described the following common major neuropathologic central nervous system findings in thallium toxicity (DeBacker et al., 1992):

1 Ganglion cell changes in the cortex, which are marked in chronic cases, but usually less severe in the more acute than might have been expected with the intensity of the clinical symptoms.

2 Degenerative changes in the ganglion cells through-out the brain stem, and particularly severe alterations in the hypothalamus. In the latter structure, the neurons exhibited granular cytoplasm with numerous large and small vacuoles. The Nissl substance was diminished in quantity and displaced toward the periphery of the cell.

3 White matter lesions consisting, most prominently, of edema and, to a lesser degree, demyelination and axonal degeneration.

4 Mild glial alterations and rather minor involvement of the spinal cord. On light microscopic examination of involved peripheral nerves, some fibers exhibit segmental myelin degeneration.

Electron microscopy of rats experimentally poisoned with thallium revealed many nerve fibers with primary neuroaxonal degeneration accompanied by mitochondrial swelling and prominent phagocytosis.

The diagnosis of thallium intoxication is based on history and urinary excretion levels. Excretion of greater than 10 mg thallium sulfate/24 h in the urine indicates severe intoxication (Rasmussen, 1981). Minimal amounts are excreted in the stool so that this latter assay is not of practical use.

Chelating agents such as BAL and diethyl-dithiocarbonate have been employed in the past. The latter agent has been controversial since animal studies demonstrate redistribution of chelated thallium from tissues into the central nervous system, with sharp increases in brain concentrations of unbound thallium. Hence, dithiocarbonate is no longer used in acute thallotoxicosis. Prussian blue (potassium ferri-hexacyanoferrate) administered via a duodenal tube has been used with success. This agent is a crystal lattice that absorbs thallium ions and is not absorbed gastrointestinally so that thallium is prevented from entering the circulation. It appears to be useful in both acute and chronic toxicity. The colloidal form is mot efficacious. A dose of 250 mg/kg/day divided into four doses dissolved in 50 ml of mannitol 15% has been used with success, especially in acute intoxication.

Potassium appears to increase the urinary excretion of thallium, either by an inhibitory effect of the ion on the reabsorption of renal tubular thallium or by a potassium-induced displacement of intracellular thallium. However, since Prick (1979) noted an increase in the severity of symptoms in thallium-intoxicated patients after potassium administration, this agent must be used extremely cautiously, especially in patients with chronic poisoning. Forced diuresis and hemodialysis have been tried, but are not associated with significant efficacy (Conradi et al., 1982). Combined hemoperfusion–hemodialysis has also been used with success (Dreisbach, 1969).

ZINC

Zinc is an abundant element that is essential to humans, with minimal toxicity compared to other metals. Although zinc deficiency is well reported and fairly common in underdeveloped countries, toxicity is rare (Fosmire, 1990). Human exposure to zinc comes predominantly through food intake. Most North Americans ingest 10–15 mg of zinc per day (National Academy of Sciences, 1989), with the major source of zinc being meat. Zinc is absorbed from the gastrointestinal tract and transported in plasma to a number of tissue sites. Excretion is predominantly via the fecal route.

At a biochemical level, zinc is required for normal functioning of many enzyme systems and binding proteins, such as metallothionene. Through these interactions, zinc can modulate synaptic transmission and hormone–receptor coupling. Zinc may play a role in the normal neurotransmission of mossy fibers in the hippocampus (Hesse, 1979). However, it is unclear how zinc may cause toxicity, especially in regards to the nervous system.

In cases of toxicity, excess zinc is usually taken orally, either as an accidental ingestion or as excessive self-supplementation. There have been cases of zinc toxicity resulting from storage of acidic food in galvanized containers (Brown et al., 1964). Occasionally the environment can be contaminated from improper waste disposal, causing elevation of zinc in drinking water and food stuffs. Occupational exposure may also occur, and is most commonly seen in welders who inhale zinc oxide fumes.

Clinically, symptoms of excess zinc ingestion are predominantly gastrointestinal, with patients often exhibiting nausea, vomiting, epigastric pain, abdominal cramping, and diarrhea. Occasionally, these individuals may have vague complaints of headache or malaise. Murphy reported lethargy and gait imbalance as primary features in a boy who accidentally took an overdose of zinc (Murphy, 1970). In addition, excess zinc may induce copper deficiency, causing anemia, leukopenia, and neutropenia (Prasad et al., 1978). Distinguishing symptoms of zinc intoxication from copper deficiency may be difficult, and generally requires laboratory evaluation.

Inhalation of zinc is usually encountered in the mining, smelting, and welding industries, and occasionally occurs with exposure to smoke bombs (Milliken et al., 1963). In these cases, zinc causes local respiratory damage. The 'metal fume fever' is characteristic of zinc poisoning and presents as a flu-like illness with cough, shaking chills, muscle aches, weakness, and hyperpyrexia (Papp, 1968). These symptoms usually resolve within one to two days and, in most cases, do not require further evaluation or treatment. Neurologic symptoms are non-specific, with patients experiencing headaches, generalized weakness, and malaise. Interestingly, workers exposed to zinc fumes do not typically demonstrate neurologic findings (Batchelor *et al.*, 1926). Although zinc has been shown to be directly toxic to neurons in animal studies (Yokoyoma *et al.*, 1986), there is a lack of evidence to support significant neurotoxicity in humans.

REFERENCES

Altmann, P., Al-Salihi, F., Butter, K. *et al.* 1987: Serum aluminum levels and erythrocyte dihydropteridine reductase activity in patients on hemodialysis. *New England Journal of Medicine*, **317**, 80–4.

Altmann, P., Hamon, C., Blair, J., Dhanesha, U., Cunningham, J. and Marsh, F. 1989: Disturbance of cerebral function by aluminum in hemodialysis patients without overt aluminum toxicity. *Lancet*, **2**, 7–12.

Anderson, A.C. 1994: Iron poisoning in children (Review). *Current Opinion Pediatrics*, **6**, 289–94.

Angle, C.R. 1993: Childhood lead poisoning and its treatment. *Annual Review of Pharmacology and Toxicology*, **32**, 409–34.

Anonymous 1971: Methionine, vitamin E, and selenium toxicity. *Nutrition Reviews*, **29**, 48–50.

Aposhian, H.V. and Aposhian, M.M. 1990: Meso-2,3-dimercaptosuccinic acid: chemical, pharmacological and toxicological properties of an orally effective metal chelating agent. *Annual Review of Pharmacology and Toxicology*, **30**, 279–306.

Arvidson, B. and Tjalve, H. 1986: Distribution of ^{109}Cadmium in the nervous system of rats after intravenous injection. *Acta Neuropathologica*, **69**, 11–16.

Baghurst, P.A., McMichael, A.J., Wiss, N.R. *et al.* 1992: Environmental exposure to lead and children's intelligence at the age of seven years (The Port Pirie Cohort Study). *The New England Journal of Medicine*, **327**, 1279–84.

Batchelor, R., Fehnel, J. and Thomson, R. 1926: A clinical and laboratory investigation of the effect of metallic zinc, of zinc oxide, and of zinc sulfide upon health of workmen. *Journal of Indian Hygiene*, **8**, 322–63.

Bates, L.W. 1912: *Mercury Poisoning in the Industries of New York City Vicinity*. New York: National Civic Federation.

Battigelli, M.C. 1960: Mercury toxicity from industrial exposure. *Journal of Occupational Medicine*, **2**, 337–44, 394–9.

Bergomi, M., Borella, P., Fantuzzi, G. *et al.* 1989: Relationship between lead exposure and neuropsychological performance in children. *Developmental Medicine and Child Neurology*, **31**, 181–90.

Binns, H.J., LeBailly, S.A., Poncher, J., Kinsella, T.R., Sanders, S.E. and The Pediatric Research Group. 1994: Is there lead in the suburbs? Risk assessment in Chicago suburban pediatric practices. *Pediatrics*, **93**, 164–71.

Bressler, J.P. and Goldstein, G.W. 1991: Mechanisms of lead neurotoxicity. *Biochemical Pharmacology*, **41**, 479–84.

Brown, M.A., Thom, J.V., Orth, G.L., Lova, P. and Juarez, J. 1964: Food poisoning involving zinc contamination. *Archives of Environmental Health*, **8**, 657–60.

Calne, D.B., Chu, N-S., Huang, C-C., Lu, C-S. and Olanow, W. 1994: Manganism and idiopathic parkinsonism: similarities and differences. *Neurology*, **44**, 1583–6.

Cash, J.M. and Klippel, J.H. 1994: Second-line drug therapy for rheumatoid arthritis. *New England Journal of Medicine*, **330**, 1368–75.

Centers for Disease Control. 1991: *Preventing Lead Poisoning in Young Children: A Statement by the Centers for Disease Control*. Atlanta, GA: United States Department of Health and Human Services.

Chan, K.W., Bond, M. and Fernandez, W. 1992: Desferrioxamine in acute iron poisoning (letter; comment). *Lancet*, **339**, 1601–2.

Chang, L.W. and Dyer, R.S. (eds) 1995: *Handbook of Neurotoxicology*. New York: Marcel Dekker.

Cheney, K., Gumbiner, C., Benson, B. and Tenenbein, M. 1995: Survival after a severe iron poisoning treated with intermittent infusions of deferoxamine. *Journal of Toxicology – Clinical Toxicology*, **33**, 61–6.

Chhutani, P.N. and Chopra, J.S. 1979: Arsenic poisoning. In *Handbook of Clinical Neurology*, Vinken, P.J. and Bruyn, G.W. (eds), pp 199–216. Amsterdam: North-Holland.

Chisolm, J.J. Jr 1968: The use of chelating agents in the treatment of acute and chronic lead intoxication in children. *Journal of Pediatrics*, **73**, 1–38.

Chisolm, J.J. Jr 1971: Treatment of lead poisoning. *Modern Treatment*, **8**, 593–611.

Choucair, A.K. and Ajax, E.T. 1988: Hair and nails in arsenical neuropathy. *Annals of Neurology*, **23**, 628–9.

Clavel, J.P., Lorrillot, M.L., Buthiau, P., Gorbet, D., Heits, F. and Galli, A. 1987: Intestinal absorption of barium during radiological studies. *Therapie*, **42**, 239–43.

Conradi, S., Ronnevi, L.O. and Norris, F.H. 1982: Motor neuron disease and toxic metals. In *Advances in Neurology: Human Motor Neuron Diseases*, Rolland, L.P. (ed.), Vol. 36, pp 201–32. New York: Raven Press.

Cook, D.G., Fahn, S. and Brait, K.A. 1974: Chronic manganese intoxication. *Archives of Neurology*, **30**, 59–64.

Cory-Slechta, D.A., Widzowski, D.V. and Pokora, M.J. 1993: Functional alterations in dopamine systems assessed using drug discrimination procedures. *Neurotoxicology*, **14**, 105–14.

Cotzias, G.C., Horiuchi, K., Fuenzalida, S. and Mena, I. 1968: Chronic manganese poisoning: clearance of tissue manganese concentrations with persistence of the neurological picture. *Neurology*, **18**, 376–82.

Cowburn, J.D. and Blair, J.A. 1987: Effect of aluminum on *in vitro* tetrahydrobiopterin synthesis in brain preparations. *Lancet*, **2**, 105.

Davis, L.E., Kornfeld, M., Mooney, H.S. and Fieldler, K.J. 1994: Methyl mercury poisoning: long-term clinical, radiological, toxicologic, and pathologic studies of an affected family. *Annals of Neurology*, **35**, 680–8.

DeBacker, W., Zachee, P. and Verpooten, G.A. 1982: Thallium intoxication treated with combined hemoperfusion-hemodialysis. *Journal Toxicology Clinical Toxicology*, **19**, 259–64.

Desenclos, J.C., Wilder, M.H. and Coppenger, G.W. 1992: Thallium poisoning: an outbreak in Florida. *Southern Medical Journal*, **85**, 1203–6.

Dreisbach, R. 1969: *Handbook of Poisoning*, 6th edn. Los Altos: Lange.

Ejima, A., Imamura, T., Nakamura, S., Saito, H., Matsumoto, K. and Momono, S. 1992: Manganese intoxication during total parenteral nutrition. *Lancet*, **339**, 426.

Fam, A.G., Gordon, D.A., Sarkozi, J. *et al.* 1984: Neurologic complications associated with gold therapy for rheumatoid arthritis. *Journal of Rheumatology*, **11**, 700–6.

Feldman, R.G. 1992: Mn as a possible eco-etiologic factor in Parkinson's disease. *Annals of New York Academy of Sciences*, **648**, 266–7.

Feldman, R.G., Niles, C.A., Kelly-Hayes, M. *et al.* 1979: Peripheral neuropathy in arsenic smelter workers. *Neurology*, **29**, 939–44.

Ferguson, D.M., Ferguson, J.E., Horwood, L.J. and Kinzett, N.G. 1988: A longitudinal study of dentine lead levels, intelligence, school performance and behavior. Part II: dentine lead and cognitive ability. *Journal of Child Psychology and Psychiatry and Allied Disciplines*, **29**, 793–809.

Fornier, L., Thomas, G., Garnier, R. *et al.* 1988: 2–3 dimercatosuccinic acid treatment of heavy metal poisoning in humans. *Medical Toxicology and Adverse Drug Experience*, **2**, 499–504.

Fosmire, G.J. 1990: Zinc toxicity. *American Journal of Clinical Nutrition*, **51**, 225–7.

Franchi, E., Loprieno, G., Ballardin, M., Petrozzi, L., Migliore, L. 1994 Jan.: Cytogenetic monitoring of fishermen with environmental mercury exposure. *Mutation Research*, **320**, 23–9.

Freeman, J.W. and Couch, J.R. 1978: Prolonged encephalopathy with arsenic poisoning. *Neurology*, **28**, 853–9.

Fulton, M., Raab, G., Thomson, G., Laxen, D., Hunter, R. and Hepburn, W. 1987: The influence of blood lead on the ability and attainment of children in Edinburgh. *Lancet*, **1**, 1221–5.

Glotzer, D.E., Freedberg, K.A. and Bauchner, H. 1995: Management of childhood lead poisoning: clinical impact and cost-effectiveness. *Medical Decision Making*, **15**, 13–24.

Goering, P.L. 1993: Lead-protein interactions as a basis for lead toxicity. *Neurotoxicology*, **14**, 45–60.

Goetz, C.G. 1985: *Neurotoxins in Clinical Practice*. New York: Spectrum Publications.

Goetz, C.G. and Cohen, M.M. 1989: Neurotoxic Agents. In *Clinical Neurology*, Joynt, R.J. (ed.), Chap. 20. Philadelphia, PA: J.B. Lippincott.

Goldstein, G.W. 1992: Neurologic concepts of lead poisoning in children. *Pediatric Annals*, **21**, 384–8.

Goldstein, G.W. 1993: Evidence that lead acts as a calcium substitute in second messenger metabolism. *Neurotoxicology*, **14**, 97–102.

Gotelli, C.A., Astolfi, E., Cox, C., Cernichiari, E. and Clarkson, T.W. 1985: Early biochemical effects of an organic mercury fungicide on Infants: 'dose makes the poison.' *Science*, **227**, 638–40.

Grandjean, P., Weihe, P. and White, R.F. 1995: Milestone development in infants exposed to methyl mercury from human milk. *Neurotoxicology*, **16**, 27–33.

Greenhouse, A.H. 1982: Heavy metals and the nervous system. *Clinical Neuropharmacology*, **5**, 45–92.

Hamilton, A. 1925: *Industrial Poisons in the United States.* New York: Macmillan.

Hansen, K. and Sharp, F. 1978: Gasoline sniffing, lead poisoning and myoclonus. *Journal of the American Medical Association*, **240**, 1375–6.

Hansen, O.N., Trillingsgaard, A., Beese, I., Lynsbye, T. and Grandjean, P. 1989: A neuropsychologic study of children with elevated dentine level: assessment of the effect of lead in different socioeconomic worlds. *Neurotoxicology and Teratolology*, **11**, 205–13.

Hatsakis, A., Kokkevi, A., Katsovanni, K., Maravolias, K. and Salamonias, F. 1987: Lead exposure and children's cognitive functions and behavior. In *International Conference on Heavy Metals in the Environment*, Lindberg, S.E. and Hutchinson, T.C. (eds), Vol. 1, pp 204–9. Edinburgh: CEP Consultants.

Hauser, R.A., Zesiewicz, T.A., Rosemurgy, A.S., Martinez, C. and Olanow, C.W. 1994: Manganese intoxication and chronic liver failure. *Annals of Neurology*, **36**, 871–5.

Herrero, F., Fernandez, E. and Gomez, J. 1995: Thallium poisoning presenting with abdominal colic, paresthesia and irritability. *Journal Toxicology and Clinical Toxicology*, **33**, 261–4.

Hesse, G. 1979: Chronic zinc deficiency alters neuronal function of hippocampal mossy fibers. *Science*, **205**, 1005–7.

Huang, C-C., Chu, N-S., Lu, C-S. *et al.* 1989: Chronic manganese intoxication. *Archives of Neurology*, **46**, 1104–6.

Huang, C-C., Lu, C-S., Chu, N-S. *et al.* 1993: Progression after chronic manganese exposure. *Neurology*, **43**, 1479–83.

Hunter, D. 1978: *The Diseases of Occupations.* London: Hodder & Stoughton.

Hurst, E.W. 1959: The lesions produced in the central nervous system by certain organic arsenical compounds. *Journal of Pathology and Bacteriology*, **77**, 523–34.

Insel, P.A. 1996: Analgesic-antipyretic and anti-inflammatory agents and drugs employed in the treatment of gout. In *Goodman and Gilman's The Pharmacologic Basis of Therapeutics*, Hardman, J., Gilman, A. and Limbird, L. (eds), pp 615–57. New York: McGraw Hill.

Iregren, A. 1990: Psychological test performance in foundry workers exposed to low levels of Mn. *Neurotoxicology Teratologogy*, **12**, 673–5.

Johnson, G.V. and Jope, R.S. 1987: Aluminum alters cyclic AMP and cyclic GMP levels but no presynaptic cholinergic markers in rat brain *in vivo*. *Brain Research*, **403**, 1–6.

Jones, H.R. 1981: Arsenic and antique copper: a potential source for intoxication and development of peripheral neuropathy. *Annals of Neurology*, **9**, 93.

Jones, M.M. and Cherian, M.G. 1990: The search for chelate antagonists for chronic cadmium intoxication. *Toxicology*, **62**, 1–25.

Josse, M., Cerf, J.A. and Hulin, G. 1965: Effects of barium ions on the resting membrane potential of striated muscle fibers. *Life Science*, **4**, 77–81.

Kaehny, W.D., Hegg, A.P. and Alfrey, A.C. 1977: Gastrointestinal absorption of aluminum from aluminum containing antacids. *New England Journal of Medicine*, **296**, 1389–90.

Kantarjiam, A.D. 1961: A syndrome clinically resembling amyotrophic lateral sclerosis following chronic mercurialism. *Neurology*, **11**, 639–44.

Kark, R.A.P. 1979: Clinical and neurochemical aspects of inorganic mercury intoxication. In *Handbook of Clinical Neurology*, Vinken, P.J. and Bruyn, G.W. (eds), Vol. 36, pp 147–98. Amsterdam: North-Holland.

Katrak, S.M., Pollock, M., O'Brien, C.P. *et al.* 1980: Clinical and morphological features of gold neuropathy. *Brain*, **103**, 671–93.

Kilness, A.W. and Hichberg, F.H. 1977: Amyotrophic lateral sclerosis in a high selenium environment. *Journal of the American Medical Association*, **237**, 2843–4.

Kitchen, I. 1993: Lead toxicity and alterations in opioid systems. *Neurotoxicology*, **14**, 115–24.

Kontoghiorghes, G.J. 1995: New concepts of iron and aluminum chelation therapy with oral Li (deferiprone) and other chelators. A review. *Analyst*, **120**, 845–51.

Landsdown, R., Urbanowicz, M.A. and Hunter, J. 1986: The relationship between blood-lead concentrations, intelligence, attainment and behavior in a school population: the second study. *International Archives of Occupational and Environmental Health*, **57**, 225–35.

Layzer, R.B. 1982: Periodic paralysis and the sodium-potassium pump. *Annals of Neurology*, **11**, 547–52.

Lemley, R.E. and Merryman, M.P. 1941: Selenium poisoning in the human. *Lancet*, **61**, 435–8.

LeQuesne, P.M. and McLeod, J.G. 1977: Peripheral neuropathy following a single exposure to arsenic. Clinical course in four patients with electrophysiological and histological studies. *Journal of the Neurological Sciences*, **32**, 437–51.

Levy, M. 1995: Dental amalgam: toxicological evaluation and health risk assessment. *Journal of Canadian Dental Association*, **61**, 667–8, 671–4.

Mahaffey, K.R. 1983: Sources of lead in the urban environment *American Journal of Public Health*, **73**, 1357–8.

Mahaffey, K.R. 1984: Toxicity of lead, cadmium, and mercury: consideration for total parenteral nutritional support. *Bulletin of the New York Academy of Medicine*, **60**, 196–209.

Mahaffey, K.R. 1990: Environmental lead toxicity: nutrition as a component of intervention. *Environmental Health Perspectives*, **89**, 75–8.

Manton, W.I. 1994: Lead poisoning from gunshots – a five century heritage. *Clinical Toxicology*, **32**, 387–9.

Mantyla, D.G. and Wright, O.D. 1979: Mercury toxicity in the dental office. *Journal American Dental Association*, **92**, 1189–92.

Marconi, M. and Catenacci, G. 1994: Biological monitoring of neurotoxic compounds. In *Occupational Neurology and Clinical Neurotoxicology*, Bleecker, M.L. and Hansen, J.A. (eds), pp 43–83. Baltimore, MD: Williams & Wilkins.

Marsh, D.G. 1979: Organic mercury. In *Handbook of Clinical Neurology*, Vinken, P.J. and Bruyn, G.W. (eds), Vol. 36, pp 73–82. Amsterdam: North-Holland.

Martyn, C.N., Osmond, C., Edwardson, J.A., Barker, D.J.P., Harris, E.C. and Lacey, R.F. 1989: Geographical relation between Alzheimer's disease and aluminum in drinking water. *Lancet*, **1**, 59–62.

Massey, E.W. 1981: Arsenic Neuropathy. *Neurology*, **31**, 1057–8.

Meco, G., Bonifati, V., Vanacore, N. and Fabrizio, E. 1994: Parkinsonism after chronic exposure to the fungicide maneb (manganese-bis-dithiocarbamate). *Scandinavian Journal of Work, Environmental Health*, **20**, 301–5.

Mena, I., Court, J., Fuenzalida, S., Papavasiliou, P.S. and Cotzias, G.C. 1970: Modification of chronic manganese poisoning: treatment with l-dopa and 5-OH tryptophane. *New England Journal of Medicine*, **282**, 5–10.

Mena, I., Marin, O., Fuenzalida, S. and Cotzias, C.G. 1967: Chronic manganese poisoning: clinical picture and manganese turnover. *Neurology*, **17**, 128–36.

Milliken, J., Waugh, D. and Kadish, M.E. 1963: Acute interstitial pulmonary fibrosis caused by a smoke bomb. *Canadian Medical Association Journal*, **88**, 36–9.

Minnema, D.J., Greenland, R. and Michaelson, J.A. 1986: Effect of *in vitro* inorganic lead on dopamine release from superfused rat striatal synaptosomes. *Toxicology and Applied Pharmacology*, **84**, 400–11.

Minnema, D.J. and Michaelson, I.A. 1986: Differential effects of inorganic lead and delta-aminolevulinic acid *in vitro* on synaptosomal gamma-aminobutyric acid release. *Toxicology and Applied Pharmacology*, **86**, 437–47.

Minnema, D.J., Michaelson, J.A. and Cooper, G.P. 1988: Calcium efflux and neurotransmitter release from rat hippocampal synaptosomes exposed to lead. *Toxicology and Applied Pharmacology*, **92**, 351–7.

Mirowitz, S.A., Westrich, T.J. and Hirsch, J.D. 1991: Hyperintense basal ganglia on T1-weighted MR images in patients receiving parenteral nutrition. *Radiology*, **181**, 117–20.

Moses, H. and Klawans, H.L. 1979: Bromide Intoxication. In *Handbook of Clinical Neurology*, Vinken, P.J. and Bruyn, G.W. (eds), Vol. 36, pp 291–312. Amsterdam: North-Holland.

Murphy, J.V. 1970: Intoxication following ingestion of elemental zinc. *Journal of the American Medical Association*, **21**, 2119–20.

Murray, J.C., Tanner, C.M. and Sprague, S.M. 1991: Aluminum neurotoxicity: a reevaluation. *Clinical Neuropharmacology*, **14**, 179–85.

Myerson, R.M. 1950: Meningitis during gold therapy. *Journal of the American Medical Association*, **143**, 1336.

National Academy of Sciences 1989: *Food and Nutrition Board Recommended Dietary Allowances*, 10th edn, pp 205–13, 284. Washington, DC: National Academy of Sciences.

Neve, J. and Favier, A. (eds) 1989: *Selenium in Medicine and Biology*. Berlin, NY: Walter de Gruyter.

Olanow, C.W., Good, P.F., Shinotoh, H. *et al.* 1996: Manganese intoxication in the rhesus monkey: a clinical, imaging, pathologic, and biochemical study. *Neurology*, **46**, 492–8.

Olson, O.E., Schulte, B.M., Whitehead, E.I., and Halverson, A.W. 1963: Effect of arsenic on selenium metabolism in rats. *Journal of Agriculture, Food and Chemicals*, **11**, 531–4.

Papp, J.P. 1968: Metal fume fever. *Postgraduate Medicine*, **43**, 160.

Papp, J.P., Gay, P.C. and Dodson, V.N. 1969: Potassium chloride treatment in thallotoxicosis. *American Journal of Internal Medicine*, **71**, 119–20.

Patocka, J. 1971: The influence of Al on cholinesterase and acetylcholinesterase activity. *Acta Biologica Medica Germanica*, **26**, 845.

Pentel, P., Fletcher, D., and Jentzen, J. 1985: Fatal acute selenium toxicity. *Journal of Forensic Sciences*, **30**, 556–62.

Prasad, A.S., Brewer, G.J., Schoomaker, E.B. and Rabbani, P. 1978: Hypocupremia induced by zinc therapy in adults. *Lancet*, **2**, 774.

Prick, J.J.G. 1979: Thallium poisoning. In *Handbook of Clinical Neurology*, Vinken, P.J. and Bruyn, G.W. (eds), pp 239–78. Amsterdam: North-Holland.

Rasmussen, O.V. 1981: Thallium poisoning: an aspect of human cruelty. *Lancet*, **1**, 1164–5.

Renes, L.E. 1953: Antimony poisoning in industry. *Archives of Industrial Hygiene and Occupational Medicine*, **7**, 99–113.

Rodier, J. 1955: Mn poisoning in Moroccan miners. *British Journal of Industrial Medicine*, **12**, 21–35.

Roels, H., Lauwerys, R. and Buchet, J.P. *et al.* 1987: Epidemiological survey among workers exposed to Mn: effects on lung, central nervous system, and some biological indices. *American Journal of Industrial Medicine*, **11**, 307–27.

Rosen, J. and Markowitz, M. 1993: Trends in the management of childhood lead poisonings. *Neurotoxicology*, **14**, 211–17.

Sato, K., Iwamasa, T., Tsuru, T. and Takeuchi, T. 1978: An ultrastructural study of chronic cadmium chloride induced neuropathy. *Acta Neuropathologica*, **41**, 185–90.

Scott, R., Mills, E.A., Fell, G.S. *et al.* 1976: Clinical and biochemical abnormalities in coppersmiths exposed to cadmium. *Lancet*, **2**, 396–8.

Selander, S. 1967: Treatment of lead poisoning: a comparison between the effects of sodium calcium edetate and penicillamine administration orally and intravenously. *British Journal of industrial Medicine*, **24**, 272.

Seto, D.S.Y. and Freeman, J.M. 1964: Lead neuropathy in childhood. *American Journal of Diseases of Children*, **107**, 337.

Shankle, R. and Keane, J.R. 1988: Acute paralysis from inhaled barium carbonate. *Archives of Neurology*, **45**, 579–80.

Shannon, M., Grace, A. and Graef, J.W. 1989: Use of penicillamine in children with small lead burdens. *New England Journal of Medicine*, **321**, 979–80.

Shannon, M., Graef, J. and Lovejoy, F.H. 1988: Efficacy and toxicity of D-penicillamine in low-level lead poisoning. *Journal of Pediatrics*, **112**, 799–804.

Sherrard, D.J., Walker, J.V. and Boykin, J.L. 1988: Precipitation of dialysis dementia by deferoxamine treatment of aluminum-related bone disease. *American Journal of Kidney Disease*, **12**, 126–30.

Shinotoh, H., Snow, B.J., Hewitt, K.A. *et al.* 1995: MRJ and PET studies of manganese-intoxicated monkeys. *Neurology*, **45**, 1199–204.

Shiraki, H. 1979: Neuropathological aspects of organic mercury intoxication. In *Handbook of Clinical Neurology*, Vinken, P.J. and Bruyn, G.W. (eds), pp 83–146. Amsterdam: North-Holland.

Siebner, H.R. and Berndt, S. 1995: Subakute Bromidintoxikation durch ein bromhaltiges 'Nerventonikum'. *Medizinische Klinik*, **90**, 173–4.

Smith, R.P. and Gosselin, R.E. 1976: Current concepts about the treatment of selected poisonings: nitrite, cyanide, sulfide, barium, and quinidine. *Annual Review of pharmacology and Toxicology*, **16**, 189–99.

Soliman, T. 1957: *A Manual of Pharmacology*. Philadelphia, PA: W.B. Saunders.

Spallholz, J.E. 1994: On the nature of selenium toxicity and carcinostatic activity. *Free Radical Biology and Medicine*, **17**, 145–64.

Tabandeh, H., Crowston, J.G. and Thompson, G.M. 1994: Ophthalmologic features of thallium poisoning. *American Journal of Ophthalmology*, **117**, 243–5.

Takeuchi, T., Matsumoto, H., Saski, M. *et al.* 1968: Pathology of Minamata disease. *Kumamoto Medical Journal*, **34**, 521–31.

Taylor, P.J. 1966: Acute intoxication from antimony trichloride. *British Journal of industrial Medicine*, **23**, 318–22.

Thompson, D.F.L. 1981: Management of thallium poisoning. *Clinical Toxicology*, **18**, 979–90.

Tokuomi, H., Okajima, T., Kanai, J. *et al.* 1961: Minamata disease. *World Neurology*, **2**, 536–48.

Trapp, G.A. 1980: Studies of aluminum interaction with enzyme and proteins. The inhibition of hexokinase. *Neurotoxicology*, **1**, 89–100.

United States Environmental Protection Agency 1991: *Strategy for Reducing Lead Exposures*. Washington, DC: United States Environmental Protection Agency.

Webb, M. 1975: Cadmium. *British Medical Bulletin*, **31**, 246–50.

Webster, W.S. and Valois, A.A. 1981: The toxic effects of cadmium on the neonatal mouse CNS. *Journal of Neuropathology and Experimental Neurology*, **40**, 247–57.

Wilson, D.N. 1988: *Cadmium – Market Trends and Influences. Cadmium 87. Proceedings of the 6th International Cadmium Conference*, pp 9–16. London: Cadmium Association.

Windebank, A.J. 1984: Metal Neuropathy. In *Peripheral Neuropathy*, Dyck, P.J. and Thomas, P.K. (eds), pp 1549–70. Philadelphia, PA: W.B. Saunders.

Wolters, E., Huang, C-C., Clark, C. *et al.* 1989: Positron emission tomography in manganese intoxication. *Annals of Neurology*, **26**, 647–51.

Yokoyama, K., Araki, S. and Abe, H. 1990: Distribution of nerve conduction velocities in acute thallium poisoning. *Muscle Nerve*, **13**, 117–20.

Yokoyama, M., Koh, J. and Choi, D. 1986: Brief exposure to zinc is toxic to cortical neurons. *Neuroscience Letters*, **71**, 351–55.

13

Noise, vibration and electromagnetic radiation

JOHN HARRISON

INTRODUCTION

The human body exists in a potentially hostile environment. Young described the body as a self-maintaining system that inevitably suffers the physical hazards imposed by a more or less tempestuous environment (Young, 1971). Such hazards include extremes of temperature, light and other parts of the electromagnetic spectrum, pressure changes, and vibration. The evolution of homeostatic mechanisms to preserve life has lead to the development of body receptors that are able to sense some of these hazards and, thereby, encourage avoidance of them. The ears, for example, detect sound via subtle pressure changes at the tympani which are then communicated to, and interpreted by, the brain. Similarly, there are vibration receptors in the skin. However, the body cannot detect other hazards, such as ultraviolet light, microwaves or gamma radiation, except indirectly when pathological changes occur.

Exposure to physical hazards occurs routinely during everyday life, but occupational exposure continues to represent the greatest risk to health because the exposure is likely to be greater and to be prolonged. Exposure to noise and vibration at work are good examples. Nonetheless, there is often greater concern about the health hazards that exist in the general environment and the continuing media coverage of the risks of living near to electric power lines bears testimony to this (Draper, 1996). Whilst there is some evidence that exposure to electric and magnetic fields might be associated with certain cancers, there is much stronger evidence that exposure to loud noise and to vibration may be causes of significant morbidity within the population. Involvement of the nervous system is common to the pathophysiological changes that occur in the respective conditions.

Noise, vibration and electromagnetic radiation: forms of energy

Sound, vibration, and electromagnetic radiation are all forms of energy. Sound is a form of energy which is detected by the hearing mechanism. Noise is the subjective appreciation of sound (Malerbi, 1993). Sound is propagated through the air by the longitudinal oscillation of individual molecules (King, 1980). Vibration, however, is the oscillation of a number of adjacent particles about a central point. The electromagnetic spectrum extends from static electric and magnetic fields through the radio frequency, microwave and infrared regions to light, ultraviolet radiation, X-rays, gamma rays, and cosmic rays (Allen et al., 1994). The part of the spectrum which has attracted considerable interest since 1979 (Theriault, 1995) is the radio frequency region. This extends from low-frequency static fields up to 300 GHz, the arbitrary lower delineating frequency of the infrared region. The radio frequency part of the spectrum can be subdivided into ten frequency bands using the nomenclature of the International Telecommunications Union (ITU). The spectrum is summarized in Table 13.1.

EFFECTS OF ENERGY ON THE BODY

The different energy forms can all have a physiological impact on the body. They can also cause pathological

Table 13.1 *Classification of radio frequencies*

Band	Abbreviation	Frequencies
Extremely low frequency	ELF	30–300 Hz
Voice frequency	VF	300–3000 Hz
Very low frequency	VLF	3–30 kHz
Low frequency	LF	30–300 kHz
Medium frequency	MF	300–3000 kHz
High frequency	HF	3–30 MHz
Very high frequency	VHF	30–300 MHz
Ultra high frequency	UHF	300–3000 MHz
Super high frequency	SHF	3–30 GHz
Extra high frequency	EHF	30–300 GHz

By convention, the ELF band is often taken to include frequencies less than 3 kHz. The UHF, SHF, and EHF bands together define the microwave part of the spectrum.

changes if exposures are either excessive and/or prolonged.

Noise

Sound is perceived when longitudinal vibrations of air molecules impact against the tympanic membrane of the ear. The function of the ear is to convert the sound waves into action potentials in the auditory (eighth cranial) nerves, which are then transmitted to the brain. Action potentials generated in the organ of Corti pass to the spiral ganglion in the cochlea and thence to the cochlea nuclei in the medulla oblongata. From there they may travel to either the inferior colliculus of the same side or that of the other side, or to the superior olivary nucleus of either side (Reid, 1978). Fibers pass from the inferior colliculus to the medial geniculate body of the thalamus and from there to part of the cerebral cortex concerned with hearing. Interconnections of fibers in the mid-brain facilitate a reflex pathway for turning the eyes and the head towards the source of a sound (Barr, 1974).

The hearing apparatus in the cochlea is the organ of Corti, where the hair cells are of particular importance. The tops of these cells are embedded in a rigid reticular lamina, whilst the hairs are embedded in the tectorial membrane. When the basement membrane moves, the tectorial membrane moves relative to the reticular lamina and bends the hairs. This generates action potentials (Ganong, 1975). The ear is a remarkably sensitive organ and is able to respond to sounds across a wide range of frequencies. The audible frequencies lie between 20–20 000 Hertz (Hz) in young people; frequencies less than 20 Hz are called infrasound and those greater than 20 000 Hz are called ultrasound. In addition, the ear may be exposed to sounds over a wide range of intensities. A measure of loudness of sound is sound power, which is the amount of sound energy per unit time. Familiar units are watts. However,

it is the sound intensity (watts/(meter)^2) which is a more important parameter clinically, as this is related to possible hearing loss. The lowest detectable sound intensity is 10^{-12} W/m^2 and this is called the threshold of hearing (*vide infra*). The main concern about exposure to loud noise is the effect that this might have on the ability to hear. It has also been suggested that continual loud noise may have adverse effects on blood pressure and on the outcome of pregnancy.

Vibration

The skin contains several types of encapsulated end organs, sensory nerve endings, which are able to detect vibration (Pelmear, 1992). The Pacinian corpuscle is a deep dermal and subcutaneous sensory receptor sensitive to vibration greater than 60 Hz. It is supplied by a single myelinated nerve. The Meissner corpuscle is found within the dermal papillary ridge and is innervated by between two and nine separate nerve fibers which lose their myelin sheaths on entering the corpuscle. This receptor is sensitive to vibration below 60 Hz. Another type of end organ is the Merkel cell–neurite complex: the Merkel cell is located in the basal layer of the epidermis. Finally, there are Ruffini end organs lying deep in the skin or in subcutaneous tissue, comprising a loose arborization of nerve fibers (Ham, 1974).

Vibration in the finger is said to stimulate four types of mechanoreceptive units (McGeoch *et al.*, 1994): slow adapting units (type I Merkel's discs and type II Ruffini end organs, SAI and SAII) and fast adapting units (type I Meissner's corpuscles and type II Pacinian corpuscles, FAI and FAII). The classification of these units is based on the properties of adaptation to constant pressure. The Pacinian corpuscles are the most sensitive of the fast-acting receptors, responding to faint displacement of the skin. Of the slow-acting receptors, Meissner's corpuscles (type I) are thought to be most potent and are valuable for both the differentiation of the shapes of objects as well as vibrotactile perception (Pyykko, 1986). These characteristics may be utilized clinically by using a moving two-point discrimination test to evaluate the function of SAI receptors. Abnormal values for two-point discrimination have been correlated with other neurological measurements of vibration-induced neuropathy (*vide infra*) (Pyykko, 1986).

The effects of vibration on the body depend on the means by which the vibration is transmitted. A major concern is the transmission of vibration to the hands from hand-held tools such as chain saws, riveting guns or grinders. The condition known as 'hand–arm vibration syndrome' may result from such exposures and has been shown to be prevalent in certain industries (Behrens and Pelmear, 1992). Estimates of workers possibly exposed to damaging degrees of hand–

arm vibration vary from 1.5 million in the USA in 1983 to 130 000 in the UK in 1986. Examples of the industries where such exposures are likely to occur are construction, car manufacturing, farming, mining, foundries, and lumbar and wood processing. The syndrome includes circulatory disturbances, sensory and motor disturbances, and musculo-skeletal disturbances (Pelmear and Taylor, 1992).

Exposure to whole-body vibration is most commonly associated with the development of low back pain and degenerative changes in the spine. However, motion sickness, an increased incidence of inguinal hernia, muscular insufficiency, scoliosis, peptic ulceration, gastritis, menstrual disorders, circulatory disorders, ischemic heart disease, hypertension, and decreased vestibular excitability have all been reported (Pelmear, 1995). Many of the studies reporting the associations lack adequate control groups, and so it is difficult to accept the relevant conclusions without reserve. Exposure to vibration in the frequency range 1–100 Hz appears to be important and intense vibration at or near 20 Hz seems critical for spinal degeneration. Osteoporosis and arthrosis of the feet has been linked to exposure to whole-body vibration in the frequency range 40–50 Hz (Pelmear, 1995).

Electromagnetic radiation

The electromagnetic spectrum is very wide and includes ionizing radiations, the effects of which have been described elsewhere (Hack, 1989). Non-ionizing radiations include ultraviolet, visible, infrared, and microwave radiation. Ultraviolet radiation may affect the skin and eyes, producing sunburn or snowburn and conjunctivitis. Visible radiation is important because of its ability to stimulate the rods and cones in the human retina, but both low and high levels of visible light may be associated with ill-health. Poor lighting is thought to be the cause of miners' nystagmus, the oscillations of which resemble congenital nystagmus (Hunter, 1957), whereas high levels may lead to retinal degeneration. High intensity light, as may be created by laser beams, can damage the eye by producing retinal burns or cataracts (Harrington, 1980). Similarly, infrared radiation may affect the eye by causing the development of posterior polar cataracts, typically in glassblowers, iron puddlers (those who stir molten pig iron on the bed of a reverberating furnace until carbon is removed), chain makers, gold smelters, tin-plate millmen, bakers, and laundresses (Hunter, 1957). Microwaves occur in the frequency range 30–300 000 MHz and can cause molecular vibration when absorbed into tissues. This leads to heating and the risk of skin and eye burns, in particular. It has also been postulated that exposure to microwaves can cause central nervous system damage expressed as intellectual impairment, insomnia, irritability, drowsiness, and loss of libido (Harrington, 1980).

Epidemiological studies have suggested that exposure to low-frequency bands of the ITU radio frequency classification are associated with the development of leukemia and brain tumors (Theriault, 1995). Most studies have been hindered by inaccurate estimations of ELF exposures. However, there is some evidence of ELF producing biological effects in cultured cells (Cridland, 1993). The photon energy of non-ionizing electromagnetic radiation is too small to affect chemical bonding directly. At 300 GHz, the infrared/microwave interface, photon energy is approximately 10^{-3} eV. This decreases linearly with decreasing frequency. This amount of photon energy is insufficient to break covalent bonds, which require an activation energy of 5 eV, and hydrogen bonds, which require 10^{-1} eV. However, possible effects of electromagnetic radiation may stem from the induction of electric fields in tissues leading to electrical charging of structures and to the creation of electric current and, hence, the absorption of energy. The effects may be classified into strong and weak field effects, the former being more likely to exert a biologically significant influence.

The development of electric charge phenomena due to strong field interactions is frequency dependent. These phenomena are termed relaxation processes. Biological tissue is characterized by four dispersion regions:

1 α dispersion (up to 10 kHz, the VLF band) and β dispersion (10 kHz–100 MHz, the VHF band) due to the movement of ions around the cell membrane and intracellular structures and from the capacitative charging of cellular membranes;
2 smaller contributions from the relaxation of asymmetrically charged molecules;
3 β dispersion due to the relaxation of water molecules bound to macro molecules;
4 γ dispersion due to the rotation of free or unbound water molecules.

The frequency ranges for 2, 3 and 4 are 1 kHz–10 MHz, 100 MHz–1 GHz and approximately 20 GHz, respectively.

For extremely low-frequency radiation ionic conduction processes are said to predominate (Cridland, 1993). It has been suggested that changes in the electric potential across cell membranes might induce conformational changes in voltage-sensitive protein 'ion channel gates,' such as in nerve or muscle cells. As frequencies increase, heating effects predominate and they are likely to be the main effect above 100 kHz (low-frequency band). However, the strengths of the electromagnetic fields required to produce such effects would have to be much greater than would be encountered in normal circumstances, in occupational or domestic settings. Similarly, weak field interactions would create insignificant electric fields in comparison to the other effects already described.

SOURCES AND MEASUREMENT

Exposure to noise, vibration, and electromagnetic radiation may be acute or chronic and may occur in a variety of settings, including occupational and domestic.

Noise

Exposure to noise is an age-old problem. Impact noise would have been expected to have occurred during the stone age and once metals started to be worked. Once gunpowder was used in munitions, noise from explosions would have occurred. Mining is an occupation dating back over centuries which would have exposed workers to noise. However, the advent of the industrial revolution and the development of mechanical industrial processes was a watershed for the chronic exposure of large groups of workers to loud noise. Many workplaces have therefore exposed workers to loud noise over the years and it is impossible to list all of them. Mining, ship building, heavy engineering, road transport, cotton mills, bottling plants, printing works, chemical works, airports, construction, and forestry are but some of the examples of environments associated with noise exposure.

MEASUREMENT OF SOUND

Measurements of sound intensity utilize the decibel scale. This is a scale of comparison (Waldron and Harrington, 1980). The sound intensity level is the intensity of interest compared to the threshold of hearing (10^{-12} W/m^2) expressed on a logarithmic scale

$$\text{sound intensity level} = 10\log_{10} I/(10^{-12})\ (\text{dB})$$

The scale has certain properties. Doubling the intensity of the sound will lead to an increase of 3 dB. On the other hand, sound intensities that are more than 10 dB different produce no increase in the higher sound intensity.

The ear responds differently to sounds of different frequencies. It is most sensitive to sounds in the 1–5 kHz range and relatively insensitive to low-frequency sound. Consequently, attempts have been made to modify the decibel scale such that sound level meters would give readings similar to the frequency responses of the ear. Using weighting networks in the meters, the responses across the hearing frequency range have been altered such that, at low frequencies, the meters are relatively unresponsive compared to their responses at 1 kHz. The usual weighting scale that is used is the A weighting scale and readings are expressed as dB(A).

Noise can be measured using a sound level meter. This is a microphone which converts sound waves into electrical impulses. There are different grades of meter available which vary in the precision of the readings and, consequently, the cost of purchase. The more advanced meters will give readings of L_{eq}, which is a measure of noise dose, and octave band analysis. The latter is useful as most noises comprise a range of frequencies and a knowledge of the sound spectrum may help in identifying sources of noise and in taking action to reduce noise exposure. By convention the octave bands are expressed as a mid-octave intensity, the frequencies being 62.5 Hz, 125 Hz, 250 Hz, 500 Hz, 1 kHz, 2 kHz, 4 kHz, and 8 kHz.

In many environments the noise levels are likely to vary with time, or work activities vary such that exposures to noise change throughout the working day. Measurement of the noise dose is performed using a noise dosimeter. This small portable instrument can be worn easily by workers throughout a shift, or part of a shift. The dose is expressed as a time-weighted average of noise energy for the period of time being studied. Thus, L_{eq} is the equivalent continuous noise level which would give the same amount of energy as the fluctuating noise. A similar expression $L_{EP,d}$ is used by the British Noise at Work Regulations (1989). This is the level of daily personal noise exposure and this has been used to set first and second action levels of 85 dB(A) and 90 dB(A), respectively. If, as a result of noise dosimetry, these levels are identified the employer in the UK has a statutory duty to designate ear protection zones, marked with signs, and to provide ear protectors.

Vibration

Workers may be exposed to vibration in many types of work. Industries with large numbers of workers potentially exposed to hand–arm vibration include construction, the motor and lorry industry, mining, steel making and foundry work, forestry and wood working, and farming. Examples of tools which cause hand–arm vibration are shown in Table 13.2.

Vibration can be measured using different methods. Exposure to hand-transmitted vibration is quantified in terms of acceleration of the surface in contact with the hand (units in m/s^2).

Vibration can be measured using an accelerometer. This measures acceleration in a single axis. However, to assess total vibration exposure, measurements should be carried out in three planes (orthogonal axes x, y, and z). The magnitude of the vibration is indicated by calculating the root-mean-square (RMS) acceleration value. This is then corrected by applying a frequency

Table 13.2 *Vibrating tools and processes*

- Pneumatic tools
  - Pneumatic riveting
  - Pneumatic caulking
  - Pneumatic fettling
  - Pneumatic drilling
  - Pneumatic clinching and flanging
  - Pneumatic hammers
  - Pneumatic rock drills
- Chipping hammers
- Holding up
- Pedestal grinders
- Hand-held portable grinders
- Flex driven grinders
- Flex driven polishers
- Rotary burring tools
- Swaging
- Chainsaws

weighting factor because low-frequency vibration (5–20 Hz) is considered to be more damaging than higher frequency vibration. (Vibration <2 Hz and >1500 Hz is not thought to be harmful.) The RMS vibration measurement is written as:

$$Ah, w$$

where, h is the hand-transmitted vibration and w is frequency weighted.

Therefore overall acceleration is:

$$Ah, w = A^2x, h, w + A^2y, h, w + A^2z, h, w$$

The daily vibration exposure (the average vibration magnitude during a working day (8 h) is defined as (Ah,w) or $A(8)$.

Health surveillance is recommended where workers' exposure regularly exceeds an $A(8)$ value of 2.8 m/s^2. Note that this value is not considered to be a 'safe' level.

Electromagnetic radiation

Electric fields are generated when an electric voltage is applied to a conductor. The difference in voltage between the surfaces gives rise to the electric field, the strength of which is measured in volts/m. The application of a potential difference across a conductor generates an electrical current. A number of effects are associated with the flow of electric current: heating, magnetic, chemical, and physiological. A magnetic field is an area where magnetic forces exist, i.e. there will be an effect on a compass needle and iron filings will be set in a pattern. The unit of strength of a magnetic field (magnetic flux density) is the tesla and magnetic fields measured in the vicinity of power cables and in

occupational settings are usually measured in microtesla (μT). Magnetic fields exist everywhere that there are electric currents, which means that they are almost ubiquitous. The characteristic of a magnetic field depends on the strength of the electric current and its frequency. The European frequency in power lines is 50 Hz, whereas in North America it is 60 Hz.

Workers exposed to static magnetic fields include electrochemical workers, staff using nuclear magnetic resonance and magnetic resonance imaging scanners, and railway workers. However, it is workers in the power industry that are likely to be exposed to the highest power-frequency electric and magnetic filed strengths. Other sources of exposure are underfloor heating, electric motors, tape erasers, and arc and spot welding. Broadcasting and telecommunications, including mobile phones, may also generate fields.

Direct measurement of electric and magnetic fields is not always straightforward. The choice of what to measure based on a known association with a biological effect remains to be determined, although certain measurements have been used more often than others in studies. Possible exposure measurements include integrated field exposures or time-weighted averages, median exposures, peak exposures, time above a specified field level, and various measures of how intermittent the exposure is. The act of measuring electric fields may affect the readings as electric fields may be perturbed by the presence of conductors, including people. There is also the problem that the fields being measured may exhibit spatial and temporal variations due to the location of the source and the possibility of power swings (Sussman, 1994). Types of instrument that have been used for measuring electric and magnetic fields include survey meters, continuous data loggers, integrating exposure meters, and computer-based data acquisition systems. Most assessments have concentrated on measuring magnetic fields. Measurements may be single axis or in three dimensions. Two commercially available instruments are the FIELDSTAR, which can be used as a hand-held survey meter, and EMDEX, which stands for electric and magnetic field digital exposure system. The AMEX (average magnetic exposure) meter is a cheaper alternative for measuring field exposures. Fixed-site systems for monitoring over an extended period of time are an alternative method of gathering data.

Unfortunately, direct measurement of fields may not be possible, or may only be possible for a small sample of the study population. Many studies have used surrogate methods of estimating exposure. In some cases the surrogate methods may be validated by performing direct measurements. Two popular surrogates have been job title and wiring configuration coding. Job title has been used in studies of occupational exposure, where generally the last job held has been chosen to represent the level of exposure. In residential studies wiring configuration coding has facilitated the ranking of potential exposures according to levels of electric current flowing in the wires. The codes classify homes according to distance from and the nature of nearby power lines and transformers. It is presumed that the codes reflect different levels of exposure to magnetic fields. Computer programs have been developed to model exposures using surrogate measures. However, it is important to appreciate that the main sources of fields (appliances, power lines, and grounding systems) produce fields which are very wide and which overlap each other.

The strength of the field diminishes with increasing distance from the source. There appears to be only a weak statistical association between measured magnetic fields and wire coding. Job titles appear to be just as imprecise. Measurements obtained in a recent large study, which were made in 11 different areas of the power industry, including offices and the headquarters site, show that there was considerable overlap of readings (Sussman, 1994; Harrington *et al.*, 1997). The term 'electrical occupation' has been used to identify a broad group of occupations where it is presumed that exposures will occur. Comparison of 'electrical' with 'non-electrical' occupations using direct measurements of exposure have suggested that task-weighted exposures for 'electrical' occupations are generally higher than in the 'non-electrical' occupations. However, even this comparison relied on estimates of the amount of time that was spent on each task. In another recent study (Savitz *et al.*, 1997) investigating the possible relationship between the incidence of lung cancer and exposures to electric and magnetic fields in the electrical utility industry, an attempt was made to refine the estimation process by combining the ranking of job exposures with random personal exposure measurements to 60 Hz magnetic fields performed during chosen work shifts. In addition, estimates of exposures to pulsed electromagnetic fields (PEMFs) were made for different job categories using data from a previous study carried out in Canada and France (Armstrong *et al.*, 1994).

In the latter study a positron meter was used to measure the proportion of time (in parts per billion) when the electric field was greater than 200 V/m in the 5–20 Hz range. Although the extrapolation of data for use in a different country can be questioned, attempts were made to validate the analysis by examining cancer mortality in relation to duration in high exposure jobs and moderate exposure jobs. High exposure jobs were defined as jobs where the percentage of workers above a 100 parts per billion (ppb) threshold was greater than 60, and moderate exposure jobs where the percentage of workers greater than 100 ppb was 25–60. Using this technique, high exposure jobs were supervisors, linemen and cable splicers, whereas moderate exposure jobs were mechanics, machinists, electricians, telecommuni-

cation technicians, and substation operators. The study did not find that the incidence of lung cancer was strongly associated with duration of employment in high exposure jobs. This method of assessing exposures has not added much to the overall understanding of disease etiology in this industry.

EFFECTS ON THE NERVOUS SYSTEM

Noise

HEARING

Noise at work and hearing loss
Exposure to loud noise at work has been shown to have a detrimental effect on hearing. Burns and Robinson in the early 1960s concluded that there was a risk to hearing from long-term exposure to noise levels greater than 85 dB(A). Since then other studies and analyses of data have suggested an alternative relationship between exposure to noise and the development of hearing loss. This suggests that occupational noise might not be as damaging as was first thought.

Of the many workplaces with noise levels leading to long-term exposures in the 85–90 dB(A) range, it has been estimated that in Australia some 500 000 workers may be exposed each day (Hogan *et al.*, 1994). A similar estimate for the UK has come from the Health and Safety Executive where 590 000 workers in manufacturing industries subject to the Factories Acts are exposed to levels of noise in excess of 90 dB(A) for at least 6 h per day. Until 1990 the legislation on noise at work only recognized 90 dB(A) as a threshold for action and there is a lot of anecdotal evidence to suggest that many companies have not taken noise-induced hearing loss seriously in the past. This is supported by the large number of compensation claims that have been paid by industry in recent times. It has been reported by Worksafe Australia that of the order of 10 000 workers seek compensation for noise-induced hearing loss each year (Hogan *et al.*, 1994).

It has been known for many years that hearing loss associated with exposure to noise is due to damage to the inner ear, specifically the hair cells and the cochlear. Pathological changes start at the basal end and spread as the hearing loss progresses. Thus, the initial changes mean that it is the higher frequencies that are affected first, but the lower frequencies become involved as the damage expands. This pattern of damage produces a characteristic pattern on audiometry.

Diagnosis
The diagnosis of occupational noise-induced hearing loss requires the performance of audiometry. This is because the loss of hearing, in the early stages, occurs at frequencies which do not affect the ability to hear the

spoken word. The onset of the hearing loss is insidious. By the time workers become aware that they cannot hear properly, considerable damage may have occurred. The features of occupational noise-induced hearing loss include the appearance of early abnormalities on the audiogram in the frequency range 3–6 kHz. The greatest hearing loss usually occurs at 4 kHz. It is usually bilateral and it is unusual for a profound hearing loss to develop solely as a result of exposure to noise. Aging must also be taken into account when reading an audiogram. Presbyacusis is also associated with high frequency hearing loss, but the pattern is different and the notch (i.e. the dip in the audiogram at 4 kHz) is not seen.

The American College of Occupational Medicine (ACOM) produced a position statement on noise-induced hearing loss in 1989. Occupational noise-induced hearing loss, as opposed to occupational acoustic trauma, is a slowly developing hearing loss over a long period (several years) as the result of exposure to continuous or intermittent loud noise. Occupational acoustic trauma is a sudden change in hearing as a result of a single exposure to a sudden burst of sound, such as an explosive blast. The diagnosis of noise-induced hearing loss is made clinically by a physician and should include a study of the noise exposure history (Dobie, 1995). Although the hearing loss is usually bilateral, the US National Institutes of Health have produced a consensus statement on noise-induced hearing loss which states that some degree of asymmetry of hearing loss is compatible with a diagnosis of noise-induced hearing loss, particularly when the noise source is a gun.

The inadequacy of scientific knowledge to predict safety from the effects of exposure to noise, on an individual basis, has been emphasized. Nonetheless, it is considered that, in stable exposure conditions, hearing losses at 3–6 kHz will plateau after about 15 years. In addition, once exposure to loud noise ceases, there should be no further loss of hearing attributable to noise-induced hearing loss. Hearing loss due to aging, or other causes, may, of course, occur. Analysis of a series of audiograms, using median threshold shifts to measure change, will reveal an accelerating high frequency loss due to aging and a decelerating loss due to noise (Dobie, 1995).

During the development of noise-induced hearing loss the initial audiometric changes will probably be temporary. A change in hearing acuity is called a threshold shift and, consequently, a temporary hearing loss following from exposure to loud noise is termed a temporary threshold shift. This is a manifestation of the protective changes that occur leading to a tightening of the eardrum and a reduction of the mobility of the ear ossicles. The time taken for the temporary threshold shift to revert to normal may be up to 48 h. Eventually the recovery from the temporary threshold shift may

become incomplete and continued exposure to noise may lead to the development of a permanent threshold shift.

Rehabilitation

Occupational noise-induced hearing loss is permanent, but the prospect of rehabilitation should be considered. Part of the rehabilitation of affected workers includes the provision of hearing aids, in the same way as any sensorineural hearing loss might be ameliorated, but other initiatives are also important.

A community-based approach to the rehabilitation of workers has been described by Getty and Hétu of the University of Montreal and Hogan et al. in New South Wales, Australia (Getty and Hétu, 1991; Hétu and Getty, 1991; Hogan et al., 1994). The program tried to overcome barriers to the prevention of hearing loss by looking at the perceptions of the effects of hearing loss by affected workers and their families, and by encouraging affected workers to accept that they have some hearing difficulty. A particular problem that may inhibit workers from seeking assistance is the stigma of being 'deaf.' In order to overcome this the program attempted to build up a trusting relationship between the worker and a professional, such as an occupational health nurse. The trusted professional introduced the worker to rehabilitation by visiting the home and talking to members of the family, as well as the worker. The program aims to change behavior and to encourage problem solving, to facilitate self-help as well as professional assistance.

BLOOD PRESSURE

The involvement of circulatory factors in the development of noise-induced hearing loss has been suggested based on experimental work (Saunders et al., 1985).

Histological and intravital microscopy techniques have been used to investigate possible mechanisms linking auditory changes with altered vascular physiology. The role of a family of peptides called endothelins has been explored in animals. In one study, rats were subjected to loud noise (100 dB) for varying periods of time (Quirk et al., 1994). Although short periods of exposure did not produce any significant changes compared to the control group, exposure for 90 min and 72 h caused significant elevations of the endothelin ET-3. Intravital microscopy is a technique which is considered to offer a number of advantages for cochlear vascular research (Quirk and Seidman, 1995).

It facilitates continuous in vivo observation of cochlear lateral wall vessels, and red blood cell velocity and capillary vasoconstriction have been observed during exposure to noise. The technique has been used to help evaluate the effect of pharmacological manipulation of the cochlear microvasculature, whereby a xanthine derivative (pentoxifylline) was shown to reduce noise-induced threshold shift, presumably by maintaining the flow of red blood cells through the capillaries. It was observed that neither vasoconstriction nor increased permeability were prevented by the drug.

Further research into identifying human susceptibility to noise has identified factors such as higher blood cholesterol and triglycerides, high blood pressure, and smoking as possible risk factors (Thomas and Williams, 1990; Cocchiarella et al., 1995). It may be the case that the converse is true, that is, for example, that exposure to noise is a risk factor for the development of hypertension. A study of the audiograms of employees from three 'noisy' companies, which was linked to a review of height, weight and blood pressure, found that hearing status (hearing loss, no hearing loss or not codable) had a minor effect on a regression model for predicting diastolic blood pressure (Sokas et al., 1995). Similarly, a prospective study of university blue collar workers identified systolic blood pressure and blood cholesterol level as independent predictors of decline in auditory sensitivity out of factors such as age, gender, occupational and non-occupational noise exposure, smoking, blood pressure, and cholesterol (Fuortes et al., 1995). However, the assessment of noise exposures did not include individual measurements. In a study of white male South African miners, where noise levels were estimated from measurements of noise levels associated with individual jobs and work areas, the results of cross-sectional and longitudinal analyses of risk factors did not show an association between blood pressure and noise exposure (Hessel and Sluiscremer, 1994). As it has been suggested that there are national differences in susceptibility to noise (Sokas et al., 1995) it would have been interesting to have conducted this study with both white South Africans and native South Africans to test this hypothesis.

PREGNANCY

It seems unlikely that exposure to noise alone has an adverse effect on the outcome of pregnancy, but the potential for noise to affect either the nervous system, and thereby cause hormonal disturbances, or the vascular system has lead researchers to investigate the possible effects of noise on pregnant workers. Outcome of pregnancy is a notoriously difficult area to research and a number of studies have been, in effect, assessing several environmental factors, of which noise was one. Recent studies have produced conflicting results, but where objective measurements of individual noise exposures have been made they do not support the proposition that noise should be considered hazardous to the fetus.

A Scandinavian study of 111 pregnant women found that noise exposures of 90 dB(A) or more ($L_{eq,8h}$) were associated with smaller birth weights than were found in a control group. This was true either when comparing absolute birth weights or when relating weights to gestational age (Hartikainen et al., 1994). Support for these findings comes from Finland (Nurminen, 1995) and the USA (Luke et al., 1995).

Exposure to 85 dB(A) ($L_{eq,8h}$) has been suggested to have an impact on both birth weight and length of gestation, but probably in association with other factors. In both studies shift work appeared to be as important, if not more important, than exposure to noise. Other factors were hours worked per week, the amount of standing in the job, physical exertion, and occupational fatigue score. If noise does affect outcome the level of impact seems likely to be small. A recent cohort study from Taiwan followed a group of 200 women from the first trimester of pregnancy to term (Wu et al., 1996).

Individual 24-h noise exposures were measured, as well as estimating possible noise exposures from traffic and occupation. No association was found between personal noise exposure and birth weight, although levels were less than 85 dB(A). Similar negative findings existed for the relationship between birth weight and estimated noise exposures. In this study, birth weight was affected by maternal weight, maternal weight gain during pregnancy, gestational age, and the sex of the baby. Further studies of women working in environments with noise levels greater than 90 dB(A) ($L_{eq,8h}$) using personal noise dosimetry are required to assess the effect of very loud noise on pregnancy. However, a large population will be necessary to allow for confounding factors and it seems unlikely that such a study will be possible.

Interaction between noise, vibration and chemicals

In many occupational settings it is usual for workers to be exposed to both noise and vibration. The sources of vibration are often the sources of loud noise. Although not the subject of much research, there is some evidence that combined exposures may potentiate the effects of noise on hearing loss. Using the amount of hearing loss at 4 kHz as an index, it has been shown that lumberjacks exposed to both noise greater than 95 dB(A) ($L_{eq,8h}$) and suffering from hand–arm vibration syndrome were associated with a greater degree of hearing loss than lumberjacks without such symptoms (Pyykko et al., 1981). The results took into account age, period of chain saw usage, and whether hearing protection was used. It may be that the underlying mechanism that might explain these findings is related to vascular changes in the cochlear.

A number of drugs are known to cause high frequency hearing loss in humans. They include quinine, acetyl salicylic acid, aminoglycosides such as streptomycin and gentamycin, and platinum. The drugs are ototoxic, i.e. they have a selective mode of action causing damage to the inner ear. Other chemicals have been shown to affect hearing although the mechanism may be either by an ototoxic effect or a neurotoxic effect. The latter is caused by the chemicals acting at the level of the brainstem or the central auditory pathways. A range of solvents have been implicated as causes of auditory impairment, including toluene, trichloroethylene, styrene, xylene, carbon disulfide, and *n*-heptane. Trimethyltin and triethyltin are also known ototoxicants.

Much of the research on the effects of solvents has been either *in vitro* or using animals, particularly rats. There is an increasing amount of evidence that toluene, which has been the subject of a lot of research, has a specific effect on the outer hair cells of the cochlear. Morata *et al.* have reviewed the effects of toluene on the auditory system (Morata *et al.*, 1995). It is clear from this and other recent papers that a battery of tests are required to identify the sub-clinical effects of solvents on the inner ear and to differentiate ototoxic effects from neurotoxic effects (Laukli and Hansen, 1995).

In the animal experiments conditioned avoidance responses, auditory brainstem responses (ABR), and distortion product otoacoustic emissions (DPOEs) were in some instances combined with morphological data. *In vitro* work has involved the micro-dissection of cochlear cells to investigate hair cell motility and length, as well as examination of the cochlear itself. Rats have usually been exposed to toluene by inhalation and the levels of exposure have been greater than might be expected in occupational settings. The OSHA (Occupational Safety and Health Administration) in the USA has set a permissible exposure limit of 100 ppm (8 h exposure). Between 12 000 and 16 000 ppm h per day over three days has been shown to impair the auditory system, whereas long-term exposure to 6000 ppm h per day for 18 months did not. The concentration threshold of toluene in the blood, which has been shown to be ototoxic to rats, is between 40 and 60 μg/ml. There is also some evidence that toluene might affect mice.

Exposure to toluene, and to trichloroethylene, styrene, and xylene, has been shown to cause mid-frequency auditory impairment, in contrast to the ototoxic drugs which cause high-frequency losses. Maximal threshold shifts in the frequency range 6.3–12.5 kHz have been found (Johnson, 1994). The ABR latency is increased but the inter-peak interval is not changed, which is interpreted to mean that the pathological effect is localized either to the cochlear or to the spinal ganglion. This interpretation has been reinforced by the measurement of reduced amplitudes of DPOEs, which are believed to originate from the cochlea. Stimulation of efferent fibers in the olivocochlear bundle, which is in contact with the outer hair cells of the cochlea, changes the DPOEs. In addition,

histological examination of the cochlea five days after exposure to toluene shows a loss of the outer hair cells.

There is evidence that exposure to solvents and some drugs might potentiate the effects of noise. Pre-exposure of rats to toluene causes a greater degree of noise-induced auditory impairment than if the rats are exposed to either toluene or noise alone. However, pre-exposure to noise did not lead to a potentiation of the effects of toluene, and the effects were additive. There may be synergistic effects on auditory loss when combining toluene and *n*-hexane and toluene and acetyl salicylic acid (aspirin). Whether combined exposures to toluene and ethanol are also synergistic remains uncertain.

The evidence about the possible effects on hearing loss in humans exists, but is not as good. Solvents are used widely in industry. Toluene, for example, is used in the manufacture of chemicals; as a carrier in paints, thinners, adhesives, inks and pharmaceutical products; in cosmetics; and in petrol. Occupations in which exposure to toluene may occur are shown in Table 13.3.

Health and safety legislation should mean that in most cases occupational exposures to solvents are well within the set exposure standards. However, it is recognized that solvents may be used inappropriately leading to high levels of exposure. Rotogravure printing is a process associated with high concentrations of airborne toluene.

Pure-tone audiometry is often the only method used in the workplace to investigate the existence of auditory impairment. More recently a battery of audiometric tests have been used to evaluate the effects of occupational exposures to solvents (Laukli and Hansen, 1995). In addition to otoscopy and pure-tone audiometry, they included extended high-frequency audiometry (8–20 kHz), speech recognition scores, a low-pass (LP) filtered version of the speech test, the acoustic stapedius reflex threshold and decay, auditory

Table 13.3 *Occupations in which exposure to toluene may occur*

- Aviation fuel blenders, petrol blenders, petrochemical workers
- Benzene makers, toluene diisocyanate makers, vinyl toluene makers
- Chemical laboratory workers
- Coke oven workers
- Lacquer workers
- Paint and paint thinner makers and users
- Perfume makers
- Rubber cement makers
- Saccharin makers
- Solvent users
- Printers

brain stem responses, and cognitive tests (Mismatch negativity; P300; N400). The stapedius reflex and the ABRs assess activity in the cochlear nerve and brainstem, and the LP-filtered speech and cognitive tests look for central effects.

Morata *et al.* (1995) report some studies in occupational settings between 1981 and 1993 that suggest that long-term exposure to high levels of toluene do cause nervous system impairment, albeit sub-clinical. However, in a cross-sectional study of rotogravure printers and painters exposed to both solvents and noise, there is some convincing evidence that the evidence of potentiation found in rats may occur in humans. Workers who were exposed to noise (88–98 dB(A)) and toluene (100–365 ppm) were compared with other groups of workers who were exposed to just noise, a mixture of solvents including toluene, or neither. Auditory function was tested using pure-tone audiometry, impedance audiometry, and stapedius reflex testing. The relative risks for hearing loss were four times greater for workers exposed just to noise, five times greater for workers exposed to the mixture of solvents, and 11 times greater for workers exposed to both agents. It is of note that the acoustic reflex findings suggested that the lesion in the noise plus toluene group was not restricted to the cochlear and was probably also in the brain stem.

More recently, the results of a study of workers in the construction industry in Germany have not supported a synergistic link between noise exposure, solvent exposure, and hearing loss (Arndt *et al.*, 1996). The study population consisted of men aged 40–64 years who had worked in different parts of the construction industry for 30 years, on average. The workers studied included carpenters and painters, who might be expected to be exposed to solvents, in addition to noise, which was considered to be a significant occupational hazard for the workers. The age-adjusted hearing loss for the painters and varnishers, which was defined as a combined hearing loss of more than 105 dB at 2, 3, and 4 kHz measured using standard audiometry, was not significantly different from white collar employees. For the carpenters, however, there was an increased level of hearing loss, but this was probably noise-related. Unfortunately, this study did not include any measurements of either noise or concentration of solvents in air and so its validity is unclear.

The evidence suggests that solvents, particularly toluene, do affect the auditory system in humans. This is based on some occupational evidence and studies that have been made on solvent abusers. It remains to be determined whether, in humans, solvents can cause damage to the inner ear and whether they have a synergistic effect when combined with noise. It is possible that, if cochlear damage is possible in humans, it will only occur at very high levels of exposure. However, in a recent study in guinea pigs, levels of exposure to toluene comparable to those that might be found in workers exposed to a concentration of 80 ppm produced shortening of the outer hair cells and an increase in free intracellular Ca^{2+} in both the outer hair cells and the spiral ganglion cells (Liu and Fechter, 1997). The latter is considered to be an important mechanism that might explain how solvents and drugs, and perhaps noise, damages the hair cells. Ca-ATPase has been shown in the outer hair cells, particularly in the middle and apical turns of the cochlear. This might explain, therefore, the finding of mid-frequency hearing loss following exposure to toluene. If these findings were to be reproduced in humans, they would have enormous significance in relation to the setting of workplace exposure standards.

There is a need for future research in this area to include more sensitive measures of hearing impairment. The inclusion of DPOEs in the assessment of workers exposed to solvents, but not noise, is thought to be a practical proposition. Acoustic reflex measurements might identify workers susceptible to hearing loss or other neurotoxic effects. These measures must be combined with better exposure data.

Vibration

HAND–ARM VIBRATION SYNDROME

Hand–arm vibration syndrome (HAVS) is a relatively new term. It replaces the older, possibly better known, term 'vibration white finger'. Other terms that have been coined for this condition include spastic anemia, vibration-induced white finger and Raynaud's phenomenon of occupational origin (McCallum, 1971; Pelmear and Taylor, 1992). The older terms reflect the focus on the vascular system as the main underlying pathology.

HAVS has been defined as a disease entity with the following components:

- circulatory disturbances;
- sensory and motor neurological disturbances;
- musculo-skeletal disturbances.

Neurological disturbances

Neurological symptoms are prevalent amongst workers exposed to hand–arm vibration and they are probably the more disabling. A review of 132 consecutive patients referred for assessment of vibration white finger (VWF) revealed that numbness, tingling, and pain were the commonest neurological symptoms accompanying the diagnosis of VWF (James *et al.*, 1989). Pyykko *et al.* have shown that among Finnish forest workers 78% complained of numbness of the hands, whereas only 40% met the criteria for Raynaud's disease of occupational origin. Numbness was commoner, however, amongst those subjects with VWF. On average, the numbness started about one year before the first attack of VWF. It was said to be particularly common at night, waking the subjects several times, when they were forced to rub and shake their hands (Pyykko *et al.*, 1986). There have been similar findings in a more recent study (Letz *et al.*, 1992). Here symptoms were very prevalent in groups of workers with both part-time and full-time exposures to hand–arm vibration.

In addition to symptoms due to vibration-induced neuropathy, workers exposed to hand–arm vibration may develop symptoms due to entrapment neuropathies. In particular, there is a recognized association between carpal tunnel syndrome and exposure to vibration. This is now a prescribed disease. Measurements taken from both the median and the ulnar nerves of rock drillers who submitted themselves to nerve conduction studies has lead to carpal tunnel syndrome being diagnosed in 44% of the exposed group, compared to only 7% of the control group (Chatterjee *et al.*, 1982). Evidence of focal blocks of sensory median nerve conduction at the wrist has also been described in a study of shipyard workers whose jobs required extensive usage of pneumatic drills (Cherniack *et al.*, 1990).

The link between carpal tunnel syndrome and work has been evaluated in what has been called the Montreal Study (Rossignol *et al.*, 1997). This was a study of cases of carpal tunnel surgery carried out in Quebec under the Quebec Health Insurance Plan. This plan funds all such surgery whether performed in public or private clinics and all Quebec residents are covered by the insurance plan independent of their employment status.

Standardized incidence ratios were computed for the 12 months June 1994–July 1995, with incidence being defined as a first lifetime surgery for carpal tunnel syndrome. The weakness of the study was the lack of information about occupation on the database. This was addressed via a telephone survey of a prospective sample of patients over the 12-month period. The standardized incidence ratio was, therefore, the number of observed cases in each occupational group in the sample interviewed, divided by the number of cases expected in that group, using the incidence of surgery for carpal tunnel syndrome for the total population of Montreal island as the reference. The annual incidence for the total population was 0.9/1000 adults with a male : female ratio of 1 : 3. Of the patients interviewed 53% reported that, at the time of onset of their symptoms, they were in a physically demanding job. The tasks described included use of force, vibrating hand-held power tools or exposure to cold. Forty percent of patients interviewed had a co-existing medical condition known to be associated with carpal tunnel syndrome, particularly diabetes (12%), thyroid disease (9%), a history of wrist fracture (8%), and pregnancy (5%). The standardized incidence ratios (SIR) for all manual workers were significantly raised,

in both men and women (SIR 1.8 (confidence interval (CI) 1.4–2.2) for women; 1.9 (CI 1.4–2.5) for men). Specific occupational groups with raised SIRs were housekeepers or cleaners, material handlers, food and beverage workers, child care (women only), and lorry and bus drivers (men only).

Where SIRs achieved statistical significance attributable fractions were computed to make the reference group more appropriate. In this case these were the fraction of surgical cases in a given occupational group in excess of that observed for all non-manual workers. For all manual workers the attributable fraction to occupation was 55% in women and 76% in men. For the specific occupational groups identified previously the attributable fractions were 75% or more. Thus, 75% of surgical cases in this population were attributable to work. However, it is of note that the study population was under-represented by workers in mining, fishing, forestry, and farming. The SIRs from these industries may be predicted to be high, with comparable attributable risks to occupation. The authors have not suggested any underlying mechanisms to explain the high incidences of surgery for carpal tunnel syndrome in occupations such as cleaning and food processing. Exposure to hand–arm vibration is unlikely and it seems probable that ergonomic factors will be important. It will be necessary to control for ergonomics in future studies on carpal tunnel syndrome in occupational groups exposed to vibration.

Diagnosis and screening

The diagnosis of the hand–arm vibration syndrome relies heavily on the history given by the patient. This is because, in the absence of an attack of finger blanching or cyanosis, clinical examination may be entirely normal. In addition, there is a lack of a single objective test that will reliably and consistently diagnose the condition.

The assessment of individual patients requires a detailed medical and occupational history to establish a diagnosis of Raynaud's phenomenon which is not due to other possible causes. Neurological symptoms must be recorded and their significance assessed. The medical history must be related to the occupational history, which will focus on activities associated with hand–arm vibration exposure, the likely significance of the exposures, and the duration of exposures. The latent period before the development of symptoms is an important part of the history as is the progression of symptoms with continuing exposure.

Recently, an international workshop, reviewing the diagnosis of hand–arm vibration and its relationship to quantitative measurements of exposure to hand–arm vibration, produced guidelines for diagnosing vibration-induced white finger and vibration-induced sensorineural disturbances (Gemne *et al.*, 1994).

With respect to the vascular symptoms, the minimal requirements for a history-based diagnosis of vibration-induced white finger were as follows:

- Raynaud's phenomenon (RP): cold provoked episodes of well-demarcated distal blanching (whiteness) in one or more fingers;
- vibration white finger (VWF): the first appearance of RP after the start of professional exposure to hand–arm vibration with no other probable causes of RP;
- current activity: VWF is currently active if episodes have been noticed during the last two years. If no episodes have occurred for more than two years, VWF has ceased, provided that there has been no significant change in cold exposure.

It was considered that Raynaud's phenomenon provoked exclusively by emotion cannot be accepted. Other symptoms such as cyanosis (blueness), numbness and throbbing of the fingers during the hyperemic (increased blood flow) recovery period are not required for the diagnosis. A history of cyanosis alone should be assessed via diagnostic discoloration of VWF and further investigation for other secondary causes and/or diseases is recommended. The duration of the latency period of vibration white finger may range from a few months after the start of vibration exposure to approximately one year after the exposure has ceased, making it difficult to give firm recommendations about its length. With respect to the subjective symptoms of VWF, these may be partly or totally reversible, if the vibration is reduced or stopped completely. This reversibility depends on the age of the subject, the duration of the exposure to vibration, and the type of vibrating tool used.

To assess the sensori-neural symptoms of hand–arm vibration syndrome the following strategy has been suggested: after obtaining the subject's medical and occupational history conduct a physical examination with special attention being paid to localized and generalized neuropathies. Based on the information obtained, perform screening tests. Depending on the results, perform additional in-depth diagnostic tests. After considering the results obtained, formulate a differential diagnosis: to what else could the diagnosis be due?

Useful screening tests include:

1 vibrotactile perception thresholds (single or multiple frequency);
2 esthesiometry (gap detection);
3 thermal detection thresholds;
4 grip and pinch strength.

The first three tests may also be used as diagnostic tests. In addition, sensory and motor nerve conduction and electromyography may be used. The latter is usually only available in specialist regional or sub-regional NHS centers in the UK, but these tests are useful for diagnosing carpal tunnel syndrome. Tests 1–3 are less well established and they are the subject of on-going research to validate their ability to identify peripheral diffusely distributed neuropathy in its early stages. However, the interpretation of nerve conduction studies when assessing workers exposed to vibration should be undertaken judiciously. Chatterjee et al. have highlighted the difficulty in comparing results with normal values. It is essential to relate the results to the overall clinical picture when they may be used to support a clinical diagnosis, rather than to suggest a previously unsuspected one (Brismar and Erkenvall, 1992).

Screening populations for the prevalence of hand–arm vibration syndrome relies on the use of questionnaires. The Faculty of Occupational Medicine in the UK have recommended such a questionnaire, which may also be found in the Health and Safety Executive publication *Hand–arm Vibration* (Faculty of Occupational Medicine, 1993; Health and Safety Executive, 1994).

The Faculty of Occupational Medicine recommend that, following an initial assessment of workers, health surveillance assessments should be repeated at six-monthly intervals for one year and annually thereafter. However, the frequency of the re-assessments of individual workers will be influenced by the rate of progression of the disease and the level of exposure to vibration.

Staging of HAVS and assessment of severity

Staging hand–arm vibration syndrome may be performed for various reasons. In the assessment of individual workers a staging system might be used to grade the severity of the symptoms and to monitor disease progression. Staging is used in epidemiological surveys of workforces to assess the prevalence of symptoms in relation to estimated or measured exposure to vibration. It is also used for medico-legal purposes. The 1975 Taylor–Pelmear classification was based mainly on the development of blanching of the fingers and the effect that this had on the ability to work, or on the interference with domestic and social activities. The limitations of this classification have been discussed widely, although it remains popular for medico-legal assessments. It is now recommended that the scales published after the 1986 Stockholm workshop, which have come to be called the Stockholm classification, should be used by physicians to stage the development of hand–arm vibration syndrome (Tables 13.1 and 13.2). This has been reinforced by the reports of two international working parties in 1994.

The relationship between the vascular and the neurological symptoms is an on-going subject for debate, although the prevailing view is that the two sets of symptoms occur independently. The original assessment of VWF, which was devised by Taylor and

Table 13.4 *The Stockholm workshop scale for the classification of cold-induced Raynaud's phenomenon in the hand–arm vibration syndrome (Gemne et al., 1987)*

Stage	Grade	Description
0		No attacks
1	Mild	Occasional attacks affecting the tips of one or more fingers
2	Moderate	Occasional attacks affecting distal and middle (rarely also proximal) phalanges of one or more fingers
3	Severe	Frequent attacks affecting all phalanges of most fingers
4	Very severe	As in stage 3, with trophic changes in the finger tips

Table 13.5 *The Stockholm workshop scale for the classification of sensorineural effects of the hand–arm vibration syndrome (Brammer et al., 1987)*

Stage	Symptoms
0sn	Exposed to vibration but no symptoms
1sn	Intermittent numbness, with or without tingling
2sn	Intermittent or persistent numbness, reduced sensory perception
3sn	Intermittent or persistent numbness, reduced tactile discrimination and/or manipulative dexterity

Pelmear, included references to neurological symptoms as evidence of an early vascular neuropathy (Pelmear and Taylor, 1992). Subjects would be placed in stages OT or ON if they complained of intermittent tingling or numbness, or both in the absence of blanching of the fingers. This is consistent with the description of these symptoms preceding the vascular symptoms. However, a new staging system was introduced following an international workshop in 1986 in Stockholm, which allowed the separate assessment of the vascular and the neurological symptoms throughout the progression of what has now become the hand–arm vibration syndrome (Brammer *et al.*, 1987; Gemne *et al.*, 1987) (Tables 13.4 and 13.5).

An assessment should be made for each hand. The grade of disorder is indicated by the stage and the number of affected fingers. It is possible to carry out both vascular and neurological investigations on the hands of affected workers. These investigations are merely supportive. Vascular investigations, such as cooling tests, are helpful if they are positive, but a negative cooling test does not rule out the diagnosis of Raynaud's phenomenon. The most supportive objective tests are visual inspection of finger colors and measurements of finger systolic blood pressure (Gemne *et al.*, 1994). The neurological tests have already been described.

The use of objective tests for the hand–arm vibration syndrome has been the subject of a recent review (Lawson and Nevell, 1997). The equipment tested included cold provocation testing and rewarming times (vascular assessment), vibrotactile thresholds, thermal thresholds, grip strength (muscular assessment), and esthesiometry. Results were obtained on 34 workers in the engineering industry known to be exposed to hand–arm vibration in the range 5.6–14 m/s² (4-h frequency weighted RMS acceleration) and known to suffer from blanching of their fingers in response to cold. The results were compared with those obtained from a control group of non-exposed workers. The subjects were initially assessed by a physician and the HAVS was staged using questionnaire data and the results of a medical examination. This staging was then compared with the ability of a derived equation to use the results of objective testing to produce a computed staging. (The final equation excluded grip strength as a significant variable.) The small numbers in the study and the predominance of subjects at stage 0 sensorineural, with few cases at stage 3 for either vascular or sensorineural symptoms, meant that the predictive power of the equation was limited. Nonetheless, the equation was able to use the results from the battery of tests to produce a single score, which would give a measure of probability of which Stockholm stage was most likely. The scoring system for the sensorineural tests is shown in Table 13.6. The degree of confidence in the probability should be increased by enlarging the study to include sufficient numbers of subjects at all stages. The results support the collective use of sensorineural and cold provocation tests to support the diagnosis of hand–arm vibration syndrome and to assess the severity. Of the individual tests, the vibrotactile thresholds were the most significant vari-

Table 13.6 *Scoring system for sensorineural results*

Test	Score 0	Score 1	Score 2
Grip test	>450 n	>200 n, 450 n	200 n
Esthesiometry	6.5 cm	>6.5 cm, 8 cm	>8 cm
Temperature neutral zone	19°C	>19°C, 24°C	>24°C
Vibrotactile threshold (31.5 Hz)	0.2 ms/s	>0.2, 0.4 ms/s	>0.4 ms/s
Vibrotactile threshold (125 Hz)	0.6 ms/s	>0.6, 1.0 ms/s	>1.0 ms/s

able out of the sensorineural tests, followed by thermal neutral zone tests and esthesiometry.

Management and prognosis

The main objectives are the avoidance of, or the reduction of, exposure to vibration and the avoidance of precipitating factors for hand–arm vibration syndrome. The systematic assessment of the disease and the identification of the probable causal factors are essential. An example of a screening program based on the above approach has been reported recently (Johnson *et al.*, 1996).

Although the numbers in the study were small the findings supported the use of a structured questionnaire and a limited number of tests to identify workers who needed a more in-depth assessment by a physician. The tests used were for vibrotactile thresholds (multiple frequency), cutaneous sensitivity, and hand and finger strength. This is more cost-effective than relying on physician-based examinations of large workforces.

Having identified workers with hand–arm vibration syndrome advice may be given about working in cold and/or wet conditions and about reducing aggravating factors such as cigarette smoking. Medication such as beta-blockers, which may be prescribed for common medical conditions such as hypertension or angina, may aggravate the symptoms and so possible alternatives should be explored.

Therapeutic measures aimed at helping workers with hand–arm vibration syndrome have not been shown to be very effective (Gemne *et al.*, 1994). Vasodilator drugs have a limited role. Calcium channel blockers are considered to be effective in the treatment of Raynaud's phenomenon (Hachulla and Devulder, 1993). The therapeutic effects have to be counter-balanced with the occurrence of side effects, such as headaches and postural hypotension, which is particularly unacceptable for patients wishing to continue working with dangerous machinery. Cervical sympathectomy has not been shown to be beneficial, probably because the fundamental pathological process is likely to be localized to the endothelium of the finger arterioles and not due primarily to an elevated sympathetic tone (Gemne, 1992; Lewis, 1929).

Consequently, the mainstay of prevention of any increase in the severity of symptoms is to avoid further exposure to vibration, where this is possible. At present, evidence about the reversibility of vibration-induced Raynaud's phenomenon must be weighed against the existence of other confounding variables, such as age and the pre-exposure level of blood flow in the fingers (Gemne *et al.*, 1994). A follow-up survey of subjects receiving treatment for hand–arm vibration syndrome has been reported recently (Ogasawara *et al.*, 1997).

This plotted the course of 353 subjects between the ages of 40 and 70 years who were receiving treatment in 1982. A comparison was made with the severity of the condition in 1988 and it was found that there was a decrease in the number of episodes of Raynaud's phenomenon, but little change in the severity of the pain and numbness in the hands. Improvement was most likely if the severity of HAVS was mild (stage 1 vascular) at the start of treatment, whereas only 17% of subjects assessed at vascular stage 3 improved. Continued use of hand-held vibrating tools was shown to reduce the likelihood of improvement. Current recommendations are that patients at Stockholm scales stages 2v, 2SN, whether singly or combined, should avoid further exposure to vibration (Faculty of Occupational Medicine, 1993).

It should not be assumed that surgery will alleviate the symptoms, if carpal tunnel syndrome is diagnosed. Patients with carpal tunnel syndrome who have a history of exposure to hand–arm vibration do not always do well after surgery. In a study of 41 male patients, contributing 55 hands for operation, there was a significant difference between the persistence of postoperative symptoms according to whether the patients were in a high-vibration exposure group or a low-exposure group (Hagberg *et al.*, 1991). All patients were assessed at follow-up via a questionnaire, physical examination by a specialist in hand surgery, and nerve conduction studies. The high-exposure group rated both their daytime and nocturnal symptoms higher than the low-exposure group. Postsurgery, recovery from nocturnal parasthesiae was reported by only 30 out of 42 patients in the high-exposure group, compared to 12 out of 13 in the low-exposure group. Thus, surgery for relief of symptoms attributable to vibration-induced carpal tunnel syndrome was shown to be only partially effective in some cases.

It has been shown that, in biopsies of dorsal interosseous nerves taken just proximal to the wrist, pathological changes, including demyelination and interstitial and perineural fibrosis, are much more prevalent in subjects who have a history of exposure to hand–arm vibration (Stromberg *et al.*, 1997).

The biopsies were taken in conjunction with resection of the nerve to assist pain relief. Consequently, these subjects represent an extreme group with respect to symptomatology. Nonetheless, these structural changes may be an explanation why carpal tunnel surgery achieves only a partial success in patients who have been exposed to hand–arm vibration.

THE AUTONOMIC NERVOUS SYSTEM

A possible explanation for the occurrence of vasospasm in vibration-induced Raynaud's phenomenon is the development of hyper-reactivity of the autonomic nervous system. Increased activity of the sympathetic nervous system can cause constriction of the arterioles in the fingers. However, were that the fundamental mechanism it would be expected that cervical sympathectomy would be more successful in alleviating the vascular symptoms of sufferers. The effect of vibration centrally on the autonomic nervous system has been the subject of research, which has been reviewed by Gemne (1992).

It has been suggested that the active mechanism for digital artery constriction involves both central and local factors, including central sympathetic reflexes and abnormal adrenergic receptor activity in smooth muscle cells or hypertrophy of vascular smooth muscle cells. Work has continued to look for evidence of altered autonomic function. Heart rate variation and the response of blood pressure to a cold pressor test has been measured in a group of Finnish railway workers and lumberjacks (Virokannas and Tolonen, 1995).

In this small study there was a relationship between exposure to hand–arm vibration and the coefficient of beat-to-beat variation in a quiet breathing test. None of the other indices showed a relationship. The use of heart rate variability (coefficient of variation of electrocardiogram R-R intervals) as an objective tool for assessing autonomic nervous system function has been reviewed recently (Murata and Araki, 1996). Although it is non-invasive it is affected by confounding factors such as age, and consumption of alcohol and tobacco. Two components of the coefficient of variation have been proposed for research purposes: respiratory sinus arrhythmia and Mayer wave-related sinus arrhythmia. It remains to be seen whether this approach will throw any new light on the involvement of the autonomic nervous system in the development of hand–arm vibration syndrome.

Low-frequency electromagnetic radiation

Research has suggested possible associations between exposure to ELF and the occurrence of a variety of cancers. The development of brain cancer is a clear example of a direct effect on the nervous system and leukemia often spreads to involve it. Other cancers may arise because of the effect of ELF on the pineal gland and the subsequent disturbance of melatonin secretion. Of these, most concern has been about the development of breast cancer (Dosemici and Blair, 1994; Cantor et al., 1995).

The possibility of a link between suicide and exposure to electric and magnetic fields has been studied in both residential and occupational settings. Once again alteration in melatonin secretion has been suggested as a possible mechanism. A recent study of a cohort of 21 744 electrical utility workers, using a combination of job histories and positron dosimeter measurements to estimate exposures, found weak evidence for a link between suicide and cumulative exposure to the geometric means of electric fields (Baris et al., 1996). The literature up to 1994 relating to epidemiological studies on the occurrence of leukemia and brain cancer has been reviewed (Ahlbom, 1994; Dab et al., 1994; Theriault, 1995). There is a greater consistency between the studies looking at residential exposures and childhood leukemia than for other cancers, including occupational exposures in adults. An association between childhood leukemia and magnetic fields assessed by using wire codes has been a key finding, rather than the direct readings chosen by the researchers. In a review of childhood nervous system cancer only studies by Wertheimer and Leeper (1979) and Tomenius (1986) have demonstrated elevated relative risks of nervous tissue cancer and 95% confidence intervals that do not include unity. Neither of these studies are recent and both have been criticized for their methods of estimating exposures. In contrast, Theriault has observed that in occupational studies the trend has been to report significant excesses of both leukemia and brain cancer since 1990. This has coincided with attempts to improve the assessment of exposure.

Recent morbidity case-control studies have failed to resolve the uncertainty about a causal relationship between electromagnetic radiation and brain cancer. A study of 261 brain cancers out of a possible 424 cases diagnosed between 1983 and 1987 amongst men aged 20–64 in Sweden showed odds ratios for brain cancer of 1.5 (CI 1.0–2.2) for exposure at the 75th percentile, compared to the least exposed 25th percentile, which was equivalent to exposures less than $0.15\,\mu T$. Odds ratios for the 50th and 90th percentiles were 1.0 and 1.4, respectively, and were not statistically significant (Floderus et al., 1993). Theriault et al. (1994) analyzed a nested case-control study amongst a cohort of approximately 223 000 male employees working for Electricité de France, Ontario Hydro, and Hydro-Québec. Between 1970 and 1989 4151 cases of cancer were observed. Exposures were estimated from job histories and sample personal dosimetry. For men exposed above the 90th percentile of cumulative magnetic field $(15.7\,\mu T)$ the odds ratio for brain cancer was 1.95 (CI 0.76–5.0).

Sahl et al. (1993) looked at a cohort of Americans who had worked for the Southern California Edison Company for at least one year between 1960 and 1988. This was a mortality study comprising three case-control studies looking at leukemia, brain cancer, and lymphoma. The cause of death was identified for 97% of the 3125 deaths. The mortality rate within the group did not show any increased risks for any cancer and the case-control studies were all negative.

Two more recent mortality studies have continued the trend of reporting either weak or no associations between brain cancer and electromagnetic radiation exposure, thus contradicting Theriault's assertion, at least for this type of cancer. A retrospective cohort study of all men who had worked full-time at five utility companies in the United States, between January 1, 1950 and December 31, 1986, contained 20 733 deaths from 2 656 436 person-years of exposure (Savitz and Loomis, 1995).

There were 144 brain cancers, 71% of which were gliomas. The overall mortality rates were lower than for the general population, as was expected. Out of a range of selected causes of death, the standardized mortality ratios for malignant neoplasm of skin, other lymphatic neoplasms, and for neoplasms of unspecified nature of the eye and brain (International Classification of Diseases, Ninth Revision, Clinical Modification (McGeogh *et al.*, 1994)) were greater than 100, but this increase was not statistically significant. Mortality by duration of employment increased for all exposed occupations, and for linemen, electricians, and power plant operators the relative risk was significantly increased for employment greater than 20 years. For brain cancer there was an increased relative risk for all exposed occupations for lengths of employment between five and 20 years, but not for greater than 20 years. However, mortality in relation to estimated exposures to magnetic fields showed no clear relationship where the duration of exposure was between 10 and 20 years, whilst there was a non-significant trend for an increase in mortality for exposures between two and 10 years and for greater than 20 years.

A British study involving a cohort of workers in the Central Electricity Generating Board failed to support the hypothesis that the risk of brain cancer is associated with occupational exposure to magnetic fields (Harrington *et al.*, 1997). The cohort studied was a more recent one, being defined as all men and women employed for at least six months between April 1, 1972 and March 31, 1984. There were 176 primary or secondary brain cancers based on death certificate information. This information was verified using the National Cancer Registry and it was possible to confirm the occurrence of 112 primary brain tumors. These cases were used to carry out a case-control study with 654 controls. Exposures were assessed by combining previously published information on measured exposures with recorded job histories. It was noted, however, that direct measurements obtained from 258 workers in various jobs revealed that there was considerable overlap of exposures for all the main job categories. The relative risk of brain cancer in relation to cumulative exposure was assessed using both time-weighted arithmetic and time-weighted geometrical means for each job category. There was no indication of a positive trend of risk of brain cancer with level of exposure.

The latter two studies took into account possible confounders (Savitz and Loomis, 1995). Savitz and Loomis (1995) assessed the potential for exposure to polychlorinated biphenyls and solvents. In the Harrington study (Harrington *et al.*, 1997) a long list of potential confounders were identified using the International Agency for Cancer Research list of carcinogens. Twenty-four separate categories of confounders were identified including ozone, caustic chemicals, ionizing radiation, methanol in bulk, O-toluidine, metallic mercury, and a variety of solvents. If there is a relationship between electromagnetic radiation and brain cancer it seems that it is unlikely to be strong and may be diluted by other factors including imprecise or inappropriate measurements. It seems likely that future studies will have to include populations with a wide variation in exposure levels and ensure that high-exposure groups are identified and followed up. The validity of future studies will also be improved if histological confirmation of the diagnoses is obtained.

Despite the conflicting results from recent studies, researchers have continued to suggest that there is a relationship between brain cancer and exposure to ELF. Exposure to magnetic fields at levels above 0.2 μT has been suggested as a possible threshold for increasing the risk of brain cancer. Another possibility is that ELF acts as a cancer promotor only at certain levels of exposure. Exposure to pulsed electromagnetic fields or even moderate rather than high levels of exposure may be more important. For example, *in vitro* studies of the effect of low-frequency magnetic fields on the proliferation rates of human (AMA) cells have shown that a 30-min exposure to 50 Hz sinusoidal field with a flux density of 80 μT resulted in a much higher increase in proliferation rate than was seen for non-exposed cells or for cells exposed for shorter or longer times (Kwee and Raskmark, 1995).

The effect of electromagnetic radiation on the pineal gland of humans is another area for more research. This gland produces low amounts of melatonin, which is an indole (*N*-acetyl-5-methoxytryptamine) and which is also found in small amounts in peripheral nerves. Melatonin may have a role in affecting the body's circadian rhythm, sleep, and in reproduction. It may also affect the immune system and, in the future, it may be used as an oncostatic drug. The pineal gland may have a role in converting environmental radiation, particularly light, into an endocrine response. Consequently, the pineal gland may be an important link that helps to explain how electromagnetic radiation might cause cancer. It has been suggested that ELF may work as 'synchronizers' or, through the action of an 'antenna' effect, transfer energy to the rest of the brain (Ronco and Halberg, 1996). Removal of the pineal gland in rats is reported to increase the incidence of tumors (Hughes, 1994). Animal studies have shown melatonin to reduce the incidence of experimentally induced breast cancer in rats and *in vitro* studies have shown it to be oncostatic and cytotoxic to breast, ovarian, and bladder cell lines (Tynes, 1993).

Melatonin secretion has its own circadian rhythm, with low amounts produced during the day and high amounts at night. Exposure to light at night (LAN) leads to a fall in the levels of circulating melatonin. Nocturnal levels of melatonin may be suppressed by exposing rats to 60 Hz electric fields. However, it remains to be determined whether similar changes will be produced by ELF in humans. A recent double-blind laboratory-based study using human volunteers evaluated the effect of exposure to magnetic fields at night (Graham et al., 1996). The first phase involved 33 men who were exposed to sham, 10 mg or 200 mg intermittent, circularly polarized magnetic fields from 2300 hours to 0700 hours. The main finding was that these exposures had no effect on melatonin levels. However, men with pre-existing low levels of melatonin seemed to be more sensitive to the effects of the magnetic fields in that there was significantly more suppression of melatonin when they were exposed to light and the 200 mg field. Further testing in a second study was unable to replicate the apparent finding of enhanced sensitivity.

In a study of occupational exposures to a visual display unit, 47 office workers volunteered blood samples for the assessment of circulating melatonin and adrenocorticotrophin (ACTH) levels (Arnetz and Berg, 1996). Levels were measured during a day at work and a day of leisure. Levels of melatonin decreased during the work-day whereas levels of ACTH increased. During the day of leisure there were no significant changes in the levels of either melatonin or ACTH. The results suggest that the work environment may suppress melatonin, although it will be important to reproduce these findings. Exposure to light does not appear to be a cause of melatonin suppression in humans, but, as this study did not measure electric or magnetic fields associated with the display units, it is not clear what, other than possibly stress, in the environment might have done so.

There is an urgent need to identify a plausible mechanism to explain how ELF might cause cancer. Until then, epidemiological studies will be limited in their ability to either alert society to its dangers or give reassurance that there is nothing to worry about.

SUMMARY

This chapter has considered how three different types of energy might affect the nervous system. Noise has been an occupational hazard for centuries, whilst vibration became important with the onset of the industrial revolution.

Electromagnetic radiation is a twentieth century phenomenon. As we approach the twenty-first century there is still much to be learnt about how all three affect the body so that we can prevent illness occurring and safeguard the public health. The main effect of noise is

on hearing, that of vibration on the peripheral vascular and nervous system, and on the spine. These are significant causes of morbidity. Electromagnetic radiation has been linked with the occurrence of brain tumors and leukemia. Both are emotive diseases and have the potential to generate anxiety amongst the public. We have reached a stage in our medical and scientific development where research must include measurement tools that are sufficiently sensitive to identify both clinical and sub-clinical effects of exposures, and must address the need for accurate and relevant exposure data. This requires an understanding of the pathophysiological processes and the mechanisms that link exposure to the development of disease. Noise, vibration, and electromagnetic radiation are all good examples of why this is important.

REFERENCES

Ahlbom, A. 1994: Cancer and residential exposure to weak extremely low-frequency magnetic fields. In Electric and Magnetic Fields and Health. Paris: CIGRE Working Group.
Allen, S.G., Blackwell, R.P., Chadwick, P.J. et al. 1994: Review of Occupational Exposure to Optical Radiation and Electric and Magnetic Fields With Regard to the Proposed CEC Physical Agents Directive. Didcot: National Radiation Protection Board.
Armstrong, B., Theriault, G., Guenel, P., Deadman, J., Goldberg, M. and Heroux, P. 1994: Association between exposure to pulsed electromagnetic fields and cancer in electric utility workers in Quebec, Canada and France. American Journal of Epidemiology, 140, 805–20.
Arndt, V., Rothenbacker, D., Brenner, H. et al. 1996: Older workers in the construction industry: results of a routine health examination and a five-year follow-up. Occupational and Environmental Medicine, 53, 686–91.
Arnetz, B.B. and Berg, M. 1996: Melatonin and adrenocorticootropic hormone levels in video display unit workers during work and leisure. Journal of Occupational and Environmental Medicine, 38, 1108–10.
Baris, D., Armstrong, B.G., Deadman, J. and Theriault, G. 1996: A case cohort study of suicide in relation to exposure to electrical and magnetic fields among electrical utility workers. Occupational and Environmental Medicine, 53, 17–24.
Barr, M.L. 1974: The Human Nervous System: An Anatomical Viewpoint, p 309. Philadelphia, PA: Harper & Row.
Behrens, V.J. and Pelmear, P.L. 1992: Epidemiology of hand–arm vibration syndrome. In Hand–arm Vibration: A Comprehensive Guide for Occupational Health Professionals, Pelmear, P.L., Taylor, W. and Wasserman, D.E. (eds), pp 105–21. New York: Van Nostrand Reinhold.
Brammer, A.J., Taylor, W. and Lundborg, G. 1987: Sensorineural stages of the hand–arm vibration syndrome. Scandinavian Journal of Work, Environment and Health, 13, 279–83.
Brismar, T. and Ekenvall, L. 1992: Nerve conduction in the hands of vibration-exposed workers. Electroencephalography and Clinical Neurophysiology, 85, 173–6.
Cantor, P., Stewart, P.A., Brinton, L.A. and Dosemici, M. 1995: Occupational exposures and female breast cancer mortality in the United States. Journal of Occupational and Environmental Medicine, 37, 336–48.
Chatterjee, D.S, Barwick, D.D. and Petrie, A. 1982: Exploratory electromyography in the study of vibration-induced white finger in rock drillers. British Journal of Industrial Medicine, 39, 89–97.
Cherniack, M.G., Letzk, R., Gerr, F., Brammer, A. and Pace, P. 1990: Detailed clinical assessment of neurological function in symptomatic shipyard workers. British Journal of Industrial Medicine, 47, 566–72.

Cocchiarella, L.A., Sharp, D.S. and Persky, V.W. 1995: Hearing threshold shifts, white cell count and smoking status in working men. *Occupational Medicine*, **45**, 179–85.

Cridland, N.A. 1993: *Electromagnetic Fields and Cancer: A Review of Relevant Cellular Studies*. Didcot: National Radiation Protection Board.

Dab, W., Lambrozo, J. and Souques, M. 1994: Magnetic fields and cancer: recent studies in adults. In *Electric and Magnetic Fields and Health*. Paris: CIGRE Working Group.

Dobie, R.A. 1995: Prevention of noise-induced hearing loss. *Archives of Otolaryngology – Head and Neck Surgery*, **121**, 385–91.

Dosemici, M. and Blair, A. 1994: Occupational cancer mortality among women employed in the telephone industry. *Journal of Occupational Medicine*, **36**, 1204–9.

Draper, G. 1996: Does electricity give you cancer? *British Medical Journal*, **312**, 517.

Faculty of Occupational Medicine 1993: *Hand-transmitted Vibration. Clinical Effects and Pathophysiology. Report of a Working Party*. London: Faculty of Occupational Medicine.

Floderus, B., Persson, T., Stenlund, C., Wennberg, A., Ost, A. and Nave, B. 1993: Occupational exposure to electromagnetic fields in relation to leukemia and brain tumors. A case-control study in Sweden. *Cancer Causes and Control*, **4**, 465–76.

Fuortes, L.J., Tang, S.H., Pomrehn, P. and Anderson, C. 1995: Prospective evaluation of associations between hearing sensitivity and selected cardiovascular risk factors. *American Journal of Industrial Medicine*, **28**, 275–80.

Ganong, W.F. 1975: *Review of Medical Physiology*, 7th edn. California: Lange Medical Publications.

Gemne, G. 1992: Pathophysiology and pathogenesis of disorders in workers using hand-held vibrating tools. In *Hand–arm Vibration: A Comprehensive Guide for Occupational Health Professionals*, Pelmear, P.L., Taylor, W. and Wasserman, D.E. (eds), pp 41–76. New York: Van Nostrand Reinhold.

Gemne, G., Brammer, A.J., Hagberg, M., Lundsdtrom, R. and Nilsson, T. (eds) 1994: *Hand–arm Vibration Syndrome: Diagnostics and Quantitative Relationships to Exposure*. Stockholm: National Institute of Occupational Health.

Gemne, G., Pyykko, I., Taylor, W. and Pelmear, P.L. 1987: The Stockholm workshop scale for the classification of cold-induced Raynaud's phenomenon in the hand–arm vibration syndrome (revision of the Taylor–Pelmear scale). *Scandinavian Journal of Work, Environment and Health*, **13**, 275–7.

Getty, L. and Hétu, R. 1991: The development of a rehabilitation program for people affected with occupational hearing loss. II: results from group intervention with 48 workers and their spouses. *Audiology*, **30**, 317–29.

Graham, C., Cook, M.R., Riffle, D.W., Gerkovich, M.M. and Cohen, H.D. 1996: Nocturnal melatonin levels in human volunteers exposed to intermittent 60 Hz magnetic fields. *Bioelectromagnetics*, **17**, 263–73.

Hachulla, E. and Devulder, B. 1993: Calcium channel blockers and Raynaud's phenomenon. *Therapie*, **48**, 707–11.

Hack, R. 1989: Ionising radiation. In *Occupational Health Practice*, Waldron, H. (ed.), 3rd edn, pp 151–74. London: Butterworths.

Hagberg, M., Nystrom, A. and Zetterlund, B. 1991: Recovery from symptoms after carpal tunnel syndrome surgery in males in relation to vibration exposure. *Journal of Hand Surgery*, **16**, 66–71.

Ham, A.W. 1974: *Histology*. Philadelphia, PA: J.B. Lippincott.

Harrington, J.M. 1980: The health effects of physical agents. In *Occupational Hygiene*, Waldron, H.A. and Harrington, J.M. (eds), pp 301–13. Oxford: Blackwell Scientific.

Harrington, J.M., McBride, D.I., Sorahan, T., Paddle, G.M. and Tongeren, M.V. 1997: Occupational exposure to magnetic fields in relation to mortality from brain cancer among electricity generation and transmission workers. *Occupational and Environmental Medicine*, **54**, 7–13.

Hartikainen, A.L., Sorri, M., Anttonen, H., Tuimala, R. and Laara, E. 1994: Effect of occupational noise on the course and outcome of pregnancy. *Scandinavian Journal of Work, Environment and Health*, **20**, 444–50.

Health and Safety Executive 1994: *Hand–arm Vibration*. Sudbury: Health and Safety Executive Books.

Hessel, P.A. and Sluiscremer, G.K. 1994: Occupational noise exposure and blood pressure – longitudinal and cross-sectional observations in a group of underground miners. *Archives of Environmental Health*, **49**, 128–34.

Hétu, R. and Getty, L. 1991: The development of a rehabilitation program for people affected with occupational hearing loss. I: a new paradigm. *Audiology*, **30**, 305–16.

Hogan, A., Ewan, C., Noble, W. and Munnerley, G. 1994: Coping with occupational hearing loss. *Journal of Occupational Health and Safety (Australia, New Zealand)*, **10**, 107–18.

Hughes, J.T. 1994: Electromagnetic fields and brain tumors – a commentary. *Teratogenesis, Carcinogenesis and Mutagenesis*, **14**, 213–7.

Hunter, D. 1957: *The Diseases of Occupations*, 2nd edn. London: English Universities Press.

James, C.A., Aw, T.C., Harrington, J.M. and Trethowan, W.N. 1989: A review of 132 consecutive patients referred for assessment of vibration white finger. *Journal of the Society of Occupational Medicine*, **39**, 61–4.

Johnson, A.C. 1994: The ototoxic effect of toluene and the influence of noise, acetyl salicylic acid or genotype – a study in rats and mice. *Scandinavian Audiology*, **23**, 1–40.

Johnson, K.L., Hans, J.C. and Robinson, M.A. 1996: Development of a vibratory white finger prevention program for shipyard workers – an exploratory study. *American Journal of Preventive Medicine*, **12**, 478–81.

King, I.J. 1980: Noise and vibration. In *Occupational Hygiene*, Waldron, H.A. and Harrington, J.M. (eds), pp 144–224. Oxford: Blackwell Scientific.

Kwee, S. and Raskmark, P. 1995: Changes in cell proliferation due to environmental non-ionizing radiation. 1 ELF electromagnetic fields. *Bioelectrochemistry and Bioenergetics*, **36**, 109–14.

Laukli, E. and Hansen, P.W. 1995: An audiometric test battery for the evaluation of occupational exposure to industrial solvents. *Otolaryngolica*, **115**, 162–4.

Lawson, I.J. and Nevell, D.A. 1997: Review of objective tests for the hand–arm vibration syndrome. *Occupational Medicine*, **47**, 15–20.

Letz, R., Cherniack, M.G., Gerr, F., Hershman, D. and Pace, P.A. 1992: Cross-sectional epidemiological survey of shipyard workers exposed to hand–arm vibration. *British Journal of Industrial Medicine*, **49**, 53–62.

Lewis, T. 1929: Experiments relating to the peripheral mechanism involved in spasmodic arrest of the circulation in the fingers, a variety of Raynaud's disease. *Heart*, **15**, 7–100.

Liu, Y. and Fechter, L.D. 1997: Toluene disrupts outer hair cell morphometry and intracellular calcium homeostasis in cochlear cells of guinea pigs. *Toxicology and Applied Pharmacology*, **142**, 270–7.

Luke, B., Mamelle, N., Keith, L. *et al.* 1995: The association between occupational factors and pregnancy – a United States nurses study. *American Journal of Obstetrics and Gynecology*, **173**, 849–62.

Malerbi, B. 1993: Noise. In *Occupational Health Practice*, Waldron, H.A. (ed.), 3rd edn, pp 113–50. London: Butterworths.

McCallum, R.I. 1971: Vibration syndrome. *British Journal of Industrial Medicine*, **28**, 90–9.

McGeoch, K.L., Gilmour, W.H. and Taylor, W. 1994: Sensorineural objective tests in the assessment of hand–arm vibration syndrome. *Occuational and Environmental Medicine*, **51**, 57–61.

Morata, C.M., Nylen, P., Johnson, A.C. and Dunn, D.E. 1995: Auditory and vestibular functions after single or combined exposure to toluene: a review. *Archives of Toxicology*, **69**, 431–43.

Murata, K. and Araki, S. 1996: Assessment of autonomic neurotoxicity in occupational and environmental health as determined by ECG R-R interval variability. *American Journal of Industrial Medicine*, **30**, 155–63.

Noise at Work Regulations 1989: *Statutory Instrument 1989*, No. 1790 ed. London: HMSO.

Nurminen, T. 1995: Female noise exposure, shift work and reproduction. *Journal of Occupational and Environmental Medicine*, **37**, 945–51.

Ogasawara, C., Sakakibara, H., Kondo, T., Miyao, M., Yamada, S. and Toyoshim. 1997: Longitudinal study on factors related to the course on vibration-induced white finger. *International Archives of Occupational and Environmental Medicine*, **69**, 180–4.

Pelmear, P.L. 1992: Anatomy and physiology of the upper limb. In *Hand–arm Vibration: A Comprehensive Guide for Occupational Health Professionals*, Pelmear, P.L., Taylor, W. and Wasserman, D.E. (eds), pp 1–17. New York: Van Nostrand Reinhold.

Pelmear, P.L. 1995: Noise and Vibration. In *Epidemiology of Work-related Diseases*, McDonald C. (ed.), pp 185–205. London: BMJ Publishing.

Pelmear, P.L. and Taylor, W. 1992: Clinical picture (vascular, neurological and musculo-skeletal). In *Hand–arm Vibration: A Comprehensive Guide for Occupational Health Professionals*, Pelmear, P.L., Taylor, W. and Wasserman, D.E. (eds), pp 26–40. New York: Van Nostrand Reinhold.

Pyykko, I. 1986: Clinical aspects of the hand–arm vibration syndrome: a review. *Scandinavian Journal of Work, Environment and Health*, **12**, 439–47.

Pyykko, I., Starck, J., Farkkila, M., Hoikala, M., Korhonen, O. and Nutriminen, M. 1981: Hand–arm vibration in the etiology of hearing loss in lumberjacks. *British Journal of Industrial Medicine*, **38**, 281–9.

Pyykko, L., Korthonen, O., Farkkila, M., Starck, J., Aatola, S. and Jantti, V. 1986: Vibration syndrome among Finnish forest workers, a follow-up from 1972–1983. *Scandinavian Journal of Work, Environment and Health*, **12**, 307–12.

Quirk, W.S., Coleman, J.K.M., Hanesworth, J.M. and Harding, J.W. 1994: Noise-induced elevations of plasma endothelin (ET-3). *Hearing Research*, **80**, 119–22.

Quirk, W.S. and Seidman, M.D. 1995: Cochlear vascular changes in response to loud noise. *American Journal of Otology*, **16**, 322–5.

Reid, C. 1978: *Primer of Neuroanatomy*, p 107. London: Lloyd-Luke.

Ronco, A.L. and Halberg, F. 1996: The pineal gland and cancer. *Anticancer Research*, **16**, 2033–9.

Rossignol, M., Stock, S., Patry, L. and Armstrong, B. 1997: Carpal tunnel syndrome: what is attributable to work? The Montreal study. *Occupational and Environmental Medicine*, **54**, 519–23.

Sahl, J.D., Kelsh, M.A. and Greenland, S. 1993: Cohort and nested case-control studies of haemopoietic cancers and brain cancer among electric utility workers. *Epidemiology*, **4**, 104–14.

Saunders, J.C., Dear, S.P. and Schneider, M.E. 1985: The anatomical consequences of acoustic injury: a review and tutorial. *Journal of Acoustical Society of America*, **78**, 833–60.

Savitz, D.A., Dufort, V., Armstrong, B. and Therialt, G. 1997: Lung cancer in relation to employment in the electrical utility industry and exposure to magnetic fields. *Occupational and Environmental Medicine*, **54**, 396–402.

Savitz, D.A. and Loomis, D. 1995: Magnetic field exposure in relation to leukemia and brain cancer mortality among electric utility workers. *American Journal of Epidemiology*, **141**, 123–34.

Sokas, R.K., Moussa, M.A.A., Gomes, J. *et al.* 1995: Noise-induced hearing loss, nationality and blood pressure. *American Journal of Industrial Medicine*, **28**, 281–8.

Stromberg, T., Dahlin, L.B., Brun, A. and Lundborg, G. 1997: Structural nerve changes at wrist level in workers exposed to vibration. *Occupational and Environmental Medicine*, **54**, 307–311.

Sussman, S.S. 1994: EMF exposure assessment. In *Electric and Magnetic Fields and Health*. Paris: CIGRE Working Group.

Theriault, G. 1995: Electromagnetic Fields. In *Epidemiology of Work-Related Diseases*, McDonald J.C. (ed.), pp 63–86. London: BMJ Publishing.

Theriault, G., Goldberg, M., Miller, A.B. *et al.* 1994: Cancer risks associated with occupational exposure to magnetic fields among electric utility workers in Ontario and Quebec, Canada and France: 1970–1989. *American Journal of Epidemiology*, **139**, 550–72.

Thomas, G.B. and Williams, C.E. 1990: Noise susceptibility: a comparison of two naval aviator populations. *Environmental International*, **16**, 363–71.

Tomenius, L. 1986: 50 Hz electromagnetic environment and the incidence of childhood tumors in Stockholm county. *Bioelectro-magnetics*, **7**, 191–207.

Tynes, T. 1993: Electromagnetic fields and male breast cancer. *Biomedicine and Pharmacotherapy*, **457**, 425–7.

Virokannas, H. and Tolonen, U. 1995: Responses of workers exposed to vibration in autonomic function tests. *International Archives of Occupational and Environmental Health*, **67**, 201–5.

Waldron, H.A. and Harrington, J.M. (eds) 1980: *Occupational Hygiene*. Oxford: Blackwell Scientific.

Wertheimer, N. and Leeper, E. 1979: Electrical wiring configurations and childhood cancer. *American Journal of Epidemiology*, **109**, 273–84.

Wu, T.N., Chen, L.J.L., Ko, G.N., Shen, C.Y. and Chang, P.Y. 1996: Prospective study of noise exposure during pregnancy on birth weight. *American Journal of Epidemiology*, **143**, 792–96.

Young, J.Z. 1971: *An Introduction to the Study of Man*. Oxford: Oxford University Press.

14

Spinal injuries and rehabilitation

JOHN R SILVER

INTRODUCTION

About 15 million people in the UK participate regularly in some form of sporting activity. Soft tissue injuries are common, but it is recognized that only about half of the injured participants will seek medical advice. The most catastrophic injury is injury to the central nervous system, and a spinal cord injury is amongst the most serious. As a result of improved methods of treatment, patients with spinal cord injury can expect a near normal life expectancy but the cost in human and financial terms is high.

There are about 300 spinal injuries per year in the UK. Most are referred to centers specializing in the management of spinal injury and the congregation of these patients at spinal centers allows detailed analysis of the clinical manifestations and mechanics of the injury, and its likely outcome.

It is important to distinguish between sport that takes place as a recreational or leisure activity, such as recreational diving into a pool or the sea, in which case more attention to preventative education is required, and sport that takes place in a supervised capacity – at school or college, in a club or competition – in which careful attention to the laws and techniques involved can have practical and medico-legal significance in preventing injury.

Epidemiology of sporting injuries

A sporting injury can be regarded as an acute illness and subject to the same methods of epidemiology. Questions that need to be asked are:

- How dangerous is the sport and which sports are most likely to result in spinal injury?
- What is the incidence of spinal injury?
- Is the incidence of spinal injury increasing or decreasing?
- What are the relative risks involved in different kinds of sport?
- Which groups of participants and what ages are most at risk?
- How can spinal injuries be prevented?
- Does a spinal injury resulting from a sporting injury differ from a spinal injury caused by trauma of a different kind?

These seemingly simple epidemiological questions cannot easily be answered because the quality of many epidemiological data is so poor. But, as explained by Silver (1994) accurate data on the incidences of serious injury is needed before it can be ascertained whether the injury can be aggravated or diminished by changes in the regulations accompanying a sport or the training methods utilized by coaches. It should also be noted that catastrophic injuries involving the spinal cord are not notifiable and not all cases are admitted to spinal units. The distinction between a serious injury that damages the ligaments and bones and does not damage the spinal cord, and an injury that does, may be fortuitous.

The data presented and discussed in this chapter are based on the personal experiences of the author, who has seen and treated some 500 sports-related injuries to the spinal cord over a period of 40 years (Silver, 1984, 1993; Silver et al., 1986a, b; Silver and Gill, 1988; Silver and Lloyd Parry, 1991).

INCIDENCE OF SPINAL INJURY

Incidence in the UK

A comparison was made between the numbers and kinds of admissions during 1951–1968 and 1984–1988, respectively, at the National Spinal Injuries Center (NSIC), Stoke Mandeville Hospital (Table 14.1). This center served a population of 18 million people in the south of England producing some 8500 traumatic admissions over the period in question. The proportion of injuries caused by road traffic accidents and falls remained constant. There was a dramatic increase in criminal injuries. Sporting injuries increased from 12% to 17.5% of the total and there was a change in the representation of different sports.

In the earlier years, for example, gymnastics and trampolining injuries were common. Many of these injuries occurred in young military personnel when National (Military) Service was compulsory in the UK. Latterly, with a more affluent society, and the abolition of National Service, horse riding, snow sports, and rugby injuries have increased. It is of interest to note that gymnastics is now extremely popular, particularly amongst young girls. Injuries are, however, rare because the sport is carefully controlled.

DISTRIBUTION OF INJURIES BY SEX

There is a preponderance of spinal injuries in males, largely due to the number of men playing high-contact sports such as rugby. The situation may change as more women participate in such sports. Injuries to women predominate in horse riding but in the UK far more women ride regularly so this may be of no statistical significance.

AGE-RELATED INJURY

Sport-related spinal injury is overwhelmingly a problem associated with young people. In the UK the major exception is spinal injury caused by riding accidents – riding is more common amongst mature adults, and, especially, mature women.

Incidence of spinal injury outside the UK

Spinal injury is a serious medical problem all over the world. Statistics from the USA covering the period 1973–1985 reported 9647 admissions to specialist units. Sport-related injury was responsible for 14.2% of the admissions.

The causes of spinal injury vary greatly from country to country, although there are few exceptions to the general rule that road traffic accidents are responsible for the vast majority all over the world. However, 'adventure sports' may soon overtake road traffic accidents as the major cause of spinal cord injuries in New Zealand (Armour *et al.*, 1997).

Deep water diving and surfing accidents are particularly common in the USA where they are popular recreational and competitive sports. Indeed leisure diving far outweighs any other cause of sport-related damage to the spine. These sports are relatively uncommon in Europe and so do not feature in the statistics relating to spinal injury

Level of injury

The majority of injuries occur in the cervical spine. In the data from the UK material, 121 out of 156 patients had injuries to the cervical spine (77%). In the American series, tetraplegia, both complete and incomplete, totaled 91.8% of all sporting injuries (Young, in Stover and Fine, 1986).

Social factors involved in the incidence of spinal injury

The collected statistics are influenced by a range of social factors. In the USA, for example, spinal injury as the result of acts of violence is far more common in the Afro-American than in the Caucasian population, and this heavily skews the data (Table 14.2).

Table 14.1 *Acute trauma admissions to the National Spinal Injuries Center*

| Period | RTA | Falls | Criminal | Sport total | Main causes of sport accidents in UK | | | | | Overall total |
					Diving	Riding	Rugby	Gymnastics	Other	
1951–1968	340 (57.8)	175 (29.8)	2 (0.3)	71 (12.1)	42 (7.1)	8 (1.4)	5 (0.85)	5 (0.85)	11 (1.9)	588 (100)
1984–1988	181 (52.7)	86 (25.1)	16 (4.7)	60 (17.5)	24 (7.0)	16 (4.7)	14 (4.1)	–	6 (Skiing) (1.7)	343 (100)

Numbers in parentheses are percentages; RTA, road traffic accidents.

Table 14.2 *Distribution of spinal injuries by race in the USA*

Causes	Caucasion population	Afro-American population
Motor vehicle accidents	52.1%	35.4%
Sports	17.0%	6.3%
Acts of violence	7.1%	36.1%
Other	23.8%	22.2%

ANATOMICAL FACTORS AND MECHANICS OF INJURY

Injuries to the thoracic and lumbar vertebrae from knocks, kicks or blows during sport or bodily contact games do not give rise to damage to the spinal cord or roots, but the cervical cord is particularly vulnerable to injury. The thoracic and lumbar spines are protected by thick muscles and large sturdy vertebrae; they are splinted by the ribs and pelvis and are relatively immobile. The cervical spine is much more mobile. The likelihood of damage occurring to the cervical vertebrae is enhanced by the disparity in the movements of the unsupported skull on the cervical spine. The skull may be likened to a heavy ball on the end of a chain. The force created by movement will fall on the two vulnerable junctions of the skull and cervical spine, as well as the relatively mobile cervical spine and fixed thoracic spine. The danger of dislocation occurring is further increased by the alignment of the facets, which in the upper cervical spine do not present such resistance to dislocation as the vertebrae lower down. This is because their facets are aligned less obliquely.

Flexion

When a force is exerted through the crown of the head it is transmitted through the skull to the cervical vertebrae. This results in a crushing of the vertebrae and extrusion of the vertebral body and disc material posteriorly into the cervical cord. Dislocation may occur without any fracture of the vertebrae but when a dislocation occurs, particularly a bifacetal one, it is inevitable that the disc will be detached from its attachment to the vertebral body and the disc will rupture. Roaf (1960), using cadaveric spines, was unable to produce dislocation without a fracture by hyperflexion alone and found that some rotation must be present. Bauze and Ardran (1978) solved this problem by showing that when the vertex is fixed (being locked on the ground, a common occurrence in rugby) far less force is required to dislocate the vertebra and dislocation can occur without fracture.

Experimental work on animals cannot readily be extrapolated to humans but may be of value when experiments on cadavers give very conflicting and misleading results. A good example of an animal-based study is that of Schneider (1985), who investigated simulated conditions of tragic soccer cases in which he studied the influence of muscle tone on cervical dislocation in anesthetized monkeys. The impact was created by a blow to the vertex of the monkey's head with the neck in flexion and extension and the cervical spine aligned to permit compression of the structure. He showed that the position of the head modified the amount of force needed to create an injury and that the state of muscular tone at the time of injury (produced by anesthesia) had a notable influence on the ability to produce a cervical lesion. Extrapolated to humans, he said that the state of muscle tone at the time of impact could modify quite significantly a dislocation. Nevertheless, biomechanical studies of the mechanisms of spinal column injury document that a bifacetal dislocation can be produced in a 70 kg person by a fall on the head from a height of 9 inches (Watkins, 1996, p 409), a force frequently generated during sporting activities.

Spearing

A blow to the head may not be transmitted to the spine but may be absorbed by the brain and result in instantaneous respiratory and cardiac arrest.

Extension

The anterior–posterior diameter of the spinal cord is reduced during extension of the cervical spine so that when the neck is forcibly extended the spinal cord is compressed between the discs, vertebral bodies anteriorly and the lamina and ligaments posteriorly. The cord can thus be injured without there being any overt fracture or dislocation – the so-called 'extension' injury. This is stable since the ligaments and bones are intact.

When the disc is already damaged due to degenerative disease, there may be tearing of an intervertebral disc and angulation of the spinal cord but, although the ligaments are disrupted, there is less likelihood of a disc extruding. This type of injury occurs with quite modest force. In contrast to the injury above, this injury is unstable. In practical terms, there is no way of determining what the pathology is, and whether the fracture is stable or unstable, without detailed X-rays and dynamic views of the injury.

Traction

In an adult the intact ligaments, disc, and vertebrae prevent traction being exerted directly on the spinal cord so it is not a source of injury, unless the column is disrupted. Only under these circumstances can traction be exerted upon the spinal cord and it is a potent source of neurological damage when the spine is manipulated following dislocation. The danger is that too much traction will be exerted, and the cord will be directly pulled upon (Brieg, 1989).

In children, SCIWORA (spinal cord injury without radiographic abnormality) is an acronym for a constellation of injuries to the pediatric spinal cord. There are several anatomic differences in the pediatric spine that make it more flexible and prone to traction-type injuries. The facet joints are more horizontal in the child. The soft tissues of the spine and, particularly the neck, are more elastic in children than in adults. No single mechanism of injury has been implicated in these injuries. The etiology of SCIWORA is not known. Longitudinal traction injury to the spinal column and cord, cord rupture, traumatic infarctions, end-plate separation, transient disc herniation, and vascular compromise have been speculated as being causative. SCIWORA constitutes 20% to 35% of spinal cord injuries in children and is particularly common in children younger than eight years of age.

Blow to the neck

A blow to the neck over the carotid artery (a common problem in high-contact, tackling sports) results in a transient spasm of the vessel and unconsciousness without any bony injury.

PATHOLOGICAL CHANGES OF THE SPINAL CORD

Contusion

The immediate consequences of a spinal cord contusion or tear, caused by trauma to the cord by a fractured vertebra or protrusion of a disc, are damaged or severed nerve fibers. The nerve fibers swell and both axonic material and myelin degenerate. The cell bodies of the neurones show disruption. This is accompanied by exudative changes of edema, red cell diapedesis and an inflammatory reaction of polymorphs, lymphocytes, and plasma cells. These changes are seen a little distance from the main site of injury where they are obscured by hemorrhage and hemorrhagic necrosis. Edema, when slight, may be perivascular but often the edematous state affects the whole cross-sectional area of the cord. The edema is seen microscopically as rounded perivascular spaces in the white matter and perineuronal spaces in the gray matter. All these changes cause swelling of the spinal cord which becomes rounded and tense within the leptomeninges and dura, the subarachnoid and subdural spaces being obliterated. This cord swelling enlarges the region of traumatic damage and the final form is often in the shape of a spindle. This comprises a fusiform region of cord softening affecting one or more segments, and ending above and below by tapering to the end as a round area, often situated in the posterior columns. This round area may be a core of damaged tissue forced up by pressure. The swelling may take 24–48 h to develop and becomes maximal over a period of several days. It will then gradually regress. The swollen cord becomes tightly adherent to the spinal canal and is more liable to further injury.

Intrinsic changes of the vertebral column

The vertebral column with its discs and ligaments may be suffering from pathological factors which may predispose to spinal cord injury.

NARROWING OF THE SPINAL CANAL

Alexander et al. (1958), Payne and Spillane (l957), and Burke (1971) suggested that when the spinal canal is narrow those patients are particularly liable to injury of the cervical cord. This has been shown in patients with chronic myelopathy (Payne and Spillane, 1957; Nurick, 1972). McMillan and Silver (1987) showed that 75 patients with extension injuries causing tetraplegia had narrower canals than a control group of normal patients and those with fracture dislocations. These observations were all made in older patients, but the significance of a narrowed canal has been explored in young fit adults during sporting activity by Torg et al. (1986). They carried out a retrospective review of 32 patients with acute transient tetraplegia from forced hyperextension of the neck. The sensory changes included burning pain, numbness, tingling, and loss of sensation, while the motor changes ranged from weakness to complete paralysis. The episodes were transient and complete recovery usually occurred, although it could take up to 48 h. Routine X-rays of the cervical spine were negative for fractures and dislocation. However, the X-rays showed developmental spinal stenosis in 17 patients, congenital fusion in five patients, cervical instability in four patients and intervertebral disc disease in six patients. When compared with 'normal' subjects there was significant stenosis in 24 of the patients. They thought there was diminution of the anterior–posterior diameter of the spinal canal and the spinal cord could, on forced hyperextension or hyperflexion, be compressed, causing transitory motor and sensory manifestations. Tory et al. (1993) suggested that those who had instability of the cervical spine or pre-existing degenerative changes should not participate in contact sports.

DISC DEGENERATION

Cervical spondylosis accompanied by disc degeneration is a normal finding as people get older. Young people show no evidence of degeneration but, by the third or fourth decade in life, there is increasing incidence and so, by the age of 55, a large percentage of the population show radiological evidence of disc degeneration (Lawrence *et al.*, 1963). Magnetic resonance imaging (MRI) has confirmed the existence of disc protrusions in asymptomatic subjects (Boden *et al.*, 1990) (see Figure 14.1).

In young athletes the question arises: what is the relationship between cervical spondylosis and trauma? Scher (1990) compared radiographs of the cervical spines of 150 rugby players with a control group of 150 male hospital patients. Rugby players showed premature and advanced changes of degenerative disease when compared with the control group. These changes were most marked in the cervical spines of the front five forwards. Rugby players so affected are therefore more likely to present with the symptoms and signs of cervical osteoarthrosis and are at greater risk of hyperextension injury to the cervical spinal cord.

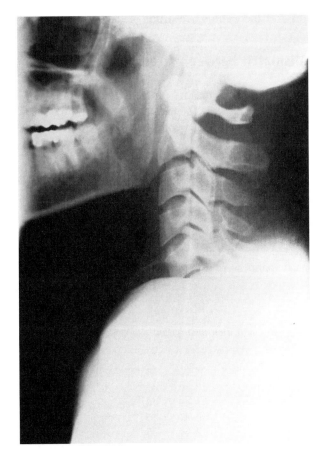

Figure 14.1 *Missed bilateral facet dislocation – lateral view shows the spine down to C5 only, but the facet dislocation at C5–C6 is just visible.*

Watkins (1986) found that in the young growing athlete there was an increased incidence of Schmorl's nodes and related compressive injuries with possible damage to the cartilaginous growth plate. These were found in 36% to 55% of all athletes participating in a wide variety of sports: football, wrestling, gymnastics, soccer, and tennis. Many athletes who did neck training exercises on a regular basis and who started young had advanced osteoarthritic changes at the lower levels.

Not only does sport cause degenerative changes but the degenerative changes are more likely to give rise to cord damage following hyperextension injury since it can further decrease the diameter of the vertebral canal. If the canal is already narrowed, then this can lead to a traumatic myelopathy.

There is, then, evidence that degenerative disease occurs at a younger age in active young sportsmen, particularly those who have experienced trauma to the neck, and that these changes can additionally narrow the cervical canal.

ROOT INVOLVEMENT

In a survey of 67 severe rugby injuries, Silver (1984) found four cases of nerve entrapment. In addition, since that series was completed, there have been two more cases of disc prolapse; one patient had a lateral disc prolapse causing severe nerve involvement and a front row rugby forward had a massive disc prolapse causing tetraplegia. In Schneider's series of 225 major trauma cases (Schneider, 1964) eight patients had ruptured cervical discs with root involvement and one had a brachial plexus lesion. All patients survived. Schneider considered that these lesions were not as serious as the head and spinal cord injuries and he was of the view that many more such injuries have remained unreported. Watkins (1986) also found many cases of nerve root entrapment.

These cases of nerve entrapment occurred in the 20–30 year age group in young fit sportsmen so that, apart from catastrophic cord injuries, severely disabling nerve root entrapment syndromes can occur as a result of premature degeneration leading to prolapse to the cervical discs.

STIFFNESS

Congenital fusion

Stiffness of the cervical spine can be caused by congenital fusion of a vertebra and, when present, this will lead to altered mechanics, loss of mobility, and additional risk of damaging the cord. Scher (1979) has shown in Klippel–Feil syndrome that tetraplegia can occur as a result of this. Damage is also more likely to occur where there has been congenital fusion.

Acquired fusion

Jaffray (in Watkins, 1996, p 574) has shown that where a surgical fusion has been carried out, the canal is narrowed and the patient is more likely to sustain spinal cord damage. He recorded an acute tetraplegia in a case of a rugby player who carried on playing after a spinal fusion.

HYPERMOBILITY

Hypermobility is a well-recognized but ill-defined syndrome and can occur idiopathically or as part of generalized disease of the mesenchyme of which Marfan's syndrome is the commonest.

The joints of the spinal column are unduly mobile so that the spine can be displaced beyond the normal range and compression of the nerve roots and the spinal cord can take place. The author has seen two cases of transient tetraplegia in rugby players both suffering from Marfan's syndrome.

COMMENT

Where the canal shows anatomical abnormalities, such as severe narrowing, either congenital or acquired, abnormalities leading to a rigid spine, severe degenerative changes, undue mobility such as Marfan's syndrome, a previously undiagnosed odontoid fracture or a cervical cord anomaly, players are at much greater risk of acquiring a traumatic injury to the spinal cord.

EXTRINSIC CAUSES OF SPINAL CORD DAMAGE

Lack of supervision

Numerous cases of serious spinal injury occur when sports and recreational games occur without adequate supervision or with disregard or ignorance of the risks involved. The following cases were all derived from the author's experiences, summarized in Table 14.3, or have been reported in clinical literature.

GYMNASTICS/TRAMPOLINING

Six of the 16 trampoline and 12 of 38 gymnastic accidents reported in Table 14.3 occurred in an unsupervised gymnasium.

RUGBY

One player was injured when someone jumped on the back of his unguarded neck while he was resting on the ground; one drunk player fell downstairs at 04.00 h while on tour; and one was tipped over someone's back in an exercise in which players' arms were linked.

SWIMMING

Frankel *et al.* (1980) have reported that two-thirds of cases studied were due to diving into the sea or rivers even though the general public was aware of the risks of diving into unknown depths of sea water and of striking submerged objects. These accidents clearly occurred during unsupervised activity.

There are similar findings by Green *et al.* (1980) who reported of 40 accidents that occurred in residential pools and a further 10 that had occurred in hotel pools. Grundy (1991) has reported that the peak incidence of injuries due to diving is in the summer and at least one-third of the victims had drunk alcohol.

Mismatch between strength and skill

This is an important problem when there is a discrepancy between the task undertaken and the ability of the performer to carry out the task, and it involves an assessment of the skills of the performers. Whereas a task may not be intrinsically dangerous to a well-trained performer, this is not the case with a beginner.

GYMNASTICS /TRAMPOLINING

Gymnastic and trampolining accidents were multi-faceted. In virtually all cases of spinal injury the participants were attempting a program beyond their abilities.

Table 14.3 Analyses of 156 sporting injuries to the spine and their distribution

Sporting activity	Date of paper	Period of study	No. of patients	Male/female	Age range	Cervical	Other
Rugby	1984	1952–1982	67	67/0	15–40	47	20
Rugby	1988	1983–1987	19	19/0	13–43	18	1
Trampolining	1986	1963–1978	16	13/3	10–43	15	1
Gymnastics	1986	1954–1984	38	33/5	12–54	35	3
Horse riding	1991	1976–1985	10	3/7	10–70	6	4
Sledding	1993	1958–1991	6	5/1	16–43	0	0
Total			156	140/16		121	

RUGBY

In rugby the clearest discrepancy of strength and skill is in the front rows of the scrum. On four occasions there was a discrepancy of skills, and on seven occasions schoolboys were playing with adults – they were unable to match them in strength – and on three occasions the scrum collapsed. On two further occasions participants were overmatched, inexpert, or playing in unfamiliar positions. This was particularly marked in those matches played at school where there was only a small pool of players available.

HANG GLIDING

Several of the participants were injured on their first excursion having been taken up to the top of a mountain and just launched. It is hardly surprising that they were injured since they did not know what they were doing and were unable to control their equipment. It is analogous to a non-swimmer being thrown into the deep end of a pool. The only difference is that if you are several hundred feet up no one can dive in to rescue you!

HORSE RIDING

The injuries sustained in horse riding were multifacetal, but seven of the riders were incapable of matching the capabilities of the horse. Whitlock (1988) studied 1554 horse riding injuries; 25% occurred during competition (Figures 14.2 and 14.3).

Competitive sports

The stress of competition can lead to errors in tasks that are undertaken easily and without error in practice.

GYMNASTICS/TRAMPOLINING

Injuries sustained by an international trampolinist participating in a major tournament were probably caused as a result of the stress of competition.

RUGBY

Of the 67 games in which injuries were sustained, three were of first class standard, 34 were club games, 12 were high school team games, four were other school games, and three were practice games. Sixteen injured schoolboys were school team players, four were not, and most injuries occurred in competitive games. Games against the fully adult 'old boys' were particularly dangerous (Figure 14.4).

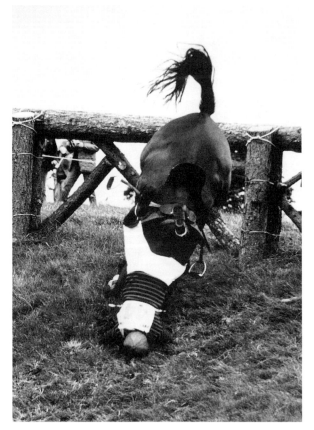

Figure 14.2 *A graphic example of the head and cervical spine being vulnerable.*

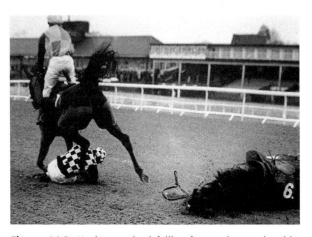

Figure 14.3 *Having survived falling from a horse, the rider may be injured by being kicked or trampled by another horse.*

Lack of fitness

GYMNASTICS /TRAMPOLINING

The general level of physical fitness of the gymnast/ trampolinist involved in an accident did not seem to be a major factor in causing accidents. However, two trampolinists had become fatigued, one accident occurred because the participant was out of practice,

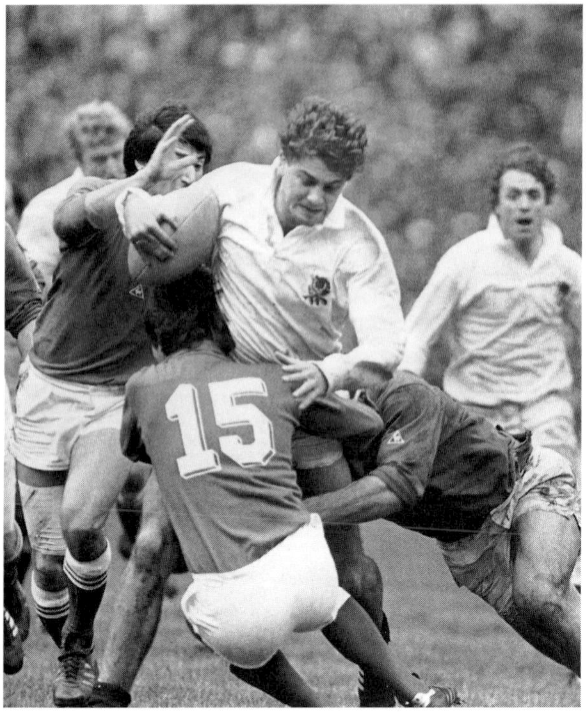

Figure 14.4 *An extremely dangerous situation. The main rugby player is being tackled by three people simultaneously and is unable to move away from the tackle.*

and another may be attributed to insufficient warm-up. One gymnast was reported as being tired, and an injured soldier had not done a certain exercise for a considerable period of time.

RUGBY

Nine rugby players were injured because they were not fit enough. Four claimed that they were not sufficiently fit to be playing any kind of sport. Five players were injured in the first game of the season. A player's failure to warm-up gave rise to an accident in the first moment of the game.

Three players were injured because they had not received sufficient specific training, i.e. they were not sufficiently fit for the particular task.

Equipment failure

This was rare. One or two accidents in trampolining could be attributed to this and one in horse riding.

Introduction of new equipment or new laws

The introduction of new equipment can have significant effects on sport-related injuries. The following cases illustrate the need for careful supervision.

GYMNASTICS/TRAMPOLINING

The trampoline was introduced into the UK in 1949. Initially all the accidents took place on unsupervised trampolines, but latterly the dangers of using equipment that can project the gymnast up to 6 m in the air have been realized. With correct supervision/coaching serious accidents have been virtually eliminated.

The trampette is an even more powerful piece of equipment enabling uncontrolled height to be achieved. It was responsible for 15 of the accidents.

WATER SPORTS

The introduction of theme parks with potentially dangerous equipment has not led to an increase in accidents at the parks because there is very careful supervision. It is where this new equipment, such as a wave machine, is introduced to swimming pools, and the appropriate level of supervision does not take place, that accidents occur; the waves can be a meter high, and children and adults can be caught unawares and flung violently to the bottom of the pool.

SURFING

Surfing may appear, at first sight, to be potentially dangerous, but an Australian study of 200 aquatic sports showed that 159 spinal injuries were due to diving, 19 were attributed to body surfing, but board surfing accounted for only two out of 200 (Watkins, 1996, p 409).

Compulsion

Compulsion in schools, prisons or the armed forces, where athletes are compelled to participate in sport, imposes significant strain on inexperienced participants. Thirteen of the patients reported in Table 14.1 were in the forces, three in the police force at one particular college, and one was in prison.

Alcohol and drugs

Any skilled performance can be adversely affected by taking drugs or drinking alcohol, thus the strict regulations with regard to driving. While a task can be carried out mechanically, judgement and insight are lost. It is difficult to obtain definitive information on the use of drugs and/or alcohol since it can lead to penalties and disqualification of the athletes; documentation is remarkably scarce. In swimming accidents, at least one-third of patients had drunk alcohol prior to their accident (Grundy, 1991). McLatchie (1986) states alcohol intoxication is responsible for 30% of all cases of tetraplegia in casual sports activities but he does not specify which sports. Firth (1985) in a study of equestrian injuries refers to the hunters having a high alcohol consumption since the 'stirrup cup' before the hunt is an integral part of the etiquette of the sport, which she considered a deadly combination. Among the rugby players, certainly one was drunk when he fell downstairs. At least one patient who was injured sledding had been drinking.

The study of 200 victims of aquatic injuries (Watkins, 1996, p 409) revealed that 150 had consumed alcohol prior to the accident.

Discussion and summary

The retrieval of detailed and reliable information on this topic was difficult. Questioning the athletes is often very time consuming. In addition some 50% of the patients, because of the nature of their accident, also had head injuries. Often they could not recall how the accident occurred. Others, either out of ignorance, shame or loyalty, were unable or unwilling to give a full account of the real cause of the accident. It is only by persistent questioning aided by experts that one can discover how these injuries have occurred.

Little attention has been paid to the question of validation of the information. Watkins (1996, pp 314–36) studied 67 neck injuries in soccer. He reported that the mechanism of injury and the nature of the incident causing the presenting complaint of neck pain were known in only 42 of the 67 players. The remaining patients could not reliably recall the direction of forces applied to the head or the position of the head at the time of injury.

Green *et al.* (1980) made a meticulous study in which they address this problem. They studied 72 swimming accidents from Florida. They noted appreciable differences between the data available from the retrospective and prospective cases. Surprisingly, the prospective patients were more difficult to interview and collect data from because of their medical condition and hesitancy on the part of the family and legal advisors to allow investigation (even when confidentiality was assured). In many cases active litigation presented a barrier to the release of information. The age group of the patients was 13–24. Forty incidents occurred in residential pools, 10 in hotels, 40 in apartment complexes, and only six in public pools. Despite these accidents happening in a hot climate in Florida, in only one patient was alcohol incriminated. This would seem to be inconceivable, and the conclusion is that the information with regard to alcohol was being withheld because of litigation.

Doctors are concerned with treating the patient's injuries and not how the injuries occurred; as a consequence it is frequently difficult to discover that a sporting accident has actually taken place. For example, in one case examined by the author, it was not clear whether the incident was a horse riding accident, or was caused by vaulting over a gymnastic horse. The causes of many sporting accidents went unrecorded when research was carried out on older records at the Spinal Center. Despite these problems, there is without doubt a relative increase in the number of sporting injuries all over the world. This may reflect the greater amount of time and wealth available for leisure activities and the even larger role sport is playing in our daily lives. The greater number of sporting accidents involving Caucasian Americans compared with the Afro-American population probably reflects the greater affluence of the former. Increasing affluence in many countries makes access to high-cost sports, such as horse riding and snow sports, easier and so accidents have increased accordingly.

The sex difference was striking. While clearly there are women who play high-contact games like rugby, they are often governed by different (and safer) rules and the numbers are small. Even in the sports where many women participate, for example, gymnastics and trampolining, more men are injured, either as a result of more aggressive behavior and a higher degree of competitiveness or, possibly, because the disciplines are different – women's gymnastics, for example, emphasizes agility, grace, and dance, whereas men's is more dependent on strength. This sex difference is supported by statistics in other sports – of 150 patients admitted to NSIC as a result of diving accidents, 142 were male (Frankel *et al.*, 1980). Only in horse riding do injuries to women predominate, reflecting the large number of women who ride. In other soft tissue injuries there is little difference between men and women. Amongst juveniles, boys over 14 years of age are three times more commonly injured than girls of the same age, which would suggest that the competitive nature of male contact sports, and the 'macho' image so important to young males, is responsible for the preponderance of severe injuries among males.

Despite the fact that during sport, particularly soccer and rugby, falls, kicks or blows are common, they rarely give rise to thoracic or lumbar spinal cord injury. Thoracic and lumbar injuries only occur when participants are flung sideways. The cervical spine however is especially at risk of injury as is shown in the figures which accompany this chapter – 121 of the cases were cervical injuries. The cervical spine is not as strong as the thoracic and lumbar spines. The cervical cord is injured in sporting activities where the head leads (for example rugby, gymnastics, and horse riding), when force is transmitted through the skull to the cervical vertebra. In the vast majority of cases such an injury is caused by direct contusion of the cord from the prolapse of the vertebra or disc. This is supported by the experimental work of Schneider (1985). In diving, unless the head strikes the bottom of the pool, river or sea the spine is not injured. It is quite extraordinary that virtually all the diving accidents seen when the bottom is struck result in a crush fracture. The author has only seen one case of a dislocation from striking the bottom. In contrast in rugby, where it would seem greater force is exerted when a scrum collapses, dislocation occurs much more frequently. A comparison of the incidence of spinal injury between soccer and rugby players is informative. From an estimated 4–5 million regular soccer players in the UK the author has only seen three broken necks (one resulting from a rugby-type tackle, one from a slip driving the head into the ground and one from diving across the goal mouth); from some 400 000 rugby players the author has seen over 100 severe spinal injuries.

It has been shown in car accidents that the force generated is directly proportional to the speed of deceleration. A car that is going slowly and strikes a tree is instantaneously decelerated and even though it is going slowly, great force is generated. If a car is moving when it is struck by another car and decelerates gradually, the occupants are far less likely to be seriously injured – that is the virtue of the seat belt which decelerates people gradually. If a rugby player is free to slide along the ground when he is tackled, he is far less likely to be injured than if there is a multiple tackle and he is immobilized by two or three other players when he is struck. It is, perhaps, surprising that, although a force of as little as a fall of 70 kg from a height of 9 inches can cause severe injury to the spine, such injuries are not seen more commonly.

It is important to distinguish between sport that takes place as a recreational or leisure activity, for example, recreational diving into a pool or the sea, in which case more attention to preventative education is required, and sport that takes place in a supervised capacity, at school, in a club or competition. The gymnasium is a dangerous place. Six of the 16 trampoline and five of the 38 gymnastic accidents occurred in an unsupervised gymnasium. The unsupervised use of equipment is hazardous – a trampoline can project the athlete 6–9 m in the air.

Supervision falls into two categories. General supervision ensures that dangerous equipment such as springboards and boxes are kept locked up and that gymnasts do not use the equipment on their own. Specific supervision ensures that dangerous exercises do not take place simultaneously, that instructors are competent and qualified to teach, and are aware of the standard of the gymnast so that over ambitious moves are not attempted. The problem exists in rugby because inadequate, or indeed no, refereeing in rugby can result in injuries. Junior players are often unskilled and lack understanding of correct and safe techniques, making up in hard contact and enthusiasm what they lack in skill. At this level a properly trained referee is often not available and this duty may be carried out by an unfit team member or a friend who has only a scant

knowledge of the laws. Illegal and unfortunate events may occur and tempers may be lost. If a game is not properly supervised, the law of negligence pertains and actions have been successfully taken against the referee and the administrators of the sport when they have failed to enforce the laws of the game. This has been upheld in the recent case of *Nolan* v. *The High Court* where the referee was found negligent for allowing persistent collapse of the scrum, as a result of which, a boy broke his neck and sustained a traumatic tetraplegia (*The Times*, 1996).

An important concept that has emerged from detailed studies of sports injuries is that of a mismatch between the skills of the sportsman and the task attempted; a relatively straightforward task could prove difficult or dangerous for an inexperienced sportsman. This is particularly common in gymnastics and trampolining where athletes can be pressed by the coach to undertake advanced maneuvers. Greater skill does not afford protection – when experts or teachers attempt a new exercise they become beginners again. In rugby the mismatch is of particular concern in the front row of the scrum where schoolboys with neither the strength nor skill are playing against adults. However, it is a problem that occurs at all levels and in all contact sports as it is particularly difficult to match players by height, weight, and age. Boys can be of the same chronological age, but there can be a great difference in their strength depending on whether they are prepuberty or postpuberty (Figure 14.5).

A potent source of injury is when equipment/rules are introduced to a sport and render even the experienced participant a beginner. When the trampo-

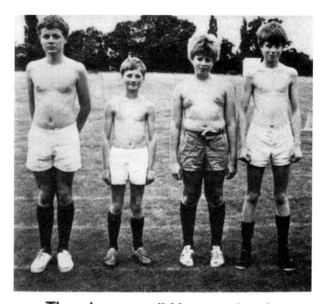

These boys are all 11 years of age!

Figure 14.5 *Difference in height and weight in 11-year-old boys. At puberty this discrepancy increases.*

line was first introduced into the UK it was regarded as a fun toy, and was used indiscriminately and without supervision. Once the dangers were appreciated virtually all trampolining accidents were eliminated. The trampette, introduced in the early 1970s, also allows uncontrolled height. It is possible to over rotate or leave the trampette at an angle causing the gymnast to miss the landing mat altogether. Catchers are also ineffective because it is impossible to catch a 70 kg+ person coming off a trampette at speed. Fifteen of the injured gymnasts had been using the trampette.

So far our discussion has hinged upon the actual trauma to the cervical spine. A difficult and controversial area is: does the cervical spine itself serve as a monitoring device in movement? Can the cervical spine itself, even though not pathologically damaged, cause injuries?

Coordination and balance, which are critical for any athletic performance, are mediated by impulses from the eyes and the otolith. In animals, the cervical spine also sends very important impulses that moderate balance. In humans these impulses from the cervical spine were not thought to be important. However, in a series of experiments reported in *Big Science* (1994), Ito *et al.* (1995) and Kanaya *et al.* (1995), and detailed clinical analysis by Cole *et al.* (1995) of a patient who had lost all posterior column impulses, have shown that the cervical spine does send impulses that monitor the position of the body in space and are of vital importance in carrying out skilled movements. It is striking (Ellis *et al.*, 1960) that many accidents in trampolining and gymnastics occur when doing somersaults. The author found 32 out of 54 cases were doing somersaults (24 forwards, eight backwards). Ellis studied five cases and found the acrobatic maneuver attempted in all but one of the cases was the backward somersault. It may well be that not only is the head stuck forward in a vulnerable position but orientation is lost due to a rotation.

TREATMENT AND MANAGEMENT

Prevention

Prevention is better than cure.

It is necessary to distinguish between social accidents, such as somersaulting on the beach, diving into the sea or shallow rivers, and organized sports because the audience to be reached is different.

SOCIAL ACTIVITIES

People who undertake social activities can be reached by:

- television;
- radio;
- word of mouth;
- peer example from parents and friends.

During hot weather in Denmark there have been epidemics of diving accidents. This has been successfully tackled by television programs warning people not to dive into shallow water. The effect of this was so successful that people would be accosted on the beach if they were seen to be doing something stupid and restrained by other members of the public.

TEACHING

With the widespread reduction of competitive sport in schools, who is to teach the children?

Parents assume a very important role in this regard, but social change and the growth of the one parent family (which account for one in five families in the UK) make it difficult to assume a major input from the parents.

Conversely, there is a very sad syndrome whereby parents try to achieve through their children what they have not achieved themselves in terms of sport. Too great encouragement, 'psyching up' from the touchline, has led to fights between parents. It does not generate the right atmosphere on the field for a skilled performance and has led to accidents.

FORMAL SPORT

Information with regard to incidents can be successful disseminate using the following forms:

- teaching in schools: lectures to schools and clubs by role models or paralyzed sportsmen may have a greater impact than the teachers at the schools themselves;
- adequate documentation – pamphlets, posters;
- demonstrations;
- teaching by people who understand the sport.

Modification of the conditions with safety in mind

The majority of diving accidents are caused by diving into shallow water. Depths of pools have been increased, safety notices have been put up, and adequate lifeguards have been employed. Separate diving pools have been introduced. Running round pools has been forbidden.

Modification of the laws

This is to ensure that potentially dangerous maneuvers are identified and eradicated. Changes to the rules of rugby have resulted in a reduction in serious injury (Noakes and Jakoet, 1995).

232 Spinal injuries and rehabilitation

Supervision

Competent people are needed to teach sport and to pass judgment on whether people are fit enough to participate in sport. Specific fitness has to be considered for a specific sport.

Resolution of conflicts of authority

It is not appreciated that all sports fall under the jurisdiction of different authorities – schools, whether public or private, are under different authorities; there are differences between the different armed forces. Competitive professional and amateur sports have their own authorities. Swimming is a particularly bad example where there is conflict between six different bodies over the safe depths of pools. Unless these problems are resolved, teachers and parents may not know where to turn for guidance.

It takes an unfortunate occurrence and a lawsuit to highlight the deficiencies of the system.

Changes in attitudes

The prime purpose of sport is to enhance health not to destroy it – you do not have to pay the price. If the attitude is that the game is governed by safety, things follow logically. If the attitude is 'win at any cost,' then accidents will, inevitably, happen.

There has to be a change in attitude towards drugs and alcohol, both of which impair judgment.

Insurance

Although not strictly preventative, since money will only be paid out if an accident has occurred, it is unfortunate that, despite repeated representations, insurance is often inadequate to meet the direct costs of an accident.

Litigation

Much as it is to be deplored, the intrusion of litigation whereby sportsmen can recover compensation if a sport has not been properly conducted has had a very salutory effect in seeing that games are conducted properly (*Van Oppen* v. *the Trustees of Bedford School* (1989); *Quinn* v. *Devon County Council* (1988); Silver and Stewart, 1994).

The very fact that insurance can exist does bring pressure to bear from insurance companies to make sure that the game is conducted properly. If the sport is not conducted properly then the insurance company will not pay out. Therefore this does have a strong

influence on ensuring that games are conducted properly.

Documentation

There is totally inadequate documentation about sporting accidents, even about fatal and catastrophic injuries. Few registers exist anywhere in the world and until such registers are established, one is left with dogmatic but inaccurately held views (Silver, 1984; Silver and Gill, 1988; Garraway *et al.*, 1991; Noakes and Jakoet, 1995). Thus, the questions posed at the beginning, which are purely epidemiological ones, cannot be answered in any sport as the information is not available.

MEDICAL ASSESSMENT

Are physicians in doctor/patient relationships with the sportsmen (in which case their interest is to prevent injury and treat any injuries) or are they employees of the sports club (in which case their interest is to win games and protect the interest of the sport)? What is the role of the physicians in preventing sporting accidents? Are the physicians responsible for assessing whether an athlete is fit enough to participate in a sporting activity? Only if they are consulted, can they make any decision. Frequently they are not consulted after sporting accidents where players are anxious to keep their places. Without the expert advice of a physician, a manager or coach may disregard an episode of concussion that can lead to a serious second injury if the person is allowed to play on. Schneider (1973) is of the opinion that someone who sustains a ruptured cervical disc should not be permitted to return to the game even if operated upon. Watkins (1996, p 409) and Jaffray (see Watkins, 1996, p 574) have similar views.

Treatment on the field of play

There should be adequate equipment on the field: a scoop stretcher and a collar to immobilize the spine. The medical attendants should know where the access gates for the ambulance are (and where the key is kept).

Who is to be the medical attendant? It is impossible for a medical attendant to be present at social activities. Even in organized games it is not always possible but there must be a chain of command whereby an appropriately trained person can attend, render first aid and seek further assistance if necessary. In practical terms, the duty falls too often to spectators, passing nurses or doctors, whose experience may not be appropriate and is always in conflict with the ambulance drivers, first aiders, boy scouts, and other experts who seem to live for such moments.

The injury must be treated appropriately on the field so that the medical attendants, whoever they may be, are aware of the dangers of spinal injury and can immobilize the patient.

When people injure their necks, if they are conscious and moving their arms and legs, they should be questioned about their symptoms and evaluated immediately by the side of the field. If the player is lying on the field, standard practice should be for the trainer to go to the player, start the evaluation, and summon more experienced help.

If doctors are involved their obligation is to diagnose a potentially unstable cervical spine that could lead to a major neurologic deficit after injury. The player on the field with neck and arm pain should be examined to determine first if there is cervical spine injury. The physician determines the potential for an unstable spine and assesses the patient's condition. This leads to a therapeutic plan, beginning with assessment of vital function and protective transportation.

An unconscious player should be treated as having an unstable cervical spine injury until it is proven otherwise. If the symptoms totally resolve, caution should still be exercised and there should be a high degree of suspicion. The player should be re-examined on the bench or taken for an immediate X-ray.

The position in which a patient is treated is a matter of controversy. Clearly the airway and saving the life takes priority. It is no good at all preserving the neck and spinal integrity if the patient dies from inhaling vomit. So, patients are vomiting or bleeding down the back of the throat, they should be turned on their face. This can be done safely if the cervical spine is controlled. Once the airway is cleared, patients can be turned onto their back and treated as an unstable spinal injury.

When people sustain a head injury, they are likely to have sustained a spinal injury. They should not be hauled to their feet nor should they be walked to the side of the field and propped up with their head lolling. They must be immobilized and lifted in one piece. It is vital that the patient is taken to an accident center where there are sufficient staff who are adequately trained.

Diagnosis in hospital

The diagnosis and management of spinal cord injuries is not easy especially if there are injuries to other organs, particularly a head injury or an injury to the chest and pelvis.

Fractures can be missed at the upper end of the cervical spine, the odontoid, through inadequate views; unifacetal dislocations can be missed at all levels;

stability can be mistaken unless careful views are taken; and damage to discs can be missed. At the lower end of the cervical spine dislocations and fractures can be missed since lateral views are difficult through the shoulders. Mid-thoracic fractures, which may be found where there is major trauma in horse riding and sledding accidents, can be missed because of the presence of fractured ribs and a hemothorax. Fractures of D12 are missed for a different reason as the fracture seems to lie in the hinterland between the thorax and the lumbar spine and may not be visible on either X-ray (Ravichandran and Silver, 1982; Jonsson et al., 1991). For this reason patients must be taken to a specialized center where properly trained staff have an awareness of these problems.

There must be adequate facilities for X-rays, computerized tomographies (CTs) and MRIs, and a Consultant Radiologist to report on the films.

A comprehensive examination should be carried out. All too frequently, subsequently, one is confronted with an inadequate examination when motor power reflexes and sensation have not been examined and, for some strange reason, patients are seldom turned on their sides so that the whole length of the spine can be palpated and the anal reflex and sacral segments, for reasons of modesty or ignorance, are not examined. Thus, medico-legal problems ensue – what was the cause of the injury, what was the situation on admission and has the patient been made worse by the treatment or lack of it?

TREATMENT

A spinal cord injury seldom occurs in isolation. It may be accompanied by head injury/chest injury. These must be investigated and appropriate treatment given by a trauma team, intensive care unit and physician. This is a large topic and outside the scope of this review.

Treatment of the fracture

The usual mechanism of injury to the cord is fracture, or a vertebra or a disc contusing the spinal cord. Such injury is at its worst at the moment of impact. Appropriate immobilization and surgical treatment may well improve the situation.

Treatment of a dislocation

A dislocation of the spine can occur and can be asymptomatic in the first instance. A dislocation can also give rise to damage to the spinal cord. This whole subject is not well understood and warrants a full discussion.

The usual mechanism of cervical dislocation has been described by Bauze and Ardran (1978). Force applied along the axis of the semi-flexed neck ruptures the posterior ligaments and causes the posterior facet or facets to slide upwards and dislocate. The forward shift of the cranial vertebra completes the rupture of the capsule of the apophyseal joint; the annulus and disc are inevitably disrupted. Primary neurological damage is caused when the cranial vertebra sweeps forward and injures the cord. If dislocation is relatively slow and gentle, particularly when it is associated with rotation, a unilateral facet dislocation may not damage the cord. More rarely a bifacetal facet dislocation occurs without neurological damage, when the spinal canal is capacious relative to the size of the spinal cord. Secondary damage may occur as swelling develops as a result of edema or evolving vascular injury. Some patients have been seen (Mahale and Silver, 1992; Mahale et al., 1993) who had minimal or no neurological damage before an attempt was made to reduce the dislocation.

The timing of the onset of paralysis in relation to the treatment can vary. Paralysis can occur during an attempt to reduce the dislocation. There may be no immediate neurological damage but paralysis can appear later on.

Damage is probably due to mechanical factors causing direct injury to the spinal cord, rather than intrinsic cord swelling. The anatomical and pathological factors that must be considered are the stability of the fracture, allowing cord injury by reproducing the acute injury, any reduction of canal diameter, disc protrusion, spondylitic changes, vascular problems, and the influence of traction and mechanical manipulation on the spinal cord.

The diameter of the spinal canal is critical, since it is recognized that a congenitally narrowed canal puts the cord at risk even when there is no complete dislocation (Payne and Spillane, 1957; McMillan and Silver, 1987). Measurements carried out on the diameter of the cord show that when there is only minimal forward displacement, no neurological damage occurs. Even when there is a bifacetal dislocation, if the diameter is large, a patient can survive without being paralyzed. However, when a person is anesthetized, the anesthesia will relax the spasm of muscles which may be protecting the cord by preventing movement of an unstable injury. When reduction is attempted, the canal diameter is reduced (Breig, 1989).

Other mechanisms may be important. Disc disruption and prolapse can occur in association with dislocation of the cervical spine (Eismont et al., 1991; Robertson and Ryan, 1992), and extruded disc material may be displaced further into the spinal canal during reduction. Patients have developed cord damage after a posterior cervical spine fusion. Disc herniation pressing on the cord has been demonstrated by myelography and CT-myelography, and there was neurological improvement after anterior discectomy and fusion with cord decompression.

The association of disc lesions with dislocations was recognized by Bohlman (1979), and MRI, which now enables one to visualize the canal and the spinal cord without the use of myelogram, has shown that this occurs in up to 50% of cases (Eismont et al., 1991). It is difficult to visualize how a bifacetal dislocation can occur without there being significant disc disruption.

Clearly the presence of spondylitic changes in the cervical spine will aggravate the situation. Elderly patients with a narrowed spinal canal are particularly at risk.

During reduction, injury to the vertebral arteries resulting in ischemic damage to the brain is possible. This is surprisingly rare, since the vertebral arteries pass through the transverse processes and must be compromised by a bilateral facet dislocation (Pratt-Thomas and Berger, 1947; Louw et al., 1990). This has been seen in patients who developed cerebellar infarction in addition to spinal cord damage. The rarity of this is probably due to the rich anastomosis between the basilar artery and the anterior cerebral circulation: in young patients the cerebral circulation can function adequately after total occlusion of one vertebral artery.

Traction

Traction, particularly if it is prolonged, excessive or applied in the wrong direction, may cause damage by stretching the cord. The commonly used method of closed reduction which involves flexion before lifting the facets clear will initially reduce the diameter of the spinal canal, potentially increasing cord compression (Breig, 1989).

Delayed paralysis

Patients can develop paralysis after an interval of 6–48 h. Where canal integrity was restored and the reduction was stable, the late deterioration was probably due to intrinsic cord factors. One recognized factor is cord edema, which may develop early. This ill-understood swelling of the cord can now be demonstrated non-invasively by MRI. Before this became available, cord edema could only be shown by myelography, which was believed to be contraindicated because of the possibility of causing cord damage, especially in the presence of blood.

Experimental work in animals shows that cord edema starts after a few minutes to 4 h, and can last for two weeks after injury (Braakman and Penning, 1971; Ducker et al., 1971, 1984). If attempts are made to reduce the dislocation within this critical period, further cord damage can develop. The swollen and edematous cord may be particularly vulnerable during this period. Any direct trauma to the cord at operation, or indirect trauma by traction, may aggravate the edema. The swollen cord may then be compressed, within a reduced bony canal, by fragments of vertebra, disc protrusion or damage to the ligamentum flavum, leading to a progression to paralysis (Mahale and Silver, 1992).

Manipulation

An operation to reduce dislocated facets inevitably causes further damage to ligaments and soft tissues, increasing any instability. It may also compromise the local blood supply to the cord, which enters along the nerve roots.

Thus, repeated unsuccessful attempts at reduction, particularly if they are later, will aggravate cord swelling.

MRI, CT, myelography, and CT-myelography are currently available to show cord compression. MRI and CT-myelography are the most appropriate investigations, and are important, especially when neurological function is intact below the level of the dislocation. The evidence (Eismont et al., 1991; Mahale and Silver, 1992; Robertson and Ryan, 1992) suggests that these investigations should be carried out before any reduction is attempted. This would help to prevent neurological complications with their attendant morbidity. Such patients should be admitted immediately after cervical injury to specialized centers where these investigations are available, and where urgent and appropriate treatment can be provided.

Final rehabilitation

The patient should be transferred to a spinal center for an appropriate period of time, up to six months, where there are specialized orthopedic surgeons, neurosurgeons, spinal consultants, chest physicians, physiotherapists, psychologists, with designated time to treat these patients so they can achieve an optimum level of rehabilitation. This is an enormous topic outside the scope of this chapter.

CONCLUSION

Medical practitioners, who are confronted with a severe spinal injury as a result of sport, since this is a rare occurrence, are unlikely to have adequate knowledge of how the sport should be conducted and they are usually so concerned with the treatment of the injury, that they will be unaware whether the sport has been carried out properly. The victim may be reticent and feel ashamed about having sustained the injury. The patient may be unaware as to how the sport should be properly conducted and many doctors have a strong sporting bias (in fact many students take up medicine as a way of continuing their sporting activities). So, for various reasons, ignorance and misguided loyalty to the sport, little enquiry is made as to how the accident has occurred. Any criticism of the techniques may be looked on as an attack upon the sport. It was Schneider (1985) who pointed out that the sports field provided a unique opportunity and a laboratory to study how spinal injuries occurred since there is likely to be a video recording of the actual game, the patient is available, witnesses are available, X-rays and, unfortunately, post mortems in many cases are available. He pursued his studies and made a unique contribution not only to our knowledge of spinal injuries but to the epidemiology of sporting injuries in the US. As a result of his research he was able to change the laws as to how American football is conducted, with a dramatic reduction in the number of spinal injuries from sport.

This chapter has concentrated not on the individual sports but on the common factors, since it is possible to elucidate a common mechanism of injury. The same faults produce injury in different sports. Unfortunately there is lack of knowledge, lack of lateral thinking, and lack of communication both within a sport and between different sports, so the lessons learnt from one sport are not applied to another.

It is only when these lessons are learnt that sport can serve to improve the quality of life rather than paralyze and despoil the human body.

> Why do we have to go over the same set of symptoms 20 times before we understand them? Why does the first statement of a new fact always leave us cold? Because our minds have to take in something which deranges our original set of ideas, but we are all like that in this miserable world.
>
> Jean Martin Charcot

REFERENCES

Alexander, E., Davis, C.H. and Field, C.H. 1958: Hyperextension injuries of the cervical spine. *Archives of Neurology and Psychiatry*, **79**, 146.
Armour, K.S., Clatworthy, B.J., Bean, A.R., Wells, J.E. and Clarke, A.M. 1997: Spinal injuries in New Zealand rugby and rugby league – a 20-year survey. *The New Zealand Medical Journal*, **110**, 462–5.
Bauze, R.J. and Ardran, G.M. 1978: Experimental production of forward dislocation in the human cervical spine. *Journal of Bone and Joint Surgery*, **60**, 239–45.
Big Science 1994: Wall to Wall. Produced by David Malone and Alexander Graham, BBC2.
Boden, S.D., McCowin, P.R., Davis, D.O., Dina T.S., Mark, A.S. and Wiesel, S. 1990: Abnormal magnetic resonance scans of the cervical spine in asymptomatic subjects. *Journal of Bone and Joint Surgery (American)*, **72**, 1178–84.

Bohlman, H.H. 1979: Acute fractures and dislocations of the cervical spine: an analysis of 300 hospitalized patients and review of the literature. *Journal of Bone and Joint Surgery (American)*, **61**, 1119–42.

Braakman, R. and Penning, L. 1971: Injuries of the cervical spine. In *Excerpta Medica*, p 172. Amsterdam

Breig, A. 1989: *Skull Traction and Cervical Cord Injury: A New Approach to Improved Rehabilitation*, p 41. Berlin: Springer.

Burke, D.C. 1971: Hyperextension injuries of the spine. *Journal of Bone and Joint Surgery*, **53**, 3.

Cole, J.D., Merton, W.L., Barrett, G., Katifi, H.A. and Treede, R.D. 1995: Evoked potentials in a subject with a large-fiber sensory neuropathy below the neck. *Canadian Journal of Physiology and Pharmacology*, **73**, 234–45.

Ducker, T.B., Bellegarrigue, R., Salcman, M. and Walleck, C. 1984: Timing of the operative care in cervical spinal cord injury. *Spine*, **9**, 525–31.

Ducker, T.B., Kindt, G.W. and Kempf, L.G. 1971: Pathological findings in acute experimental spinal cord trauma. *Journal of Neurosurgery*, **5**, 700–8.

Eismont, F.J., Arena, M.J. and Green, B.A. 1991: Extrusion of an intervertebral disc associated with traumatic subluxation or dislocation of cervical facets. Case report. *Journal of Bone and Joint Surgery (American)*, **73**, 1555–60.

Ellis, W.G., Green, D., Holzaepfel, B.S. and Sahs, A.L. 1960: The trampoline and serious neurological injuries. *Journal of the American Medical Association*, **174**, 1673–6.

Firth, J.L. 1985: *Sports Injuries, Mechanisms, Prevention and Treatment*. Baltimore, MD: Williams & Wilkins.

Frankel, H.L., Montero, F.A. and Penny, P.T. 1980: Spinal cord injury due to diving. *Paraplegia*, **18**, 118–22.

Garraway, W.M., Macleod, D.A.D. and Sharp, J.C.M. 1991: Rugby injuries, the need for case registers. *British Medical Journal*, **303**, 1082–3.

Green, B.A., Gabrielsen, M.A., Hall, W.J. and O'Heir, J. 1980: Analysis of swimming pool accidents resulting in spinal cord injury. *Paraplegia*, **18**, 94–100.

Grundy, D. 1991: Diving into the unknown. *British Medical Journal*, **302**, 670–1.

Ito, Y., Corna, S., von Brevern, M., Bronstein, A., Rothwell, J. and Gresty, M. 1995: Neck muscle responses to abrupt free fall of the head, comparison of normal with labyrinthine-defective human subjects. *Journal of Physiology*, **489**, 911–16.

Jonsson, H., Bring, G., Rauschning, W. and Sahlstedt, B. 1991: Hidden cervical spine injuries in traffic accident victims with skull fractures. *Journal of Spinal Disorders*, **4**, 251–63.

Kanaya, T., Gresty, M.A., Bronstein, A.M., Buckwell, D. and Day, B. 1995: Control of the head in response to tilt of the body in normal and labyrinthine-defective human subjects. *Journal of Physiology*, **489**, 895–910.

Lawrence, J.S., de Graaf, R. and Laine, V.A.I. 1963: In *The Epidemiology of Chronic Rheumatism*, Kellgren, J.H., Jeffrey, M.R. and Ball, J. (eds), Vol. 1, p 98. Oxford: Blackwell.

Louw, J.A., Mafoyane, N.A., Small, B. and Neser, C.P. 1990: Occlusion of the vertebral artery in cervical spine dislocations. *Journal of Bone and Joint Surgery (British)*, **72**, 679–81.

Mahale, Y.J. and Silver, J.R. 1992: Progressive paralysis after bilateral facet dislocation of the cervical spine. *Journal of Bone and Joint Surgery (British)*, **74**, 219–23.

Mahale, Y.J., Silver, J.R. and Henderson, N.J. 1993: Neurological complications of the reduction of cervical spine dislocations. *Journal of Bone and Joint Surgery (British)*, **75**, 403–9.

McLatchie, G.R. 1986: *Essentials of Sports Medicine*, pp 159–69. Edinburgh: Churchill Livingstone.

McMillan, B.S. and Silver, J.R. 1987: Extension injuries of the cervical spine resulting in tetraplegia. *Injury*, **18**, 224–33.

Noakes, T. and Jakoet, I. 1995: Spinal cord injuries in rugby union players. *British Medical Journal*, **310**, 1345–6.

Nurick, S. 1972: The pathogenesis of the spinal cord disorder associated with cervical spondylosis. *Brain*, **95**, 87–100.

Payne, E.R. and Spillane, J.D. 1957: The cervical spine. An anatomico-pathological study of 70 specimens (using a special technique) with particular reference to the problem of cervical spondylosis. *Brain*, **80**, 571.

Pratt-Thomas, H.R. and Berger, K.E. 1947: Cerebellar and spinal injuries after chiropractic manipulation. *Journal of the American Medical Association*, **133**, 600–3.

Ravichandran, G. and Silver, J.R. 1982: Missed injuries of the spinal cord. *British Medical Journal*, **284**, 953–6.

Roaf, R. 1960: A study of the mechanics of spine injuries. *Journal of Bone and Joint Surgery*, **42**, 810–23.

Robertson, P.A. and Ryan, M.D. 1992: Neurological deterioration after reduction of cervical subluxation. *Journal of Bone and Joint Surgery (British)*, **74**, 224–7.

Scher, A.T. 1979: Cervical spine fusion and the effects of injury. *South African Medical Journal*, **56**, 525–7.

Scher, A.T. 1990: Premature onset of degenerative disease of the cervical spine in rugby players. *South African Medical Journal*, **77**, 557–8.

Schnieder, R.C. 1964: Serious and fatal neurosurgical football injuries. *Clinical Neurosurgery*, **12**, 226–36.

Schneider, R.C. 1973: *Head and Neck Injuries in Football. Mechanisms, Treatment and Prevention*. Baltimore, MD: Williams & Wilkins.

Schneider, R.C. 1985: Football. In *Sports Injuries: Mechanisms, Prevention, and Treatment*, Schneider, R.C., Kennedy, J.C. and Plant, H.L. (eds), pp 1–44. Baltimore, MD: Williams & Wilkins.

Silver, J.R. 1984: Injuries of the spine sustained in rugby. *British Medical Journal*, **288**, 37–43.

Silver, J.R. 1993: The dangers of sledging. *British Medical Journal*, **307**, 1602–3.

Silver, J.R. 1994: Methods of recording statistics in rugby football: the experience in the United Kingdom. *Sports Exercise and Injury*, **1**, 46–51.

Silver, J.R. and Gill, S. 1988: Injuries of the spine sustained during rugby. *Sports Medicine*, **5**, 328–34.

Silver, J.R. and Lloyd Parry, M.A. 1991: Hazards of horse riding as a popular sport. *British Journal of Sports Medicine*, **25**, 105–10.

Silver, J.R., Silver, D.D. and Godrey, J.J. 1986a: Trampolining injuries of the spine. *Injury*, **17**, 117–24.

Silver, J.R., Silver, D.D. and Godfrey, J.J. 1986b: Injuries of the spine sustained during gymnastic activities. *British Medical Journal*, **293**, 861–3.

Silver, J.R. and Stewart, D. 1994: The prevention of spinal injuries in rugby football. *Paraplegia*, **32**, 442–53.

Stover, S.L. and Fine, P.R. (eds) 1986: *Spinal Cord Injury: The Facts and Figures*, p 35. Alabama: The University of Alabama.

The Times 1996: *Smoldon* v. *Whitworth and another.*

Torg, J.S., Pavlov, H. and Genuario, S. 1986: Neuropraxia of the cervical spinal cord with transient quadriplegia. *Journal of Bone and Joint Surgery*, **68**, 1354.

Watkins, R.G. 1986: Neck injuries in football players. *Clinics in Sports Medicine*, **5**, 215.

Watkins, R.G. (ed.) 1996: *The Spine in Sports*, pp 314–36, 409, 574. St Louis, MO: Mosby.

Whitlock, N.R. 1988: *Horse Riding is Dangerous for your Health. Proceedings of the Second International Conference on Emergency Medicine, Brisbane, Australia*. Australian College for Emergency Medicine.

15

Neurotoxicology of organophosphates, with special regard to chemical warfare agents

PETER G BLAIN

INTRODUCTION AND BACKGROUND

Chemical poisons have a long history in political intrigue as a tool of the assassin. However, it was on April 22, 1915 when the military use of mass chemical poisoning as a weapon was most crudely demonstrated. The Algerian division of the French army was attacked at Ypres with 150 tons of chlorine released from 6000 cylinders over a front of 4 miles by the German army. The first British troops to be attacked with a chemical weapon were the 1st Battalion of the Dorset Regiment on May 1, 1915. The effects were devastating and starkly demonstrated the military potential of such weapons. On one day, March 9, 1918, German forces fired some 200 000 shells containing sulfur mustard.

After World War I there was a widespread campaign to ban chemical warfare but even as late as the Italian campaign in Ethiopia (1935–36) sulfur mustard was used on a large scale against unprotected forces, producing many casualties. More recently, Iraq used chemical weapons (sulfur mustard and the organophosphate nerve agents) on a large scale against Iranian troops during the Iran–Iraq War (1981–86). Even now there are estimated to be some 30 000 casualties of these attacks still requiring medical support in Iran. In a particularly horrific incident, at Halabja in Iraq, some 5000 civilians were killed. Other alleged uses of chemical and biological warfare include 'yellow rain' in south-east Asia (Seagrave, 1981) and the use of 'knock-down agents' and 'black-body agents' by USSR forces in Afghanistan. US forces used defoliants and irritants on a large scale during the war in Vietnam, some of which may have been genotoxic.

Although most of these chemicals are regarded as weapons of mass destruction (WMD) some are specifically seen as a means of incapacitating individuals. The recent use of CS tear gas (2-chlorobenzylidene malononitrile) by UK police forces against civilians has been criticized as the inappropriate deployment of a chemical weapon. However, despite universal condemnation of these past uses, expansion of the capacity to wage chemical and biological warfare continues in many countries, including both the industrialized and the newly industrializing countries of the world.

Many of the chemical and biological weapons currently, or recently, in production are vesicants, attacking either the skin and/or lungs, or bacterial toxins (for example, *Bacillus anthracis*) attacking the same targets. The organophosphates are the only agents that were specifically developed as warfare agents because of their lethal neurotoxicity. The recent uses of organophosphates during military conflicts in the Middle East and in terrorist attacks in Japan has heightened interest in these agents. For this reason, this chapter will discuss exclusively the neurotoxicology of anticholinesterases (AChEs), such as the organophosphates, with special reference to the compounds developed specifically as agents for use in war.

Organophosphates are very widely used now as plasticizers, expanders, antioxidants, and flame retardants in a variety of industries. In addition, their widespread use as insecticides results in low levels of exposure for huge numbers of people. The majority of organophosphates have a relatively low capacity to cause damage to the nervous system but some are highly toxic. It is important to note that the essential difference between the 'warfare agents', sarin, tabun, soman and VX, and the commonly used sheep-dip agents, such as diazinon, is that the former are much more highly toxic to humans.

The typical industrial worker and home gardener may be exposed chronically to low levels of organophosphates, the sheep dipper to occasional high levels but the serviceman to single exposures at extremely high levels. It is important, therefore, to distinguish between the effects of chronic low-level exposure and acute high-level exposure. As will be seen, this poses very considerable problems in the formal description of the effects of organophosphates on physical and mental functions in humans.

Chemical nature and distinguishing features

Most organophosphates are either phosphates (esters of phosphoric acid), phosphonates (esters of phosphonic acid), or phosphinates (esters of phosphinic acid). Some have sulfur, fluorine or nitrogen attached to the phosphorus and are named accordingly. Carbamates, organophosphorus pesticides, and warfare agents inhibit cholinesterases in general and acetylcholinesterases in particular. Most of the commonly used anticholinesterases are either organophosphates or carbamates (esters of carbamic acid). Inhibition by carbamates is, in most cases, spontaneously reversible whereas that by organophosphates is relatively irreversible and functional recovery following exposure is the result of the synthesis of new enzyme. Monitoring of blood AChE or cholinesterase (ChE) has been used as a marker of exposure in humans and up to 60–70% inhibition of red blood cell AChE can occur before clinical signs are detectable.

The organophosphate warfare agents (also called nerve agents) are chemically similar to organophosphate pesticides, but have a much higher acute toxicity for humans by ingestion, inhalation or via the percutaneous route. However, the clinical toxicology of the nerve agents and pesticides is broadly similar and treatment of acute poisoning is the same. The nerve agents tabun, sarin, and soman were developed in Germany before and during World War II (UK Ministry of Defence, 1972; Maynard and Beswick, 1992) and other nerve agents, such as the binary agents, were developed later by the USA (Le Chene, 1989).

The 'classical' nerve agents are:

- sarin (isopropyl methylphosphonofluoridate);
- soman (pinacolyl methylphosphonofluoridate);
- tabun (ethyl *N,N*-dimethylphosphoramidocyanidate);
- VX (*O*-ethyl-*S* (2(diisopropylarnino)ethylmethylphosphonothioate).

Although they show similar 'group' toxicity effects they have different physical properties; VX is not very volatile and so can be used for terrain denial or canalizing troop movements.

It is difficult to extrapolate the civilian experience with organophosphate pesticides directly to exposure to warfare agents; the clinical findings in nerve-agent poisoning can only be inferred from experimental poisonings in animals and human poisoning with organophosphate pesticides. Battlefield poisoning with nerve agents (in contrast to pesticides) has only rarely been seen by civilian clinicians (Sidell, 1974; Maynard and Beswick, 1992) but these rare cases, and low-dose human volunteer studies with nerve agents, do not suggest that there are any significant qualitative differences between the effects in humans and other animals. The difference between organophosphate warfare agents and those for 'normal' civilian use is that the former are designed to be highly toxic and used at very high concentrations. As a result, the medical emphasis is on acute toxicity rather than delayed toxicity.

Organophosphate insecticides are in general characterized by their low acute mammalian toxicity and high acute insect toxicity. This selective toxicity has been designed into the molecule and exploits differences in the metabolism of organophosphates between mammals and insect pests. Structurally, most commercial pesticides are phosphates or phosphorothioates with O,O-dimethyl or O,O-diethyl substituents on the phosphorus atom. To exploit further metabolic differences between species, some organophosphates are delivered as 'pro-pesticides' which are, generally, thiophosphate derivatives that are metabolically activated to the proximate phosphate inhibitors by the target animal species. Organophosphate pesticide are, in general, inhibited enzymes readily reactivated by oxime reactivators of AChE. Most commercial pesticides have acute toxicities (LD_{50}) within the range $1\,mg\,kg^{-1}$ to $1–2\,g\,kg^{-1}$ and dose–effect curves which are notably shallower than those of the chemical warfare organophosphates

Chemical warfare organophosphates have a different chemical structure. In general, these are phosphonates, or phosphoramidates, in which there is a direct chemical bond between the alkyl substituent and the phosphorus atom. This P–C bond confers a high degree of stability to the organophosphate-inhibited cholinesterase *in vivo* and is, in large part, responsible for the high toxicity of the nerve agents. Nerve agents have acute toxicities (LD_{50}) within the range $5–500\,\mu g\,kg^{-1}$ and are characterized by having extremely steep dose–effect curves with slopes above 10.

Reactivity of carbamates and organophosphates

Historically carbamates were the first recognized inhibitors of cholinesterases to be used for pharmacological purposes. They are reversible inhibitors of AChE with half-lives of inhibition ranging from 15 min to several hours, depending on the structure of the molecule. Physostigmine (eserine), the toxic alkaloid of the Calabar bean (*Physostigma venenonsum*), was for many years the drug of choice for the treatment of the atonic gastrointestinal tract and for the induction of miosis. Pyridostigmine, a synthetic carbamate, has been used for many years in the treatment of myasthenia gravis and, more recently, as a pretreatment drug (nerve agent protection set (NAPS)) for protection against the lethal effects of chemical warfare organophosphates. Research since World War II has led to the development of carbamates for use as drugs and pesticides.

The toxicity of organophosphates is based on their ability to act as substrates for a number of ester-hydrolyzing enzymes. Thus the anticholinesterases mimic the effects of ACh and act as pseudo-substrates for cholinesterases and a number of other related enzymes. Inhibition of the enzyme results from phosphorylation. The process is illustrated in Figure 15.1. The formation of the enzyme/substrate complex (stage 1) is followed by the elimination of a 'leaving group' (stage 2) and then, either the reactivation of the enzyme (stage 3), or its 'aging' (stage 4). The aging stage involves the covalent cleavage of the enzyme-substrate adduct and the formation of a stabilizing

negative charge which prevents entry into stage 3. The difference in toxicity of the various organophosphate anticholinesterases is determined largely by the relative speed and efficiency of the two processes of reactivation and aging. Reactivation is very fast for natural substrates, and tends to be very rapid for the carbamates (for example, physostigmine). On the other hand, reactivation is very slow with nerve agents and so the enzyme ages. The enzyme is almost irreversibly blocked when aging is complete. An equally important outcome of aging is that end-point toxicity is dependent upon both organophosphate concentration and exposure time.

A second, extremely important target for some of the organophosphate anticholinesterases is the enzyme neuropathy target esterase (NTE). This is a membrane-bound neuronal protein of unknown function (Johnson, 1990). It is the phosphorylation and aging of this enzyme that appears to be associated with, and possibly causally related to, the onset of an organophosphate-induced polyneuropathy but often without any evidence of cholinergic hyperactivity (Zech and Chemnitius, 1987). Those organophosphates that do not interact with NTE do not cause the polyneuropathy, however potent they may be as cholinesterase inhibitors.

It has also been shown that *in vitro* some organophosphate anticholinesterases are potent inhibitors of a number of tissue proteases (Mantle *et al.*, 1997) and have the potential for a wide range of other interactions (Figure 15.2). The significance of these various interactions has not been demonstrated, but tissue

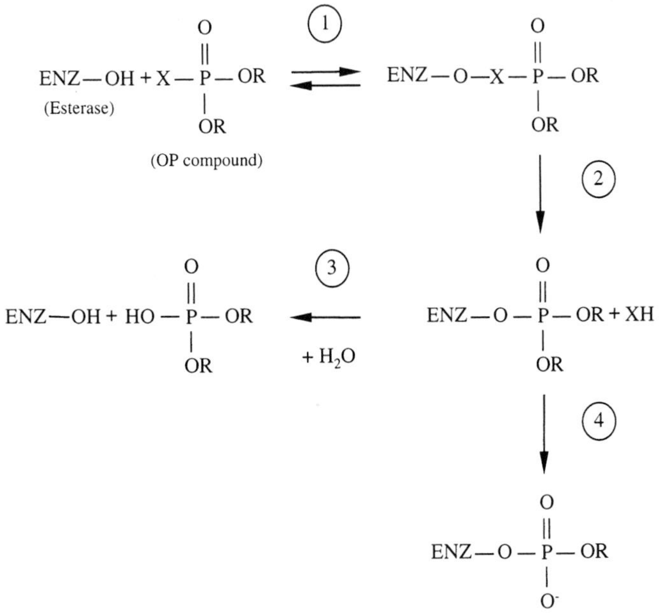

Figure 15.1 *Inhibition of an esterase by an organophosphate compound.*

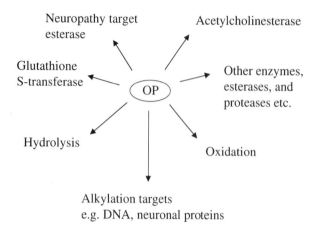

Neuropathy target esterase

Acetylcholinesterase

Glutathione S-transferase

OP

Other enzymes, esterases, and proteases etc.

Hydrolysis

Oxidation

Alkylation targets e.g. DNA, neuronal proteins

Figure 15.2 *Potential interactions of organophosphate compounds.*

proteases are such important regulators of cellular function that the finding that some organophosphates are potent inhibitors of proteases deserves more attention.

Metabolism and detoxification of organophosphates

Some of the factors involved in determining the toxicity and pharmacological profiles of the anticholinesterases include uptake via the skin, ingestion or inhalation, the metabolic capacity for detoxification, and the speed of degradation when distributed in the environment. As a general rule, the resistance or sensitivity of humans to the organophosphate anticholinesterases is primarily dependent upon the rate of detoxification; the corollary is that there is little evidence that susceptibility is primarily determined by the sensitivity of the target proteins. This is a particularly important factor in the sulfur-containing organophosphates because these compounds need to be oxidized *in vivo* before they become activated. If they are metabolized rapidly, metabolism may detoxify the agents before the process of activation can occur. If, however, the oxidized form is produced (the oxon product), detoxification may be slow and the oxon may then continue to inhibit the appropriate esterase for a number of days.

Most organophosphates are rapidly metabolized and excreted in the urine so the presence of hydrolysis products in the urine can be used as a marker of exposure. Some anticholinesterases may be excreted unchanged. For example, pyridostigmine (a carbamate), when administered by intravenous injection, has an elimination half-life of less than 2 h, and between 75% and 90% is excreted unchanged in the urine. When taken by mouth however, it is poorly absorbed and only 20% of the absorbed material is excreted unchanged.

Organophosphates are typically detoxified by aryl-dialkylphosphatases (for example, paraoxonase), carboxylesterases or cytochrome P450. There is a great deal of variation both in the sensitivity of various organophosphates to the major detoxification systems and in the individual detoxifying enzymes. For example, carboxylesterase binding is particularly important for the detoxification of organophosphate nerve agents since those with a P–N bond, such as tabun, are poor substrates for paraoxonase. In rodents, on the other hand, the rapid binding of soman to plasma carboxylesterase prevents it from reaching the target organs (Gaustad *et al.*, 1991; Due *et al.*, 1994; Jokanovic *et al.*, 1996).

Human serum paraoxonase (PON1) has an amino-acid polymorphism at position 191. The variant PON1 (type R), which has arginine at position 191, has eight times the activity of PON 1 (type Q) that has glutamine at that position. Fifty percent of Caucasians are homozygous (i.e. QQ) for the Q allozyme, 40% are QR heterozygotes, and the rest are RR homozygotes (La Du, 1996). The organophosphates differ in their relative affinity for these variants. The variants Q and R both hydrolyze chlorpyrifos oxon at the same rate. However, the polymorphic forms appear to have differential specificities for the hydrolysis of diazinon oxon, sarin, and soman compared to paraoxon. The Q variant hydrolyzes diazinon oxon, sarin and soman, and conversely the R variant hydrolyzes paraoxon (Davies *et al.*, 1996).

In those organophosphates that require activation, oxidation to the toxic oxon is accompanied by detoxification by cytochrome p450 enzymes (mainly cyp 3A, one of the abundant isoforms). Metabolism is mainly in the liver but may occur locally in the brain. Cyp 3A expression has wide interindividual differences due to variability in cyp 3A4 and the presence or absence of cyp 3A5, which may be under genetic control in humans (Mutch *et al.*, 1992, 1996a; Butler and Murray, 1997). Differences in these pathways may contribute to interindividual differences in susceptibility in humans to those organophosphates which require activation.

Pharmacological activity and toxic mechanisms

Most of the pharmacological consequences of poisoning by organophosphate anticholinesterases are easily explained. AChE breaks down ACh, a chemical neurotransmitter, at many neuronal synapses and neuromuscular junctions. Inhibition of the enzyme leads to an accumulation of ACh at muscarinic and nicotinic sites in the central and peripheral nervous systems (CNS and PNS). The excess ACh causes excitation, followed by inhibition of cholinergic transmission from depolarization block, and desensitization (although other mechanisms may also be involved). The expression of the acute CNS- and PNS-related symptoms depends upon the degree of AChE inhibition. Organophosphates that cross the blood–brain barrier (for example, mipafox and paraoxon) inhibit central cholinesterases and can produce transient changes in brain AChE activity but whether the organophosphate anticholinesterases directly cause significant changes in CNS function is unclear and highly contentious. Many organophosphates do not cross the blood–brain barrier. For those that do, it is important that the effects on the CNS, particularly of chronic exposure to low doses of organophosphates, are more thoroughly examined.

The neurotoxic effects of anticholinesterases should be considered in the context of the known biochemical activities of this group of compounds. Anticholinesterases may be direct-acting and irreversible (for example, organophosphate nerve agents), direct-acting but reversible (for example, carbamates) or require activation (for example, organophosphate pesticides). The effects of acute poisoning with an organophosphate (nerve agent or pesticide) or a carbamate are associated with inhibition of acetylcholinesterase which, by hydrolyzing acetylcholine, regulates the transmission of nerve impulses across specific nerve/nerve synapses or neuromuscular junctions. The primary biochemical event associated with inhibition of acetylcholinesterase is the phosphorylation of the serine residue of the active site of the enzyme. The nature of the biochemical reaction with AChE is similar to that of the natural substrate, acetylcholine. The principal difference between anticholinesterase compounds is the rate constant for enzyme reactivation. This is fast for the natural substrate, but extremely slow for organophosphate nerve agents, and the phosphorylated enzyme complex ages very quickly. Carbamates act as reversible inhibitors and so the enzyme reactivates much faster than with most organophosphates. Consequently, organophosphates vary widely in their potency to inhibit AChE as well as their rates of spontaneous reactivation or aging. Inhibition of acetylcholinesterase by 50–70% may be associated with acute central and peripheral cholinergic clinical effects due to excess acetylcholine.

There is significant variability between organophosphtes in terms of sensitivity in both the central and peripheral nervous systems (Ligtenstein, 1984; Churchill et al., 1987; Misulis et al., 1987). There is evidence that much of this variability may reflect the differences in the sensitivity of the many different molecular forms of acetylcholine esterases (Sellstrom et al., 1985). Neuronal acetylcholinesterase, for example, exists in functional and non-functional pools of several molecular forms. The functional forms are located extracellular in the cleft of the neuromuscular junction and comprise the lipophilic asymmetric form (A12, collagen-tailed) which is bound to the basal lamina and some water-soluble globular AChE (G4) present in the extracellular matrix in the cleft (Younkin et al., 1982). The non-functional precursor pool containing G1 and G4 is found intracellular. AntiAChE compounds differentially affect the AChE molecular forms (Ogane et al., 1992; Taylor et al., 1994). There is also a difference in aggregation of the monomeric globular forms between slow and fast muscle, diaphragm, and certain areas of the brain. Several studies have shown that A12 is absent from brain synapses where G4 may be the functional form.

The structural components of the organophosphorus compounds that produce anticholinesterase properties have been determined (Maxwell and Lenz, 1992). Anticholinesterase organophosphates are derivatives of phosphoric acids (not phosphinic) and structurally contain a leaving group and two alkyl groups. For sarin and soman, the leaving group is a fluorine atom, for tabun it is a cyanide moiety, and with VX it is a (diisopropylamino) ethyl moiety. Reactivation of the inhibited enzyme is slow and aging occurs if dealkylation of the dialkylphosphoryl enzyme produces a much more stable monoalkylphosphoryl complex (Marrs, 1993). AChE inhibited by soman ages rapidly after the loss of a pinacolyl group and recovery of any enzyme function only follows synthesis of new AChE (Gray, 1984). The correlation between CNS, neuromuscular junction, and red blood cell antiacetylcholinesterase activity is poor, probably because the kinetics of inhibition, and the concentrations, differ at the various sites.

A single dose of a carbamate causes a reversible inhibition of acetylcholinesterase. Carbamates are widely used as insecticides and therapeutic agents (for example, in the treatment of myasthenia gravis). However, pyridostigmine is used as a prophylactic medical countermeasure against organophosphate chemical warfare agents (as NAPS). The dose used results in an unstable equilibrium between inhibited AChE and pyridostigmine in blood and peripheral tissues. A prophylactic dosage of pyridostigmine is achieved when the activity of red cell AChE is reduced by between 20% and 40% of normal. The standard dose to produce an adequate level of reserved enzyme is an oral dose of 30 mg pyridostigmine bromide every 8 h. Pyridostigmine, a quaternary ammonium compound, does not penetrate the CNS but a recent study has suggested that stress may compromise the integrity of the blood–brain barrier and allow ingress of excluded compounds (Friedmann et al., 1996). However, this concept is not widely accepted. Physostigmine, another carbamate, crosses the blood–brain barrier and inhibits acetylcholinesterase in the CNS. In humans, pyridostigmine has an elimination half-life of less than 2 h and between 75–90% of the absorbed dose is excreted in the urine unchanged after an intravenous dose. It is poorly and irregularly absorbed from the gastrointestinal tract with first pass metabolism and less than 20% of the dose is excreted unchanged. The metabolites include 3-hydroxymethylpyridinium. Physostigmine is also rapidly hydrolyzed and most of a dose is eliminated within 2 h.

The studies using organophosphates are consistent with the results of Lintern et al. (1997) with carbamates. Multiple low doses of carbamates have not been shown to produce overt adverse effects in humans, although they induce biochemical changes in mice (Lintern et al., 1995; Smith et al., 1997). The effects of pyridostigmine administered as single and multiple doses on total AChE and the relative activity against the multiple forms of AchE were studied in the mouse. It was shown that there were increased total levels, possibly due to the selective up-regulation of expression of globular forms of AchE following pyridostigmine inhibition of functional AChE at the basal lamina. It was suggested that feedback control followed increased levels of acetylcholine in the cleft. In the diaphragm, pyridostigmine (500 μg/kg) produced an inhibition at 3 h, followed by an increase, which, when enzyme activity had apparently returned to normal, sensitized the muscle to a subsequent challenge with a single dose of pyridostigmine. Smith et al. (1997) studied the profile of multiple forms of acetylcholinesterase in the guinea pig and the tissue differences (diaphragm vs brain) following a single dose of soman (27 μg/kg). They showed differential inhibition of the molecular isoforms in the different tissues and differential rates of recovery. Milatovic and Dettbarn (1996) showed that rats develop a tolerance to low doses of paraoxon that is associated with changes in affinity for paraoxon and phosphorylation of acetylcholinesterase in brain and diaphragm (Dettbarn and Milatovic, 1994; Milatovic and Dettbarn, 1994, 1996). Similarly, continuous injections of diisopropyl phosphofluoridate (DFP) for up to 14 days did not produce additional inhibition of AChE but a recovery of the enzyme in the diaphragm (Gupta et al., 1986).

For mipafox and paraoxon, which cross the blood–brain barrier, inhibition of brain acetylcholinesterase is similar to the diaphragm. Following multiple doses there is an increase in brain acetylcholinesterase at 3 h following each dose. Ecothiopate, a quaternary ammonium salt, does not cross the blood–brain barrier and probably remains extracellularly at the neuromuscular junction. Consistent with this, ecothiopate does not inhibit brain acetylcholinesterase following a single dose in vivo, although there were non-significant increases in brain enzyme activity at 7 and 28 days. Ecothiopate did inhibit brain acetylcholinesterase in vitro (Mutch et al., 1996b).

Elevated acetylcholine levels may exert feedback control on transmitter synthesis, reduce receptor density, and produce secondary effects on other transmitters and enzymes. For example, functional AChE was measured in whole hemidiaphragm from animals exposed to sarin in parallel with other biochemical markers such as adenosine triphosphate (ATP), cyclic adenosine monophosphate (cAMP), cyclic guanosine monophosphate (cGMP), and calcium. Functional AChE was reduced, which resulted in increased levels of ACh. cAMP and cGMP were elevated, possibly due to ACh activation of guanylate and adenylcyclases in an inhibitory feedback loop. Internal levels of calcium were elevated and proteases activated leading to myofibril damage and a myopathy. It has been reported that neurotoxicity is associated with an increased autophosphorylation of calcium/calmodulin kinase II and enhanced phosphorylation of cytoskeletal proteins. The effects were produced by neuropathic organophosphates but also hexane and acrylamide and so probably do not reflect acetylcholinesterase inhibition (Gupta and Abou-Donia, 1995).

Central biochemical effects of those anticholinesterases that can enter the central nervous system have been clearly summarized by Lotti (1992). The number of cholinergic muscarinic receptors decreases following exposure to organophosphates, nicotinic receptors decrease with carbamates. Excessive cholinergic stimulation gradually reduces the effect at cholinergic muscarinic receptors, possibly by adaptation at the receptor level from desensitization or reduction in receptor density. There is a correlation between central neurotransmitter changes and incapacitation produced by soman. An increasing amount of experimental evidence suggests that excitatory amino acids (EAAs) are involved in the brain lesions observed after severe intoxication with soman. Jacobsson et al. (1997) studied the acute actions of soman, and the glutamatergic receptor agonists, kainic acid and N-methyl-d-aspartate (NMDA), on striatal release of dopamine and amino acids. The compounds were administered in high (10 mM) concentrations by unilateral intrastriatal microdialysis perfusion and the rats were observed for toxic signs related to convulsions. The glial fibrillary acidic protein (GFAP) was monitored as a marker of neurotoxicity in parts of the prefrontal cortex, hippocampus, striatum, and cerebellum. Acetylcholinesterase inhibition in six brain regions was measured after soman perfusion in order to assess the cerebral distribution. The soman perfusion induced a major release of dopamine, gamma-aminobutyric acid (GABA) and aspartate in the striatum. Kainic acid also induced a release of dopamine and aspartate. NMDA was not as potent an inducer of striatal neurotransmitter release as soman and kainic acid. Soman and kainic acid perfusion produced convulsive behavior in the rats. The main neurochemical event in the striatum during soman- and kainate-induced convulsions is the release of dopamine. Jacobsson et *al.* (1997) suggested that this major dopamine release might be as important as an increase in EAAs in the cascade of pathological events leading to the brain damage in the striatum observed after soman intoxication.

Deshpande *et al.* (1995) used primary neuronal cultures to evaluate the intrinsic toxicity of soman and the efficacy of potential countermeasures. The association between soman toxicity, glutamate hyperactivity and neuronal death in the central nervous system was investigated in primary dissociated cell cultures from rat hippocampus and cerebral neocortex. Exposure of cortical or hippocampal neurons to glutamate for 30 min produced neuronal death in almost 80% of the cells examined at 24 h. Hippocampal neurons exposed to soman for 15–120 min at 0.1 μM concentration caused almost complete inhibition ($\geq$90%) of acetylcholinesterase but there was no evidence of a loss in cell viability, suggesting a lack of direct cytotoxicity. Neither acetylcholine (0.1 mM), alone nor a combination of ACh and soman potentiated glutamate toxicity in hippocampal neurons. Memantine, a drug used in the treatment of Parkinson's disease, spasticity, and other brain disorders significantly protected hippocampal and cortical neurons in culture against glutamate and NMDA excitotoxicity. In rats, a single dose of memantine (18 mg/kg) administered 1 h prior to a subcutaneous injection of a 0.9 LD$_{50}$ dose of soman reduced the severity of convulsions and increased survival, but was accompanied by neuronal loss in the frontal cortex, piriform cortex, and hippocampus.

Acute pretreatment with physostigmine and hyoscine prevents changes in brain neurochemistry induced by organophosphates, measured as acetylcholine, noradrenaline, dopamine turnover (DOPAC/DA), 5HT turnover (5HIAA/5HT), aspartate transaminase (AST) and GABA. Increases in neurotransmitters are probably a secondary effect in response to the raised acetylcholine levels.

A number of biochemical effects do occur as the result of acute, severe AChE inhibition, but it has not been confirmed whether these also occur following low-level chronic exposure to specific anticholinesterases, when the level of inhibition is low. Confirmation of these toxic effects in humans and their implications for the health risks following prolonged low-level exposure to these compounds are more difficult to determine. Similarly, it is not clear whether the biochemical changes that produce electrophysiological or histological changes are associated with clinical effects.

Electrophysiological aspects of toxicity

The acute electrophysiological effects on the nervous system following exposure to organophosphates are well recognized and have been documented in great detail. The central and peripheral nervous systems are both affected, the effects probably mediated by inhibition of AChE. Initially, excess ACh causes excitation, followed by inhibition of cholinergic transmission, from depolarization block, although other mechanisms may also be involved. The expression of the acute CNS- and PNS-related symptoms depends on the degree of AChE inhibition. It is not yet clear whether repeated exposure to small amounts of organophosphorus compounds can produce delayed neurotoxic effects. A study by Stålberg *et al.* (1978) would seem to suggest that repeated low-dose exposure in workers using organophosphorus pesticides can produce a mild motor and sensory neuropathy.

An increase in jitter is also commonly seen in both humans and animals. Stålberg *et al.* (1978) studied subjects exposed to organophosphate insecticides. They found no consistent changes in jitter within 1–24 h postexposure, although some cases did have abnormal values. Four out of 11 cases had increased fiber density before exposure and no significant change afterwards. An increase in fiber density may indicate previous denervation and subsequent re-innervation. A reduction in sensory conduction velocities after occupational exposure was seen in seven subjects and was thought to suggest a mild sensory neuropathy in some of the workers. This study did not demonstrate significant disturbance of neuromuscular transmission associated with exposure but did suggest a subclinical motor and sensory axonal neuropathy in subjects repeatedly exposed to organophosphate pesticides. There is evidence from animal studies that necrosis may be induced in some muscle fibers, but this is unlikely to account for an abnormality in jitter persisting for up to 28 days in some animal studies (see below). The duration probably reflects the time needed to replace the inhibited acetylcholinesterase. However, there could be other secondary changes occurring, presynaptic or postsynaptic, affecting the physiological events controlling transmitter release, or structural components of the postsynaptic complex.

The functional significance of the myopathic changes and the relationship to any electrophysiological abnormalities seen after exposure to certain organophosphates is not clear. There is some evidence that organophosphate-induced myopathy is more severe with those organophosphates whose effects are mainly peripheral, such as DFP, than those with predominantly central effects (Dettbarn, 1992). It has been suggested that muscle necrosis is a contributor to the 'intermediate syndrome' (see below) but there is no direct evidence. The degeneration of muscle fibers typically begins at the end plate and is recognized as localized hypercontraction, segmental necrosis and an increase in plasma and urinary creatine kinase (Hughes *et al.*, 1991; Dettbarn, 1992; Vanneste and Lison, 1993). It is generally thought that the elevated ACh in the cleft causes a prolonged depolarization of the muscle fiber, the entry of Ca^{2+} ions and the initiation of Ca^{2+}-activated proteolysis (Inns et al., 1990).

Previous studies have reported long-term changes in the electoencephalograms (EEGs) of individuals exposed to organophosphorus compounds. These take the form of a relative increase in β- and θ-activities and a reduction in other activity (Duffy et al., 1979). The changes were found to persist for up to a year or more after a single large dose of sarin or repeated smaller doses (Burchfiel et al., 1976). In contrast, chronic administration of sarin resulted in a shift from high-frequency β to low-frequency θ-activity. However, these changes are rather non-specific and their functional significance is unknown. Nevertheless they do indicate that organophosphates can have a long-term effect on the central nervous system, and further studies are needed to determine the possible pathophysiological mechanisms.

In the acute toxic phase of organophosphate poisoning a repetitive muscle response is seen following a single shock to the nerve. Repetitive nerve stimulation produces an immediate drop in amplitude of the first and succeeding responses, particularly at relatively high rates of stimulation. Single fiber electromyography (SFEMG) also reveals abnormal jitter in these circumstances, both in humans and in vitro animal models. Studies on mouse diaphragm muscle preparations, pretreated in vivo with sarin and soman, show variation in the latency, or jitter, of muscle action potentials following stimulation of the nerve. The effects are seen maximally three days postsoman administration and seven days postsarin administration, and the effects may last for up to 28 days. They can be reduced by pyridostigmine pretreatment and prevented by treatment with oximes. These findings suggest that the early changes may be due to the acetylcholinesterase inhibition.

Single doses of ecothiopate (a pure anticholinesterase) or mipafox (a known neuropathic, weak anticholinesterase, slowly reversible) have differential effects on electrophysiological 'jitter' in the mouse hemi-diaphragm (Kelly et al., 1994). The effects on jitter, after a single dose, appear to relate to inhibition of total acetylcholinesterase and neuropathy target esterase (NTE) measured in brain and diaphragm homogenate at early times (Mutch et al., 1996b; Williams et al., 1997).

Multiple low doses of both mipafox and ecothiopate, and paraoxon, which do not inhibit NTE or produce a delayed neuropathy in the hen, produce similar effects on electrophysiology. This suggests that some long-term effects of organophosphate exposure may result from prolonged acetylcholinesterase inhibition (Kelly et al., 1997). The organophosphates also produce additive inhibition of diaphragm acetylcholinesterase suggesting that some electrophysiological effects may be elicited following additive inhibition. It is likely that the effect on the nerve is related to the time/degree profile of inhibition of acetylcholinesterase and so may be shared by many other organophosphates. The relevance of these findings to humans is suggested by a report of similar effects on the SFEMG in human volunteers following a single dose exposure to sarin at a dose which inhibited acetylcholinesterase by about 40% (Baker and Sedgwick, 1996). Similar effects may be produced in the central nervous system and cause some of the psychological symptoms reported by people exposed to organophosphates.

The studies by Baker and Sedgwick (1996) showed that a single exposure of human volunteers to a low dose of sarin can produce slight but significant increases in jitter. These may persist for up to 30 months, but eventually return to normal. The long-term effects are unlikely to be due to continuing inhibition of any cholinesterase since replacement enzyme should have been resynthesized de novo within a few weeks after the initial exposure. In the congenital myasthenia syndrome, which is associated with an acetylcholinesterase deficiency, secondary myopathic damage to the motor end-plate has been reported, associated with reduction of the postsynaptic folds. The postsynaptic folds contain an abundance of voltage-dependent sodium channels responsible for magnifying the effects of sodium influx through the acetylcholine receptor (AChR) channel and the production of the end-plate potential. It is possible that excessive calcium influx (which is a recognized mechanism for local muscle fiber damage) at the motor end-plate could be considered as a secondary toxic mechanism. This would damage muscle but not nerve. Morphological studies are needed on single identified muscle fibers from which the jitter was recorded.

Pathology

There is remarkably little reliable information on the neuropathology caused by exposure to organophosphate anticholinesterases. It is generally acknowledged that the acute and intermediate effects of organophosphates are largely defined in terms of their actions at peripheral cholinergic neuro-effector junctions. It is surprising, therefore, that there have been no complete studies of the changes to the terminal innervation or the presynaptic or postsynaptic structure of any peripheral synapse as a result of organophosphate poisoning. As a result, there are no morphological data to help interpret any of the physiological or pharmacological observations that have been made relating, for example, to neuromuscular transmission.

It is probable that one of the reasons for such a lack of good neuropathology is that the most commonly used animal for testing for overt neurotoxicity is the hen – an unusual experimental laboratory animal – but, whatever the reason, there remains a significant gap in our knowledge and understanding of the pathophysiology of organophosphate poisoning.

The effects of the neurotoxic organophosphates (i.e. those causing organophosphate-induced polyneuropathy) are better defined, although not at the molecular level. Wallerian degeneration of proximal motor axons, and degeneration of long spinal tracts are now recognized neuropathological signs of severe poisoning (Cavanagh, 1982). The pathogenic mechanism has not been determined but may be non-cholinergic and involve phosphorylation of unidentified neuronal sites. Pathological changes in muscle fibers adjacent to the motor end-plate have been described in experimental animals (Preusser, 1967; Ariens et al., 1969; Wecker and Dettbarn, 1976; Wecker et al., 1978; Leonard and Salpeter, 1979; Dettbarn, 1984; Bright et al., 1991; Hughes et al., 1991; Vanneste and Lison 1993). Gupta et al. (1987a, b) showed that tabun and soman exposure could produce a myopathy. Bright et al. (1991) and Hughes et al. (1991) showed that sarin had similar effects as the carbamate anticholinesterases (Rash et al., 1985), which may, paradoxically, be protective against an organophosphate-induced myopathy (Kawabuchi et al., 1989).

The severity of pathological changes correlate with high-frequency repetitive discharges generated peripherally rather than with centrally generated discharges (Misulis et al. 1987). The changes start near the motor end-plate and spread along the muscle fiber. Light microscopy shows loss of sarcoplasm, nuclear pyknosis, and mononuclear infiltration. Ultrastructural changes include hypercontraction and gross disruption of sarcomeres with loss of A and Z bands (Hughes et al., 1991). In studies on nerve agents only a small number of fibers are affected. The morphological changes of segmental necrosis are reversible and repair starts within five days and is completed at 14 days. The morphology is associated with certain biochemical changes including an increase in plasma and urine creatine phosphokinase (CPK) activity, increased urinary creatinine and increased urinary calcium-activated neutral protease (Dettbarn, 1992; Vanneste and Lison, 1993). These events may be initiated by calcium influx, caused by acetylcholine accumulation at the neuromuscular junction (Inns et al., 1990; Marrs et al., 1990). The pathological changes have been implicated in the intermediate syndrome (see below) (Senanayake and Karalliedde, 1992; Karalliedde and Henry, 1993).

Large single doses of soman (McLeod et al., 1984) or sarin (Kadar et al., 1995) may produce progressive neuropathological lesions in experimental animals. The sites of cerebral damage with these two compounds are different but similar in type. In the study by Kadar et al. (1995), rats were injected with $1 \times LD_{50}$ of sarin (95 μg/ kg; IM) and surviving animals were sacrificed at varying time intervals postexposure (4 h–90 days). Cerebral damage was found in 70% of the surviving animals, mainly in the hippocampus, piriform cortex and thalamus, and was most marked in those that had prolonged seizures. At 4 h following the injection of sarin significant changes were present in the hippocampus and thalamus, and later degeneration, vacuolar necrosis, hemorrhage, gliosis, ventricular enlargement, calcification, and hyaline plaques were seen in the piriform cortex, hippocampus, amygdaloid nucleus, and thalamus. Morphometric analysis revealed a significant decline in the area of CA1 and CA3 hippocampal cells as well as in the number of CA1 cells. The cerebral damage was exacerbated with time and at three months postexposure extended to regions which were not initially affected. Minimal lesions were found in animals with convulsions lasting less than 2 h. The cortical pathology was less marked than with soman and frontal cortex damage was specific to soman poisoning. Kadar et al. (1995) concluded that the changes could be related to the duration and severity of the seizures. If seizures did not occur the neuropathological changes could have been be prevented, although seizures and neuropathological changes are independent indices of severity of poisoning, and not causally related. Comparable evidence is not available for humans but, although there may be important species differences in susceptibility to organophosphate-induced cerebral damage, these studies indicate that cerebral damage might result from low-level exposure to organophosphates. The neuropathological changes described by Kadar et al. (1995) suggest that at low doses nerve agent organophosphates may induce neurochemical change which progresses and eventually results in morphological change. The review in Chapter 3 of the neuropsychological and neuropsychiatric evidence in relation to organophosphates is of particular importance in this context.

In studies with acute lethal doses of nerve agents histopathological changes are not seen in the CNS (Anzueto et al., 1986) but the situation may be different if the animals survive. In severe but sublethal poisoning, changes may be seen as early as 24 h after exposure. Following exposure to soman, for example, the initial changes seen are edema, particularly astrocytic edema, perivascular hemorrhages, and early indicators of cerebral ischemia. Neuronal degeneration or necrosis, which may be diffuse, is seen and in the hippocampus and piriform cortex discrete infarcts, with necrosis of all cell types, are found (McLeod, 1985). These pathological changes do not appear to correlate with areas where the blood–brain barrier is compromised and may be followed by an encephalopathy. The regions frequently affected are the cerebral cortex, hippocampus, and thalamic nuclei, suggesting that anoxia is a likely cause (McLeod, 1985; McDonough et al. 1986, 1989). In a study reported by Petras (1981) other regions, including the basal ganglia, hypothalamus, fornix, septum and superior colliculi, were also affected. The correlation with seizure activity, and the response to anticonvulsants, suggests that hypoxia secondary to convulsions is the probable cause (Martin *et al.*, 1985; Anzueto *et al.*, 1986).

CLINICAL EFFECTS OF ANTICHOLINESTERASES

The majority of available clinical literature relates to incidents of poisoning following exposure to insecticidal organophosphates. The acute neurological effects of organophosphates principally reflect abnormalitites of neuromuscular function, but more severe incidents of poisoning might result in the intermediate syndrome or a delayed neuropathy. There is inadequate evidence to confirm the existence of long-term physical damage to the CNS following exposure to either organophosphates insecticides or related nerve agents. However, sequential EEG studies in animals have demonstrated definite, if subtle, chronic changes after exposure to organophosphate nerve agents and, although the significance of these changes is unclear, the findings have suggested that nerve agents may be capable of producing irreversible CNS damage.

The clinical neurological effects of pesticides or nerve agent organophosphates can be classified into four groups:

- acute toxic effects;
- delayed polyneuropathy;
- intermediate syndrome;
- chronic central pathology.

Acute toxicity

Inhibition of AChE by an organophosphate causes the rapid accumulation of ACh at cholinergic synapses. The symptoms and signs of acute organophosphate poisoning can be grouped into muscarinic (largely parasympathetic), nicotinic (sympathetic and motor), and CNS effects (see Table 15.1). The latency between exposure and onset of symptoms depends on the route of exposure, dose, and specific chemical properties of the organophosphate.

The muscarinic effects result from parasympathetic overactivity and include miosis, excessive salivation and bronchial secretions, bradycardia, and abdominal colic (Grob and Harvey, 1953). The nicotinic effects at autonomic ganglia produce pallor, tachycardia, and hypertension so that the overall effect on the cardiovascular system depends on the balance between

Table 15.1 *Cholinergic signs in organophosphate poisoning*

Nicotinic	
Skeletal muscle:	Weakness
	Muscle twitching, fasciculation
	Aches and cramps
	Respiratory paralysis
Sympathetic nervous system:	Pallor
	Hyperglycemia
	Tachyarrhythmias
	Hypertension
Muscarinic	
Eye:	Miosis
	Difficulty with accommodation
	Lachrymation
Lungs:	Bronchoconstriction and dyspnoea
	Increased bronchial secretion
	Pulmonary edema
Gastrointestinal tract:	Nausea, vomiting and colic
	Diarrhea and tenseness
	Fecal incontinence
Cardiovascular:	Bradycardia and hypotension
	Atrial and ventricular Tachyarrhythmias
Bladder:	Urinary frequency and incontinence
Other:	Hyperhidrosis
	Hypersalivation
Central effects	
Confusion	Dizziness
Anxiety	Headache
Apathy	Hypothermia
Convulsions	Impaired concentration
Depersonalization	Irritability
Respiratory depression	Restlessness
Circulatory collapse	Tremor
Drowsiness	Cognitive impairment
Emotional lability	Dysarthria
Generalized weakness	Opsoclonus

muscarinic and nicotinic effects. At the neuromuscular junction, nicotinic effects include muscle fasciculation and eventually paralysis.

Acute intoxication with organophosphates has major clinical effects and includes convulsions, respiratory failure, and cardiac arrhythmias. Each of these may be associated with anoxia (Lebeda *et al.*, 1988; Millis *et al.*, 1988) and it is, therefore, predictable that serious poisoning could be associated with long-term CNS changes, both in experimental animals (Anzueto *et al.*, 1986) and in humans (Holmes and Gaon, 1956; Tabershaw and Cooper, 1966; Korsak and Sato, 1977; Hirshberg and Lerman, 1984; Rosenstock *et al.*, 1991).

Biological monitoring of acetylcholinesterase or cholinesterase has been used as a marker of exposure in humans and up to 70% inhibition can occur before serious clinical signs are seen. The clinical signs and symptoms of poisoning by organophosphate nerve agents also result from acetylcholine accumulation. Respiratory paralysis is often the cause of death in fatal poisonings (Chang *et al.*, 1990) but if a patient survives the acute cholinergic crisis, the effects are mostly reversible provided there has been no significant hypoxia. Cholinesterases have different levels of sensitivity to inhibition but whilst plasma cholinesterase is most sensitive, red cell acetylcholinesterase seems to mirror better the inhibition of neuromuscular junction AChE than plasma cholinesterase. Detoxification of organophosphates may occur by spontaneous breakdown or binding to carboxylesterases (Mutch *et al.*, 1999) and monitoring the rate of detoxification enzymes may be a predictive marker of susceptibility to severe poisoning in an individual.

Intermediate syndrome

An intermediate syndrome was described by Senanayake and Karalliedde in 1987 and is associated with a marked weakness of proximal muscles and cranial nerve palsies (Senanayake and Karalliedde, 1987). It occurs after an episode of acute acetylcholinesterase inhibition and may last for about 18 days. The clinical findings are consistent with a proximal neuropathy and, significantly, include involvement of the cranial nerves and brain stem. The patient develops paralysis of proximal muscles, of muscles innervated by cranial nerves, and respiratory muscles 24–96 h after poisoning. There may be acute ventilatory failure due to paralysis of the respiratory muscles. Respiratory failure is not seen in classical delayed organophosphate neurotoxicity (see below) in which the distal muscles are most affected. Pyramidal signs and dystonia developed in some of the patients described by Senanayake and Karalliedde (1987).

The pathological mechanisms underlying the intermediate syndrome are not understood but may involve a combination of neuropathic and myopathic toxic effects and changes at the neuromuscular junction. Electrophysiological studies suggest that there is a postsynaptic abnormality but the site has not been determined. Neurophysiological studies showed normal motor and sensory nerve conduction, with marked fade with tetanic stimulation, but not to low-frequency stimulation, indicative of a postsynaptic defect at the neuromuscular junction (Senanayake and Karalliedde, 1987). Muscle necrosis peaks after a few days with recovery in 3–4 weeks (Karalliedde and Senanayake, 1989). It is suspected that the necrosis is caused by excessive calcium ions influx into muscle cells following prolonged transmitter–receptor interaction. The intermediate syndrome is more common in severe organophosphate poisoning assessed by the severity of the initial cholinergic phase (Karalliedde and Henry, 1993).

Organophosphate-induced delayed polyneuropathy

A delayed polyneuropathy may follow exposure to a specific group of neurotoxic organophosphates (Johnson, 1975). Not all organophosphates have this property although some, which are considered safe for general use as pesticides (for example, chlorpyrifos), may produce a polyneuropathy (Kaplan *et al.*, 1993). Organophosphate-induced delayed polyneuropathy (OPIDN) is a symmetrical mixed sensory and motor polyneuropathy most severe in long neurones. Clinical signs appear about 1–3 weeks after exposure and mainly affect the lower limbs. A disabling feature may be a paraplegia, although in less severe cases there is a high stepping gait. Severely affected cases may develop a flaccid paralysis. An interesting finding is the apparent improvement of the patient from the acute cholinergic effects before the onset of OPIDN (Cavanagh, 1982). Recovery may occur although there is no specific treatment (Barrett *et al.*, 1985) and residual disability is common.

It is now commonly thought that the delayed peripheral neuropathy (OPIDN) is associated with phosphorylation and aging at the active site of a membrane-bound protein neuropathy target esterase (NTE) (Johnson, 1990; Lotti, 1990). Organophosphates, such as the lubricant triorthocresylphosphate (TOCP), inhibit NTE and produce OPIDN but do not inhibit acetylcholinesterase (Zech and Chemnitius, 1987). The histological changes seen in peripheral nerves resemble Wallerian degeneration with disintegration of axons, hypertrophy of Schwann cells, and macrophage infiltration (Cavanagh, 1954). Axonal degeneration is also observed in long spinal tracts. Neuropathy target esterase is present in many peripheral tissues including blood lymphocytes and platelets, and inhibition of the enzyme in lymphocytes has been used as a marker of exposure to the neuropathic organophosphates (Mutch *et al.*, 1992). Recovery from enzyme inhibition does appear to parallel clinical recovery following an overdose of chlorpyrifos (Lotti *et al.*, 1986). Other organophosphate insecticides are capable of causing a delayed peripheral polyneuropathy following suicidal or accidental ingestion of large doses (Minton and Murray, 1988; Karalliedde and Senanayake, 1989).

Recovery from OPIDN is highly variable and often prolonged beyond two years (Morgan and Penovich, 1978). Randall *et al.* (1997) have shown that some compounds that are not inherently neurotoxic can potentiate the neuropathic activity of organophosphates. The clinical significance of this finding is difficult to assess but it is probably noteworthy that no commonly used compound has been shown to be a promoter and the degree of potentiation of toxicity is slight.

Chronic effects of exposure to organophosphates

It is not clear whether doses not causing acute clinical effects may still be capable of producing long-term damage in the CNS. Petras (1981) suggested from the pathology found in rats injected with soman that EEG changes and neurobehavioral effects would occur and several studies have shown behavioral, psychological or electrophysiological changes after organophosphate exposure in humans (Gershon and Shaw, 1961; Dille and Smith, 1964; Durham et al., 1965; Rodnitzky et al., 1975; Levin et al., 1976; McDonough et al., 1986; Maizlish et al. 1987; Savage et al., 1988). Behavioral effects with subtle EEG changes were described in humans by Duffy et al. (1979) after exposure to sarin severe enough to cause acute symptoms of clinical poisoning. The EEG changes were not sufficiently well marked to enable immediate classification into exposed or control groups, and only became apparent after complex computer analysis of wave forms. In this study it is not clear if the authors excluded cases of severe poisonings. Burchfiel et al. (1976) described changes in the EEGs of rhesus monkeys that persisted for a year after exposure to varying doses of sarin. The changes after the larger dose were anticipated since the animals had convulsions. However, the group size was small (three per group; two controls). Similar EEG changes, a relative increase in activity, were seen after exposure to the organochlorine dieldrin. Burchfiel and Duffy (1982) described a relative increase in β-activity that persisted for over a year in the EEG of rhesus monkeys after a single large dose ($5 \mu g/kg$) or repeated small doses ($1 \mu g/kg$ weekly to a total dose $10 \mu g/kg = 7\%$ LD$_{50}$) of sarin. The analysis of data such as these is difficult because implanted electrodes were used. It is important to ensure that long-term implantation of electrodes in such animal experiments are not associated with moderate changes in the EEG activity.

Follow-up studies of individuals poisoned by very high levels of organophosphates suggest that neurobehavioral changes may develop. These include drowsiness, confusion, anxiety, emotional lability, depression, fatigue, and irritability. The studies are limited by the non-specific nature of many of the symptoms and the reliability, validity, repeatability, and sensitivity of the various neuropsychological and neurophysiological tests used (see Chapter 3).

Chronic exposure to low levels of organophosphates

There are increasing reports of chronic health problems following multiple exposures to low levels of organophosphates (Blain, 1992; Steenland, 1996). These problems include reductions in conduction velocity in peripheral nerves and supposed CNS involvement not necessarily accompanied or preceded by acute clinical signs of poisoning at the time of exposure, but the evidence in favor of long-term sequelae of acute organophosphate exposure is conflicting. Some animal studies have suggested that organophosphate nerve agents, administered in doses many times in excess of their LD$_{50}$, can produce chronic neurotoxic effects in animals that survive only because they were protected by the prior administration of atropine and an oxime. However, such experiments have no clinical relevance unless humans exposed to organophosphate nerve agents, such as sarin, survive severe acute poisoning by therapeutic intervention (Willems et al., 1983).

Many people exposed to organophosphates complain of impaired cognition, weakness and fatigue but it is difficult to identify a clear syndrome. The possibility that neurobehavioral changes may follow organophosphate exposure is a major but highly contentious issue (see Chapter 3). Similarly, observations of reduced tactile responses to vibration, reduced sensory nerve conduction velocities, abnormal EMG activity, etc. are inconsistent and minimal, and do not conform to any clear pattern (Rodnitzky et al., 1975; Levin et al., 1976; Kaplan et al., 1993; McConnell et al., 1994).

Despite the lack of firm evidence in favor of long-term consequences following exposure to organophosphates, it seems unwise to reject the possibility. It may be that some long-term effects are mediated by cholinergic mechanisms but phosphorylation of neuronal protein sites may contribute to the underlying disorder (Duffy et al., 1979). Genetic differences in the rate and degree of activation of detoxification enzymes may account for some of the inter-individual variations in susceptibility to anticholinesterases (Mutch et al., 1999). It is not inconceivable therefore that the development of long-term effects may have a genetic component or involve altered gene expression.

The situation with organophosphate nerve agents is rather different. Doses of these agents below the LD$_{50}$ can cause markedly degraded performances in behavioral studies in animals (Brimblecombe, 1974; Wolthuis and Vanwersch, 1984; D'Mello and Duffy, 1985) but individual nerve agents differ in their ability to promote such changes. Wolthuis and Vanwersch (1984) found that doses of sarin and tetraethyl pyrophosphate (TEPP) at up to 30% LD$_{50}$ in rats did not cause any changes in a variety of behavioral paradigms involving higher CNS functions. Soman, at

3% of the LD_{50}, did have a detectable effect on performance. Wolthuis *et al.* (1990) reported also that tolerance occurred after low doses of DFP, but not of soman, and there was no cross tolerance between the two compounds. These behavioral effects of exposure to single doses of nerve agents may be prolonged (McDonough *et al.*, 1986) and the clear implication is that the degradation of human performance may occur at low doses of particular organophosphates.

It is commonly stated that a delayed neuropathy is not seen following exposure to low doses of the organophosphate nerve agents (for example, Anderson and Dunham, 1985; Parker *et al.*, 1988; Hodgetts, 1991; Maynard *et al.*, 1991; Henderson *et al.*, 1992; Maynard and Beswick, 1992). One reason, it is suggested, may be that the concentrations of nerve agent required to produce AChE inhibition are low compared to those required for inhibition of NTE. This is not the case with the neuropathic organophosphates, such as mipafox or DFP, and is not always the case with organophosphate nerve agents. Husain *et al.* 1995 found that hens treated with equipotent doses of mipafox (10 mg/kg, sc), sarin (50 μg/kg, sc) or parathion (1 mg/kg, sc) daily for 10 days exhibited severe, moderate and no ataxia, respectively, on the 14th day after the start of exposure. The activity of NTE was significantly inhibited in the brain, spinal cord, and platelets of hens treated with the mipafox or sarin, whereas no change was noticed with parathion treatment. All three compounds significantly inhibited AChE activity in the platelets. The spinal cord of hens treated with mipafox, sarin or parathion showing axonal degeneration was marked, moderate and none, respectively. It is concluded that repeated administration of equitoxic doses of mipafox, sarin and parathion to hens cause marked, moderate and no delayed polyneuropathy, respectively.

Gordon *et al.* (1983) measured the concentrations of various organophosphates required to produce 50% inhibition *in vitro* of AChE and NTE. The ratio AChE:NTE was 1.8 for mipafox, 1.1 for DFP, but 0.0056 for sarin, 0.0012 for soman, 0.0005 for tabun, and 10^6 for VX. Johnson *et al.* (1985) have shown that a negligible proportion of soman-inhibited NTE from hen brain and spinal cord undergoes the necessary aging reaction and soman-dosed birds do not develop a delayed polyneuropathy. Indeed, soman protected hens against the neuropathic effects of DFP.

Baker and Sedgewick (1996) have observed abnormal values of EMG jitter in military volunteers following a very low exposure to sarin. The exposure resulted in the inhibition of acetylcholinesterase activity by around 40%. These changes had returned to normal within two years.

A degree of tolerance to organophosphates occurs (for example, DFP) (Lim *et al.*, 1987) which may be due to down regulation of postsynaptic receptors or reduced sensitivity of presynaptic functions. However,

most of the differences in symptoms between the main nerve agents are probably due to differences in kinetics and distribution. Kinetic differences between the different stereoisomers of soman have been reported (Benschop *et al.*, 1987). Consequently, formulations of nerve agents from different sources may differ significantly in their toxicity.

Chronic ophthalmological effects

The recognized acute effect of an organophosphate on the eye is miosis. However, some long-term effects have been reported in experimental animals and humans. Chronic exposure to organophosphates can produce changes in the ciliary muscle and optic nerve (Ishikawa, 1973; Uga *et al.*, 1977), reduced retinal sensitivity (Ohto, 1974), and a form of macular degeneration (Misra *et al.*, 1982). There is no evidence that long-term ophthalmological damage may follow an acute exposure to organophosphate nerve agents but the evidence with chronic organophosphate exposure to the eye suggests that irreversible damage can occur to retina and optic nerve.

Neurotoxic effects of pyridostigmine and oximes

It has been demonstrated that significant protection against the action of organophosphates nerve agents is provided by carbamates, such as pyridostigmine. It is, therefore, important to determine if short- or long-term exposure to carbamates has any significant acute or long-term toxic effects on the central and peripheral nervous systems.

An anticholinergic drug, such as atropine, and an enzyme reactivator, such as the oximes pralidoxime or obidoxime, are used in the treatment of acute organophosphate poisoning (Marrs, 1991; Bismuth *et al.*, 1992; Heath and Meredith, 1992). A sedative (such as diazepam) may be used to manage convulsions or muscle fasciculation (Sellstrom, 1992). The choice of which oxime to use is difficult in nerve-agent poisoning because pralidoxime is relatively ineffective against tabun and obidoxime may have hepatotoxic side effects Also there are three salts of pralidoxime, the chloride in the USA, the methanesulfonate in the UK, and the methylsulfate in France, which may have differing potencies. A serious problem is the relative ineffectiveness of atropine and an oxime to treat the acute cholinergic phase of soman poisoning since rapid aging of the inhibitor/enzyme complex means that the oximes cannot reactivate the enzyme.

Lintern *et al.* (1998) studied the effects of carbamates on acetylcholinesterase activity in mouse muscle. They showed an increase, at 120 h postexposure to pyridostigmine, in the activity of various molecular forms of the enzyme. It is possible that excessive acetylcholinesterase activity at some neuromuscular junctions could reduce the normal safety factor and produce an increase in jitter.

Physostigmine, a carbamate which crosses the blood–brain barrier, has been shown to induce an increase in β_2 activity in one of four rhesus monkeys exposed to subcutaneous physostigmine given over 14 days. This effect was noted after seven days and persisted for up to 12 months. The other three monkeys showed no significant changes in the EEG.

The potential neurotoxicity of pyridostigmine in short-term (up to four weeks) administration to human volunteers has been studied by psychometry, personality assessment, subject diaries, and tests of performance. No adverse effects were identified in 305 subjects. However, there are no published studies of long-term clinical neurological damage, either peripheral or central, with prolonged administration of pyridostigmine, although the drug has been used routinely, and often for periods of many years, in the treatment of patients with myasthenia gravis. Patients with myasthenia gravis who are treated with pyridostigmine do have an increase in fiber density which is more marked than found in myasthenics who have not been given this drug (Hilton-Brown et al., 1982). This may indicate the presence of denervation and reinnervation changes in their muscles, although other toxic mechanisms may be responsible.

The toxicity of the oximes used in the treatment of organophosphate poisoning is reviewed by Marrs (1991). In most cases treatment is for short periods although some patients may need longer term treatment. Little information exists of long-term adverse clinical neurological effects. There is no evidence that oximes or atropine have any use in the treatment of OPIDN.

Gulf War illnesses

Three-quarters of a million service personnel were involved in the Persian Gulf War (1991). It is estimated that 30 000 have complained subsequently of neurological symptoms of unknown nature and causation. One contributing factor may have been simultaneous exposure to the many compounds used as prophylactics, in particular, pyridostigmine bromide (in nerve agent pretreatment set (NAPS)), the insect repellent DEET (N,N-diethyl-m-toluamide), and the insecticide permethrin (3-(2,2-dichloro-ethenyl)-2,2-dimethylcyclopropanecarboxylic acid (3-phenoxyphenyl) methyl ester) (Abou-Donia et al., 1996). Neurotoxicity in hens following individual or simultaneous exposure to these agents (five days per week for two months to 5 mg/kg/day PB in water, po; 500 mg/kg/day DEET, neat, sc.;

and 500 mg/kg/day permethrin in corn oil, sc.) was reported by Abou-Donia et al. (1996). At these doses, exposure to the single compounds caused minimal toxicity but combinations of two agents produced greater neurotoxicity that was further enhanced following concurrent administration of all three agents. It was suggested that competition for liver and plasma esterases by these three compounds leads to decreased breakdown and increased transport to nervous tissue. Carbamylation of peripheral esterases by pyridostigmine would reduce hydrolysis of DEET and permethrin and increase their bioavailability. The hens exposed to a combination of the three agents exhibited neuropathological lesions with characteristics similar to those previously reported in studies with near-lethal doses of DEET and permethrin. The study also suggested that individuals with low plasma esterase activity may be predisposed to develop neurological damage following exposure to such mixtures.

The conclusions drawn from this study and the relevance proposed to the etiology of 'Gulf War Illness' has not been widely accepted. Indeed, it is difficult to determine a single causative agent or mechanism for the variety of symptoms, signs and illnesses reported by Gulf War veterans.

CONCLUSION

There is evidence from experimental research and, more recently, human volunteer studies that exposure to organophosphates can have long-term toxic effects on the peripheral nervous system and skeletal muscle in animals and humans (Marrs, 1993). The toxic mechanisms have not been clearly established for any of these effects but probably involve more than just inhibition of cholinesterases. Information about long-term toxic effects on the central nervous system is more limited but evidence does exists of neurobehavioral changes following repeated exposures and some functional and pathological changes (Lotti, 1992).

The implications of potential long-term adverse health effects of any organophosphate is of considerable concern and is most serious for individuals, such as sheep dippers, exposed to these compounds on a regular basis. Chemical weapons are deployed with the intention of producing a lethal outcome but the increasing effectiveness of medical countermeasures and resuscitation techniques suggests that many military personnel exposed to an organophosphate nerve agent may well survive and make a full recovery. Unfortunately, there is now also an increased risk of exposure to non-lethal concentrations of nerve agent from terrorist use as occurred in Japan. Exposed civilians may only develop symptoms of mild poisoning before recovering. In both of these situations it will be very important to assess the risks and clinical significance of any long-term adverse health effects.

REFERENCES

Abou-Donia, M.B., Wilmarth, K.R., Jensen, K.F., Oehme, F.W. and Kurt, T.L. 1996: Neurotoxicity resulting from coexposure to pyridostigmine bromide, deet, and permethrin: implications of Gulf War chemical exposures. *Journal of Toxicology and Environmental Health*, **48**, 35–56.

Anderson, R.J. and Dunham, C.B. 1985: Electrophysiologic changes in peripheral nerve following repeated exposure to organophosphorus agents. *Archives of Toxicology*, **58**, 97–101.

Anzueto A., Berdine G.G., Moore, G.T. *et al.* 1986: Pathophysiology of soman intoxication in primates. *Toxicology and Applied Pharmacology*, **86**, 56–68.

Ariens, A.T., Wolthuis, O.L. and Van Bentham R.M.J. 1969: Reversible necrosis at the end-plate region in striated muscles of the rat poisoned with cholinesterase inhibitors. *Experientia*, **1**, 57–9.

Baker, D.J. and Sedgwick, E.M. 1996: Single fiber electromyographic changes in man after organophosphate exposure. *Human and Experimental Toxicology*, **15**, 369–75.

Barrett, D.S., Oehme, F.W. and Kruckenberg, S.M. 1985: A review of organophosphorus ester-induced delayed neurotoxicity. *Veterinary and Human Toxicology*, **27**, 22–37.

Benschop, H.P., Bijleveld, E.C., de Long, L.P.A., van der Wiel, H.J. and van Helden, H.P.M. 1987: Toxicokinetics of the four stereoisomers of the nerve agent soman in atropinized rats – influence of a soman simulator. *Toxicology and Applied Pharmacology*, **90**, 490–500.

Bismuth, C., Inns, R.H. and Marrs, T.C. 1992: Efficacy, toxicity and clinical use of oximes in anticholinesterase poisoning. In: *Clinical and Experimental Toxicology of Organophosphates and Carbamates*, Ballantyne, B. and Marrs, T.C. (eds), pp 555–77. Oxford: Butterworth-Heinemann.

Blain, P.G. 1992: Long-term effects of organophosphate pesticides. *Human and Experimental Toxicology*, **11**, 560–1.

Bright, J.E., Inns, R.H., Tuckwell, N.J., Griffiths, G.D. and Marrs, T.C. 1991: A histochemical study of changes observed in the mouse diaphragm after organophosphate poisoning. *Human and Experimental Toxicology*, **10**, 9–14.

Brimblecombe, R.W. 1974: *Drug Actions in Cholinergic Systems*, pp 64–132. New York: MacMillan.

Burchfiel, J.L. and Duffy, F.H. 1982: Organophosphate neurotoxicity: chronic effects of sarin on the electroencephalogram of monkey and man. *Neurobehavioural Toxicology and Teratology*, **4**, 767–78.

Burchfiel, J.L., Duffy, F.H. and Sim, V.M. 1976: Persistent effects of sarin and dieldrin upon the primate electroencephalogram. *Toxicology and Applied Pharmacology*, **35**, 365–79.

Butler, A.M. and Murray, M. 1997: Biotransformation of parathion in human liver: participation of CYP3A4 and its inactivation during microsomal parathion oxidation. *Journal of Pharmacology and Experimental Therapeutics*, **280**, 966–73.

Cavanagh, J.B. 1954: The toxic effects of tri-ortho-cresyl phosphate on the nervous system *Journal of Neurology, Neurosurgery and Psychiatry*, **17**, 163–72.

Cavanagh, J.B. 1982: Mechanisms of axon degeneration in three toxic 'neuropathies': organophosphorus, acrylamide and hexacarbon compared. In: *Recent Advances in Neuropathology*, Smith, W.T. and Cavanagh, J.B. (eds), Vol. 2, pp 213–41. Edinburgh: Churchill-Livingstone.

Chang, F.C., Foster, R.E., Beers, E.T., Rickett, D.L. and Filbert, M.G. 1990: Neurophysiological concomitants of soman-induced respiratory depression in awake, behaving guinea pigs. *Toxicology and Applied Pharmacology*, **102**, 233–50.

Churchill, L., Pazdernik, T.L., Cross, R.S., Giesler, M.P., Nelson, S.R. and Samson, F.E. 1987: Cholinergic systems influence local cerebral glucose use in specific anatomical areas: diisopropyl phosphorofluoridate versus soman. *Neuroscience*, **20**, 329–39.

Davies, H., Richter, M.F., Broomfield, C.A., Sowalla, J. and Furlong, C.E. 1996: The effect of the human serum paraoxonase polymorphism is reversed with diazoxon, soman and sarin. *Nature Genetics*, **14**, 334–6.

Deshpande, S.S., Smith, C.D. and Filbert, M.G. 1995: Assessment of primary neuronal culture as a model for soman-induced neurotoxicity and effectiveness of memantine as a neuroprotective drug. *Archives of Toxicology*, **69**, 384–90.

Dettbarn, W.D. 1984: Pesticide-induced muscle necrosis: mechanisms and prevention. *Fundamental and Applied Toxicology*, **4**, S18–S26.

Dettbarn, W.D. 1992: Anticholinesterase induced myonecrosis. In: *Clinical and Experimental Toxicology of Organophosphates and Carbamates*, Ballantyne, B. and Marrs, T.C. (eds), pp 151–60. Oxford: Butterworth-Heinemann.

Dettbarn, W.D. and Milatovic, D. 1994: Changes in acetylcholinesterase kinetics following prolonged treatment with paraoxon. Abstract SOT Dallas, TX.

Dille, J.R. and Smith, P.W. 1964: Central nervous system effects of chronic exposure to organophosphate insecticides. *Aerospace Medicine*, **6**, 475–8.

D'Mello, G.D. and Duffy, E.A.M. 1985: The acute toxicity of sarin in marmosets (*Callithrix jacchus*): a behavioral analysis. *Fundamental and Applied Toxicology*, **5**, S169–74.

Due, A.H., Trap, H.C., Langenberg, J.P. and Benschop, H.P. 1994: Toxicokinetics of soman stereoisomers after subcutaneous administration to atropinized guinea pigs. *Archives of Toxicology*, **68**, 60–3.

Duffy, F.H., Burchfiel, J.L., Bartels, P.H., Gaon, M. and Sim, V.M. 1979: Long-term effects of an organophosphate upon the human electroencephalogram. *Toxicology and Applied Pharmacology*, **47**, 161–76.

Durham, W.F., Wolfe, H.R. and Quinby, G.E. 1965: Organophosphorus insecticides and mental alertness. Studies in exposed workers and in poisoning cases. *Archives of Environmental Health*, **10**, 55–66.

Friedman, A., Kaufer, D., Shemer, J., Hendler, I., Soreq, H. and Tur-Kjaspa.I. 1996: Pyridostigmine brain penetration under stress enhances neuronal excitability and induces early immediate transcriptional response. *Nature Medicine*, **2**, 1282–5.

Gaustad, R., Johnsen, H. and Fonnum, F. 1991: Carboxylesterases in guinea pig. *Biochemical Pharmacology*, **42**, 1335–43.

Gershon, S. and Shaw, F.H. 1961: Psychiatric sequelae of chronic exposure to organophosphorus insecticides. *Lancet*, **i**, 1371–4.

Gordon, J.J., Inns, R.H., Johnson, M.K. *et al.* 1983: The delayed neuropathic effects of nerve agents and some other organophosphorus compounds. *Archives of Toxicology*, **52**, 71–82.

Gray, A.P. 1984: Design and structure-activity relationships of antidotes to organophosphorus anticholinesterase agents. *Drug Metabolism Reviews*, **15**, 557–89.

Grob, D. and Harvey, A.M. 1953: The effects and treatment of nerve gas poisoning. *American Journal of Medicine*, **14**, 52–63.

Gupta, R.C., Patterson, G.T. and Dettbarn, W.D. 1986: Mechanisms of toxicity and tolerance to diisopropylphosphorofluoridate at the neuromuscular junction. *Toxicology and Applied Pharmacology*, **84**, 541–50.

Gupta, R.C., Patterson, G.T. and Dettbarn, W.D. 1987a: Acute tabun toxicity; biochemical and histochemical consequences in brain and skeletal muscles of rats. *Toxicology*, **46**, 329–41.

Gupta, R.C., Patterson, G.T. and Dettbarn, W.D. 1987b: Biochemical and histochemical alterations following acute soman intoxiciation in the rat. *Toxicology and Applied Pharmacology*, **87**, 393–402.

Gupta, R.P. and Abou-Donia, M.B. 1995: Neurofilament phosphorylation and calmodolin binding by Ca/calmodulin-dependent protein kinase in the brain subcellular fractions of DFP-treated hen. *Neurochemical Research*, **20**, 1095–105.

Heath, A.J.W. and Meredith, T. 1992: Atropine in the management and anticholinesterase activity. In: *Clinical and Experimental Toxicology of Organophosphates and Carbamates*, Ballantyne, B. and Marrs, T.C. (eds), pp 543–54. Oxford: Butterworth-Heinemann.

Henderson, J.D., Higgins, R.J., Dacre, J.C. and Wilson, B.W. 1992: Neurotoxicity of acute and repeated treatments of tabun, paraoxon, diisopropyl fluorophosphate and isofenphos to the hen. *Toxicology*, **72**, 117–29.

Hilton-Brown, P., Stalberg, E.V. and Osterman, P.O. 1982: Signs of reinnervation in myasthenia gravis. *Muscle and Nerve*, **5**, 215–21.

Hirshberg, A. and Lerman, Y. 1984: Clinical problems in organophosphate poisoning: the use of a computerized information system. *Fundamental and Applied Toxicology*, **4**, S209–14.

Hodgetts, T.J. 1991: Update box. *British Medical Journal*, **302**, 398.

Holmes, J.H. and Gaon, M.D. 1956: Observations on acute and multiple exposure to anticholinesterase agents. *Transactions of the American Clinical and Chemical Association*, **68**, 86–103.

Hughes, J.N., Knight, R., Brown, R.F.R. and Marrs, T.C. 1991: Effects of experimental sarin intoxication on the morphology of the mouse diaphragm: a light and electron microscopical study. *International Journal of Experimental Pathology*, **72**, 195–209.

Husain, K., Pant, S.C., Raza, S.K., Singh, R. and Das Gupta, S. 1995: A comparative study of delayed neurotoxicity in hens following repeated administration of organophosphorus compounds. *Indian Journal of Physiology and Pharmacology*, **39**, 47–50.

Inns, R.H., Tuckwell, N.J., Bright, J.E. and Marrs, T.C. 1990: Histochemical demonstration of calcium accumulation in muscle fibres after experimental organophosphate poisoning. *Human Experimental Toxicology*, **9**, 242–50.

Ishikawa, S. 1973: Chronic optico-neuropathy due to environmental exposure of organophosphate pesticides (Saku disease). Clinical and experimental study. *Acta Society of Ophthalmology, Japan*, **77**, 1835–86.

Jacobsson, S.O., Casse, G.E., Karlsson, B.M., Sellstrom, A. and Persson, S.A. 1997: Release of dopamine, GABA and EAA in rats during intrastriatal perfusion with kainic acid, NMDA and soman: a comparative microdialysis study. *Archives of Toxicology*, **71**, 756–65.

Johnson, M.K. 1975: The delayed neuropathy caused by some organophosphorus esters: mechanism and challenge. *Critical Reviews in Toxicology*, **3**, 289–316.

Johnson, M.K. 1990: Organophosphate and delayed neuropathy – is NTE alive and well? *Toxicology and Applied Pharmacology*, **102**, 385–99.

Johnson, M.K., Willems, J.L., de Bisschop, H.C., Read, D.J. and Beschop, H.P. 1985: Can soman cause delayed neuropathy? *Fundamental and Applied Toxicology*, **5**, S180–1.

Jokanovic, M., Kosanovic, M. and Maksimovic, M. 1996: Interaction of organophosphorus compounds with carboxylesterase in the rat. *Archives of Toxicology*, **70**, 444–50.

Kadar, T., Shapira, S., Cohen, G., Sahar, R., Alkalay, D. and Raveh L. 1995: Sarin-induced neuropathology in rats, *Human Experimental Toxicology*, **14**, 252–9.

Kaplan, J.G., Kessler, J., Rosenberg, N., Pack, D. and Schaumberg, H.H. 1993: Sensory neuropathy associated with Dursban (chlorpyriphos) exposure. *Neurology*, **43**, 2193–6.

Karalliedde, L. and Henry, J.A. 1993: Effects of organophosphates on skeletal muscle. *Human Experimental Toxicology*, **12**, 289–96.

Karalliedde, L. and Senanayake, N. 1989: Organophosphorus insecticide poisoning. *British Journal of Anaesthetics*, **63**, 736–50.

Kawabuchi, M., Boyne, A.F., Deshpande, S.S. and Albuquerque, E.X. 1989: The reversible carbamate, (−)physostigmine, reduces the size of synaptic end-plate lesions induced by sarin, an irreversible organophosphate. *Toxicology and Applied Pharmacology*, **97**, 98–106.

Kelly, S.S., deBlaquiere, G., Williams, F.M. and Blain, P.G. 1997: Effects of multiple doses of organophosphates on evoked potentials in mouse diaphragm. *Human and Experimental Toxicology*, **16** 72–8.

Kelly, S.S., Mutch, E., Williams, F.M. and Blain, P.G. 1994: Electrophysiological and biochemical effects following single doses of organophosphates in the mouse. *Archives of Toxicology*, **68**, 459–66.

Korsak, R.J. and Sato, M.M. 1977: Effects of chronic organophosphate pesticide exposure on the central nervous system. *Clinical Toxicology*, **11**, 83–95.

La Du, B.N. 1996: Structural and functional diversity of paraoxonases. *Nature Medicine*, **2**, 1186–7.

Lebeda, F.J., Wierwille, R.C., Vanmeter, W.G. and Sikora-vanmeter 1988: Acute ultrastructural alterations induced by soman and hypoxia in rat hippocampal CA$_3$ pyramidal neurons. *Neurotoxicology*, **9**, 9–22.

Le Chene, E. 1989: *Chemical and Biological Warfare – Threat of the Future*. Mackenzie Paper. Toronto: The Mackenzie Institute.

Leonard, J.P. and Salpeter, M.M. 1979: Agonist-induced myopathy at the neuromuscular junction is mediated by calcium. *Journal of Cell Biology*, **82**, 811–19.

Levin, H.S., Rodnitzky, R.L. and Mick, D.L. 1976: Anxiety associated with exposure to organophosphate compounds. *Archives of General Psychiatry*, **33**, 225–8.

Ligtenstein, D.A. 1984: *On the Synergism of the Cholinesterase Reactivating Bispyridinium-Aldoxime HI-6 and Atropine in the Treatment of Organophosphate Intoxications in the Rat. MD Thesis.* The Netherlands: University of Leyden.

Lim, D.K., Hoskins, B. and Ho, I.K. 1987: Evidence for the involvement of presynaptic cholinergic functions in tolerance to diisopropyl fluorophosphate. *Toxicology and Applied Pharmacology*, **90**, 465–76.

Lintern, M.C., Smith, M.E. and Ferry, C.B. 1995: The effect of repeated treatment with pyridostigmine on the activity of acetylcholinesterase molecular forms in mouse skeletal muscle. *British Journal of Pharmacology*, **116**, 814.

Lintern, M.C., Smith, M.E. and Ferry, C.B. 1997: Effect of repeated treatment with pyridostigmine on acetylcholinesterase in mouse muscles. *Human and Experimental Toxicology*, **16**, 158–255.

Lintern, M.C., Wetherell, J.R. and Smith, M.E. 1998: Differential recovery of acetylcholinesterases in guinea pig muscle and brain regions after soman treatment. *Human and Experimental Toxicology*, **17**, 157–62.

Lotti, M. 1990: Scientific basis for risk assessment and biological monitoring for organophosphorus-induced polyneuropathy. In: *Basic Science in Toxicology, Proceedings of the 5th International Congress of Toxicology, Brighton*, Volans, G.N., Sims, J., Sullivan, F.M. and Turner, P. (eds), pp 133–42. London: Taylor and Francis.

Lotti, M. 1992: Central neurotoxicity and behavioural effects of anticholinesterases. In: *Clinical and Experimental Toxicology of Organophosphates and Carbamates*, Ballantyne, B. and Marrs, T.C. (eds), pp 75–83. Oxford: Butterworth-Heinemann.

Lotti, N., Moretto, A., Zoppellari, R., Dianese, R., Rizzutto, N. and Barusco, G. 1986: The inhibition of lymphocyte NTE predicts the development of OPIDN. *Archives of Toxicology*, **59**, 176–80.

Maizlish, N., Schenker, M., Weisskopf, C., Seiber, J. and Samuels, S. 1987: A behavioral evaluation of pest control workers with short-term, low-level exposure to the organophosphate diazinon. *American Journal of Industrial Medicine*, **12**, 153–72.

Mantle, D., Saleem, M.A., Wilkins, R.M. and Williams, F. M. 1997: Effect of pirimiphos-methyl on proteolytic enzyme activities in rat heart, kidney, brain, and liver tissues *in vivo*. *Clinica Chimica Acta*, **262**, 89–97.

Marrs, T.C. 1991: Toxicology of oximes used in treatment of organophosphate poisoning. *Adverse Drug Reactions and Toxicological Reviews*, **10**, 61–72.

Marrs, T.C. 1993: Organophosphate poisoning. *Pharmacology and Therapeutics*, **58**, 51–66.

Marrs, T.C., Bright, J.E., Inns, R.H. and Tuckwell, N.J. 1990: Histochemical demonstration of calcium influx into mouse diaphragms induced by sarin. *Toxicologist*, **10**, 132.

Martin, L.J., Doebbler, J.A., Shih, T-M. and Anthony, A. 1985: Protective effect of diazepam pretreatment of soman-induced brain lesion formation. *Brain Research*, **325**, 287–9.

Maxwell, D.M. and Lenz, D.E. 1992: Structure-activity relationships and anticholinesterse activity. In: *Clinical and Experimental Toxicology of Organophosphates and Carbamates*, Ballantyne, B. and Marrs, T.C. (eds), pp 47–58. Oxford: Butterworth-Heinemann.

Maynard, R.L. and Beswick, F.W. 1992: Organophosphorus compounds as chemical warfare agents. In: *Clinical and Experimental Toxicology of Organophosphates and Carbamates*, Ballantyne, B. and Marrs, T.C. (eds), pp 373–85. Oxford: Butterworth-Heinemann.

Maynard, R.L., Marrs, T.C. and Johnson, M.K. 1991: Organophosphorus poisoning (letter). *British Medical Journal*, **302**, 963.

McConnell, R., Keifer, M. and Rosenstock, L. 1994: Elevated quantitative vibrotactile threshild among workers previously poisoned with methamidophos and other organophosphate pesticides. *American Journal of Industrialized Medicine*, **25**, 325–34.

McDonough, J.H., Jaax, N.K., Crowley, R.A., Mays, M.Z. and Modrow, H.E. 1989: Atropine and/or diazepam therapy protects against soman-induced neurla and cardiac pathology. *Fundamental and Applied Toxicology*, **13**, 256–76.

McDonough, J.H., Smith, R.F. and Smith, C.D. 1986: Behavioural correlates of soman-induced neuropathology: deficits in DRL acquisition. *Behavioral Toxicology and Teratology*, **8**, 179–87.

McLeod, C.G. 1985: Pathology of nerve agents: perspectives on medical management. *Fundamental and Applied Toxicology*, **5**, S10–16.

McLeod, C.G., Singer, A.W. and Harrington, D.G. 1984: Acute neuropathology in soman-poisoned rats. *Neurotoxicology*, **5**, 53–8.

Milatovic, D. and Dettbarn, W.D. 1994: Changes in affinity and phosphorylation constants regulating inhibition of acetylcholinesterase in paraoxon tolerant rats. Abstract SOT, Dallas, TX.

Milatovic, D. and Dettbarn, W.D. 1996: Modification of acetylcholinesterase during adaptation to chronic, subacute paraoxon application in rat. *Toxicology and Applied Pharmacology*, **136**, 20–8.

Millis, R.M., Archer, P.W., Whittaker, J.A. and Trouth, C.O. 1988: The role of hypoxia in organophosphorus intoxication. *Neurotoxicology*, **9**, 273–86.

Minton, N.A. and Murray, V.S.G. 1988: A review of organophosphate poisoning. *Medical Toxicology*, **3**, 350–75.

Misra, V.K., Nag, D., Misra, N.K. and Krishna Murti, C.R. 1982: Macular degeneration associated with chronic insecticide exposure. *Lancet*, **1**, 288.

Misulis, K.E., Clinton, M.E., Dettbarn, W.D. and Gupta, R.C. 1987: Differences in central and peripheral neural actions between soman and diisopropyl fluorophosphate, organophosphorus inhibitors of acetylcholinesterases. *Toxicology and Applied Pharmacolology*, **89**, 391–8.

Morgan, J.P. and Penovich, P. 1978: Jamaica ginger paralysis: 47-year follow-up. *Archives of Neurology*, **35**, 530–2.

Mutch, E., Blain, P.G. and Williams, F.M. 1992: Interindividual variations in enzymes controlling organophosphate toxicity in man. *Human Experimental Toxicology*, **11**, 109–16.

Mutch, E., Blain, P.G. and Williams, F.M. 1996a: Cytochrome p450 isozymes involved in parathion metabolism in the rat. *Human and Experimental Toxicology*, **15**, 689.

Mutch, E., Blain, P.G. and Williams, F.M. 1999: Involvement of cytochrome p450 3A in the metabolism of parathion by human liver (in press).

Mutch, E., Kelly, S.S., Blain, P.G and Williams, F.M. 1996b: Comparative studies of two organophosphorus compounds in the mouse. *Toxicology Letters*, **81**, 45–53.

Ogane, N., Giacobini, E. and Messamore, E. 1992: Preferential inhibition of acetylcholinesterase molecular forms in rat brain. *Neurochemical Research*, **17**, 489–95.

Ohto, K. 1974: Long-term follow-up study of chronic organophosphate pesticide intoxication (Saku disease) with special reference to retinal pigmentary degeneration. *Acta Society of Ophthalmology, Japan*, **78**, 237–43.

Parker, R.M., Crowell, J.A., Bucci, T.J. and Dacre, J.C. 1988: Negative delayed neuropathy study in chickens after treatment with isopropyl methylphosphonofluoridate (sarin type1). *Toxicologist*, **8**, 248.

Petras, J.M. 1981: Soman neurotoxicity. *Fundamental and Applied Toxicology*, **1**, 242.

Preusser, H.J. 1967: Ultrastruktur der motorischen Endplatte im Zwerchfell der Ratte und Veranderungen nach Inhibierung der Acetylcholinesterase. *Zeitschrift fur Sellforsch*, **80**, 436–57.

Randall, J.C., Ambroso, J.L., Groutas, W.C., Brubaker, M.J. and Richardson, R.J. 1997: Inhibition of neurotoxic esterase *in vitro* by novel carbamates. *Toxicology and Applied Pharmacology*, **143**, 173–8.

Rash, J.E., Morita, M., Giddings, F.D. *et al.* 1985: Physostigmine toxicity: acute and delayed effects on neuromuscle junctions. In: *United States Army Medical Research Institute of Chemical Defense Bioscience Review*, pp 121–3. Washington, DC: Department of Defense.

Rodnitzky, R.L., Levin, H.S. and Mick, D.L. 1975: Occupational exposure to organophosphate pesticides. A neurobehavioral study. *Archives of Environmental Health*, **30**, 98–103.

Rosenstock, L., Keifer, M., Daniell, W.E., McConnell, R., Claypoole, K. and the Pesticide Health Effects Study Group 1991: Chronic central nervous system effects of acute organophosphate pesticide intoxication. *Lancet*, **338**, 223–7.

Savage, E.P., Keefe, T.J., Mounce, L.M., Heaton, R.K., Lewis, J.A. and Burcar, P.J. 1988: Chronic neurological sequelae of acute organophosphate pesticide poisoning. *Archives of Environmental Health*, **43**, 38–45.

Seagrave, S. 1981: *Yellow Rain: A Journey Through the Terror of Chemical Warfare.* New York: M. Evans.

Sellstrom, A. 1992: Anticonvulsants in anticholinesterase poisoning. In: *Clinical and Experimental Toxicology of Organophosphates and Carbamates*, Ballantyne, B. and Marrs, T.C. (eds), pp 578–86. Oxford: Butterworth-Heinemann.

Sellstrom, A., Alglers, G. and Karlsson, B. 1985: Soman intoxication and the blood–brain barrier. *Fundamental and Applied Toxicology*, **5**, S122–6.

Senanayake, N. and Karalliedde, L. 1987: Neurotoxic effects of organophosphorus insecticides. An intermediate syndrome. *New England Journal of Medicine*, **316**, 761–3.

Senanayake, N. and Karalliedde, L. 1992: The intermediate syndrome in anticholinesterase neurotoxicity. In: *Clinical and Experimental Toxicology of Organophosphates and Carbamates*, Ballantyne, B. and Marrs, T.C. (eds), pp 126–34. Oxford: Butterworth-Heinemann.

Sidell, F.R. 1974: Soman and sarin: treatment of accidental poisoning. *Clinical Toxicology*, **7**, 1–17.

Smith, M., Lintern, M. and Wetherell, J. 1997: Studies on functional AChE and its induction after inhibition (internal presentation).

Stålberg, E., Hitton-Brown, P., Kolmodin-Hedman, B., Holmstedt, B. and Augustinsson, K.B. 1978: Effect of occupational exposure to organophosphorus insecticides on neuromuscular function. *Scandinavian Journal of Work, Environment and Health*, **4**, 255–61.

Steenland, K. 1996: Chronic neurological effects of organophosphate pesticides. *British Medical Journal*, **312**, 1312–13.

Tabershaw, I.R. and Cooper, W.C. 1966: Sequelae of acute organic phosphate poisoning. *Journal of Occupational Medicine*, **8**, 5–20.

Taylor, J.L., Mayer, R.T. and Himel, C.M. 1994: Conformers of acetylcholinesterase: a mechanism of allosteric control. *Molecular Pharmacology*, **45**, 74–83.

Uga, S., Ishikawa, S. and Mukuno, K. 1977: Histopathological study of canine optic nerve and retina treated by organophosphate pesticide. *Investigative Ophthalmology*, **16**, 877–81.

UK Ministry of Defence 1972: *Medical Manual of Defence Against Chemical Agents* JSP 312 A/24/Gen/4392, pp 7–12. London: Her Majesty's Stationery Office.

Vanneste, Y. and Lison, D. 1993: Biochemical changes associated with muscle fiber necrosis after experimental organophosphate poisoning. *Human Experimental Toxicology*, **12**, 365–70.

Wecker, L. and Dettbarn, W.D. 1976: Paraoxon-induced myopathy: muscle specificity and acetylcholine involvement. *Experimental Neurology*, **51**, 281–91.

Wecker, L., Kiauta, T. and Dettbarn, W.D. 1978: Relationship between acetylcholinesterase inhibition and the development of a myopathy. *Journal of Pharmacology and Experimental Therapeutics*, **206**, 393–402.

Willems, J.L., Palate, B.M., Vranken, M.A. and de Bisschop, H.C. 1983: Delayed neuropathy by organophosphorus nerve agents. In: *Proceedings of the International Symposium on Protection Against Chemical Warfare Agents*, Stockholm, 6–9 June, pp 95–100.

Williams, F.M., Charlton, C., De Blaquiére, G.E., Mutch, E., Kelly, S.S. and Blain, P.G. 1997: The effects of multiple low doses of organophosphates on target enzymes in brain and diaphragm in the mouse. *Human and Experimental Toxicology*, **16**, 67–71.

Wolthuis, O.L. and Vanwersch, R.A.P. 1984: Behavioural changes in the rat after low doses of cholinesterase inhibitors. *Fundamental and Applied Toxicology*, **4**, S195–208.

Wolthuis, O.P.L., Philippens, I.H.C.H.M. and van-Wersch, R. 1990: On the development of behavioral tolerance to organophosphates. III. Behavioral aspects. *Pharmacological and Biochemical Behaviour*, **35**, 561–5.

Younkin, S.G., Rosenstein,C., Collins,P.L. and Rosenberry, T.L. 1982: Cellular localization of the molecular forms of acetylcholinesterase in rat diaphragm. *Journal of Biological Chemistry*, **257**, 13630–7.

Zech, R. and Chemnitius, J.M. 1987: Neurotoxicant sensitive esterase. *Progress in Neurobiology*, **29**, 193–218.

The investigation of neurotoxicity

16

The neuropsychological investigation

JOHN M GRAY

INTRODUCTION

This chapter is concerned with the role of neuropsychological assessment in detecting the long-term neuropsychological impairments resulting from the self-administration of, or the accidental or environmental exposure to, neurotoxins in individual clients. The areas of neuropsychological function typically assessed include cognition, emotion, executive control of behavior, personality, and social interaction style. The methods used when examining patients include interview, behavioral observation, questionnaires, and, of course, cognitive tests. Cognitive testing is central to clinical neuropsychology and this chapter is concerned largely with the use of cognitive tests in neuropsychological toxicology. Nevertheless frequent reference is made to other sorts of data. Indeed, one of the recurrent themes in this chapter will be the advantages of combining behavioral data from a number of sources.

To conduct any sort of systematic neuropsychological examination, some provisional inventory of the various dimensions and components which comprise mental function is needed. Traditionally, mental functions are conceived of as cognitive, conative, and emotional. The word conative means concerned with the will. The modern term 'executive functions' subsumes the selection, initiation, continuation, termination, and inhibition of physical and mental action, and thus, covers much the same area. Most psychologists and neuropsychologists have followed this tripartite division. For instance Lezak (1995) acknowledges cognitive and executive functions, and emotionality. Luria (1966) has a very similar tripartite division.

He saw the brain as organized into three systems concerned with information processing (i.e. cognition), mental and behavioral control (i.e. conation or executive function), and arousal modulation (concerned with the intensive if not the qualitative aspects of emotionality). Cognition, conation, and emotion are involved in all behaviors, but each can be conceptualized and measured separately.

Basic sensory functions (such as visual and auditory acuity, color vision, and pitch perception) are sometimes taken for granted in the neuropsychological examination, as are the chemical senses. However, they are affected in some forms of toxic exposure. Basic motor functions such as grip strength and dexterity may also be affected and so both these are discussed where relevant.

Higher cognitive process may be subdivided into higher level perceptual processes, language processes, mnemonic functions, thinking, and the more cognitive aspects of executive function. The higher perceptual and language skills at least are mediated by a large number of semi-autonomous systems or modules, each of which is capable of separate impairment. Higher visual perceptual processes include the visual perception of objects (and visual patterns) and of space. These two aspects of visual perception are processed separately, and should be examined separately. Auditory perception of language is also divided into two broad streams of processing, one dealing with segmental aspects such as the perception of speech sounds and words, and the other with suprasegmental aspects such as intonation and prosody. Segmental processing has a hierarchical structure, with separate modules for the perception of phonemes, the recognition of words, and the retrieval of semantic information. The special use of visual perception in reading combines aspects of both visual object perception and language processing.

Mnemonic functions can be split into procedural memory (including motor skills) and declarative memory (such as knowledge of facts, word meanings, etc.). Acquired functions (for example single word reading, writing or forming grammatical sentences) represent forms of procedural memory. In Luria's (1966) scheme, a functional process may be achieved in one of a number of ways, each of which employs a number of structures, some of which are activated in all ways and some of which are particular to a subset of ways. Single word reading, for instance, may be seen as the product of selecting and tuning a set of modular functions and assembling them into functional systems (Ellis and Young, 1988).

Declarative memory is the store of facts and personal memories which we can call into consciousness and communicate to others on demand. It can be conceived of as consisting of two sorts of memory: semantic memory, or our store of facts and concepts about the world in general; and episodic memory, which refers to our individual time- and context-specific memories. Both semantic and episodic memory have separate verbal and visuo-spatial components, separately capable of suffering impairment. In addition, both have separate learning, storage, and retrieval functions. It is not at all uncommon for the learning of new material to be impaired while the storage and retrieval of previously learned material remains intact.

Thinking, including all active, goal-directed, controlled information processing such as involved in problem solving, is not modular. Certain aspects of thinking are covered in the notion of intelligence. There is substantial evidence that humans have at least two intelligences, verbal and visuo-spatial. Active thinking and problem solving is by definition open to higher level discretionary control, and so there is no definite boundary between thinking and executive function. Executive functions, at least as they refer to the control of attention, mental set, mental fluency, etc., are integral to active thinking. Hence, tests like the category test (Reitan and Wolfson, 1993) are sometimes referred to as tests of abstraction (a type of thinking), and sometimes as tests of executive function. Certain aspects of personality, such as behavioral and emotional control, may be explained in terms of cognitive control processes, and may be assessed by these or other frontal tasks. However, other aspects of executive dysfunction, particularly as they relate to emotional and motivational aspects may best be captured by history and behavioral observation and reports.

There are important cognitive aspects to emotion, such as sensitivity to emotional expressions of others, accuracy of reading others' emotional states, fineness of discrimination, and so on. Nevertheless there remain certain qualitative and subjective aspects of emotion which are not captured in information processing models. The mental state examination, behavioral reports, and observation as well as structured self-reports would normally be used to capture these.

MEASUREMENT

Virtually all clinical neuropsychological examinations involve administering neuropsychological tests, i.e. formal, standardized procedures designed to measure the client's performance across a range of specified cognitive functions. There are several different types or levels of measurement: nominal, ordinal, fixed interval, and fixed ratio. Fixed ratio scales represent the highest level of measurement. These are the numbers we use to count objects with. Apart from simple frequency counts – how often this or that behavior occurred – this level of measurement is rarely achieved in psychology. At the other end of the scale, nominal measurement means simply allocating the object or event you are measuring to one of a number of categories. (For this reason, these kinds of data are often referred to as categorical.) Although numbers may well be used as shorthand for the description of particular categories (for example 1 = Christian, 2 = Moslem, 3 = Buddhist or 4 = other) this level of measurement is not really numeric or quantitative at all. For instance, it would make no sense to ask of a set of 20 people allocated to categories 1–4 on the basis of their religious affiliation as above, what was their average score on religion. Ordinal measurement exists when a set of values, such as performance by different individuals on a specific neuropsychological test, can be organized into ascending or descending order. So it is possible to tell of two scores which is more or less, but not how much more or less. Fixed interval scales, as their name suggests, do have a defined interval between adjacent values, and so it does become possible to ask how much more or less x scored than y on a particular dimension.

For a value to be meaningful it must relate to some standard. Neuropsychological tests differ on the sort of norm or standard against which the data are compared. Certain tests are designed to reveal the presence or absence of certain neuropsychological features or signs characteristic of brain damage, or of a specific sort of brain damage. These tests rely on there being human, species-wide characteristics which can be used as standards, any deviation from which is pathological. For example, all normal humans over the age of, say, four years speak a language with a (specifiable) minimal level of grammatical complexity. Only if there is some neuropsychological impairment will this not be the case. These tests yield nominal, usually dichotomous data. One example of this sort of test would be Luria's clinical examination (see later).

Other tests take as their starting point the variability that is evident in normal cognitive performance. These tests measure the performance of an individual client against the average performance of a comparable group of people of the same age, sex, language, and culture. Pathological states or impairments are seen as extreme deviations from the mean on dimensions of normal human function, rather than as distinct states. Population norms allow the comparisons of an individual's performance on a specific test against the performance of a particular defined population. In fixed interval measurement, the individual score is compared to the average for that population and deviation above or below that average is expressed using one of the various conventions for standard scoring, for example T scores or z scores. Examples of this sort of test include the Wechsler adult intelligence scale (WAIS-R) (Wechsler, 1981). In some cases fixed interval measurement is not possible or appropriate and ordinal measurement is used. In the most common system, the score is expressed in percentiles; that is the percentage of the population scoring equal to or lower than the individual in question. Ordinal scaling has the advantage that it does not require the data from the standardization sample to conform to any specific distribution.

Which type of scaling is appropriate depends in part on how the function being measured is organized. If a particular function either serves adequately or fails, thereby producing a qualitatively distinct pattern of response, a sign approach may be appropriate. One example might be drawing a symmetrical simple figure such as a star. Patients will normally be able to do this, or they will fail, showing one of a number of patterns, for example unilateral neglect. Another function, say verbal list learning, may vary continuously in power or efficiency; in this case ordinal or fixed interval scales may be more appropriate. Cutting score, of course, can be used to translate ordinal or fixed interval data to nominal (pass/fail) data.

In any case, the measure needs to be reliable. An instrument is reliable if any two (or more) measures of the same real value taken using that instrument yield the same observed value. There are a number of different kinds of reliability, two of which are important here: inter-rater and test–retest. Both imply that the instrument is applied (at least) twice to the same object to be measured. In the case of inter-rater reliability, it is applied by a different tester on each occasion. The reliability is the correlation between the scores. For nominal data the equivalent measure is 'concordance'. Concordance is the extent to which any two (or more) attempts to allocate the same set of real objects to a number of categories actually allocates the same objects to the same categories.

The measure also needs to be a valid measure of what it purports to measure. There are several sorts of validity, each corresponding to a particular sort of evidence used to establish the correspondence of the measure to the underlying trait. 'Face validity' is when a scale is held to measure a particular trait because its content makes it seem reasonable that it should do so. Of course, this is not really a guarantee of validity at all, but unfortunately, there are many neuropsychological assessments which rely entirely on face validity. Two different sorts of items may go wrong. First, the underlying trait may not be unitary – it may decompose into a number of unrelated competencies. Attention is one such construct in psychology, where difficulties in speed of information processing and in sustaining attention turn out to be quite separate. Second, the trait may be viable, but the measure may not adequately tap it, because it measures a group of traits (as in the WAIS-R arithmetic sub-test which can be affected by impairment in a number of factors including auditory–verbal immediate memory, executive function, and knowledge of arithmetic rules). An instrument has construct validity when it can be demonstrated unequivocally to measure the trait in question. Construct validity is essentially a judgement, but it can be based on a number of more formalized measures such as convergent validity, demonstrated when it correlates with other measures of the same construct; or divergent validity, when it fails to correlate with measures of different but related constructs.

For a measure to have criterion validity it must correlate with some criterion variable, such as success in a rehabilitation program. The criterion variable is measured either at the same time (concurrent validity) or in the future (predictive validity). Where the criterion variable is a dichotomous variable (such as brain damaged or not) criterion validity is measured by sensitivity, specificity, and correct classification rate.

Selection of tests

There are three ways in which neuropsychological examination of the individual client can contribute to clinical management: description, monitoring change, and diagnosis. If the assessment is primarily diagnostic, the stress will be on the pattern of deficits. However, if it is intended to guide management, a description of the neuropsychological functioning of an individual patient, stressing particularly those deficits which are most persistent and most disruptive to the client's social, recreational, interpersonal and vocational life, may be useful. What matters here is the shape and degree of the client's strengths and weaknesses irrespective of how they have come about, and there is nothing in this sort of examination that is particular to neurotoxicology. Monitoring change can help to chart therapeutic or natural recovery, to monitor deterioration, and aid diagnosis. Diagnosis in neuropsychology covers a number of issues: detection and quantification of brain disease, organic versus functional, syndromic, localization and lateralization, and even selecting among categories in differential diagnosis.

The purposes for which an instrument is intended relates to the kinds of validity that are relevant. In neurotoxicology the main issue is the detection and quantification of brain damage in the case of an individual client who has been exposed or may have been exposed to a known or potential neurotoxin, and to determine whether any brain damage is a consequence of exposure. To this end tests are selected on the basis of their criterion, and in particular their concurrent validity.

There are many hundreds of neuropsychological tests in the literature. It would not be particularly useful to consider each of the tests separately. Instead, the literature on neuropsychological toxicology is briefly reviewed, and those tests which seem to have proved useful are described afterwards. The literature is reviewed under two headings: drugs, whether therapeutic or recreational; and environmental neurotoxins, including metals and industrial and agricultural chemicals. Single and repeated acute events are covered, as is chronic sub-acute exposure. The focus is on the effects after the exposure has terminated, and any acute or, in the case of chronic exposure as in drug abuse, any acute withdrawal effects have dissipated. The assumption is that these long-term changes in behavior and cognition reflect underlying changes in brain function which may in turn relate to structural changes. Only the effects of adult exposure on adult neuropsychological performance is considered.

One advantage of neuropsychological testing is that it allows the detection and measurement of relatively subtle effects, which may nevertheless have profound consequences for everyday life. Dramatic and obvious neuropsychiatric syndromes do occur in neurotoxicology, but they are by no means the whole story. There is a danger of considering the more florid syndromes as central, and the less severe levels of impairment as a *forme fruste* of the full-blown syndrome. For instance, alcohol abuse may be associated with obvious and dramatic neuropsychiatric consequences in the form of Korsakoff's psychosis with its profound anterograde amnesia. However, the most usual cognitive consequence of long-term alcohol abuse is not memory impairment at all, but impairment in processing complex visuo-spatial stimuli. In general, both acute intoxication and the severe end of long-term effects are diagnosed on clinical medical examination. In both these cases a neuropsychological examination may be useful in describing and quantifying the impairment and in monitoring the course of recovery or decline. However, it is in detecting and measuring the chronic

non-syndromic impairment that the neuropsychological examination is crucial in the investigation.

DRUGS

This section is concerned with exposure to drugs whose primary action is on the central nervous system, and whose primary function is to change some aspect of mental state. All these drugs have both therapeutic and recreational uses. The main categories of drug discussed are benzodiazepines, cocaine and amphetamines, ecstasy, hallucinogenic drugs (including cannabis and LSD), and opiates.

The issue as to whether and which drugs when abused cause cognitive impairment is fraught with methodological difficulties. Recreational use of drugs is associated with alcohol abuse and other lifestyle factors which may compound any toxic effects, and confound any attempt to sort out the contributions of the individual substances. Also, there may be genetic and developmental factors which underlie both the tendency to substance abuse and the observed pattern of cognitive impairment. To some extent these effects can be accounted for. For instance, chronicity, unlike, say, frequency or peak daily use, is not obviously related to predisposing factors. Where studies of chronic drug abuse have shown cognitive deficits in the drug user that are related to chronicity of use, this is at least consistent with the view that drug abuse may cause cognitive impairment independently of lifestyle and predisposing factors.

It is probable that specific drugs will cause different patterns of cognitive impairment. Nevertheless, the consensus is that there is a core syndrome of poor memory for new material, perhaps especially visuo-spatial material, and poor non-verbal abstraction. There are a number of reasons why a common neuropsychological profile across many drugs could occur. First, not all neuropsychological functions are equally vulnerable to acquired brain damage. Some cognitive functions, mainly overlearned crystallized knowledge or skills such as single word reading, tend to be resistant to the effects of brain damage. To some extent the common profile might represent the same pattern of 'hold' and 'don't hold' tests evident in diffuse brain damage due to other causes such as traumatic brain injury (TBI) or aging. Second, there may be general non-psychopharmacological effects. Although each different drug may have specific acute psychopharmacological effects due to its actions on different neurotransmitter systems in the brain, this need not underpin any cognitive impairment observed. Changes in blood supply, damage to blood vessels, infections, etc. may all play a part. This is certainly the case in cocaine abuse, where at least some of the damage is due to ischemia and vasculitis. Third, any common profile might also reflect a widespread tendency to abuse a number of drugs or both drugs and alcohol.

Polydrug abuse

Polydrug abuse and/or concomitant drug and alcohol abuse are the norm rather than the exception. For instance, when Rosselli and Ardila (1996) set out to compare cocaine abusers with polydrug abusers, they found that, in their cocaine abuser group, 'most ... had also used other substances including alcohol and marihuana.' Polydrug abusers might be expected to be especially at risk. However, not all studies of polydrug abuse have found evidence for cognitive impairment in currently drug-free long-term users. Bruhn and Maage (1975) found no differences on a variety of neuro-psychological tests, including verbal and visuo-spatial learning and memory tasks, the category test and reaction time (RT), among different categories of drug user and between drug user and non-user in 87 male prisoners. The authors were confident that their subjects were currently drug free, making this a study of genuinely postacute effects. On the other hand, Grant et al. (1976) used blind ratings of the Halstead–Reitan battery (HRB) (Reitan and Wolfson, 1993) test profiles to show that 41 to 64% of polydrug users (drug free for an average of 60 days) were impaired, compared to 11 to 26% of medical patients, and 84 to 89% of neurologic patients. The high rates of impairment among neuro-logic patients may be taken as implying that the authors were picking up on genuine organic cognitive impair-ment, suggesting that there was an excess of such impairment in the drug abuser group compared to normal controls. The most sensitive sub-tests were the picture completion and object assembly sub-tests of the WAIS and the category test from the HRB. Grant and Judd (1976) performed neuropsychological evaluations, again using the HRB, of 66 drug users three weeks after admission to the polydrug study unit and found 45% to be impaired, a figure very similar to that found in the Grant et al. study cited above. Note, however, that in all these studies around half of the drug abuser group were not rated as impaired.

There are two possible reasons for the disagreement between Bruhn and Maage, and Grant et al. The first concerns the means of assessing impairment. Grant et al. allocated individuals to impaired or non-impaired on the basis of clinicians' ratings of their performance across the range of tests, and then compared the number of individuals impaired in each group. In this procedure, group means on any single test do not need to be different to produce significant differences between groups in the number of individuals with overall impairment indices in the impaired range. Bruhn and Maage compared group mean scores. If a number of

Bruhn and Maage's subjects were impaired, but this impairment was on different tests for each subject, this might not be exposed by the comparison of means. In addition, while Grant et al. used an extensive battery (the HRB), Bruhn and Maage selected a small number of tests selected for their hypothesized sensitivity to drug effects. Thus, if drug-induced impairment does manifest itself in different ways in different subjects, Grant et al. would have a better chance of picking it up. A second possibility relates to possible differences in the sub-stances involved. Brahn and Maage do not mention sedatives, while this class of drugs is heavily represented in both the Grant et al. studies.

Thirty of Grant and Judd's (1976) patients were followed up five months later, using the same evaluation procedure. Only 25% were impaired (com-pared to 45% at withdrawal). Although there was no guarantee that subjects were drug free at follow-up, drug involvement was, in general, less at the later period, suggesting a percentage of formerly impaired drug users will improve with abstinence.

The Collaborative Neuropsychological Study of Polydrug Abuse (CNSP) (Grant et al., 1977, 1978) also used clinician ratings to dichotomise Halstead–Reitan protocols into impaired and non-impaired, and looked at the previous 10-year history of use of several categories of drug. Polydrug users were more likely to be impaired, with two categories of drug – sedatives and opiates – being associated with impairment. The most common impairments were on perceptual and visuo-motor skills, and on motor strength.

Rosselli and Ardila (1996) found differences between polydrug users and controls across a wide range of neuropsychological tests, but also found evidence of pre-existing neurodevelopmental and psychosocial differences. However, a number of test variables were related to chronicity of use. These included WAIS-R digit symbol and block design, logical memory, Rey complex figure delayed recall, and Wisconsin card sort test (WCST) errors. Despite similar methodologies (group comparisons of mean scores), these results are at variance with those of Bruhn and Maage, perhaps because the subjects in this group were current users.

There is, then, considerable evidence that polydrug use is associated with neuropsychological impairment. Opiates and sedatives, especially when combined together or with alcohol, are perhaps more closely implicated. Where there is drug-related impairment, it most commonly manifests in test of perceptual and visuo-motor function (including block design and digit symbol), of new learning, and of non-verbal abstraction (category test, WCST). However, host factors play a considerable part, and not all chronic users will manifest impairment. Abstention may cause reduction of impairment in some cases, although host factors may again be involved in determining whether any effects are reversible or not.

Benzodiazepines

Benzodiazepines are in widespread if declining use as minor tranquillizers and anxiolitics. They are also drugs of abuse with both iatrogenic dependence supported by repeat prescribing and widespread recreational use. They are central nervous system (CNS) depressants and, thus, there is particular anxiety about their cognitive effects (see above). This concern is all the greater because a large number of patients have been prescribed various benzodiazepines over time periods stretching to years and, in some cases, decades. Much work has concentrated on delineating the effects of this long-term use in patients still taking the drug. Other studies have concentrated on effects immediately post-withdrawal, with few studies on long-term effects of chronic use after use has stopped.

Petursson et al. (1983) studied 22 patients during withdrawal from therapeutic benzodiazepines, comparing them to normal healthy drug-free volunteers recruited from the community, and from the staff of the research institute. Four weeks after withdrawal, patients were impaired on the digit symbol substitution test (DSST), symbol copying, and decision time. In contrast Lukki et al. (1986) found no effect on these variables in 43 long-term therapeutic users still taking diazepam, and no effect on 17 of them during withdrawal.

Golombok et al. (1988) found impairment in tasks involving visuo-spatial ability and sustained attention in patients on benzodiazepines for more than one year. Scores returned to normal on withdrawal, at least for low-dose users. Tata et al. (1994) studying current long-term users once more found impairment in psycho-motor speed as measured by DSST, as well as in verbal memory. In contrast to Golombok et al. they found that impairment persisted after six months' withdrawal. Gorenstein et al. (1995) confirmed the effects on psychomotor speed and verbal memory both in current users and after withdrawal, 10 months after. They also found effects on manual dexterity for both current and withdrawn groups.

In summary, there is substantial evidence for impairment in manual dexterity, psychomotor speed, and verbal memory in current long-term users, and some evidence for specific impairment in visuo-spatial processing. There is some evidence that while the impairments in psychomotor speed and in verbal memory remits somewhat, they are still detectable up to 10 months after withdrawal.

Cocaine and the amphetamines

Amphetamines and cocaine are both CNS stimulants, acting in the short term to increase synaptic concentrations of dopamine and noradrenaline. Cocaine has short- and long-term effects on cerebral blood flow (Volkow et al., 1988) and is a risk factor for both hemorraghic and ischemic strokes. Indeed in one study in San Francisco (Kaku and Lowenstein, 1989), cocaine abuse was the most prevalent risk factor for strokes in patients under 40. The neuropsychological effects, of course, depend on the extent and location of the damage rather than the ultimate cause. Cerebral vasculitis is also reported in cocaine abuse (Kaye and Fainstat, 1987).

One view is that long-term users currently drug free and with no complications such as stroke or vasculitis do not show neuropsychological impairment. However, long-term use of cocaine may also cause neuropsychological impairment through intermittent changes in cerebral blood flow, or other mechanisms. Certainly, Rosselli and Ardila (1996) showed substantial impairment in cocaine users in WAIS-R arithmetic, picture completion, and block design, in WCST, in logical memory and in visuo-spatial memory (RCF recall). Long-term anhedonia and anergia are also reported. Of course, anhedonia or anergia arising from constitutional or other factors may predispose towards stimulant use.

Ecstasy/MDMA

Although derived from amphetamine and closely akin to it in molecular structure, MDMA has quite different pharmacological properties. Acute subjective effects include increased sensory-perceptual sensitivity, increased depth of emotion, and feelings of increased openness to people and to ideas. MDMA acts on the serotonergic system, and, at least in the short term, has neurotoxic effects on serotonergic neurones resulting in decreased levels of serotonin in several brain regions. Assessment of neuropsychological function in nine chronic users revealed no intellectual deficits, but mild to moderate verbal memory impairment in some subjects (Krystal and Price, 1992).

Hallucinogenic drugs

This group includes cannabis, mescaline, psilocybin, lysergic acid diethylamide (LSD) and DOM. These drugs have similar acute effects including hallucinations, illusions, changes in color, depth and size perception, and disturbances of body image. Long-term effects have been suggested, at least so far as LSD is concerned. These can include a variety of visual perceptual disturbances including 'trailing' and post-hallucinogenic perception disorder. There is little evidence of any long-term cognitive impairment.

Opiates

Strong and Gurling (1991) found that most long-term users of pharmaceutical heroin showed both psychometric impairment and signs of brain damage on computerized tomography (CT) scan. However, some showed neither. Where psychometric impairment was found, it was most common in verbal memory and in symbol digit test. Fields and Fullerton (1974) examined a group of heroin users (mean length of addiction = 4.9 years) on the Halstead–Reitan test battery and compared them to a non-drug using group matched for age, sex, and education. They found no deleterious effect of the drug on group comparison. Hill *et al.* (1979), however, did find opiate addicts impaired on certain sub-tests of the Halstead–Reitan test battery (tactual performance test, tapping and category), as well as on Raven's standard progressive matrices (1988) and the Peabody picture vocabulary test (Dunn and Dunn, 1981). However, the differences on the Peabody test may be interpreted as suggesting pre-existing differences between the groups, in this case pre-existing differences stretching back to schooldays or early childhood. Since vocabulary is closely related to intelligence, it may be that the differences detected by the application of Raven's matrices in particular are suspect. More proximate differences between heroin using and non-using groups, including alcohol and other drug abuse, nutrition, and general health status, may also have an effect. One study which attempted to control for these was the CNSP. As already discussed, this massive study did implicate opiates in damage to visuo-motor functions, but perhaps only when combined with alcohol and/or sedative use.

Long-term users of sedatives and of opiates (especially if combined with alcohol) are at risk of cognitive impairment. Cocaine users are also at risk, but the mechanism may be different. In any case, the impairment need not occur in all subjects. Where it does occur, it is best detected by examining individual subjects across a wide range of functions. However, tests of motor and psychomotor speed, dexterity, visuo-spatial processing, new learning (perhaps especially of visuo-spatial material), and non-verbal abstraction are most likely to show impairment. Impairment on these measures is generally at least partially reversible with abstinence.

INDUSTRIAL AND AGRICULTURAL CHEMICALS

Potential neurotoxins are in common use in industry and agriculture. In industry, most concern has focused on the issue of organic solvents and metals, although other areas of concern include industrial gases, such as hydrogen sulfide, and fuels, such as petrol. In agriculture, most concern has focused on pesticides.

Solvents

Solvents are virtually ubiquitous in modern industry. Many workers in many industries are exposed to a large number of different varieties of organic solvent, and it is clear that at least some of them are neurotoxic. In addition, solvents are readily available and have become relatively widely abused as recreational drugs.

There have been many reports of impaired sensory abilities including reduced vibration sense, reduced auditory acuity, and impaired color discrimination as an outcome of solvent exposure. Braun *et al.* (1989) compared the performance of 29 print-shop workers exposed to a variety of solvents with closely matched controls on a wide range of neuropsychological tests and on a test of color discrimination. None of the neuropsychological tests revealed differences between the groups (on comparison of means). However, performance on the color discrimination task was significantly poorer in the exposed group, with degree of impairment related to level of exposure.

A number of studies have used a computerized battery, the neurobehavioral evaluation system (NES). Spurgeon *et al.* (1992) reported two cross-sectional studies of solvent-exposed workers. Taking both studies together, compared to controls, workers with more than 30 years' exposure showed a significant effect on a range of cognitive functions and workers with more than 10 years' showed a significant decrement in new learning. There was no indication of increased psychiatric symptomatology. On the other hand, Spurgeon *et al.* (1994) found no effects of chronic low-level solvent exposure on cognitive functioning or psychiatric symptomatology in 110 paintworkers. In this study, records allowed the calculation of exposure levels, which were generally below current recommended occupational limits, suggesting that their previous positive findings may have been due to excessive exposure. Broadwell *et al.* (1995), using a range of tests including those from the NES, found workers involved in the manufacture of microcircuits and chronically exposed to low levels of industrial solvents with intermittent acute exposure differed from closely matched controls on mood and symptoms scales and on three cognitive tests: finger tapping, simple reaction time, and symbol digit. Danielle *et al.* (1993) found that in car body shop workers older workers with a history of solvent exposure showed a decrement on tests of visual perception (pattern recognition) and memory (serial digit learning and pattern memory). Symptom scores were also greater in exposed groups, but, contrary to Broadwell's findings, there was no effect on mood, motor speed or visuo-motor performance.

Using the WHO neurobehavioral core test battery (NCTB) (Johnson, 1987), Chia *et al.* (1993) studied workers in a videotape factory exposed to a number of solvents including toluene, and found them impaired on the Santa Ana pegboard, digit span test and Benton visual retention test. There was some evidence that safe exposure levels had been exceeded. Ng *et al.* (1992) reported differences between solvent exposed and non-exposed workers on a neurobehavioral symptom list, pursuit aiming, and on the Benton visual retention test. Those with higher scores on the symptom list also did poorly on the digit symbol test. This study followed a single case investigation of a worker from the same location who had suffered several episodes of acute intoxication. The implication is that exposure may once again have exceeded recommended levels. Kishi *et al.* (1993) found a relationship between duration of solvent exposures in industrial painters and performance on digit span and block design, with those workers also exposed to toluene also showing reduced scores on the Santa Ana pegboard and the Benton visual retention test. There were also differences between painters and controls on a symptom checklist, including differences on items relating to depression and irritability. Escalona *et al.* (1995) found differences on similar variables (mood states, simple reaction time, and digit symbol) between Venezuelan workers exposed to organic solvents in an adhesive factory and their matched controls. With a slightly modified battery (adding finger tapping, omitting simple reaction time (SRT), and substituting the grooved pegboard for the Santa Ana). Foo *et al.* (1994) found paint formulators in Singapore poor on digit span and on the grooved pegboard.

Colvin *et al.* (1993) combined tests from both the NES and the NCBT and found workers in a paint manufacturers poor on continuous performance test, digit span and pursuit aiming, with performance related to a cumulative exposure index. Reinvang *et al.* (1994) combined tests from the NCTB, NES and other tests in a study of workers exposed to solvents for a minimum of 10 years (mean exposure was 24.5 years). They again found differences in digit symbol and digit span, as well as on memory tests including paired associate learning (PAL). There were no differences on pegboard, block design, or RT, and no differences on profile of mood state (POMS).

Eskelinen *et al.* (1986) were able to distinguish between groups of patients with organic solvent intoxication and other diffuse brain damage from cerebral trauma, as well as among organic solvent intoxication, vertebrobasilar insufficiency, and headache. Optimal discrimination used both cognitive test variables (block design and digit span) and scales measuring subjective features (fatigue, sleep disturbance, and neurovegetative disturbance).

Rasmussen *et al.* (1993) used a customized battery consisting of the WAIS, paced auditory serial addition test (PASAT), and selected tests from Luria in their examination of 96 degreasers. They were careful to allow for confounding factors and found many of their effects disappeared. However, the close response relationship between cumulative exposure and acoustic motor function (from the Luria), and PASAT survived, as it did for the visual gestalt test.

Morrow *et al.* (1992) examined performance on a number of attention and memory tasks in subjects with a history of solvent exposure and their demographically similar controls. Exposed subjects had reduced digit spans, heightened interference on Brown–Peterson, and sharp vigilance decrement on the continuous performance test (CPT). Relatively poor performance on learning tasks was attributed to impaired allocation of attention.

In summary, in a number of different studies, workers with history of moderate exposure to solvents demonstrated adverse neurobehavioral effects including fatigue, emotional changes, and cognitive impairment. Performance is reduced on tests of motor, psychomotor, and information processing speed (digit symbol, finger tapping, reaction time, PASAT). Visuo-motor coordination (aiming, pursuit rotor) and dexterity (grooved pegboard) may also be affected. Visual memory (Benton visual retention test, BVRT) and certain attentional variables (digit span, CPT) are less reliably affected. A number of these studies illustrate the value of combining subjective and performance measures. Mood effects may be related to psychomotor speed. Toluene exposure may be particularly likely to cause neuropsychological impairment. Different findings are perhaps due to different levels and durations of exposure, with the different levels due to different industrial hygiene practices.

Pesticides

A number of studies have examined the longer-term effects of acute poisoning with organophosphates. Savage *et al.* (1988) compared individuals with a history of acute poisoning to matched controls. There were no differences on ophthalmic or audiometric examination. Neuropsychological examination on the HRB, however, revealed differences across a range of functions from simple motor skills to general intellectual function. Twice as many of the postacute group were overall impaired compared to the controls. The exposed group also differed on subjective and emotional features, showing greater levels of drowsiness, confusion, fatigue, emotional lability, anxiety, depression, and irritability. Rosenstock *et al.* (1991) studied workers who had suffered a single episode of poisoning an average of two years before, again using the Halstead–Reitan test. They found deficits on neuropsychological tests of motor speed and dexterity, visuo-motor speed, visuo-motor tracking (Trails A), visuo-spatial memory (BVRT), and visuo-spatial problem solving (block design).

As regards the neuropsychological effects of chronic sub-acute exposure, Rodnitzky *et al.* (1975) found no effect on memory, vigilance, language or proprioceptive feedback. Danielle *et al.* (1992) found no convincing evidence of adverse neuropsychological effects of a single season's work applying organophosphate pesticide. Even where the pesticide exposure resulted in measurable cholinesterase inhibition, Ames *et al.* (1995) found no adverse effects. On the other hand, one large and well-controlled study (Stephens *et al.*, 1995) found farmers exposed to pesticides in sheep dip were impaired compared to controls on sustained attention and information processing speed, with the impairment greatest for complex tasks. There was also some evidence of a dose–response relationship, again for more complex tasks.

Acute poisoning may have long-term adverse effects on cognitive abilities, perhaps especially in speeded tasks and those involving complex visuo-spatial processing. Studies on chronic sub-acute exposure have been much more equivocal, but with some evidence of the same sort of impairments.

METALS

Mercury

Behavioral changes are common after acute exposure to mercury, and, indeed, the behavioral syndrome known as 'erethysm' may be considered the cardinal feature of mercury poisoning. Mercury has a special affinity for the cerebellum and the primary sensory cortices, with MRI studies of victims of mercury poisoning showing particular damage to these areas (Korogi *et al.*, 1994). It is not surprising, then, that the longer-term effects of acute intoxication include prominent sensory and motor features. Motor slowness, clumsiness, tremor, loss of visual acuity, constricted visual fields, and impaired hearing may all occur.

Chronic exposure at levels not sufficient to cause the acute syndrome causes mood disturbance, social withdrawal, and fatigue. The mood disturbance is frequently characterized as depression, but irritability and subjective anger seem to be more typical and anxiety, obsessiveness, and paranoia have all been reported. Personality disturbance is common, particularly shyness and sensitivity. Obsessive–compulsive features have also been reported.

Chronic low-level exposure also causes motor slowing and incoordination, as well as cognitive changes including psychomotor slowing and reduced auditory–verbal immediate memory (digit span) (Kishi

et al., 1994). There is some evidence for a specific vulnerability to impairment of visuo-spatial memory and praxis of the left hand (Uzzell and Oler, 1986). This differential right hemisphere impairment may be based on an affinity of mercury for myelin, and the greater amount of white matter in the right hemisphere.

Lead

Like mercury, lead selectively targets the cerebellum, hence the motor symptoms. However, it also tends to cause damage in sub-cortical and basal ganglia structures. The subjective effects of chronic sub-acute exposure to lead include fatigue, headache, restlessness, irritability, and poor emotional control. The neuropsychological effects include poor coordination, reduced motor and psychomotor speed, and impaired attention, learning and visuo-spatial processing (Hanninen, 1982). Bolla-Wilson (1988) found levels of lead in blood correlated negatively with verbal and visuospatial learning, word usage, and construction. Bellinger *et al.* (1994) found impairments in certain aspects of frontal and attention function in young adults. However, although Braun and Daigneult (1991) found motor deficits related to lead exposure, they found no attentional impairment in lead smelter workers with six times the average urban blood level. The apparent contradiction may be due to different effects of developmental versus adult exposure.

Aluminum

Aluminum has long been implicated in Alzheimer's disease due to its presence in the neural plaques and tangles which characterize this disease. Also, one form of exposure (during renal dialysis) can result in a form of Alzheimer's. However, whether normal environmental exposure is involved in the etiology of Alzheimer's disease or cognitive impairment more generally is controversial. The Camelford incident provided an unfortunate naturalistic experiment on the effects of short-term exposure to high levels of aluminum when the drinking water supply in an area of Cornwall was contaminated. The official enquiry into the incident reported that no neurological damage had been caused. However, in a recent neuropsychological study, McMillan *et al.* (1993) reported that a small group of individuals exposed to the contamination showed impairment of information processing (PASAT) and of learning of verbal material (Rey auditory–verbal learning test) and non-verbal material (Rey complex figure).

Neuropsychological studies have demonstrated a relatively consistent pattern of cognitive impairment related to heavy metal exposure which comprises deficits in attention, visuo-spatial processing, abstract reasoning, new learning, and motor abilities, with relative sparing of language skills and long-term memory. Other subjective, emotional, and behavior changes are also common, perhaps especially irritability and reduced motivation. However, within this broad pattern, there are more specific abnormalities associated with specific metallic toxins.

THE NEUROPSYCHOLOGICAL EXAMINATION

There are three components of the neuropsychological examination: background information, description of the present state, and formal testing. Background information in the form of demographic details such as age, sex, educational and occupational status, and ethnicity is important in the context of scoring standardized tests. Performance on many neuropsychological tests, especially where speed of information processing is involved, decline markedly with age, and so raw scores are generally converted to standard scores using different norms for different age groups. Alternatively an adjustment is made to the raw score before comparing to the standardization sample. In some cases, there are important sex differences in performance, and separate norms for males and females are not uncommon. Performance on many cognitive tests is highly correlated with educational and occupational status. This is especially true of those measuring verbal skills, but, surprisingly, even tests of basic visuo-spatial functions such as judgement of line orientation require correction for years schooling. The appropriate norms may vary from one country or cultural group to another. Handedness should be assessed, preferably using one of the standard instruments, such as the Edinburgh Handedness Inventory (Oldfield, 1971).

Relevant medical history emphasizes those prior events with the greatest likelihood of affecting central nervous system function. Strub and Black (1985) give a good outline. This history may come in large part from referral letter, medical notes, etc., although as part of the neuropsychological examination the patient should be questioned on the neurocognitive sequelae of each episode.

An accurate and detailed history of alcohol and drug use/abuse is important. Drinkers tend to under-report their consumption, and some methods are known to give more accurate estimates than others. Both therapeutic and recreational use of psychotropic drugs should be noted. Recreational use may be particularly important since substance abuse coexists with a number of other vulnerability factors for neuropsychological impairment (Wilson and Wiedman, 1992). Substance abusers, perhaps especially alcohol abusers, are more likely to suffer head injury. Chronic high levels of substance abuse may coexist with poor nutrition, and with poor self-care of health in general. All of these may, of course, have there own neuropsychological outcomes.

Alcohol is, of course, an important neurotoxin in its own right, and its effects may confound attempts to discern the effects of, say, industrial exposure to other neurotoxins. There is some evidence that alcohol interacts with environmental neurotoxins, and that a high combined load plays a part in the genesis of a number of common neuropsychiatric syndromes (Cherry et al., 1992). It is likely that this is also the case in less severe non-syndromic cognitive and other mental impairment.

Alcohol interacts with psychotropic drugs, especially sedative drugs. Alcohol abuse and drug abuse overlap to a very large degree. Indeed the more severe the alcohol abuse, the more likely it is to co-exist with drug abuse, and the more severe the drug abuse, the more likely – and the relationship is ever stronger this way around – it is to co-exist with the alcohol abuse. It is likely therefore that this interaction plays an important part in cognitive impairment among substance abusers.

The personal history should concentrate on neuro-developmental and neurobehavioral factors, such as delay in achieving language or other milestones, clumsiness, etc. Educational and vocational history are relevant in a number of ways. The highest educational and vocational level achieved will be relevant in the estimation of premorbid intellectual and social functioning. Decline in occupational status is also important, as it may represent the effects of some pre-existing neurological or psychiatric history, or may point to history of substance abuse. Any specific educational strengths or weaknesses should be noted. The history of relationships with others at school and at work is important for assessing putative emotional and behavioral change, as are relationships with society in general, including any forensic history.

The mental state examination

Information on the current state of the patient comes from a number of sources including interview with the patient, interview where possible with a relative or carer, and behavioral observation during interview and testing. The main focus of the interview with the client will be on subjective, emotional, behavioral, and adaptive function changes. Episodic features may not manifest during interview or testing, and it is important that these are not omitted entirely from the account. For each effect, the time of onset and its relation to exposure history is crucial, as is the mode of onset as sudden, gradual or stepwise.

Where possible, both the patient and an informant (close relative or partner) should be interviewed. The addition of an informant interview not only gives a more complete cover by relying on two different sources, but allows these two sources to be contrasted. Commonly neurologically impaired persons underestimate their deficits. Extreme denial is fairly rare, but it can occur with, for example, frank denial of hemiplegia. More commonly, clients tend to underreport problems. For instance, in head injury there are systematic differences between the reports of relatives and patients with good agreement as regards physical and sensory difficulties, modest disagreement over cognitive abilities, and major differences over emotional and behavioral changes (McKinlay and Brooks, 1984). There is some evidence that relatives' reports are usually nearer the truth, at least as regards memory problems (Sunderland et al., 1983).

Different causes of brain injury produce different patterns of deficit. Motor and language disorders are common after stroke; emotional, behavioral, and cognitive changes as well as slowness and tiredness after head injury (Brooks and Mckinlay, 1983; Thomsen, 1984). In the neurotoxicological examination, particular attention needs to be paid to subtle aspects of sensory and motor function, attention, visuo-spatial processing, and emotional and personality changes.

The data should be organized in terms of the traditional mental status examination.

APPEARANCE AND BEHAVIOR

The examiner should note the patient's dress, grooming, carriage, eye contact, level of activity, mannerisms, and any unusual movements. In a neuropsychological examination particular attention should be paid to the level of consciousness, continuity of rapport, gait, posture, facial expression, hemiplegia, involuntary movements, and motor restlessness. Some problematic behaviors may not be manifest in the relatively formal and structured setting of a clinical interview. If these are to be recorded and given due consideration, this will depend on questioning the client and informant. Positive behavioral signs such as disinhibition and aggression are unlikely to be missed, but negative signs and symptoms including apathy, lack of interest in previous activities and lack of social interest, although equally important to the client's overall adaptive functioning, may not be reported spontaneously.

SPEECH

Observations are made of both delivery and form of speech. The examiner is looking for relatively low-level problems such as dysarthria, dysphonia, and dysprosody, as well as specific language problems like aphasia.

THINKING

Problems to do with the content and control of speech arising, perhaps, from disinhibition, frontal lobe syndrome, etc. are dealt with here. The examiner should note, for instance, any difficulty in shifting mental set flexibly from one task to another. One is also looking for such things as confusion, poverty of speech, perseveration, circumstantiality, incoherence, and stickiness.

ATTENTION AND CONCENTRATION

These are assessed formally, but episodic features which may be missed in formal testing are noted here.

ORIENTATION/MEMORY

Orientation is explicitly assessed in the mini mental state examination (Folstein et al., 1975) (see later) if this is used. Memory will be more formally and fully tested later but you really need to know, in order to have a sensible conversation with someone, whether they have sufficient memory to keep track of what you are saying and what they themselves have said. Also, the examiner should note how information supplied incidentally (for example examiner's name, reason for the assessment) is retained and used.

EMOTIONAL FUNCTIONING

Both the mood (patient's prevailing emotional tone) and affect (the range and the appropriateness of the patient's responses on this background) are relevant. High levels of anxiety may disrupt test performance. Depression may mimic frontal lobe syndrome. In examinations of neuropsychological mental state, particular consideration must be given to the issues of emotional lability and control. Some quantification, or at least structured description, should be attempted. POMS is the most common measure of emotional factors in neuropsychological toxicology. This self-rating instrument gives results on six dimensions (tension/anxiety; depression/dejection; anger/hostility; vigor; fatigue/inertia; and confusion/bewilderment). Norms are available for a range of comparison groups. However, neither direct questioning or self-report instruments are substitutes for observation, since any mismatch between responses to formal questioning and behavioral manifestations may be illuminating.

OTHER SUBJECTIVE PROBLEMS

Other subjective problems such as headache, dizziness, irritability, slowness, tiredness, and increased need for sleep, insomnia and fatigue should be covered using, where possible, one of the questionnaires specifically designed for neurotoxicology.

ABNORMAL EXPERIENCES

Exposure to some neurotoxins, perhaps especially metals, may cause characteristic psychiatric symptoms, including paranoia. Frank psychiatric symptomatology may be captured using any one of a number of psychiatric screening instruments, but the one most commonly used in neurotoxicology is the symptom question list – revised (SQL-90-R) (Derogatis and Cleary, 1977). In this instrument, subjects are asked to rate themselves over the last week on each of 90 symptoms. Results are reported for nine symptom dimensions: somatization, obsessive-compulsive, interpersonal sensitivity, depression, anxiety, hostility, phobic anxiety, paranoia, and psychoticism; and three global indices: severity, distress, and total number of symptoms. There is a short form (brief symptom inventory (BSI)) which generates the same symptom dimensions. Direct questioning is also used to reveal aspects of the patient's experience including the content of thoughts. Just as in other areas, direct questioning and formal measures may be at variance with non-verbal expression or behavior.

INSIGHT

The extent of any mismatch between what the client reports and what the examiner observes, or between the relatives' and the impaired person's accounts may help estimate the client's degree of insight.

Formal testing

ere are basically three approaches to test selection: fixed batteries, flexible batteries, and hypothesis testing. Fixed batteries are ready-made comprehensive batteries intended to be used with all but the most special populations (such as the blind or prelinguisticly deaf) and are intended to provide a more or less comprehensive description of the client's neuropsychological status. At one time, fixed batteries, including the various versions of Luria's clinical examination and the Halstead–Reitan, dominated neuropsychological testing.

LURIA'S CLINICAL EXAMINATION

Luria's clinical examination is the best known example of a battery using the clinical approach. Luria (1966) described a large number of procedures which he deployed in a flexible, individualized manner with an initial hypothesis which is formulated on the basis of the presentation and history, and tested, refined and re-tested by administration of the appropriate tests. Essentially each procedure is intended to determine whether a particular sign is present or absent. Christensen (1979) provided a standard administration and materials for each item, but retained the clinical hypothesis-driven features. Golden (1985) organized the material into 14 scales, with proven reliability, discriminant validity, etc. to produce in the Luria–

Nebraska battery. Of course, these 'psychometricized' scales lack the flexibility of the original. Although not widely used in neurotoxicology, some individual items have proved useful.

HALSTEAD–REITAN NEUROPSYCHOLOGICAL TEST BATTERY

The Halstead–Reitan neuropsychological test battery (Reitan and Wolfson, 1993) is among the most widely used batteries in both general neuropsychological practice and in the neuropsychological evaluation of the effects of substance abuse. There are a number of versions but all include: the Reitan–Klove sensory-perceptual examination; grip strength; the finger tapping or finger oscillation test; the tactual performance test; the speech sounds perception test; the seashore rhythm test; the Reitan–Indiana aphasia screening test; the category test; the trail making test; the Wechsler adult intelligence scale; and the Minnesota multiphasic personality inventory (MMPI). Some of these (the sensory-perceptual examination, the WAIS-R) are batteries in themselves.

The whole battery takes about 8 h to administer. Given its manifest weakness in the area of memory, it is normally supplemented with the Wechsler memory scale – revised (WMS-R) (Wachster, 1987), adding another 2 h to the time taken to perform the complete examination. Yet it by no means provides comprehensive coverage of neuropsychological functions. The psychometric properties of some of its components, the aphasia component, for instance, have been criticized, and are probably best considered as providing materials and structure for a clinical examination, rather than as a standardized test. Nevertheless the Halstead–Reitan battery as a battery has proved useful in detecting the effects of substance use. Also, individual tests from the battery, grip strength, finger tapping, and the category test have all proved separately useful in neurotoxicological neuropsychology.

WECHSLER ADULT INTELLIGENCE SCALE – REVISED

The Wechsler adult intelligence scale – revised (Wechsler, 1981) is the best known and most used neuropsychological instrument. It consists of a battery of 11 sub-tests divided into a verbal scale consisting of six sub-tests (vocabulary, information, arithmetic, digit span, similarities, and comprehension), and a performance scale consisting of five (picture completion, picture arrangement, block design, object assembly, and digit symbol). Taken together the 11 sub-tests yield a measure of psychometric intelligence. Verbal and performance intelligence quotients are also calculable. The full scale, the verbal and performance scales, and the 11 sub-scales all have known and adequate psychometric properties, and are standardized against normative samples for the USA, the UK, and a number of other countries where it is used. Although originally intended as measure of intelligence, the sub-tests are increasingly used individually to represent different aspects of information processing. Vocabulary (as a measure of premorbid function), digit span, arithmetic, similarities, picture completion, block design, and digit symbol have all proved useful in neurotoxicology. Those are described in the subsequent text.

FLEXIBLE BATTERIES

The flexible battery approach involves the production of customized batteries for particular purposes. This approach is now in favor if only because increasingly articulated schemes of cognitive architecture make truly comprehensive examination impossible. A number of batteries have been developed specifically for neurotoxicological applications.

Neurobehavioral test battery (NBTB) (Baker *et al.*, 1983)

This battery was developed specifically to measure neuropsychological effects of industrial neurotoxins. A wide range of neuropsychological tests were applied to a sample of blue collar workers who had been exposed to industrial neurotoxins, mainly heavy metals. Those which successfully discriminated exposed from non-exposed workers were included. The resulting battery consisted of 10 instruments: Santa Anna dexterity test, continuous performance test, digit symbol (WAIS), digit symbol recall, digit span (WMS), paired associates learning (WMS), block design (WAIS), similarities (WAIS), vocabulary (WAIS), and the profile of mood states (POMS).

National Institute of Occupational Health and Safety battery (Johnson, 1987)

Much of the work on the NBTB was used in the formulation of the joint World Health Organization (WHO) and National Institute of Occupational Health and Safety (NIOSH) battery. Four instruments (Santa Anna, digit symbol, digit span, and the profile of mood states) were retained from the NBTB. Verbal learning was replaced by the BVRT to allow cross-cultural comparison. Another three tests (pursuit aiming, simple reaction time, and Benton visual retention task) were added to produce this battery of seven instruments, now amongst the most widely used instruments in occupational neurotoxicology.

Neurobehavioral evaluation system (Baker *et al.*, 1985)

This is an automated microcomputer delivered battery of automated testing. Five of the tests (asterisked below) consist of modified versions of the NIOSH battery. It consists of:

1 *Hand-eye coordination replaces pursuit aiming as a test of visuo-motor skills.

2 *Symbol-digit substitution. This variant of the WAIS digit symbol test is more suitable for automated administration, since each response is numeric rather than a special symbol. It is assumed to tap the same underlying abilities as the digit symbol. This and *simple reaction time test psychomotor speed.

3 Continuous performance test tests sustained attention or vigilance.

4 *Digit span and the memory scanning test examine auditory verbal working memory, while the pattern memory test taps into visuo-spatial working memory.

5 A test of learning and memory for new verbal material, paired associate learning, was reintroduced. The pattern recognition test and the *visual retention test were used for non-verbal.

6 A vocabulary test was reintroduced.

7 Mood scales were reintroduced.

The strengths and weaknesses of automated batteries have been discussed elsewhere. However, greater standardization of presentation and scoring clearly encourages higher inter-rater reliability. Also, real time operation affords the possibility of easily collected, accurate performance data.

Pittsburgh occupation exposure test (POET) (Ryan *et al.*, 1987)

This battery contains measures of motor function (grooved pegboard), psychomotor speed (WAIS-R digit symbol), general intelligence (WAIS-R sub-tests: information, similarities, digit span, picture completion, block design), visuo-spatial processing (Boston embedded figures, mental rotation, WMS visual reproduction copy trial), learning and memory (WMS visual reproduction 30-min recall, paired associate learning, continuous word recognition, symbol digit learning), and executive abilities (trails A and B). This is a considerably more extensive battery than the WHO/NIOSH battery. It contains less on basic motor and visuo-motor skills and more on general intelligence, on higher level visual information processing, and on learning and memory. It is probably better able to produce the sort of cognitive profile which would be useful in predicting adaptation in the real world and in guiding rehabilitation. Its main strength, however, is the normative data which have been collected on blue collar industrial workers, providing appropriate comparisons, at least in the USA, for the most likely patients.

California neuropsychological screening battery (Bowler *et al.*, 1986)

Like the POET, this battery tests a relatively wide range of functions and is used, not only in detection and diagnosis, but to provide a profile of the patient's cognitive strengths and weaknesses. It includes a number of tests from the Halstead–Reitan (grip strength/dynamometer, finger tapping test and WAIS-R vocabulary, digit symbol, digit span, arithmetic, block design), the Purdue pegboard, a visual information processing test, the Wechsler memory scale and Benton visual retention test, the trail making test A and B, and a neurotoxic anxiety scale.

The hypothesis testing approach

In a hypothesis testing approach, tests are selected on the basis of their ability to examine specific hypotheses formulated on the basis of the history and the earlier components of the examination. Traditionally, the mental status examination includes a brief examination of basic cognitive function involving observation of the client's performance in simple tasks. This is best done with a standard instrument such as the mini mental state examination (Folstein *et al.*, 1975). Observation of the client's behavior, the client interview, and the informant interview will provide information not available from formal testing, including information about specifically cognitive aspects, such as social information processing and executive control. This information is used to guide the selection of formal neuropsychological tests in two ways. First, it allows the examiner to be sure that the tests can in fact be administered to the patient. It is clearly no good administering a test which is dependent on a set of highly complex verbal instructions to someone who is confused or aphasic. Second, it may reveal specific areas of concern, which guides the selection of further tests and investigations. In this way testing is adjusted to the strengths and weaknesses of the individual client as revealed in the mental state examination.

Neuropsychological testing also needs to be adjusted to the particular reasons for testing. The examination needs to cover those domains most likely to be affected by the particular exposure history. Whilst different neurotoxins have different effects, it is possible to give certain general guidelines.

1 The following domains should be covered: basic sensory and motor abilities including motor speed and dexterity, psychomotor and information processing speed, attentional and executive function, visuo-spatial processing, and new learning of verbal and visuo-spatial material.
2 Where possible, tests and combinations of tests (batteries) which are widely used for the substance or group of substances in question should be included. This has two functions: first, to allow the use of previously acquired knowledge; and second to ensure that useable knowledge does accumulate.
3 Basic sensory and motor features examined should include, on the motor side, grip strength, finger tapping and Purdue pegboard. On the sensory side, the color saturation test should be included.
4 Performance tests (i.e. those where in both normal and abnormal populations the results form a

continuous function) should be included. WAIS-R digit symbol and digit span have become more or less mandatory. Arithmetic, block design, similarities, and picture completion might also be included.
5 There is no need to do the complete WMS or WMS-R. However, new learning of both verbal and visuo-spatial material should be examined. For verbal learning, PAL should be included. For non-verbal learning and memory, the BVRT is probably best, although WMS-R visual reproduction or Rey complex figure recall can both be used.
6 Tests of attentional control and speed of information processing should include PASAT and/or Stroop. Tests of executive function should include FAS and trail making test.
7 Where possible results are interpreted in terms of premorbid estimates. The NART should be used instead of a vocabulary scale. If a vocabulary scale is used, a multiple choice format is to be preferred.

Sensory, motor, and cognitive tests

LANTHONY 15-HUE DESATURATED PANEL

The Lanthony 15-hue desaturated panel (D-15d) (Mergler and Blain, 1987) comprises 15 pastel colored discs presented in standard lighting which the subject is asked to order in terms of chromatic similarity.

GRIP STRENGTH/DYNAMOMETER

This test from the Halstead–Reitan battery is intended to measure simple grip strength. Generally, three trials are given for each hand, and with multiple trials, quite high reliabilities are achieved. However, it depends on effort. Deploying voluntary effort may be compromised independently of strength.

FINGER TAPPING TEST

Intended as a test of manual dexterity, this test consists of a counter and an attached key which has to be pressed repeatedly as quickly as possible using the forefinger. In the standard administration, three trials of 10 s are given for each hand, the score being the average of these trials. High reliabilities are achieved in most studies, but there is the occasional report of low or nil reliability.

PEGBOARD TESTS

The Santa Ana is one of a number of pegboard tasks all measuring aspects of motor speed and dexterity. In the Purdue pegboard task, subjects are presented with a board with a number of lines of holes, and with a set of small pegs. They are required to place the pegs in the holes as quickly as possible. There are three trials each lasting 30 s, one with the dominant hand, one with the non-dominant, and one with both hands. The score for each trial is the number of pegs placed.

REY COMPLEX FIGURE

This is perhaps the most commonly used non-object drawing test. Again, there are a number of scoring systems, although that by Taylor (1959) is by far the most common. Usual practice is to use the Taylor scheme to provide some numerical estimate, and to supplement with qualitative analysis according to one of the standard systems, or simply on the basis of clinical experience. With the Taylor or other formalized scoring procedures, very high inter-rater reliability can be achieved.

NATIONAL ADULT READING TEST (NART) (NELSON, 1982)

This is ostensibly a test of reading and pronunciation of irregular words. However, these skills are both highly correlated with general intelligence in the normal population, and are relatively resistant to many forms of diffuse brain damage, making scores on this test a good basis for estimating premorbid cognitive function. Inter-rater reliabilities of around 0.96 can be achieved. Test–retest reliability is highly satisfactory at 0.98 (Crawford *et al.*, 1989).

WAIS-R VOCABULARY

This sub-test measures established knowledge. Like the NART, its main use in neurotoxicology is to allow estimates of premorbid function. Vocabulary measures declarative knowledge, which may be less resistant than procedural skills to diffuse brain damage. On the other hand, the reading and pronunciation of irregular words may be more bound to middle class upbringing and formal education. Test–retest reliability is high at around 0.91 to 0.93.

WAIS-R DIGIT SPAN

Subjects are asked to repeat increasingly long strings of digits in the order given (forward span) or in reverse order (backward span). Test–retest reliability is high at around 0.82 to 0.89.

WAIS-R ARITHMETIC

Subjects are given a series of arithmetic problems of increasing difficulty. Test–retest reliability is high at around 0.80 to 0.90.

WAIS-R SIMILARITIES

Subjects are given a series of pairs of words referring to items, and for each pair are asked to say what makes them alike. Pairs are organized in increasing order of difficulty from 'orange and banana' (both fruit) through 'egg and seed' (both the beginnings of life) to 'fly and tree' (both living things). Test–retest reliability is high at around 0.82 to 0.86.

WAIS-R PICTURE COMPLETION

This test requires subjects to examine 20 printed pictures one at a time, and say which essential feature is missing from each picture. Test–retest reliability is high at around 0.86 to 0.89.

WAIS-R BLOCK DESIGN

In this test, the subject uses blocks colored red, white, or half red and half white to copy designs from either a block model or a printed card. Easier items use four blocks, more difficult, nine. Test–retest reliability is high at around 0.80 to 0.91.

WAIS-R DIGIT SYMBOL

This WAIS-R sub-test consists of a key that pairs each digit from one to nine arbitrarily with a symbol, and four rows of random digits with spaces for the symbol. The task is simply to enter the appropriate symbol under each digit as quickly as possible making as few errors as possible. This is a test of psychomotor performance, that is of visuo-motor coordination, complex scanning response speed, and sustained attention. Test–retest reliability is high at around 0.82–0.86.

PAIRED ASSOCIATE LEARNING

This WMS-R sub-test consists of eight pairs of words, four easy (for example metal–iron) and four hard (for example cabbage–dark). In each trial, pairs are first read out in a different random (but specified) order, then again in random order, the first word of each pair is given and the subject asked to recall the second. Reported test–retest reliabilities vary widely. For the standardization sample, a modest reliability of 0.60 is quoted, but most subsequent studies have reported higher values, for example Youngjohn *et al.* (1992) report a value of 0.72.

VISUAL REPRODUCTION

This WMS-R sub-test tests immediate and delayed recall of four relatively simple (much simpler than the Rey) figures. Test–retest reliability is modest to high at around 0.56 to 0.80 for immediate recall, and 0.58 to 0.80 for delayed.

BENTON VISUAL RETENTION TEST

This is a test of visuo-spatial memory. Ten cards are presented in a variety of administrations. Each card contains a number of open or closed figures. Administration A requires a 10-s exposure of each card, followed by immediate recall, whilst administration D requires a 15-s delay. The test is sensitive to unilateral neglect, visuo-spatial, and constructional as well as visual memory impairment, and is among the more sensitive to organic brain damage. There are three forms of more or less equal difficulty.

SYMBOL-DIGIT LEARNING

This test is given after the DSST. Subjects are presented with the 10 symbols and asked to recall the digit associated with each (the key having been removed). Since no warning is given, this is a test of incidental learning.

TRAILS A AND B (REITAN, 1958)

This widely used test is in two parts. Part A measures visuo-motor speed and tracking. Part B measures complex visuo-motor tracking, mental tracking, and mental flexibility. Both parts are sensitive to diffuse brain damage. Disproportionate impairment of part B indicates frontal/executive impairment. Unfortunately, there are a number of administrations, and care must be taken to apply published norms to the appropriate administration. For most administrations, test–retest reliability is satisfactory at between 0.7 and 0.9. However, these figures come from studies within the same laboratories; given the rather loose instructions for administration, reliabilities measured between independent administrators may be lower than for most neuropsychological tests.

PACED AUDITORY SERIAL ADDITION TASK (PASAT) (GRONWALL, 1977)

In this task, subjects are presented aurally with a string of single digits at a set rate (usually 1.2 and 2.4 s inter-stimulus interval (ISI)). After each digit, subjects are asked to respond with the sum of the two immediately previously presented digits. Frequently cited as the most sensitive indicator of attentional dysfunction after TBI, it must be a strong candidate for measuring attentional dysfunction in possible toxic encephalopathy. However, there have been suggestions that its utility in this role depends on a familiarity with number rules that can no longer be taken for granted.

REACTION TIME

Reaction time measures both central processing speed and motor speed associated with making a simple motor reaction to the occurrence of a simple stimulus. The two components can be separately assessed by requiring the subject to maintain a continuous response (for example lever press) until stimulus onset, allowing for measurement of stimulus onset to movement initiation (central processing time), and initiation onset to response completion (motor time). Unfortu-

nately, performance depends crucially on apparatus and administration. Any published norms apply only to the precise circumstances under which they were collected. Test–retest reliability is generally low.

CONTINUOUS PERFORMANCE TEST (CPT)

A set of stimuli are presented. Some of these are designated targets; the others are distractors. The subjects must respond to the targets as in reaction time, and ignore the distractors. The focus on this test is on changes in detection rate or response latency over time.

INTERPRETATION AND INTEGRATION

Neuropsychological test results of individuals are open to damaging misinterpretation. In general, neuropsychological examination of individual clients should be undertaken by, or under the supervision of, a suitably trained and experienced neuropsychologists. The following is only an outline of the procedures for interpreting individual test data.

Individual test scores

Scoring a neuropsychological test consists of reducing relatively complex behaviors across a range of items to a single numerical value. Generally this is done in two stages, calculation of raw scores and conversion to standardized scores. Raw (as well as standardized) scores are summary measures and may be misleading when they obscure meaningful differences in the observations. The very act of allocating a score to any one item may disregard important qualitative information. For instance, in the Rey complex figure, calculation of the quantitative score on the basis of presence and correct placement of the elements disregards some configural and all-process (order of execution) information, which may be relevant to the type of problem and the localization of the lesion. Similarly, in the graded naming test, the scoring of each individual item as correctly named or not discards important information on whether any errors were visual, semantic or phonological. Also, when the raw score represents the sum of several individual items, information about consistency is lost. For instance, where items are ordered in terms of difficulty, as in WAIS-R sub-tests, scoring correctly on the first five of 10 items is quite different from scoring correctly on every second item, although the raw score would be the same.

Each raw score is intended to represent performance on a single dimension. For instance, forward and backward digit span can be combined to produce a single meaningful score only if performances in the two components are similar. For example, if someone consistently scores correctly up to a maximum span of seven forward and five backward and another consistently scores correctly up to a maximum span of nine forward and three backwards, both will achieve the same average raw score. However, the latter clearly represents a specific abnormality in the manipulation of material in working memory.

The main problem with calculating standard scores is to select adequate and appropriate norms. Inadequate norms are those relying on small or unrepresentative samples. Inappropriate norms are where the standardization sample is not relevant to the person undergoing examination. For instance, tests developed for use in industrial toxicology might be best standardized on industrial workers from the same country and language group. Of course the point about any single score being intended to represent performance on a single dimension applies equally to standard scores: compound standard scores, WAIS-R IQs for instance, are meaningless when sub-scale scatter is high.

Comparison of scores across tests

Most neuropsychological examinations involve the administration of a number of different tests of diverse behaviors such as handwriting and memory. Diagnostic decisions often rest on comparisons between these different behaviors. For instance, diffuse brain injury may be said to be typified by slowed information processing and difficulty in learning new information in the context of intact basic language and visuo-spatial skills. Meaningful comparisons among these tests can only be made if they are reduced to a common currency, such as standard scores. The probability of any two standard scores differing by more than a set amount by chance depends on the correlation between the two scales. Problems with this approach are minimized if all the tests form part of an integrated battery standardized on the same sample. The intercorrelation matrix will be available for battery, rendering such calculations relatively easy. Also empirical data may be available. However, in most neuropsychological examinations the different tests of different functions will have been devised or developed by different authors using different types of measurement and different standardization samples. In this case, an estimate of the probability of any difference in standard scores occurring by chance may be made by assuming zero correlation, but this may be inaccurate, although generally conservative. In addition, tests may cover different ranges of ability, and floor and ceiling effects may make comparisons invalid where one of the scores is at the limit.

Comparison with estimates of premorbid function

Neuropsychological testing for the detection and quantification of brain damage implies a focus on impairment. For test scores to be useful in the evaluation of impairment in individual clients, they need to be compared to individual standards. Obviously, the best individual standard would be the results on the same measure administered prior to the event presumed to underlie any neuropsychological impairment. Of course, this is only rarely available.

In the absence of any other information, the population mean for the particular test is often used. This is of very limited value. On a standard IQ scale such as the WAIS-R, a relatively large drop of 15 points will leave 84% of a truly representative sample scoring in the normal range (IQ 70+), and 66% of them in the average range or above. This means many cases with a clinically and personally significant decline in performance might still produce scores within the normal range, making detection and quantification of impairment in individual clients at best unreliable.

Most attempts to find satisfactory premorbid estimates have been concentrated in this area of general intellectual function or intelligence. An estimate can be based either on background data or on some aspect of present performance. The most common background methods include using demographic characteristics, personal history, or old achievement tests (including public examination results). A number of background variables, such as socio-economic class, occupational level or educational level, tend to correlate with IQ. It is possible to reverse the correlation and, using a combination of these variables, predict IQ within certain specifiable confidence limits. Present data methods include hold tests (including current achievement scores), modal scores, and best scores. Hold test methods depend on there being some skills, and therefore some areas of test performance which are resistant to certain forms of brain damage. Generally, tests of overlearned procedural skills are best. Single word reading is utilized in the NART. Best score methods rely on the existence of a large amount of covariance between cognitive measures. They are most appropriate for focal damage; generally these procedures will produce lower bound estimates. If a number of discrepant estimates are produced, the higher should be accepted in most cases. Other cognitive measures tend to correlate positively with IQ, and also independently with achievement. To the extent to which this is true, this procedure also leads to estimates of these measures. For instance the NART gives satisfactory estimates not only of WAIS-R intelligence, but of verbal fluency.

Avoiding false positives/over interpretation of findings

The frequency of 'abnormal' neuropsychological scores in the population is frequently underestimated. Abnormal scores are usually defined as scores in the bottom 2% of the population, although some authors include the bottom 5%. Crawford and Allan (1996) found 37% of their sample to exhibit at least one abnormal sub-test score, i.e. a sub-test score in the bottom 5% of their sample. Similarly, the frequency of 'abnormal' discrepancies between scores is often underestimated. Again empirical data are often available. Where it is not, the same principles apply as underly Bonferronni corrections for multiple comparisons in analysis of variance (ANOVAs). Wedding and Faust (1989) discuss the operation in neuropsychology of confirmation bias, 'a tendency to seek and value supportive evidence at the expense of contrary evidence.' Failure to apply such corrections is a special case of this common error.

In general overinterpretation of single scores should be avoided, especially where a single mistake, perhaps due to fatigue or boredom, can reduce the score significantly (Wedding and Faust, 1989; Lezak, 1995). The simplest way to increase reliability is repeat testing of positive findings. Alternatively, one can compare other measures of the same construct.

Increasing sensitivity/avoiding false negatives

Absence of evidence is not evidence of absence. Many clinical examinations fail to reveal evidence of brain damage, when genuine brain damage with devastating real life consequences is in fact present. This is most often due to failure to test the appropriate cognitive domains. Clinical neurological examinations can fail to reveal even gross cognitive impairment. Standard cognitive testing often means the Wechsler intelligence and memory scales, which can fail to reveal impairment of attentional, executive, and social information processing functions.

Integration

Finally, the neuropsychological data must be integrated with the history and with the other present state data. The important questions here are whether the neuropsychological impairment arises from causes other than acquired brain damage; and whether any brain damage arises from causes other than toxic exposure. The argument that because a certain neuropsychological sign, say poor new learning, is often present in cases of, say, head injury, then the presence of poor new learning implies head injury has been caused seductive inference

(Miller, 1983; Walsh, 1987). In fact, impaired new learning is found in a number of conditions including most other sorts of permanent organic brain damage. It is also found in functional psychiatric illness such as depression, and indeed in more transient states such as fatigue or intoxication.

Background information is crucial to the interpretation of neuropsychological test scores. Demographic information, such as age, affects the interpretation of present state data including test results (quite independently of its use in calculating standard scores). This is because neuropsychological test results, like other clinical data, need to be interpreted in the light of base rates. Base rates for a whole host of neurological conditions vary across the age range. Also, certain ethnic groups are more likely than others to suffer adverse reactions to certain substances. Personal and medical history is crucial in the interpretation of neuropsychological impairment. The observation that scores are low on tests measuring new learning and information processing speed, compared to those measuring vocabulary, takes on an entirely different significance in the context of an earlier serious head injury.

Finally, there is the question of the possibility of brain damage affecting the client's adaptive function and enjoyment of life in the absence of neuropsychological impairment. The consensus in neuropsychological toxicology is that there exists a syndrome characterized by subjective features, such as fatigue, in the absence of definite neuropsychological impairment which is the result of permanent alteration of brain function due to neurotoxic exposure.

REFERENCES

Ames, R.G., Steenland, K., Jenkins, B., Chrislip, D. and Russo, J. 1995: Chronic neurologic sequelae to cholonesterase inhibition among agricultural pesticide applicators. *Archives of Environmental Health*, **50**, 440–4.

Baker, E.L., Feldman, R.G., White, R.F., Harley, J.P., Dinse, G. and Berky, C.S. 1983: Monitoring neurotoxins in industry: Development of a neurobehavioral test battery. *Journal of Occupational Medicine*, **25**, 125–30.

Baker, E.L., Letz, R.E. and Fidler, A.T. 1985: A computer-administered neurobehavioral evaluation system for occupational and environmental epidemiology. Rationale, methodology and pilot study results. *Journal of Occupational Medicine*, **27**, 206–12.

Bellinger, D., Hu, H., Titlebaum, L. and Needleman, H.L. 1994: Attentional correlates of dentin and bone lead levels in adolescents. *Archives of Environmental Health*, **49**, 98–105.

Bolla-Wilson, K., Bleecker, M.L., and Agnew, J. 1988: Lead toxicity and cognitive functions: A dose responsive relationship (abstract). *Journal of Clinical and Experimental Neuropsychology*, **10**, 88.

Bowler, R.M., Thaler, C.D. and Becker, C.E. 1986: California neuropsychological screening battery. *Journal of Clinical Psychology*, **42**, 946–55.

Braun, C.M. and Daigneult, S. 1991: Sparing of cognitive executive functions and impairment of motor functions after industrial exposure to lead: a field study with control group. *Neuropsychology*, **5**, 179–93.

Braun, C.M., Daigneult, S. and Gilbert, B. 1989: Color discrimination testing reveals early printshop solvent neurotoxicity better than a neuropsychological test battery. *Archives of Clinical Neuropsychology*, **4**, 1–13.

Broadwell, D.K., Darcey, D.J., Hudnell, H.K., Otto, D.A. and Byes, W.K. 1995: Worksite clinical and neurobehavioral assessment of solvent exposed microelectronics workers. *American Journal of Industrial Medicine*, **27**, 677–98.

Brooks, D.N. and McKinlay, W.W. 1983: Personality and behavioral change after severe blunt head injury – a relative's view. *Journal of Neurology, Neurosurgery and Psychiatry*, **46**, 336–44.

Bruhn, P. and Maage, N. 1975: Intellectual and neuropsychological functions in young men with heavy and long-term patterns of drug abuse. *American Journal of Psychiatry*, **132**, 397–401.

Cherry, N.M., Labreche, F.P. and McDonald, J.C. 1992: Organic brain damage and occupational solvent exposure. *British Journal of Industrial Medicine*, **49**, 776–81.

Chia, S.E., Ong, C.N., Phoon, W.H., Tan, K.T. and Jeyeratnam, J. 1993: Neurobehavioral effects on workers in a videotape manufacturing factory in Singapore. *Neurotoxicology*, **14**, 51–6.

Christensen, A-L. 1979: *Luria's Neuropsychological Investigation*, 2nd edn. Copenhagen: Munksgaard.

Colvin, M., Myers, J., Nell, V., Reed, D. and Cronje, R. 1993: A cross-sectional survey of neurobehavioral effects of chronic solvent exposure on workers in a paint manufacturing plant. *Environmental Research*, **63**, 122–32.

Crawford, J.R. and Allan, K.M. 1996: WAIS-R sub-test scatter: base rates from a healthy UK sample. *British Journal of Clinical Psychology*, **35**, 235–47.

Crawford, J.R., Parker, D.M., Stewart, L.E. *et al.* 1989: Prediction of WAIS IQ with the national adult reading test: cross-validation and extension. *British Journal of Clinical Psychology*, **28**, 267–73.

Danielle, W., Barnhart, S., Demers, P. *et al.* 1992: Neuropsychological performance among agricultural pesticide applicators. *Environmental Research*, **59**, 217–28.

Danielle, W., Stebbins, A., O'Donnell, J., Horstman, S.W. and Rosenstock, L. 1993: Neuropsychological performance and solvent exposure among car body repair shopworkers. *British Journal of Industrial Medicine*, **50**, 368–77.

Derogatis, L.R. and Cleary, P.A. 1977: Confirmation of the dimensional structure of the SCL-90. A study in construct validation. *Journal of Clinical Psychology*, **33**, 981–9.

Dunn, L.M. and Dunn, L.M. 1981: *Peabody Picture Vocabulary Test – Revised*. Circle Pines, MN: American Guidance Service.

Ellis, A., and Young, A. 1988: *Human Cognitive Neuropsychology*. Hove: Lawrence Erlbaum Associates.

Escalona, E., Yanes, L., Feo, O. and Maizlish, N. 1995: Neurobehavioral evaluation of Venezuelan workers exposed to organic solvent mixtures. *American Journal of Industrial Medicine*, **27**, 15–27.

Eskelinen, L., Luisto, M., Tenkanen, L. and Mattei, O. 1986: Neuropsychological methods in the differentiation of organic solvent intoxication from certain neurological conditions. *Journal of Clinical and Experimental Neuropsychology*, **8**, 239–56.

Fields, S. and Fullerton, J. 1975: Influence of heroin addiction on neuropsychological functioning. *Journal of Consulting and Clinical Psychology*, **43**, 114.

Folstein, M.F., Folstein, S.E. and McHugh, P.R. 1975: Mini-mental state. A practical method of grading the cognitive state of patients for the clinician. *Journal of Psychiatric Research*, **12**, 189–98.

Foo, S.C., Lwin, S., Chia, S.E. and Jeyaratnam, J. 1994: Chronic neurobehavioral effects in paint formulators exposed to solvents and noise. *Annals of the Academy of Medicine, Singapore*, **23**, 650–4.

Golden, C.J. 1981: A standardized version of Luria's neuropsychological tests. In *Handbook of Clinical Neuropsychology*, Filskov, S. and Boll, T.J. (eds). New York: John Wiley.

Golombok, S., Moodley, P. and Lader, M. 1988: Cognitive impairment in long-term benzodiazepine users. *Psychological Medicine*, **18**, 365–74.

Gorenstein, C., Bernik, M.A., Pompeia, S., and Marcourakis, T. 1995: Impairment of performance associated with long-term use of benzodiazepines. *Journal of Psychopharmacology*, **9**, 313–8.

Grant, I., Adams, K.M., Carlin, A.S. and Rennick, P.M. 1977: Neuropsychological deficit in polydrug users. A preliminary report of the findings of the collaborative neuropsychological study of polydrug users. *Drug and Alcohol Dependence*, **2**, 91–108.

Grant, I., Adams, K.M., Carlin, A.S. *et al.* 1978: Organic impairment in polydrug users: risk factors. *American Journal of Psychiatry*, **132**, 178–84.

Grant, I. and Judd, L.I. 1976: Neuropsychological and EEG disturbances in polydrug users. *American Journal of Psychiatry*, **133**, 1039–42.

Grant, I., Mohns, L., Miller, M. and Reitan, R. 1976: A neuropsychological study of polydrug users. *Archives of General Psychiatry*, **33**, 973–8.

Gronwall, D.M.A. 1977: Paced auditory serial addition task: a measure of recovery from concussion. *Perceptual and Motor Skills*, **44**, 367–73.

Hanninen, H. 1982: Behavioral effects of occupational exposure to mercury and lead. *Acta Neurologica Scandinavica*, **66**, 167–75.

Hill, S.Y., Reyes, R.B., Mikhael, M. and Ayre, F. 1979: A comparison of alcoholics and heroin abusers: computerized transaxial tomography and neuropsychological functioning. *Currents in Alcoholism*, **5**, 187–205.

Johnson, B.L. (ed.) 1987: *Prevention of Neurotoxic Illness in Working Populations*. New York: John Wiley.

Kaku, D.A. and Lowenstein, D.H. 1989: Recreational drug use: a growing risk factor for stroke in young people. *Neurology*, **39**, 161.

Kaye, B.R. and Fainstate, M. 1987: Cerebral vasculitis associated with cocaine abuse. *Journal of the American Medical Association*, **258**, 2104–6.

Kishi, R., Harabuchi, I., Katakura, Y., Ikeda, T. and Miyake, H. 1993: Neurobehavioral effects of chronic occupational exposure to organic solvents among Japanese industrial painters. *Environmental Research*, **62**, 303–13.

Kishi, R., Rikuo, R., Fukuchi, Y. *et al.* 1994: Residual neurobehavioral effects associated with chronic exposure to mercury vapor. *Occupational and Environmental Medicine*, **51**, 35–41.

Korogi, Y., Takahashi, M., Shinzato, J. and Okajima, T. 1994: MR findings in seven patients with organic mercury poisoning (Minamata disease). *American Journal of Neuroradiology*, **15**, 1575–8.

Krystal, J.H. and Price, L.H. 1992: Chronic MDMA use: effects on mood and neuropsychological function. *American Journal of Drug and Alcohol Abuse*, **18**, 331–41.

Lezak, M.D. 1995: *Neuropsychological Assessment* 3rd edn. New York: Oxford University Press.

Lukki, I., Rickels, K. and Geller, A.M. 1986: Chronic use of benzodiazepines and psychomotor and cognitive test performance. *Psychopharmacology*, **88**, 426–33.

Luria, A.R. 1966: *Higher Cortical Functions in Man*. New York: Basic Books.

McKinlay, W.W. and Brooks, D.N. 1984: Methodological problems in assessing psychosocial recovery following severe head injury. *Journal of Clinical Neuropsychology*, **6**, 87–99.

McMillan, T.M., Freemomt, A.J., Herxheimer, A. *et al.* 1993: Camelford water poisoning accident: serial neuropsychological assessment and further observations on bone aluminum. *Human and Experimental Toxicology*, **12**, 37–42.

Mergler, D. and Blain, L. 1987: Assessing color vision loss among solvent-exposed workers. *American Journal of Industrial Medicine*, **12**, 195–203.

Miller, E. 1983: A note on the interpretation of data derived from neuropsychological tests. *Cortex*, **19**, 131–2.

Morrow, L.A., Robin, N., Hodgson, M.J. and Kamis, H. 1992: Assessment of attention and memory efficiency in persons with solvent neurotoxicity. *Neuropsychologica*, **30**, 911–22.

Nelson, H.E. 1982. *National Adult Reading Test (NART): Test Manual*. Windsor: NFER-NELSON.

Nelson, H.E. and O'Connel, A. 1978. Dimentia: the estimation of premorbid intelligence levels using the new adult reading test. *Cortex*, **14**, 234–44.

Ng, T.P., Lim, L.C. and Win, K.K. 1992: An investigation of solvent-induced neuropsychiatric disorder in spray painters. *Annals of the Academy of Medicine, Singapore*, **21**, 797–803.

Oldfield, R.C. 1971: The assessment and analysis of handedness: the Edinburgh Inventory. *Neuropsychologia*, **9**, 97–113.

Petursson, H., Gudjonsson, G.H. and Lader, M.H. 1983: Psychometric performance during withdrawal from long-term benzodiazepine treatment. *Psychopharmacology*, **81**, 345–9.

Rasmussen, K., Jeppesen, H.J. and Sabroe, S. 1993: Psychometric tests for assessment of brain function after solvent exposure. *American Journal of Industrial Medicine*, **24**, 553–65.

Raven, J.C., Court, J.H. and Raven, J. 1988: *Manual for Raven's Progressive Matrices and Vocabulary Scales: Section 3: Standard Progressive Matrices.* London: H.K. Lewis.

Reinvang, I., Borchgrevink, H.M., Aaserud, O. *et al.* 1994: Neuropsychological findings in a non-clinical sample of workers exposed to solvents. *Journal of Neurology, Neurosurgery and Psychiatry*, **57**, 614–6.

Reitan, R.M. 1958: Validity of the trail making test as an indicator of organic brain damage. *Perceptual and Motor Skills*, **8**, 271–6.

Reitan, R.M. and Wolfson, D. 1993: *The Halstead–Reitan Neuropsychological Test Battery: Theory and Clinical Interpretation.* Tucson, AZ: Neuropsychology Press.

Rodnitzky, R.L., Levin, H.S. and Mock, D.L. 1975: Occupational exposure to organophosphate pesticides: a neurobehavioral study. *Archives of Environmental Health*, **30**, 98–103.

Rosenstock, L., Keifer, M., Daniell, W.E., McConnell, R. and Claypole, K. 1991: Chronic central nervous system effects of acute organophosphate pesticide intoxication. *Lancet*, **338**, 223–7.

Rosselli, M. and Ardila, A. 1996: Cognitive effects of cocaine and polydrug abuse. *Journal of Clinical and Experimental Neuropsychology*, **18**, 122–35.

Ryan, C.M., Morrow, L.A. and Bromet, E.J. 1987: Assessment of neuropsychological dysfunction in the workplace: normative data from the Pittsburgh occupational exposure test battery. *Journal of Experimental and Clinical Neuropsychology*, **9**, 665–79.

Savage, E.P., Keefe, T.J., Mounce, L.M. *et al.* 1988: Chronic neurological sequelae of acute organophosphate pesticide poisoning. *Archives of Environmental Health*, **43**, 38–45.

Spurgeon, A., Glass, D.C., Calvert, I.A., Cunningham-Hill, M. and Harrington, J.M. 1994: Investigation of dose-related neurobehavioral effects in paintmakers exposed to low levels of solvents. *Occupational and Environmental medicine*, **51**, 626–30.

Spurgeon, A., Gray, C.N., Sims, J. *et al.* 1992: Neurobehavioral effects of long-term occupational exposure to organic solvents: two comparable studies. *American Journal of Industrial Medicine*, **22**, 325–35.

Stephens, R., Spurgeon, A., Calvert, I.A. *et al.* 1995: Neuropsychological effects of long-term exposure to organophosphates in sheep dip. *Lancet*, **345**, 1135–9.

Strong, J. and Gurling, H. 1991: Psychometric testing and CT scans of long-term opiate addicts. In *Physiopathology of illicit drugs*, Nahas, and Latar, (eds).

Strub, R.L. and Black, F.W. 1985: *Mental Status Examination in Neurology*, 2nd edn. Philadelphia, PA: F.A. Davis.

Sunderland, A., Harris, J.E. and Baddeley, A. 1983: Assessing everyday memory after severe head injury. In *Everyday Memory, Actions and Absentmindedness*, Harris, J.E. and Morris, P.E. (eds). London: Academic Press.

Tata, P.R., Rollings, J., Collins, M., Pickering, A. and Jacobson, R.R. 1994: Lack of cognitive recovery following withdrawal from long-term benzodiazepine use. *Psychological Medicine*, **24**, 203–13.

Taylor, E.M. 1959: *Psychological Appraisal of Children with Cerebral Defects.* Cambridge, MA: Harvard University Press.

Thomsen, I.V. 1984: Late outcome of very severe blunt head trauma: a 10–15 year second follow up. *Journal of Neurology, Neurosurgery and Psychiatry*, **47**, 260–8.

Uzzell, B.P. and Oler, J. 1986: Chronic low-level mercury exposure and neuropsychological functioning. *Journal of Clinical and Experimental Neuropsychology*, **8**, 581–93.

Volkow, N.D., Mulani, N., Gould, K.I. *et al.* 1988: Cerebral blood flow in chronic cocaine users. *British Journal of Psychiatry*, **152**, 641–8.

Walsh, K.W. 1987: *Neuropsychology*, 2nd edn. Edinburgh: Churchill-Livingstone.

Wechsler, D. 1981: *WAIS-R Manual.* New York: The Psychological Corporation.

Wechsler, D. 1987: *Wechsler Memory Scale – Revised Manual.* San Antonio, TX: The Psychological Corporation.

Wedding, D. and Faust, D. 1989: Clinical judgement and decision making in neuropsychology. *Archives of Clinical Neuropsychology*, **4**, 233–65.

Wilson, J.T.L. and Wiedmann, K.D. 1992: Neuropsychological assessment in alcohol, drug abuse and toxic conditions. In *A Handbook of Neuropsychological Assessment*, Crawford, J.R., Parker, D.M. and McKinlay, W.W. (eds). Hove: Lawrence Erlbaum Associates.

Youngjohn, J.R., Larrabee, G.J. and Crook, T.N. 1992: Test-retest reliability of computerized everyday memory measures and traditional tests. *The Clinical Neuropsychologist*, **3**, 276–86.

17

The electrophysiological investigation

MASASHI NAKAJIMA AND ANDREW EISEN

INTRODUCTION

This chapter explores how a variety of electrophysiological techniques can be used to investigate toxic impact on the somatic sensory and motor systems. In particular the fundamentals involved in the pathophysiology of toxic neuropathies and myelopathies will be followed by descriptions of specific electrophysiological abnormalities seen in individual disorders affecting the peripheral nervous system, neuromuscular junction, and the spinal cord. We will not discuss the role of electroencephalography (EEG), or techniques designed to specifically evaluate the visual, auditory, and vestibular systems. However, EEG is particularly useful in the diagnosis of metabolic encephalopathies, which result from exposure to, or ingestion of, a variety of toxins. Similarly, toxicity-induced visual, auditory or vestibular disease may occur in isolation or in combination, and there are a variety of electrophysiological techniques which are helpful in their evaluation. Electrophysiological investigations should be used as an extension of the neurological examination. When regarded this way, the techniques described are of diagnostic and prognostic value, and are helpful in determining the site of the lesion(s) and the mode of neuronal injury. They can also be employed as screening techniques in individuals at risk who work in a potentially neurotoxic environment. Since the range of normal values for most electrophysiological measurements is broad, the results taken outside the clinical context may be misinterpreted. On the other hand, normal electrodiagnostic studies do not exclude toxicity-related diseases. For example, most neurotoxic substances that affect the peripheral nervous system produce axonal degeneration. The result is only a slight change in maximum motor nerve conduction velocity, one of the most frequently employed measurements. Motor conduction may be normal, even when the condition is severe. Detection of a toxic neuropathy often requires a specifically designed electrophysiological investigation beyond the daily routine of the laboratory. Table 17.1 lists the different types of electrophysiological investigation which are briefly described, followed by a discussion of how these techniques help the diagnosis of different toxic disorders.

ELECTROPHYSIOLOGICAL TECHNIQUES

Nerve conduction studies

Electrical stimulation of a nerve discloses the conduction characteristics of the motor, sensory, or mixed nerves to be examined. For motor conduction studies, the nerve is stimulated at two or more points along its course while recording from a muscle innervated by the motor nerve. The compound muscle action potential (CMAP) is recorded with a pair of surface electrodes (belly-tendon technique). The usual measurements include amplitude, duration, and latency of the response. Conduction velocity is calculated from the difference in latency between two stimulus points. Most motor nerves in the upper limbs conduct at about 55 m/s; lower limb nerves conduct about 5 m/s slower.

Sensory nerve conduction studies are performed by stimulating a cutaneous nerve and recording over it at some proximal (orthodromic method) or distal (antidromic method) site. Sensory conduction of the median or ulnar nerve is studied orthodromically with stimulation of the digital nerve and recording

Table 17.1 *Electrophysiological techniques employed in the diagnosis of toxic disorders*

Toxic disorders	Action potential from sensory conduction studies		Action potential from motor conduction studies				SEP	MEP
	Amplitude	Velocity	Amplitude	Velocity	F-wave	EMG		
Axonal neuropathy								
Acrylamide	+++	+	+	+	+	+	++	
Organophosphate	+++	−	++	−	−	+++	++	
Axonal neuropathy with secondary demyelination								
Hexacarbon	++	+++	++	+++	+++	++	+++	
Dorsal root ganglion neuronopathy								
Pyridoxine	+++	++	−	−	−	−	+++	
CNS disorders								
Konzo, lathyrism	−	−	−	−	−	−	−	+++
Organic mercury	−	−	−	−	−	−	+++	

EMG: electromyography; SEP: somatosensory evoked potential; MEP: magnetic evoked potential.
+++: abnormal, sensitive; ++: abnormal, less sensitive; +: abnormal in advanced cases; −: normal.
No data are available for empty spaces in the MEP column.

along the nerve trunk at the wrist, or antidromically with stimulation of the nerve trunk at the wrist and recording at the digital nerve. With the use of surface electrodes, the amplitude of the compound sensory nerve action potential (SNAP) is greater in the antidromic than the orthodromic mode. Velocity is determined from the absolute latency of the SNAP. In conduction studies of the mixed nerve, sensory nerve conduction is assessed since large diameter sensory fibers have a lower threshold and a faster conduction velocity than motor fibers. However, disease states that affect different fibers selectively would preclude differentiation between the sensory and motor components of mixed nerve potentials.

Focal nerve disease is best revealed by short segment conduction studies with stimuli being applied at 1 cm intervals over about 10–15 cm of nerve length (the 'inching technique'). In motor nerve conduction studies of focal or multifocal neuropathies, stimulation below the lesion may elicit a normal response from a paretic or paralyzed muscle, even though proximal stimulation above the lesion evokes a response of reduced amplitude or no response. The reduction in amplitude is proportional to the number of axons that are inexcitable and is referred to as conduction block. Persistent normal excitability of paralyzed muscle after distal nerve stimulation indicates neurapraxia or demyelinative conduction block, and is predictive of complete recovery in most patients. Loss or reduction in amplitude of CMAP or SNAP after stimulation distal to the lesion occurs when there is discontinuity of the nerve sheath (neurotmesis) or of the axon (axonotmesis), resulting in permanent dysfunction or incomplete recovery commonly associated with nerve trauma.

Evaluating conduction abnormalities along the proximal segments and roots of peripheral nerves requires very proximal stimulation that is technically difficult. This can be achieved for motor nerves using F-wave recording, originally described by Magladery and McDougal (1950). The F-wave, so called because it was first recorded from the small foot muscles, is a long-latency compound action potential which can be evoked intermittently from a muscle by supramaximal electrical stimulation to the innervating motor nerve. The pathway for the F-wave involves antidromic excitation of all stimulated motor axons travelling to the spinal cord, which activates the axon hillock of the anterior horn cells, and thus incorporates very proximal conduction segments. It is produced by the antidromic activation of a variable, but normally small, proportion of the anterior horn cells that innervate the muscle. Sequential supramaximal stimuli evoke F-waves that are variable in their configuration and latency due to the activation of different anterior horn cells.

In general, axonal damage or dysfunction results in the diminished amplitude of the compound action potential rather than a reduction of conduction velocity, reflecting a reduction in the number of functioning axons. Mild conduction slowing, up to 20% below normal, occurs when large numbers of the fast-conducting, large-diameter fibers are impaired as occurs, for example, in acrylamide neuropathy. In contrast, conduction slowing due to demyelination is marked, usually less than 60% of the normal lower limit, but may remain normal if enough fast-conducting fibers are preserved. However, even then, a mixture of normal, demyelinating, and remyelinating fibers gives rise to increase in duration of the evoked response (abnormal temporal dispersion) or conduction block, or both.

Needle electromyography

The electrical activity of muscles is studied by inserting a recording electrode directly to the muscle to be examined. Muscles are selected for examination on the basis of the patient's symptoms and signs. In general proximal and distal muscles of one arm and leg are examined if the disease is bilaterally symmetrical (polyneuropathy, myopathy or a diffuse anterior horn cell disease). For radiculopathy, plexopathy and isolated peripheral nerve lesions, muscles are chosen so as to confirm the apparently restricted distribution of these lesions. Needle electromyography compliments nerve conduction studies. It gives information about the severity of disease, rate of progression, and likelihood and extent of recovery. Spontaneous activity recorded in a relaxed muscle may be due to nerve-muscle discontinuity. This type of activity takes the form of fibrillation and positive sharp waves. They reflect the spontaneous activity of a single muscle fiber that is deprived of its nerve supply. Fibrillation is only visible in skinned muscle, which in humans translates into the tongue musculature. Fibrillation or positive sharp waves may occur in any situation depriving the muscle fiber of its innervation and it should not be equated with 'neurogenic disease.' For example, if the muscle undergoes segmental necrosis with fiber splitting, portions of the muscle fiber may no longer be connected to its terminal axon so that it becomes functionally denervated. The time to onset of fibrillation and positive sharp waves is axon-length dependent. The shorter the distal stump the less time it takes for the spontaneous activities to commence.

There are many other types of spontaneous activity that can be recorded by needle electromyography (EMG), but they are all prejunctional in origin and some of them have little, if any, relevance to the subject at hand. Fasciculation is referred to visible twitching of muscle bundles and is typically, but not exclusively, seen in diseases of anterior horn cells. Fasciculation potentials result from spontaneous discharges of a group of muscle fibers representing either a whole or possibly part of a motor unit. In contrast to isolated discharges of one motor unit, more complex bursts of repetitive discharges cause vermicular movement of the skin, called myokymia. Myokymic discharges are repetitive firing of the same motor units (recurrent trains of motor unit potentials). Electromyography allows detection of clinically invisible fasciculation and myokymia in the depth of muscles.

The motor unit is comprised of a single anterior horn cell and the muscle fibers supplied by its terminal branches. When the anterior horn cell fires, or the axon that arises from it is stimulated, all of the muscle fibers that belong to that motor unit are excited. The electrical activity from all of these muscle fibers summate to produce a motor unit action potential (MUAP). The muscle fibers constituting a single motor unit are interspersed randomly with the muscle fibers of the other motor units so that five to 10 different motor units share a territory of 4–6 mm in circumference. During voluntary contraction, motor units are recruited in a fixed order from weakest to strongest. This was identified and first described by Henneman et al. (1965) and became known as the Henneman size principle, and is readily appreciated on needle EMG. Smaller motor neurons have a lower threshold and fire earlier than larger, higher threshold motor neurons. With increased contraction the first-recruited smaller motor units increase their firing rate and then larger motor units are gradually recruited. Only at full force is interference complete. The firing frequency of the first recruited motor unit divided by the number of other motor units that can be recognized is called the recruitment ratio. Thus, if the first motor unit fires at a frequency of 16 Hz when four others can be identified the recruitment ratio would be $16/4 = 4$. The normal value ranges from three to five. This measure is useful in detection of an early stage of diseases that cause loss of functioning anterior horn cells or their axons. With a fallout of functioning motor units there are fewer units to achieve force–function than normal. They compensate by firing more frequently. As a result interference at full force is reduced. This type of recruitment is referred to as reduced recruitment or decreased recruitment, or better still discrete interference. Recruitment ratios are also increased as a secondary response to ischemia, and temporarily during recovery from local and general anesthetics.

Several characteristics of the MUAP itself can be studied; the amplitude, duration, number of phases or complexity, presence of satellites, and stability. Peak MUAP amplitude reflects synchronized activity of single muscle fibers within a diameter of 0.5 mm or less of the electrode's recording surface. The duration depends on the length of the terminal axons (spatial dispersion), and conduction velocities of themselves and of the muscle fibers they innervate (temporal dispersion). The propagated nerve action potential enters each axon terminal to excite a single muscle fiber. Those fibers innervated by the shortest terminals will be the first to depolarize and a triphasic waveform will begin travelling along the muscle. Muscle fibers innervated through terminals of increasing lengths will be excited sequentially. The action potentials from all of the single muscle fibers belonging to one motor unit summate to yield a MUAP, which is usually triphasic, positive–negative–positive.

The morphology of the MUAP should be considered in terms of its complexity (number of turns and phases) and stability. These characteristics of the MUAP can only be analyzed qualitatively if a delay line and raster recording is performed. This is readily available on all modern equipment. The voltage summation often results in a MUAP with small serration or turns superimposed on the main waveform. These can be accentuated by narrowing the recording band pass to 200 or 500 Hz–10 kHz from an ordinary 2 Hz–10 kHz. The restricted band pass is that used in single fiber electromyography (SFEMG) that picks up activity of single muscle fibers within a diameter of 0.02 mm of the electrode recording surface. However, much of the information that is gleaned quantitatively by SFEMG can be achieved qualitatively by conventional EMG with a monopolar or concentric electrode using the narrow band pass. Recording with the narrow band pass will reduce the amplitude and duration of MUAPs and will increase the phase. The phase is defined as the number of baseline crossings plus one, and is usually less than four. The stability of a motor unit is a qualitative measure of variation in time of firing of individual muscle fibers belonging to the unit, that is called jitter. Providing the recording electrode is held steadily, the identical MUAP recorded on sequential sweeps is very stable and superimposes very well. Instability can occur in any situation that renders the neuromuscular junction insecure. Newly formed terminal sprouts, disease of the neuromuscular junction, and regenerating muscle fibers can all cause instability of the MUAP. Instability is a valuable 'measure' because it clearly indicates that there is an ongoing, active pathological process.

In neurogenic disease, changes in the motor unit are time dependent and the processes of denervation and reinnervation usually occur together. Axonal injury causes fibrillations and positive sharp waves after a latent period of two to three weeks. Within two to six weeks, depending on the length of the distal stump, immature terminal sprouts become functional, increasing the number of muscle fibers belonging to intact motor units (reinnervation). With reinnervation, fibrillation potentials and positive sharp waves decrease. The terminal sprouts are initially immature and insecure, producing asynchronous summation of electrical activity within the motor unit. Conduction along the immature terminal axon may be blocked completely. These pathophysiological changes result in MUAPs that are complex (increased fiber density), unstable (increased jitter), and prolonged in duration (more temporal and spatial dispersion). Over the ensuing months the newly formed terminal sprouts mature and their conduction stabilizes accompanied by an increased velocity. The electrical summation of all motor unit action potentials increases with an associated decrease in the number of phases detected in the reinnervated MUAP. The configuration of the MUAP will also stabilize and jitter will decrease. Reinnervation following profound or complete denervation results in asynchronous electrical summation of the relatively few muscle fibers producing small, highly polyphasic, and usually short-duration MUAPs. A characteristic sputtering

sound results from action potentials of the temporally dispersed single muscle fibers within the motor unit. These potentials are sometimes referred to as nascent potentials. Thus, in polyneuropathies, findings of denervation and/or reinnervation implies axonal injury. Recruitment of motor units showing reinnervating activity in a clinically paralyzed muscle may predict a recovery. A lack of signs of denervation in patients with definite muscle weakness suggests conduction block due to demyelination. Electromyographic evidence of denervation/reinnervation can be detected in muscles with clinically normal strength. Subclinical distal axonopathy can be disclosed by examination of the distal muscles. In focal neuropathy, the distribution of denervated muscles localizes the lesion.

In myopathies muscle fibers are randomly involved throughout the whole motor unit, resulting in a reduction in the number of muscle fibers comprising each MUAP. As a result, the MUAPs in myopathies are usually short in duration and small in amplitude. The remaining fibers demonstrate an increased variation in fiber diameter. The combination of fiber loss and change in size reduces the motor unit territory. There is some spatial collapse of the motor unit territory so that intact muscle fibers of one motor unit become closer in proximity (packing). This tends to increase the MUAP amplitude. However, the fiber loss in myopathy is usually sufficiently uniform so that the reduced number of muscle fibers in all of the motor units is more than enough to offset the electrical summation induced by packing. These effects result in complex, unstable MUAPs with increased fiber density and jitter, the same as is seen in neurogenic processes. In myopathies, the random loss of muscle fibers results in a reduction of the net force output from each motor unit. This is compensated for by multiple motor units firing simultaneously at high rates. The interference is increased or full and often there is recruitment of many MUAPs when the patient is unaware of any muscle contraction. The recruitment ratio is decreased. At minimal contraction, the first recruited motor unit may only fire at a rate of 5 Hz before additional motor units are added. If five other MUAPs are recognized at this time, the recruitment ratio would only measure one.

Somatosensory evoked potentials

Sensory responses from the central nervous system can be evoked by stimulation of a peripheral mixed or cutaneous nerve; these are called somatosensory evoked potentials (SEPs). They are smaller in amplitude than sensory nerve action potentials, and require averaging techniques to be recorded. Conventional studies of sensory nerve conduction velocity only evaluate the distal portions of the peripheral nerve, whereas the SEP assesses the entire afferent system. The electrical stimulus to the sensory or mixed nerve activates predominantly large-diameter, fast-conducting group Ia muscle and group II cutaneous afferents, and these contribute predominantly to the resulting SEPs (Burke *et al.*, 1981; Gandevia *et al.*, 1984; Eisen and Aminoff, 1986). The central pathway that carries most information responsible for SEPs is the large-fiber dorsal column-lemniscal system (Eisen and Aminoff, 1986; Chiappa, 1990).

Magnetic evoked potentials

The remarkable discovery by Merton and Morton (1980) that it was possible to stimulate the awake and intact human motor cortex opened a new era of human neurophysiological investigation. These initial experiments were performed using high voltage, short duration electrical stimuli applied to the scalp overlying the motor cortex. This procedure was tolerable but uncomfortable and has been largely replaced by transcranial magnetic stimulation (TMS). Compound muscle action potentials evoked after magnetic stimulation are called magnetic evoked potentials (MEPs). This method is virtually free of any discomfort. It also appears very safe in both the short and long term (Rossini and Caramia, 1988; Murray, 1991). TMS activates the corticomotoneuronal system presynaptically through the apical dendrites of the corticomotoneuron. It is not possible to stimulate descending motor tracts directly because the current density induced by the magnetic coil is insufficient. In the awake subject, many laboratories use TMS routinely to provide an indirect estimate of the fast conducting (primarily) direct corticomotoneuronal tract passing

through the spinal cord. Motor cortex and spinal roots (to account for the peripheral component) are stimulated in turn whilst recording MEPs from the same target muscle. The latency difference between cortical and root stimulation reflects central motor conduction through the spinal cord (Cusik *et al.*, 1979).

Assessment of neuromuscular transmission

The neuromuscular junction, being a synaptic structure, is remarkably sensitive to pharmacologically active substances. A variety of natural toxins and synthesized chemicals exert their paralytic action on presynaptic or postsynaptic structures, or sometimes both. The presynaptic ending contains many minute vesicles containing acetylcholine (ACh) molecules. Depolarization of the presynaptic ending at the axon terminal triggers an influx of calcium (Ca^{2+}), initiating the calcium-dependent release of vesicles into the junctional space. Liberated ACh molecules generate an end-plate potential (EPP) through binding to the postsynaptic ACh receptor, and are subsequently degraded by acetylcholinesterase. The EPP opens the voltage-gated Na^+ channels. The resulting depolarization exceeds the excitability threshold of the muscle cell membrane and a propagated action potential ensues, activating the contractile elements through excitation–contraction coupling. There are several proven mechanisms for interfering with successful neuromuscular transmission by a variety of drugs (Figure 17.1). They include:

1 interference with the movement of Ca^{2+} ions into and within the nerve terminal;
2 failure of release of ACh from the presynaptic membrane;

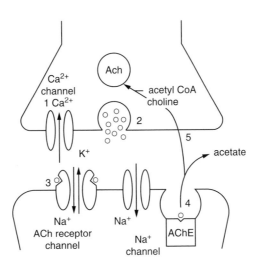

Figure 17.1 *Vulnerability of neuromuscular transmission exposed to natural and synthetic chemicals.*

3 competition by drugs or toxins for the binding site of ACh receptor;

4 inhibition of acetylcholinesterase, which would result in depolarization blockade form an over-activity of Ach;

5 interference with reuptake of choline into the nerve terminal for resynthesis into ACh.

REPETITIVE NERVE STIMULATION

Neuromuscular transmission is readily tested by repetitive nerve stimulation in which the nerve is stimulated at supramaximal intensity repetitively at a rate of one to five per second. Quantal release of ACh falls gradually with each stimulus so that the amplitude of EPP progressively decreases until the fifth stimulus. The ratio of the 'amount' of EPP to the threshold for action potential generation is called the 'safety factor' for neuromuscular transmission. In normal muscle, this factor is great enough to ensure that each nerve impulse, even with a falling EPP, is followed by a muscle contraction and maximum compound muscle action potential (CMAP). Decremental responses after a train of stimuli at slow rates will develop in myasthenia gravis and Lambert–Eaton myasthenic syndrome, and other conditions that impair either presynaptic release of ACh or postsynaptic sensitivity to ACh. When presynaptic ACh release is blocked, the CMAP is small after a single stimulus and increases dramatically after maximum voluntary contraction or after repetitive stimulation at fast rates (post-tetanic potentiation). After exercise, a transient potentiation is followed by decreased excitability of the neuromuscular junction in 2–4 min after exercise (post-tetanic exhaustion). In myasthenia gravis, neuromuscular block worsens during post-tetanic exhaustion, indicating a reduced margin of safety. In premature infants and some newborns with limited neuromuscular reserve, the amplitude of the compound muscle action potential progressively declines at high rates of stimulation.

SINGLE FIBER ELECTROMYOGRAPHY

Variation in the amplitude of EPP causes a delay or a failure in generation of the action potential. The variation in time between nerve impulse and muscle action potential is called neuromuscular jitter, and a failure to evoke action potential is called neuromuscular blocking. Both phenomena can be recorded on needle electromyography with a restricted band-pass, and more precisely with single fiber electromyography which separates the electrical activity of individual muscle fibers (Stålberg and Trontelj, 1979). When the safety factor is reduced for any reason, the neuromuscular jitter increases. In myasthenia gravis, single fiber electromyography has higher sensitivity for the detection of abnormal neuromuscular transmission than repetitive nerve stimulation (Stålberg, 1980). Increased

jitter is not specific to the disorders of neuromuscular junction and also occurs in immature sprouting of nerve terminals, which have insecure conduction, and newly regenerated muscle fibers in which the end plate is also insecure.

ELECTROPHYSIOLOGICAL APPROACHES TO DIAGNOSIS

Generalized peripheral neuropathy (polyneuropathy)

Polyneuropathies of toxic origin can be classified into three pathologic classes, axonopathies, neuronopathies, and myelinopathies (Nielsen and Wright, 1987).

AXONOPATHIES

These are the most frequent type of polyneuropathy and involve the axons of motor, sensory, and autonomic nerves. One or other may be affected predominantly, or even in isolation, but usually all components are affected. Axonal degeneration starts distally in most axonal neuropathies and progresses toward the cell body, a phenomenon referred to as 'dying-back.' In toxic neuropathies, Spencer and Schaumburg (1976) and Schaumburg and Spencer (1979) showed a multifocal process that initially affects distal portions of axons not only in the peripheral axons but also in selected tracts of the central nervous system, and they introduced a term 'central–peripheral distal axonopathy.' The susceptibility of nerve fibers depends on their length and diameter. Sumner (1975) and Sumner and Asbury (1975) showed that for the same fiber length, large-diameter fibers were more vulnerable than smaller diameter fibers in acrylamide neuropathy. They also observed that dorsal root muscle afferent fibers were several times more susceptible than motor efferent fibers. The susceptibility of nerve fibers depends on the size of their parent neurons ('neuron size principle'). Although this is irrespective of whether the axons are central or peripheral (Spencer and Schaumburg, 1977) in most human examples and experimental animal models with these conditions, the clinical presentation is one of a peripheral neuropathy. The onset of clinical symptoms or signs due to the central axonopathy, for example spasticity or dorsal column features, may lag behind or even follow partial recovery of paralysis due to the peripheral axonopathy. Not all axonotoxic substances have a selective affinity for larger-diameter nerve fibers. In experimental triorthocresyl phosphate (TOCP) neuropathy in the baboon, fibers of all diameters are affected, and some of the largest diameter fibers are preserved (Hern, 1973).

Acrylamide neuropathy

Acrylamide neuropathy is a prototype of central–peripheral distal axonopathy. Sensory symptoms and signs are a prominent clinical manifestation. The amplitude of sensory nerve action potentials is usually markedly reduced in upper and lower extremities (Fullerton, 1969; Takahashi et al., 1971). In a series of 71 acrylamide workers and 51 unexposed referents, He et al. (1989) showed that electrophysiological abnormalities, including a decrease in the sensory action potential amplitude, electromyographic evidence of denervation, and prolongation of the ankle tendon reflex latency can precede the neuropathic symptoms and signs. In animal experiments, the maximum motor conduction velocities eventually become reduced by up to 20% during development of severe neuropathy (Fullerton and Barnes, 1966; Hopkins and Gilliatt, 1971). However, most individuals with acrylamide neuropathy are less severely affected clinically, and display only slight slowing of sensory and motor conduction velocity. Thus, in seeking minimal or subclinical acrylamide neuropathy, estimation of sensory nerve action potential amplitude would be the most appropriate measurements (Le Quesne, 1978). This is also applicable to neuropathies that are dominated by distal sensory symptoms and a loss of ankle jerk in the initial stages. As has been shown by Arezzo et al. (1982), somatosensory evoked potentials (SEPs) can provide evidence of early disease affecting the gracile fasciculus in animal experiments. In clinical settings, cervicomedullary potentials can be separated with a dipolar recording technique in median nerve stimulation (Kaji and Sumner, 1987; Nakajima and Hirayama, 1995). However, with lower limb testing, activity in the medulla cannot be routinely recorded in human subjects. Recordings can be made from needle electrodes or using large numbers of stimulus repetitions (Lueders et al., 1981; Chiappa, 1990).

To examine sensory conduction through the most distal segments, Casey and Le Quesne (1972a) developed a technique for recording potentials from digital nerves after applying electrical stimulation at the tip of the finger. With this technique, they examined 16 alcoholic subjects who had minimal or no evidence of peripheral neuropathy (Casey and Le Quesne, 1972b). Reduction of digital sensory potentials were much more sensitive than the routine procedure of recording sensory action potentials at the wrist after digital stimulation at the interphalangeal joint. They also demonstrated a subclinical neuropathy in patients receiving vincristine for hematological malignancies (Casey et al., 1973). All patients showed a reduction in amplitude of the digital potentials within four to six weeks after onset of treatment. The reduction of sensory action potentials recorded at wrist was less pronounced. Guiheneuc et al. (1980) showed that a reduction in the ratio of the size of the soleus CMAP elicited by tapping the Achilles tendon (T reflex) to the CMAP from the same recording after electrical stimulation of the posterior tibial nerve (H reflex) was the most sensitive index in vincristine neuropathy. This might be explained by a distal axonopathy, probably affecting the Ia afferent terminals in the muscle spindle first, which was the earliest change in the experimental acrylamide neuropathy (Sumner, 1975; Sumner and Asbury, 1975).

Nitroimidazoles

Nitroimidazoles were first developed as an antiprotozoal agent in 1960s. Misonidazole (2-nitroimidazole) was introduced in the mid-1970s as a radiosensitizer for cancer chemotherapy, and metronidazole is used in long-term treatment of patients with Crohn's disease. Both nitroimidazoles cause a dose-dependent sensory neuropathy. Stahlberg et al. (1991) showed no significant abnormalities in neurophysiologic investigations of patients with Crohn's disease receiving metronidazole up to 800 mg for at least one year. Because of its long-term use in Crohn's disease, further investigation with the most sensitive electrophysiological techniques would be expected to monitor the toxicity.

Organophosphate-induced delayed polyneuropathy

Organophosphate-induced delayed polyneuropathy arises one to three weeks after exposure to some organophosphorus compounds. The best-known compound causing toxic peripheral neuropathy is triorthocresyl phosphate (TOCP). The organophosphate neuropathy shows different clinical and electrophysiologic characteristics from acrylamide neuropathy. In this condition, sensory disturbances are usually mild, but distal wasting and weakness may be profound. Later, pyramidal signs become apparent as the peripheral neuropathy regresses. There are few neurophysiologic studies of organophosphate-induced neuropathy in humans. In one patient who had marked distal weakness and wasting with mild sensory disturbances in the lower limbs, an axon innervating a single surviving motor unit in the hand showed normal conduction velocity (Le Quesne, 1978). Sensory nerve action potentials were markedly reduced in amplitude, or absent. In experimental TOCP neuropathy on baboons, Hern (1973) showed that conduction velocities were unaffected at a time when a profound reduction in muscle action potential amplitude had occurred. Histometric measurement showed that TOCP affects fibers of all diameters equally, some large-diameter fibers being spared enough to preserve a normal conduction velocity.

Motor axonal involvement

The primary findings of motor axonal involvement are denervation potential activity in distal muscles, low amplitudes of compound muscle action potentials, increased distal motor latencies, and normal or mildly slowed conduction velocities. One or more of these changes were described in toxic neuropathies due to lead (Oh, 1975; Butchthal and Behse, 1979), Gold (Chamberlain and Bruckner, 1970), mercury vapor (Albers *et al.*, 1982), and carbon disulfide (Seppäläiren and Tolonen, 1974; Gilioli *et al.*, 1979). Lead neuropathy causes bilateral radial nerve palsies without sensory loss in adults due to predominant involvement of motor fibers innervating the extensor muscles of the upper extremities. Catton (1970) detected subclinical neuropathy in a group of workers exposed to lead with temporally dispersed compound muscle action potentials but normal maximal conduction velocity. Gold-induced neuropathy is only known as a complication of chrysotherapy in rheumatoid arthritis. Gold therapy causes symmetrical sensorimotor polyneuropathy, and patients with gold neuropathy may present with myokymia.

NEURONOPATHIES

When the disease starts in the cell body (anterior horn cell, dorsal root ganglion cell or autonomic ganglion cell) the process is a 'dying forward' axonopathy and is best referred to as a neuronopathy. Although there are many experimental models of anterior horn cells disease, some of which are induced by chemical toxicity, a synthetic neurotoxin, β,β-iminodipropinonitrile (IDPN), and ammonium salts for example, there are no known toxins that unquestionably result in anterior horn cell disease in humans. A syndrome clinically resembling amyotrophic lateral sclerosis has been reported in association with lead intoxication (Boothby *et al.*, 1974) and chronic exposure to mercury vapor (Kontarjian, 1961).

Dorsal root ganglion neuronopathy clinically presents with marked ataxia due to profound impairment of proprioceptive modalities of sensation, whereas motor function is conspicuously spared. Sensory nerve action potentials are usually absent while motor conduction studies are normal. Paraneoplastic sensory neuronopathy is a representative disorder. A similar clinical disorder has been described in patients with Sjögren's syndrome and in other patients with an undefined lymphoproliferative condition. Predominantly sensory polyneuropathy caused by a chemotherapeutic agent, cisplatin, is often confused with paraneoplastic sensory neuronopathy. However, electromyography occasionally shows acute or chronic denervation (Roelofs *et al.*, 1984).

Among toxic neuropathies, Schaumburg *et al.* (1983) described seven patients who developed pure sensory polyneuropathy following taking as much as 2–6 g/day of pyridoxine for several months to years. No sensory action potentials could be elicited, whereas motor nerve conduction and electromyogram were normal. The

sural nerve from one patient showed severe fiber loss and some degenerating myelinated fibers. Somatosensory evoked potentials revealed, in contrast to distal axonopathy, impaired proximal conduction of tibial or median nerves. In one patient who had no SEPs after tibial nerve stimulation, definite improvement in central conduction was obtained seven months after withdrawal from pyridoxine. Substantial improvement occurred in all cases in months after the withdrawal. They referred to histological examination of the nervous system in dogs receiving high doses of pyridoxine hydrochloride, which revealed selective degeneration of the sensory neurons of the dorsal root and gasserian ganglion. Parry and Bredesen (1985) reported 16 patients with pure sensory neuropathy with low-dose pyridoxine (0.2–5 g/day for months to years). Lhermitte's sign in eight patients suggested central afferent tract involvement. In pyridoxine intoxication, toxicity directed against the dorsal root ganglion neurons may cause conditions ranging from central–peripheral axonal degeneration to neuronal loss.

MYELINOPATHIES

In myelinopathies there is primary paranodal or segmental demyelination, or demyelination secondary to impairment of the Schwann cells or, in the central nervous system, the oligodendrocytes. Axonopathy and myelinopathy can coexist because of secondary changes, i.e. primary axonal degeneration with secondary demyelination (Dyck *et al.*, 1971), or extensive demyelination with eventual axonal degeneration. Therefore, electrodiagnostic distinction of these pathological types is occasionally difficult. The chronological sequence of the pathological processes should be taken into account to interpret the electrophysiological findings. Lead intoxication is a model of segmental demyelination in some animal species (Gombault, 1880; Fullerton, 1966). There are several lines of evidence to suggest that this change is primary due to impairment of Schwann cells and not secondary to axonal degeneration (Windebank and Dyck, 1984). However, lead toxicity does not produce segmental demyelination in humans (Buchthal and Behse, 1979). Diphtheritic neuropathy is the classical example of a toxic neuropathy in which segmental demyelination is the primary nerve pathology (Veith, 1949; Fisher and Adames, 1956). Perhexiline malleate, 2-(2,2-dicyclohexylethyl) piperidine, is a unique pharmacological agent that causes segmental demyelination (Said, 1978). The drug was introduced for the long-term prophylactic treatment of angina pectoris in the early 1970s. Cytoplasmic inclusions, probably of lysosomal origin, are seen in many different cells including Schwann cells (Fardeau *et al.*, 1979).

Guillain–Barré syndrome and chronic inflammatory demyelinating polyneuropathy are a prototype of demyelinating polyneuropathies. They have immune-mediated pathogenesis and have been successfully treated with immunoregulatory or immunosuppressive procedures. Paradoxically, in patients with bone marrow or solid organ transplantation, vigorous immunosuppression with total body irradiation or chemotherapeutic agents may precipitate the onset of demyelinating polyneuropathy (Amato et al., 1993). Yoshiyama et al. (1997) reported a patient with demyelinating brachial plexus neuropathy complicating syngeneic graft–versus–host disease that was induced by cyclosporin A (CyA). A similar multifocal demyelinating polyneuropathy occurred in patients receiving FK 506 after liver transplantation (Wilson et al., 1994). FK 506 closely resembles CyA in its mechanisms of immunosuppression. Interference with regulatory T cells by these agents may have a role in developing demyelinating polyneuropathy.

AXONAL DEGENERATION WITH SECONDARY DEMYELINATION

The initial ultrastructural changes in experimental acrylamide neuropathy was an accumulation of neurofilaments at the distal ends of peripheral nerves (Prineas, 1969). Paranodal accumulations of neurofilaments may cause axonal swelling and subsequent retraction of myelin. This may yield an appearance of paranodal demyelination (Hopkins, 1970). However, as mentioned before, electrophysiological findings in the earlier stages of most distal axonopathies are those of distal axonal degeneration. In the neuropathy caused by hexacarbons, marked conduction slowing may predominate even when the neuropathy is minimal (Allen et al., 1975). Kuwabara et al. (1993) described multifocal conduction block in a patient with n-hexane neuropathy, in which the proximal conduction blocks were likely responsible for the early clinical motor deficits. Pathologic changes in hexacarbon-solvent neuropathy are characterized by the term 'giant axonal neuropathy' (Korobkin et al., 1975; Spencer et al., 1975). Although giant axonal swellings filled with neurofilaments develop initially in the distal ends, paranodal myelin retraction along the course of nerves causes demyelinative features in electrophysiological investigation.

Neurotoxins that primarily involve the central nervous system

Organic mercury compounds, such as methyl and ethyl mercury, caused two pollution catastrophes, in the 1950s around Minamata Bay in Japan and in 1971–1972 in Iraq. Each compound is primarily neurotoxic to the central nervous system (CNS). A peripheral toxic neuropathy had also been suspected since distal paresthesiae are among prominent symptoms. Methyl mercury in rats affects the dorsal root ganglion, causing secondary degeneration of sensory axons (Somjen et al.,

1973). However, in patients with sensory disturbances, normal sensory nerve conduction was reported in Iraq, (Le Quesne et al., 1974) and absent cortical somatosensory evoked potentials in the presence of normal peripheral conduction time was reported in Japan (Tokuomi et al., 1982).

Lathyrism and Konzo are two examples of toxic myelopathy in which magnetic stimulation studies are helpful. Lathyrism is due to toxicity from the consumption of Lathyrus sativus (the chickling pea). The responsible ingredient, β-N-oxalylamino-L-alanine (BOAA), is an excitotoxic amino acid. Lathyrism is endemic in geographic areas subject to famine and drought, such as Bangladesh, China, Ethiopia, and India. The chickling pea, a drought resistant crop, becomes a cheap and often the only source of nutrition at times of famine and drought. For unknown reasons the disease affects men more frequently than women and characteristically induces pyramidal leg weakness. The arms are typically much less involved (Spencer et al., 1991). Use of transcranial magnetic stimulation in lathyrism has demonstrated prolonged central conduction to the lumbar spinal cord in patients in whom a leg MEP could be recorded, although no response could be elicited in most patients. MEPs recorded from hand muscles are usually normal (Hugon et al., 1993).

Konzo has many similarities to lathyrism. It too causes an acute onset spastic paraparesis, particularly in young malnourished males, during dry seasons in Tanzania, Zaire and other parts of East Africa (Howlett et al., 1990; Tylleskär et al., 1991). The disease spectrum varies from hyper-reflexia in the legs to severe spastic paraparesis with weakness in the arms. There is good evidence that konzo results from ingestion of insufficiently processed cassava roots used to make flour. Short-soaking of the cassava root leads to residual cyanohydrins in the flour, and it is likely that this is responsible for the neurological deficit (Tylleskär et al., 1992). Long-standing high cyanide levels result in reactions between cyanide and cysteine residues in albumin-yielding aminothiazolidine carboxylic acid which has structural similarities to BOAA (Rosling, 1986). A recent study from Uppsala (Tylleskär et al., 1993) carried out extensive electrophysiolgical testing in two patients with konzo disease that were previously seen in Tanzania (Howlett et al., 1990). In both patients motor and sensory nerve conductions, EMG (including SFEMG), autonomic testing, somatosensory, visual and auditory brainstem evoked potentials, and EEG were all normal. However, repeated efforts to stimulate the motor cortex with the magnetic coil at 100% output, with and without facilitation, failed to elicit any MEPs from either hand or leg muscles. Stimulation of the cervical roots with the coil elicited normal responses.

Based upon clinical findings and motor evoked potential studies, they might be better referred to as toxic disorders of the motor pathways in which the corticomotoneuronal axons are primarily involved. The exact site of the lesion could be further elucidated by comparing the ability to evoke responses by electrical versus magnetic transcranial stimulation. If the primary lesion involves the corticomotoneuron, it should be possible to elicit a response by direct activation of the axons with electrical stimulation. On the other hand, if the lesion is in the motor tracts, then both transcranial magnetic and electrical stimulation will fail to elicit a response.

Focal neuropathy (mononeuropathy or multiple neuropathy) due to physical agents

These may result from physical, usually repetitive, trauma producing compression, angulation or stretching of individual nerves. They may occur after irradiation and are also associated with burn injuries. The electrophysiological investigation helps to localize the site of the individual nerve injury and also gives an indication of severity and likelihood of recovery.

Traumatic nerve lesions are classified into neurapraxia, axonotmesis, and neurotmesis that provide a basis for therapeutic approaches (Seddon, 1942, 1943; Mumenthaler and Schliak, 1991). In neurapraxia, or conduction loss without structural change of the axon, recovery takes place within days or weeks after the removal of the cause. Causes of conduction block can be ranged from transient trauma-related disturbance of the blood–nerve barrier with changes in the endoneurial environment and resulting compromise of conductive function to morphologically recognizable damage that is paranodal or segmental demyelination. The disturbance of function can last hours or weeks, rarely up to several months (Denny-Brown and Brenner, 1944). Axonotmesis is defined as a nerve lesion which leads to transection of the axons while the nerve sheaths remain intact. The axons lose continuity, with subsequent Wallerian degeneration. With the structure of the nerve coverings remaining intact, regeneration can take place slowly over months or years at a rate of 1–3 mm/day. A nearly complete recovery is possible after reinnervation of the end organ without surgical intervention (Weiss and Taylor, 1944). Neurotmesis is a nerve lesion with complete transection of the nerve fiber, including the nerve sheaths. The elastic properties of the nerve sheaths causes the dehiscence between the nerve stumps. In the case of short dehiscence spontaneous regeneration is possible, yet it usually leads to imperfect healing. When the dehiscence is large, surgical reunion of the two ends with sutures or an autologous nerve graft is the treatment of choice, but complete restoration of lost function cannot be expected after neurotmesis.

ENTRAPMENT OR COMPRESSION NEUROPATHIES

Genetic, metabolic, and environmental factors all predispose to entrapment or compression neuropathies. Of the environmental factors, repetitive and forceful movements or pressures are the commonest, and a major concern in occupational and sports medicine. However, Buckle (1994) cautioned researchers in the field of ergonomic stressors on the upper limbs to bear in mind that the scientific literature in this field does not usually report the validity or reliability of the methods used for either diagnosis or for exposure to hypothesized risk factors. This section refers to disorders of the upper limb nerves in which, among a variety of causes, ergonomic stressors may also have an important etiological role.

Carpal tunnel syndrome
This is by far the most common form of a median nerve lesion. The median nerve runs in the carpal tunnel after giving off the palmar branch, together with the tendons and tendon sheaths of the long flexors in the tight space between the carpal bones and the flexor retinaculum. A constitutional tightness of the canal predisposes to symptoms. Phalen (1966, 1972) suggested that nonspecific tenosynovitis resulting from work tasks probably contribute the major proportion of carpal tunnel syndrome (CTS) cases, and many recent studies support this view (Buckle, 1994). An increased prevalence of carpal tunnel syndrome is found in certain occupational groups that involved repetitive movements of the hand and wrist (Jarvinen and Kuorinka, 1979; Punnett et al., 1985). The conventional determination of distal motor latency between the wrist and the abductor pollicis brevis or sensory conduction velocity between the lateral fingers and the wrist afford a valuable contribution to the diagnosis. Diagnostic sensitivity is further increased with the determination of nerve conduction in the wrist-to-palm segment for both motor and sensory fibers (Kimura, 1979; Mills, 1985). The electrophysiologic procedure has become so sensitive that it may detect an incidental finding in some asymptomatic subjects, and one must interpret test results in the context of the patient's symptoms, and clinical findings to avoid unnecessary or premature surgical intervention (Kimura, 1989).

Other disorders of the median nerve
Pronator teres syndrome can be caused by entrapment of the median nerve at the site where the nerve passes under the pronator teres muscle, particularly with specific activities that require repetitive grasping or pronation, or both (Hartz et al., 1981). The clinical features include tenderness over the pronator teres, paresthesias of the lateral fingers, weakness of the flexor pollicis longus and abductor pollicis brevis, and preservation of forearm pronators. Sensory change

over the thenar eminence help differentiate this disorder from carpal tunnel syndrome. The conduction studies may reveal mild slowing in the median nerve trunk at the forearm in conjunction with a normal distal latency and normal sensory nerve action potentials at the wrist.

The anterior interosseous nerve arises from the median nerve some 5–8 cm distal to the lateral epicondyle and is pure motor supplying the flexor pollicis longus, flexor digitorum profundus, and the pronator quadratus muscles. The isolated dysfunction of this nerve was first described by Kiloh and Nevin (1952), and has since been reported repeatedly. Approximately one-half of the cases had occurred spontaneously, and less frequently in association with various etiologies including a fracture of the forearm. There are cases that have been recorded among those involved in occupations or strenuous exercise requiring elbow flexion and pronation of a repetitive nature (O'Brien and Upton, 1972; Nakano et al., 1977; Rask, 1979). Electromyography shows selective denervation in the muscles described above. Ordinary median nerve conduction studies reveal no abnormalities (O'Brien and Upton, 1972). A delayed proximal latency of the median nerve to the pronator quadratus muscle compared to the latency to the abductor pollicis brevis muscle is helpful for the diagnosis (Meya and Hacke, 1983).

Ulnar nerve

Ulnar nerve entrapment at the elbow is frequently referred to as cubital tunnel syndrome, and results from widely varying causes (Levy and Apfelberg, 1972; Hagstrom, 1977). This is also considered an occupational disorder in workers who must support themselves on their elbow or those who work with their arms in flexed and restricted postures. Motor or mixed nerve conduction study across the elbow is diagnostic, when showing a drop in compound muscle action potential amplitude greater than 25%, (Pickett and Coleman, 1984) or slowing of conduction velocity by greater than 10 m/sec as compared with the more proximal or distal segments (Eisen, 1974; Eisen and Danon, 1974). Electromyography may demonstrate denervation in the first dorsal interosseous muscle which is the most consistently affected muscle in ulnar nerve lesion at any level. In cases in which the ulnar nerve is trapped at the constriction by the aponeurosis of the flexor carpi ulnaris, denervation can be seen in the ulnar half of the flexor digitorum profundus, sparing the flexor carpi ulnaris which receives nerve supply proximal to the aponeurosis.

The palmar branch of the ulnar nerve tends to suffer from compression due to chronic repetitive trauma to the base of the hypothenar eminence. Many factors, including repetitive work tasks and sports injuries, are associated with this disorder (Sunderland, 1991), which is sometimes named according to the task such as cyclist palsy (Noth et al., 1980) or video-game palsy (Friedland and St John, 1984). Exposure to vibration, usually for several years, is a well-recognized risk factor for both carpal tunnel syndrome (Cannon et al., 1981) and injury to the palmar branch of the ulnar nerve (Dawson et al., 1983), as well as for vibration white finger (Raynaud's phenomenon). Sensory deficit, if present, spares the dorsum of the hand innervated by the dorsal cutaneous branch, which arises proximal to the wrist. Damage of the deep motor branch distal to the origin of the superficial sensory branch gives rise to no sensory abnormality and spares motor branches supplying the hypothenar muscle. Electromyography shows selective abnormalities of the intrinsic hand muscles innervated by the ulnar nerve except for abductor digiti minimi. The compound muscle action potential recorded from the abductor digiti minimi is routinely normal, whereas that recorded from the first dorsal interosseous may show a prolonged latency and reduced amplitude.

Radial nerve

Pressure palsies on the upper arm are the most common radial nerve palsies and the most frequent among sleep palsies. The sleep was usually particularly deep (paralysie des ivrogens, Saturday night palsy), or in addition the arm lay unfavorably on a hard surface (park bench palsy). Besides sleep palsies, such tasks as the carrying of heavy loads in the Near East (Kirchof et al., 1962) or the pressure resulting from a tight rifle sling (Munz et al., 1955; Burke, 1957) may compress the radial nerve on the inner aspects of the arm. Strenuous muscular effort was considered to be the problem leading to the condition (Lotem et al., 1971; Dawson et al., 1983). The most impressive and typical sign is the drop hand. The most proximal motor deficit in these cases is the paralysis of the brachioradialis muscle. Electromyographic exploration of paralyzed muscles and sensory conduction study of the superficial radial nerve are useful to differentiate between neurapraxia and axonotmesis, although these two types of injury coexist to a varying degree in most cases.

Posterior interosseous syndrome results from nerve entrapment distal to the elbow joint, where the deep branch enters the supinator muscle. Among a variety of causes, tasks that require repeated pronation and supination or forceful extension of the arms seemed to be associated with the onset (Feldman et al., 1983). Even the emergence of a lateral epicondylitis (tennis elbow) supposedly is an expression of this disorder in some cases (Thompson and Kopell, 1959; Capener, 1966; Comtet et al., 1976; Werner, 1979). The patient complains of pain over the lateral aspect of the elbow but experiences no sensory loss. Despite the weak extensor carpi ulnaris, normal contraction of the extensor carpi radialis longus and brevis innervated by the radial nerve proper results in characteristic radial deviation of the wrist on attempted dorsiflexion. In an individual case it is quite possible that a different extensor muscle will be affected first. The differential diagnosis includes rupture of the extensor tendon(s), in which passive palmar flexion of the wrist induces no extension of the metacarpophalangeal joints. Electromyographic findings of denervation confirm the diagnosis.

Thoracic outlet syndrome

The lower trunk of the brachial plexus tends to be compressed in several anatomical conditions in the posterior scalene triangle that is bordered by the scalenus anterior muscle, the scalenus medius muscle, and the first rib. A rudimentary cervical rib or a fibrous band attaching to the first rib may compress the lower trunk and the subclavian artery, especially in women with 'droopy' shoulders (Swift and Nichols, 1984). This syndrome is frequently reported to result from repetitive movements of the shoulder and arm, especially where abduction and adduction are involved. Musicians are susceptible to the syndrome due to maintaining their shoulders in abducted or extended positions for many hours, along with the need for precise digit control (Lederman, 1989). A frequent subjective complaint is diffuse pain in the arm, predominantly on the ulnar side of the hand and the forearm, which is position dependent. The neurological deficits are those of a lower brachial plexus palsy, i.e. sensory and motor deficits distributing C8 and T1 segments. The electrodiagnostic findings include a reduced or absent ulnar but normal median sensory action potential, a small median compound muscle action potential, and a prolonged ulnar F-wave latency. Electromyography shows evidence of denervation in the intrinsic hand muscles, especially the abductor pollicis brevis. Patients without neurological deficits have none of these abnormalities even when they have signs of position and movement-dependent circulatory compromise in the subclavian artery (Daube, 1975).

RADIATION NEUROPATHY

The peripheral nervous system is much less sensitive to the deleterious effects of radiation than is the central nervous system. For example, there are no acute sequels to radiation therapy on peripheral nerves; they are all subacute and more frequently chronic. The brachial and lumbar-sacral plexus are much the commonest sites of involvement. Radiation affecting individual peripheral nerves is most unusual. Salner et al. (1981) described a brachial plexopathy resulting from radiation occurring within a few weeks of treatment (early delayed brachial plexopathy) that was characterized by paresthesias in the hand and forearm, sometimes associated with pain which was occasionally accompanied by weakness and atrophy distributed

between myotomes C6 to T1. Spontaneous recovery over a few weeks or months is a usual course. Nerve conduction studies in these patients showed slowing of conduction in keeping with focal demyelination, a neurophysiological finding which correlates with the benign clinical course. More commonly postradiation brachial or lumbosacral plexopathy develops months to years after radiation treatment and has a progressive course (late delayed radiation plexopathy). The main differential diagnosis of radiation brachial plexopathy, most commonly occurring after therapy for breast cancer, is carcinomatous infiltration (Thomas and Colby, 1972). Radiation plexopathy usually affects the upper trunk, is painless, and associated with lymphedema (Kori et al., 1981). This contrasts with painful lower trunk lesions with a Horner's syndrome which usually imply tumor infiltration, best confirmed by computerized tomography (CT) scan or magnetic resonance imaging (MRI) of the plexus. In a series of 50 patients reported by Thomas et al. (1985), radiation lumbosacral plexopathy caused painless leg weakness early, often bilaterally. In contrast, tumor patients typically had painful unilateral weakness. Sciatic neuropathy has also been reported after intraoperative irradiation (Kinsella et al., 1985).

In late delayed radiation plexopathy, features of axonal injury predominate and these are most readily detected by needle electromyography. Motor nerve conduction studies are usually normal, but sensory nerve action potentials may be of reduced amplitude or even absent (Eisen, 1993). A rather unique type of spontaneous electromyographic discharge, myokymia, can be recorded in about 30% of radiogenic nerve lesions (Stöhr, 1982). It is not specific to radiation, but when recorded, myokymic discharges (recurrent trains of motor unit potentials) are a diagnostic clue to radiation neuropathy; it is not seen as a result of carcinomatous infiltration (Albers et al., 1981a; Eisen, 1993).

BURN-ASSOCIATED NEUROPATHY

Multiple mononeuropathy after thermal burn covering greater than 20% total body surface area has been reported (Dagum et al., 1993; Marquez et al., 1993). In a series of 16 patients with peripheral neuropathy from a tertiary care burn center, Marquez et al. (1993) identified 13 patients with multiple mononeuropathy (12 patients) or mononeuropathy (one patient). The upper limb (36 nerves) were more commonly involved than lower limb (11 nerves). Nerve conduction studies showed that only two of these lesions appeared to be compressive with conduction block and the remainder were axonal without segments of slow conduction. Of 13 patients, nine (69%) had axonal lesion in the area of maximal thermal burn, two (15%) had lesions only in unburned areas and two (15%) had lesions in burned and unburned areas. The extent of the patient's burn (full thickness burns) and total body surface burns correlated to the number of nerves affected. Pathophysiology and etiologic mechanisms are unknown, although vascular occlusion of the vasa nervorum, direct thermal injury, or disseminated neurotoxin are postulated.

DISORDERS OF NEUROMUSCULAR JUNCTION

Botulinum toxin inhibits calcium-dependent ACh release, causing failure of neuromuscular transmission, possibly by blocking exocytosis at the release sites (Kao et al., 1976; Maselli et al., 1992). Organophosphorus compounds inhibit acetylcholinesterase and cause a depolarizing block of neuromuscular transmission. Aminoglycoside antibiotics interfere with both presynaptic ACh release and postsynaptic transmission. In patients being treated with antibiotics, the most frequently encountered clinical syndrome is postoperative respiratory depression. Argov and Mastaglia (1979) listed a variety of drugs used in clinical practice that may interfere with neuromuscular transmission by causing a postsynaptic block or through an additional presynaptic effect (Figure 17.1). The clinical manifestation of neuromuscular block, however, occurs only when the safety margin of neuromuscular transmission is reduced, as in hypocalcemia or other electrolyte disturbances, or in patients with subclinical myasthenia gravis.

In diagnosis of botulism, electrophysiologic investigations have a limited value because the abnormalities tend to evolve with time and may not be present early in the disease. The amplitude of the compound muscle action potential is small in affected muscles, although the muscles that are affected first, such as the ocular and oropharyngeal muscles, are inaccessible for this study. There may be a decremental pattern to low-frequency repetitive nerve stimulation in some muscles, but this is not seen in all patients (Gutmann and Pratt, 1976). Post-tetanic potentiation of 30–100% is seen in some muscles at some time in more than 60% of patients (Cherington, 1974). Since single fiber EMG demonstrates markedly increased jitter and blocking, (Schiller and Stålberg, 1978) its application to oropharyngeal muscles may provide evidence for an early disease.

In infantile botulism, Gutierrez et al. (1994) reviewed the literature on the electrophysiologic features and concluded that low compound muscle action potential amplitude in combination with tetanic and post-tetanic potentiation and absence of post-tetanic exhaustion support the diagnosis.

D-Penicillamine, which is used in the treatment of rheumatoid arthritis and Wilson's disease, can induce myasthenia gravis that is clinically, immunologically, and electrophysiologically indistinguishable from idiopathic myasthenia gravis. Penicillamine-induced myasthenia is usually mild and may be restricted to the ocular muscles, in which case repetitive nerve stimulation tests may be normal. However, singe fiber EMG demonstrates increased jitter, and the degree of jitter shows a positive correlation with the duration of administration but not the dosage of penicillamine (Albers et al., 1981b).

Besides their well-known anticholinesterase action resulting in a typical cholinergic crisis, organophosphorus compounds are capable of producing several subacute or chronic neurological syndromes. Transmission abnormalities in acute cholinergic crisis is produced by an excess effect of ACh (depolarization block). Electrophysiological studies of a 10-year-old girl with cholinergic crisis who had an unsuspected accidental cutaneous exposure showed repetitive compound muscle action potentials in response to a single stimulation. With repetitive stimulation at higher rates, an initial decrement at the second response was followed by subsequent progressive facilitation (Maselli et al., 1986). Organophosphate-induced delayed neuropathy that arises one to three weeks after exposure to some compounds was described before. The intermittent syndrome (Senanayake and Karalliedde, 1987), is a rapid deterioration of strength appearing after apparent recovery from the cholinergic crisis and before the usual onset of delayed neuropathy. A similar paralytic syndrome was described earlier by Wadia et al. (1974). The most threatening symptom is a sudden respiratory failure requiring re-intubation. Kuwabara et al. (1990) showed characteristic transmission abnormalities in five patients with the intermediate syndrome. Repetitive stimulation of the median nerve at 20 and 50 Hz showed an initial small CMAP amplitude and a progressive decrement of subsequent potentials up to 70 to 90%, which was correlated to clinical weakness.

An acute generalized weakness associated with the use of non-depolarizing muscle blocking agents such as pancuronium and vecuronium, often in combination with glucocorticoid administration, has been increasingly reported in intensive care unit patients. Electrophysiological findings of these patients include prolonged neuromuscular transmission blockade, reduced CMAP amplitude, and a 'myopathic' motor unit potential with or without fibrillation (Zochodne et al., 1994). A lack of abnormalities in conduction velocities and sensory action potentials differentiate this condition from 'critical illness polyneuropathy' that is another important cause of acute paralysis in intensive care unit patients. Fibrillations and positive sharp waves may arise immediately after onset of paralysis, which cannot be expected in the case of polyneuropathy. Histological changes are myofiber necrosis and severe cases are associated with high serum creatinine kinase (CK) levels, myoglobinuria, and acute renal failure (Sitwell et al., 1991; Zochodne et al., 1994). Prolonged neuromuscular transmission deficit may also have a role in the onset of paralysis in less severe cases. Zochodne *et al.* (1994) showed decremental responses with repetitive stimulation in three patients from 3 to 16 days following vecuronium withdrawal, and found a persistently elevated level of 3-desacetyl-vecuronium, a metabolite nearly as active as its parent.

REFERENCES

Albers, J.W., Allen, A.A., Bastron, J.A. and Daube, J.R. 1981a: Limb myokymia. *Muscle Nerve*, **4**, 494–504.

Albers, J.W., Beals, C.A. and Levine, S.P. 1981b: Neuromuscular transmission in rheumatoid arthritis, with and without penicillamine treatment. *Neurology*, **31**, 1562–4.

Albers, J.W., Cavender, G.D., Levine, S.P. and Langolf, G.D. 1982: Asymptomatic sensorimotor polyneuropathy in workers exposed to elemental mercury. *Neurology*, **32**, 1168–74.

Allen, N., Mendell, J.M., Billmaier, D.J., Fontaine, R.E. and O'Neil, J. 1975: Toxic polyneuropathy due to methyl *n*-butyl ketone. *Archives of Neurology*, **32**, 209–18.

Amato, A.A., Barohn, R.J., Sahenk, Z., Tutschka, P.J. and Mendell, J.R. 1993: Polyneuropathy complicating bone marrow and solid organ transplantation. *Neurology*, **43**, 1513–8.

Arezzo, J.C., Schaumburg, H.H., Vaughan, Jr H.G., Spencer, P.S. and Barna, J. 1982: Hind limb somatosensory evoked potentials in the monkey. The effects of distal axonopathy. *Annals of Neurology*, **12**, 24–32.

Argov, Z. and Mastaglia, F.L. 1979: Disorders of neuromuscular transmission caused by drugs. *New England Journal of Medicine*, **301**, 409.

Boothby, J.A., De Jesus, P.V. and Rowland, L.P. 1974: Reversible form of motor neuron disease: lead 'neuritis'. *Archives of Neurology*, **31**, 18–23.

Buchthal, F. and Behse, F. 1979: Electrophysiology and nerve biopsy in men exposed to lead. *British Journal of Industrial Medicine*, **36**, 135–47.

Buckle, P. 1994: Ergonomic stressors related to neurological disorders of the upper limbs. In *Occupational Neurology and Clinical Neurotoxicology*, Bleecker, M.L. (ed.), pp 253–67. Baltimore, MD: Williams & Wilkins.

Burke, D., Skuse, N.F. and Lethlean, A.K. 1981: Cutaneous and muscle afferent components of the cerebral potential evoked by electrical stimulation of human peripheral nerves. *Electroencephalography and Clinical Neurophysiology*, **51**, 579.

Burke, E.L. 1957: Rifle sling palsy in Marine Corps recruits. *United States Armed Forces Medical Journal*, **8**, 1189–94.

Cannon, L.J., Bernacki, E.J. and Walter, S.D. 1981: Personal and occupational factors associated with carpal tunnel syndrome. *Journal of Occupational Medicine*, **23**, 255–8.

Capener, N. 1966: The vulnerability of the posterior interosseous nerve of the forearm. *Journal of Bone and Joint Surgery*, **48**, 770–3.

Casey, E.B., Jellife, A.M., Le Quesne, P.M. *et al.* 1973: Vincristine neuropathy: clinical and electrophysiological observations. *Brain*, **96**, 69–86.

Casey, E.B. and Le Quesne, P.M. 1972a: Digital nerve action potentials in healthy subjects and in carpal tunnel and diabetic patients. *Journal of Neurology, Neurosurgery and Psychiatry*, **35**, 612–23.

Casey, E.B. and Le Quesne, P.M. 1972b: Evidence for a distal lesion in alcoholic neuropathy. *Journal of Neurology, Neurosurgery and Psychiatry*, **35**, 624–30.

Catton, M.J., Harrison, M.J.G., Fullerton, P.M. and Kazantzis, G. 1970: Subclinical neuropathy in lead workers. *British Medical Journal*, **2**, 80–2.

Chamberlain, M.A. and Bruckner, F.E. 1970: Rheumatoid neuropathy. Clinical and electrophysiological features. *Annals of the Rheumatic Diseases*, **29**, 609–16.

Cherington, M. 1974: Botulism. Ten-year experience. *Archives of Neurology*, **30**, 432.

Chiappa, K.H. 1990: *Evoked Potentials in Clinical Medicine*, 2nd edn. New York: Raven Press.

Comtet, J.J., Cahmbaud, D. and Généty, J. 1976: La compression de la branche postérieure du nerf radial. Une étiologie méconnue de certaines paralysies et de certaines épicondylalgies rebelles. *Nouvelle Presse médicale*, **5**, 1111–14.

Cusik, J.F., Myklebust, J.B., Larson, S.J. and Sances, A. Jr 1979: Spinal cord evaluation by cortical evoked responses. *Archives of Neurology*, **36**, 140.

Dagum, A.B., Peters, W.J., Neligan, P.C. and Douglas, L.G. 1993: Severe multiple mononeuropathy in patients with major thermal burns. *Journal of Burn Care and Rehabilitation*, **14**, 440–5.

Daube, J.R. 1975: Nerve conduction studies in the thoracic outlet syndrome. *Neurology*, **25**, 847.

Dawson, D.M., Halett, M. and Millender, L. 1983: *Entrapment Neuropathies*. Boston, MA: Little, Brown & Co.

Denny-Brown, D. and Brenner, C. 1944: Lesion in peripheral nerve resulting from compression by spring clip. *Archives of Neurology*, **52**, 1–19.

Dyck, P.J., Johnson, W.J., Lambert, E.H. and O'Brien, P.C. 1971: Segmental demyelination secondary to axonal degeneration in uremic neuropathy. *Mayo Clinic Proceedings*, **46**, 400.

Eisen, A. 1974: Early diagnosis of ulnar nerve palsy: an electrophysiologic study. *Neurology*, **24**, 256–62.

Eisen, A. 1993: The electrodiagnosis of plexopathies. In *Clinical Electromyography*, Brown, W.F. and Bolton, C.F. (eds), 2nd edn, pp 211–25. Boston, MA: Butterworth-Heinemann.

Eisen, A. and Aminoff, M.J. 1986: Somatosensory evoked potentials. In *Electrodiagnosis in Clinical Neurology*, Aminoff, M.J. (ed.), 2nd edn, pp 535–73. New York: Churchill Livingstone.

Eisen, A. and Danon, J. 1974: The mild cubital tunnel syndrome: its natural history and indication for surgical intervention. *Neurology*, **24**, 608–13.

Fardeau, M., Tomé, F.M.S. and Simon, P. 1979: Muscle and nerve changes induced by perhexiline maleate in man and mice. *Muscle Nerve*, **2**, 24–36.

Feldman, R.G., Goldman, R. and Keyserling Monroe, W. 1983: Peripheral nerve entrapment syndromes and ergonomic factors. *American Journal of Industrial Medicine*, **4**, 661–81.

Fisher, C.M. and Adames, R.D. 1956: Diphtheric polyneuritis – a pathological study. *Journal of Neuropathology and Experimental Neurology*, **15**, 243.

Friedland, R.P. and St John, J.N. 1984: Video-game palsy. Distal ulnar neuropathy in a video game enthusiast. *New England Journal of Medicine*, **311**, 58–9.

Fullerton, P.M. 1966: Chronic peripheral neuropathy produced by lead poisoning in guinea-pigs. *Journal of Neurology, Neurosurgery and Psychiatry*, **25**, 218–36.

Fullerton, P.M. 1969: Electrophysiological and histological observations on peripheral nerves in acrylamide poisoning in man. *Journal of Neurosurgery and Psychiatry*, **32**, 186–92.

Fullerton, P.M. and Barnes, J.M. 1966: Peripheral neuropathy in rats produced by acrylamide. *British Journal of International Medicine*, **23**, 210–21.

Gandevia, S.A., Burke, D. and McKeon, B. 1984: The projection of muscle afferents from the hand to cerebral cortex in man. *Brain*, **107**, 1.

Gilioli, R., Bulgheroni, C., Bertazzi, P.A. *et al.* 1979: Study of neurological and neurophysiological impairment in carbon disulfide workers. *Medicina del Lavoro*, **69**, 130–43.

Gombault, A. 1880: Contribution a l'etude anatomique de la nevrite parenchymateuse subaigue et chronique – nevrite segmentaire peri–axile. *Archives of Neurology (Paris)*, **1**, 11.

Guiheneuc, P., Ginet, J., Grouleau, J.Y. *et al.* 1980: Early phase of vincristine neuropathy in man. *Journal of the Neurological Sciences*, **45**, 355–66.

Gutierrez, A.R., Bodensteiner, J. and Gutmann, L. 1994: Electrodiagnosis of infantile botulism. *Journal of Child Neurology*, **9**, 362–5.

Gutmann, L. and Pratt, L. 1976: Pathophysiologic aspects of human botulism. *Archives of Neurology*, **33**, 175.

Hagstrom, P. 1977: Ulnar nerve compression at the elbow. Results of surgery in 85 cases. *Scandinavian Journal of Plastic and Reconstructive Surgery*, **11**, 59–62.

Hartz, C.R., Linscheid, R.L., Gramse, R.R. and Daube, J.R. 1981: The pronator teres syndrome, compressive neuropathy of the median nerve. *Journal of Bone and Joint Surgery*, **63**, 885–90.

He, F.S., Zhang, S.L., Wang, H.L. *et al.* 1989: Neurological and electroneuromyographic assessment of the adverse effects of acrylamide on occupationally exposed workers. *Scandinavian Journal of Work Environment and Health,* **15**, 125–9.

Henneman, E., Somjen, G. and Carpenter, D.O. 1965: Functional significance of cell size in spinal motoneurons. *Journal of Neurophysiology,* **28**, 560–80.

Hern, J.E.C. 1973: Tri-ortho cresyl phosphate neuropathy in the baboon. In *New Developments in Electromyography and Clinical Neurophysiology,* Desmedt, J.E. (ed.), Vol. 2, pp 181–7. Basel: Karger.

Hopkins, A.P. 1970: The effect of acrylamide on the peripheral nervous system of the baboon. *Journal of Neurosurgery and Psychiatry,* **33**, 805.

Hopkins, A.P. and Gilliatt, R.W. 1971: Motor and sensory nerve conduction velocity in the baboon, normal values and changes during acrylamide neuropathy. *Journal of Neurosurgery and Psychiatry,* **34**, 415–26.

Howlett, W.P., Brubaker, G.R., Milingi, N. and Rosling, H. 1990: Konzo: an epidemic upper motor neuron disease studied in Tanzania. *Brain,* **113**, 223–35.

Hugon, J., Ludolph, A.C., Spencer, P.S., Gimenz-Roldan, S. and Dumas, J.L. 1993: Studies on the etiology and pathogenesis of motor neuron diseases III – magnetic cortical stimulation in patients with lathyrism. *Acta Neurologica Scandinavica,* **88**, 412–6.

Jarvinen, T. and Kuorinka, I. 1979: Prevalence of tenosynovitis and other occupational injuries of upper extremities in repetitive work. *Arhiv za Higijenu Rada I Toksikologiju,* **30**, 1281–4.

Kaji, R. and Sumner, A.J. 1987: Bipolar recording of short-latency somatosensory evoked potentials after median nerve stimulation. *Neurology,* **37**, 410–8.

Kao, I., Drachman, D.B. and Price, D.L. 1976: Botulinum toxin: mechanism of presynaptic blockade. *Science,* **193**, 1256–8.

Kiloh, L. and Nevin, S. 1952: Isolated neuritis of the anterior interosseous nerve. *British Medical Journal,* **1**, 850–1.

Kimura, J. 1979: The carpal tunnel syndrome. Localization of conduction abnormalities within the distal segment of the median nerve. *Brain,* **102**, 619–35.

Kimura, J. 1989: *Electrodiagnosis in Diseases of Nerve and Muscle, Principle and Practice,* 2nd edn. Philadelphia, PA: F.A. Davis.

Kirchhof, J.K.J., Kumral, K. and Ertekin, C. 1962: Doppelseitige Radialislähmung infolge lastentragens auf dem Rücken (Druckläsion). *Nervenarzt,* **33**, 536–8.

Kinsella, T.J., Sindelar, W.F., DeLuca, A.M. *et al.* 1985: Tolerance of peripheral nerve to intraoperative radiotherapy, clinical and experimental studies. *International Journal of Radiation, Oncology, Biology and Physics,* **11**, 1579.

Kontarjian, A.D. 1961: A syndrome clinically resembling amyotrophic lateral sclerosis following chronic mercurialism. *Neurology,* **11**, 639–44.

Kori, S.H., Foley, K.M. and Posner, J.B. 1981: Brachial plexus lesions in patients with cancer, 100 cases. *Neurology,* **31**, 41–50.

Korobkin, R., Asbury, A.K., Sumner, A.J. *et al.* 1975: Glue-sniffing neuropathy. *Archives of Neurology,* **32**, 158–62.

Kuwabara, S., Ito, N., Watanabe, S. and Hirayama, K. 1990: Dysfunction of neuromuscular junction in acute organophosphate poisoning. A serial study of repetitive stimulation test. *Neurologica Medico (Tokyo),* **33**, 377–80.

Kuwabara, S., Nakajima, M., Tuboi, Y., Hirayama, K. 1993: Multifocal conduction block in n-hexane neuropathy. *Muscle Nerve,* **16**, 1416–7.

Le Quesne, P.M. 1978: Neurophysiological investigation of subclinical and minimal toxic neuropathies. *Muscle Nerve,* **1**, 392–5.

Le Quesne, P.M., Damluji, S.F. and Rustam, H. 1974: Electrophysiological studies of peripheral nerves in patients with organic mercury poisoning. *Journal of Neurosurgery and Psychiatry,* **37**, 333–9.

Lederman, R.J. 1989: Peripheral nerve disorders in instrumentalists. *Annals of Neurology,* **26**, 640–6.

Levy, D.M. and Apfelberg, D.B. 1972: Results of anterior transposition for ulnar neuropathy at the elbow. *American Journal of Surgery,* **123**, 304–8.

Lotem, M., Fried, A., Levy, M. *et al.* 1971: Radial palsy following muscular effort. *Journal of Bone and Joint Surgery,* **53**, 500.

Lueders, H., Andrish, J., Gurd, A. *et al.* 1981: Origin of far-field subcortical potentials evoked by stimulation of the posterior tibial nerve. *Electroencephalography and Clinical Neurophysiology,* **52**, 336–44.

Magladery, J.W. and McDougal, D.B. Jr 1950: Electrophysiological studies of nerve and reflex activity in normal man. 1. Identification of certain reflexes in the electromyogram and the conduction velocity of peripheral nerve fibers. *Bell Johns Hopkins Hospital,* **86**, 265–90.

Marquez, S., Turley, J.J. and Peters, W.J. 1993: Neuropathy in burn patients. *Brain,* **116**, 471–83.

Maselli, R.A., Burnett, M.E. and Tonsgard, J.H. 1992: *In vitro* microelectrode study of neuromuscular transmission in a case of botulism. *Muscle Nerve,* **15**, 273–6.

Maselli, R.A., Jacobsen, J.H. and Spire, J-P. 1986: Edrophonium, an aid in the diagnosis of acute organophosphate poisoning. *Annals of Neurology,* **19**, 508–10.

Merton, P.A. and Morton, H.B. 1980: Stimulation of the cerebral cortex in the intact human subject. *Nature,* **285**, 227.

Meya, U. and Hacke, W. 1983: Anterior interosseous nerve syndrome following supracondylar lesions of the median nerve, clinical findings and electrophysiological investigations. *Journal of Neurology,* **229**, 91–96.

Mills, K.R. 1985: Orthodromic sensory action potentials from palmar stimulation in the diagnosis of carpal tunnel syndrome. *Journal of Neurosurgery and Psychiatry,* **48**, 250–5.

Mumenthaler, M. and Schliack, H. (eds) 1991: *Peripheral Nerve Lesions.* New York: Thieme.

Munz, H.H., Coonrad, R.W. and Murchison, R.A. 1955: Rifle sling palsy. *United States Armed Forces Medical Journal,* **6**, 353.

Murray, N.M.F. 1991: The clinical usefulness of magnetic cortical stimulation. *Electroencephalography and Clinical Neurophysiology,* **85**, 81–5.

Nakajima, M. and Hirayama, K. 1995: Midcervical central cord syndrome, numb clumsy hands due to mid-line cervical disc protrusion at the C3–4 intervertebral level. *Journal of Neurosurgery and Psychiatry,* **58**, 607–13.

Nakano, K.K., Lundergan, C. and Okihiro, M.M. 1977: Anterior interosseous nerve syndromes. Diagnostic methods and alternative treatments. *Archives of Neurology,* **34**, 477–80.

Nielsen, V.K. and Wright, K.C. 1987: Toxic polyneuropathies. In *Clinical Electromyography,* Brown, W.F. and Bolton, C.F. (eds), pp 285–303. Boston, MA: Butterworth-Heinemann.

Noth, J., Dietz, V. and Mauritz, K.H. 1980: Cyclist's palsy, neurological and EMG in four cases with distal ulnar lesions. *Journal of Neurological Sciences,* **47**, 111–16.

O'Brien, M.D. and Upton, A.R. 1972: Anterior interosseous nerve syndrome. A case report with neurophysiological investigation. *Journal of Neurosurgery and Psychiatry,* **35**, 531–16.

Oh, S.J. 1975: Lead neuropathy. Case report. *Archives of Physical Medicine and Rehabilitation,* **56**, 312–17.

Parry, G.J. and Bredesen, D.E. 1985: Sensory neuropathy with low-dose pyridoxine. *Neurology,* **35**, 1466–8.

Phalen, G.S. 1966: The carpal-tunnel syndrome. Seventeen years' experience in diagnosis and treatment of six hundred and fifty-four hands. *Journal of Bone and Joint Surgery,* **48**, 211–28.

Phalen, G.S. 1972: The carpal tunnel syndrome. *Clinical Orthopedics and Related Research,* **83**, 29–40.

Pickett, J.B. and Coleman, L.L. 1984: Localizing ulnar nerve lesions to the elbow by motor conduction studies. *Electromyography and Clinical Neurophysiology,* **24**, 343–60.

Prineas, J. 1969: The pathogenesis of dying-back polyneuropathies. Part II. An ultrastructural study of experimental acrylamide intoxication in the cat. *Journal of Neuropathology Experimental Neurology,* **28**, 571.

Punnett, L., Robins, J.M., Wegman, D.H. and Keyserling, W.M. 1985: Soft tissue disorders in the upper limbs of female garment workers. *Scandinavian Journal of Work and Environmental Health,* **11**, 417–25.

Rask, M.R. 1979: Anterior interosseous nerve entrapment (Kiloh–Nevin syndrome): report of seven cases. *Clinical Orthopedics and Related Research,* **142**, 176–81.

Roelofs, R.I., Hrushesky, W., Rogin, J. and Rosenberg, L. 1984: Peripheral sensory neuropathy and cisplatin chemotherapy. *Neurology,* **34**, 934.

Rosling, H. 1986: Cassava, cyanide, and epidemic spastic paraparesis. A study in Mozambique on dietary cyanide exposure. *Acta Universitatis Upsaliensis,* **19**, 1–52.

Rossini, P.M. and Caramia, M.D. 1988: Methodological and physiological considerations on the electric or magnetic transcranial stimulation. In *Non-invasive Stimulation of the Central Nervous System, Methodological and Physiological Aspects*, Rossini, P.M. and Marsden, C.D. (eds), pp 37–65. New York: Alan R. Liss.

Said, G. 1978: Perhexiline neuropathy: a clinicopathological study. *Annals of Neurology*, **3**, 259–66.

Salner, A.L., Botnick, L.E., Herzog, A.G. *et al.* 1981: Reversible brachial plexopathy following primary radiation therapy for breast cancer. *Cancer Treatment Report*, **65**, 797.

Schaumburg, H.H., Kaplan, J., Windebank, A. *et al.* 1983: Sensory neuropathy from pyridoxine abuse. A new megavitamin syndrome. *New England Journal of Medicine*, **309**, 445–8.

Schaumburg, H.H. and Spencer, P.S. 1979: Toxic neuropathies. *Neurology*, **29**, 429–31.

Schiller, H.H. and Stålberg, E. 1978: Human botulism studied with single fiber electromyography. *Archives of Neurology*, **35**, 346.

Seddon, H.J. 1942: Classification of nerve injuries. *British Medical Journal*, **2**, 237–9.

Seddon, H.J. 1943: Three types of nerve injury. *Brain*, **66**, 237–88.

Senanayake, N. and Karalliedde, L. 1987: Neurotoxic effects of organophosphorus insecticides. *New England Journal of Medicine*, **316**, 761–3.

Seppäläinen, A.M. and Tolonen, M. 1974: Neurotoxicity of long-term exposure to carbon disulfide in the viscose rayon industry. A neurophysiological study. *Work and Environmental Health*, **11**, 45–153.

Sitwell, L.D., Weinshender, B.G., Monpetit, V. and Reid, D. 1991: Complete ophthalmoplegia as a complication of acute corticosteroid- and pancuronium-associated myopathy. *Neurology*, **41**, 921–2.

Somjen, G.G., Herman, S.P. and Klein, R. 1973: Electrophysiology of methyl mercury poisoning. *Journal of Pharmacology and Experimental Therapeutics*, **186**, 579–92.

Spencer, P.S., Allen, C.N., Kisby, G.E., Ludolph, A.C., Ross, S.M. and Roy, D.N. 1991: Lathyrism and Western Pacific amyotrophic lateral sclerosis. Etiology of short and long latency motor system disorders. In *Advances in Neurology, Amyotrophic Lateral Sclerosis and Other Motor Neuron Diseases*, Rowland, L.P. (ed.), Vol. 56, pp 287–299. New York: Raven Press.

Spencer, P.S. and Schaumburg, H.H. 1976: Central-peripheral distal axonopathy – the pathogenesis of dying-back polyneuropathies. In *Progress in Neuropathology*, Zimmerman, H. (ed.), Vol. 3, p 253. New York: Grune & Stratton.

Spencer, P.S. and Schaumburg, H.H. 1977: Ultrastructural studies of the dying back process. IV. Differential vulnerability of PNS and CNS fibers in experimental central-peripheral exonopathies. *Journal of Neuropathology and Experimental Neurology*, **36**, 300–20.

Spencer, P.S., Schaumburg, H.H., Raleigh, R.L. and Terhaar, C.J. 1975: Nervous system degeneration produced by the industrial solvent methyl *n*-butyl ketone. *Archives of Neurology*, **32**, 219–22.

Stahlberg, D., Barany, F., Einarsson, K., Ursing, B., Elmqvist, D. and Persson, A. 1991: Neurophysiologic studies of patients with Crohn's disease on long-term treatment with metronidazole. *Scandinavian Journal of Gastroenterology*, **26**, 219–24.

Stålberg, E. and Trontelj, J. 1979: *Single Fiber Electromyography*. Old Woking, Surrey: Mirvalle Press.

Stålberg, E. 1980: Clinical electrophysiology in myasthenia gravis. *Journal of Neurosurgery and Psychiatry*, **43**, 622–33.

Stöhr, M. 1982: Special types of spontaneous electrical activity in radiogenic nerve injuries. *Muscle Nerve*, **5**, 78–83.

Sumner, A.J. 1975: Early discharge of muscle afferents in acrylamide neuropathy. *Journal of Physiology (London)*, **246**, 277–88.

Sumner, A.J. and Asbury, A.K. 1975: Physiological studies of the dying-back phenomenon. Muscle strength afferents in acrylamide neuropathy. *Brain*, **98**, 91–100.

Sunderland, S. 1991: *Nerve Injuries and their Repair*. New York: Churchill Livingstone.

Swift, T.R. and Nichols, F.T. 1984: The droopy shoulder syndrome. *Neurology*, **34**, 212–5.

Takahashi, M., Ohara, T. and Hashimoto, K. 1971: Electrophysiological study of nerve injuries in workers handling acrylamide. *International Archives of Arbeits Medicine*, **28**, 1–11.

Thomas, J.E., Cascino, T.L. and Darle, J.D. 1985: Differential diagnosis between radiation and tumor plexopathy of the pelvis. *Neurology*, **35**, 1.

Thomas, J.E. and Colby, M.Y. Jr 1972: Radiation-induced or metastatic brachial plexopathy? A diagnostic dilemma. *Journal of the American Medical Association*, **222**, 1392–5.

Thompson, W.A.L. and Kopell, H.P. 1959: Peripheral entrapment neuropathies of upper extremity. *New England Journal of Medicine*, **260**, 1261–5.

Tokuomi, H., Uchino, M., Imamura, M., Yamanaga, H., Nakanishi, R. and Ideta, T. 1982: Minamata disease (organic mercury poisoning), neuroradiologic and electrophysiologic studies. *Neurology*, **32**, 1369–75.

Tylleskär, T., Banea, M., Bikangi, N., Cooke, R.D., Poulter, N.H. and Rosling, H. 1992: Cassava cyanogens and konzo, an upper motoneuron disease found in Africa. *Lancet*, **339**, 208–11.

Tylleskär, T., Banea, M., Bikangi, N., Fresco, L., Persson, L.A. and Rosling, H. 1991: Epidemiological evidence from Zaire for a dietary etiology of konzo, an upper motor neuron disease. *Bull World Health Organization*, **69**, 581–9.

Tylleskär, T., Howlett, W.P., Rwiza, H.T. *et al.* 1993: Konzo, a distinct disease entity with selective upper motor neuron damage. *Journal of Neurosurgery and Psychiatry*, **56**, 638–43.

Veith, G. 1949: Untersuchunger uber die Histologie der Polyneuritis diphtherica. *Beitrage Pathology and Anatomy*, **110**, 567.

Wadia, R.S., Sadgopan, C., Amin, R.B. *et al.* 1974: Neurological manifestation of organophosphorus insecticides poisoning. *Journal of Neurology, Neurosurgery and Psychiatry*, **37**, 841.

Weiss, P. and Taylor, A.C. 1944: Impairment of growth and myelinization in regenerating nerve fibers subject to constriction. *Proceedings of the Society for Experimental Biology*, **55**, 77–80.

Werner, C.O. 1979: Lateral elbow pain and posterior interosseous nerve entrapment. *Acta Orthopedica Scandinavica*, **suppl 174**.

Wilson, J.R., Conwit, R.A., Eidelman, B.H. *et al.* 1994: Sensorimotor neuropathy resembling CIDP in patients receiving FK506. *Muscle Nerve*, **17**, 528–32.

Windebank, A.J. and Dyck, P.J. 1984: Lead intoxication as a model of primary segmental demyelination. In *Peripheral Neuropathy*, Dyck, P.J., Thomas, P.K., Lambert, E.H. and Burge, R. (eds), 2nd edn, p 650. Philadelphia, PA: W.B. Saunders.

Yoshiyama, Y., Nakajima, M., Kuwabara, S. and Kawano, E. 1997: Demyelinating brachial neuropathy complicating syngeneic graft-versus-host disease. *Neurology*, **48**, 287–8.

Zochodne, D.W., Ramsay, D.A., Saly, V., Shelley, S. and Moffatt, S. 1994: Acute necrotzing myopathy of intensive care. Electrophysiological studies. *Muscle Nerve*, **17**, 285–92.

18

The neuropathological investigation

M ANTHONY VERITY

INTRODUCTION

Definitions of neurotoxicity are still open to argument, but usually refer to an adverse change in structure or function of the nervous system following exposure to chemical, biological or physical agents. Whether such toxicity reflects reversible or irreversible neuro-injury is open to debate but most investigators identify the critical role of altered morphology in the recognition of toxicity. In this discussion we will identify the major methods and technologies used in recognizing toxicant-induced pathological change, identify and provide examples of special methods, and discuss the use of numerous *in vivo* and *in vitro* systems of value in investigating dose-response and pathogenetic mechanisms.

Broadly speaking, the basic objectives of anatomic neuropathology are:

1 to identify the existence and locality of pathological change within the central or peripheral nervous system;
2 describe the nature of the pathological alteratiom;
3 provide for correlation between the abnormal clinical and/or the behavioral state with its appropriate anatomical correlate;
4 allow for analysis of dose–response correlations as a function of lesion development and magnitude; and
5 by specific molecular target examination, for example cytoskeleton, ribosome integrity, specific target proteins, suggest possible mechanisms for the underlying neurotoxicity.

The extrapolation of the basic tenets and objectives of neuropathology (see above) to clinical neurotoxicology appears well established. For instance, the recognition of major clinical neurological syndromes induced by various neurotoxins invokes the necessity to identify specific regions of preferential neuro-injury and their associated behavioral/clinical correlation.

Table 18.1 presents an abbreviated list of clinical syndromes based upon regional selectivity and appropriate intoxicants. Unfortunately, the use of neuropathological findings in risk assessment requires a reliable classification of neuropathological change. This is rarely observed in central nervous system (CNS) injury but has been categorized and evaluated in examples of toxicant-induced polyneuropathy. In this case the primary injury may be considered to affect the cell body, axon, end plate or myelin. In addition, there is the recognition that neurotoxicity preferentially induces a distal axonopathy, for example *n*-hexane is characterized by a sensory-motor distal symmetric neuropathy concordantly associated with the distal axonopathy and Wallerian change. Dose–response relationships used to evaluate neuroanatomical injury are amenable to quantitative analysis and may be incorporated into risk assessment protocols. Finally, an understanding of the pathogenesis of neurotoxicity may be initially suggested through the use of neuromorphological strategies. The characterization of cellular and subcellular alterations may provide critical information in devising hypotheses concerning pathogenesis. In particular, silver impregnation and immunohistochemical studies may identify early cytoskeletal alterations, or glial fibrillary acidic protein (GFAP) immunohistochemistry may identify an early glial reaction.

Table 18.1 *Clinical neurological syndromes induced by specific neurotoxins*

Syndrome	Neurotoxicant
Encephalopathy	Antidepressants
	Alcohol
	Aluminum
	Solvents
Cerebellar dysfunction	Methotrexate
	Narcotics
	Methyl mercury
	Toluene
Polyneuropathy	Alcohol
	cis-Platinum
	n-Hexane
	Arsenic
Seizures	Antidepressants
	Amphetamine
	Lead
	Carbon monoxide
Extrapyramidal movement syndrome	Neuroleptics
	MPTP
	Manganese
	Carbon monoxide

GENERAL NEUROANATOMICAL TECHNIQUES

The visual nature of neuropathology demands use of tissue preparations which allow for fixation or stabilization of tissue elements prior to performance of procedures whereby cellular elements are defined. Optimum staining procedures for visualization rest upon optimum tissue fixation. Such fixation may be performed by immersion of small segments of brain tissue, but is more optimally performed by perfusion. Appropriate perfusion fixatives include 10% buffered formalin, 4% buffered paraformaldehyde, and 2.5% buffered glutaraldehyde, the latter being optimum for transmission electron microscopy. Perfusion fixation avoids 'dark neuron' artifacts, maintains optimum cellular relationships, and identifies vascular structures easily.

Routine

For general purposes, hematoxylin and eosin (H&E) serves as a standard procedure, has been recognized for many years, is routine, easy to perform, and provides good nuclear detail (Figure 18.1A and Figure 18.11A (color plate section)). Routine use allows for recognition of nuclear change, pyknosis, apoptosis, mitotic activity, abnormal inclusions, nerve cell loss, vacuolization and edema, abnormal cellular infiltration, and major regional areas of hemorrhage, infarction, etc. Early changes in myelin, axons or dendrites are not specifically identified. While the H&E method provides

a powerful nuclear and chromatin stain (Lillie, 1965) the use of Nissl stains has provided a routine method based upon the metabolic integrity of the polysomes comprising the highly structured endoplasmic reticulum (Nissl bodies) characteristic of neurons (Peters *et al.*, 1991). Toluidine blue and Cresyl violet have been used in this respect often combined with the Luxol-fast blue (Kluver) reaction allowing for simultaneous demonstration of neuronal endoplasmic reticulum and myelin (Figure 18.1B and Figure 18.11B (color plate section)). A characteristic change occurs in the Nissl substance following axonal injury. This retrograde response, called chromatolysis or the axonal reaction, reflects an early response including swelling of the perikaryon, dispersion of Nissl granules leaving a peripheral rim of ribonucleic acid (RNA), nuclear displacement, and often enlargement of nucleolus. While commonly appearing following axonal injury, similar changes have been recognized in segmental demyelination, neuromuscular blockade with botulinum toxin (Duchen, 1992), and trimethyl lead intoxication.

Silver impregnation

The use of silver impregnation procedures stems from the ability to reveal early details of axonal injury especially in the classic studies of Ramon Y. Cajal (1928). Bielschowsky (1935) described the method of staining axons in formalin-fixed frozen sections. Bodian (1936) improved on these methods which have been further developed with physical developers (Gallyas and Zoltay, 1992). The Bodian method for axonal processes is valuable in detecting axonal atrophy, swelling or Wallerian degeneration. The Bielschowsky method is relatively more selective for high and low molecular weight neurofilament protein within axons and nerve cell bodies (Figure 18.1C, D, E) (Abou-Donia and Gupta, 1994). The ability to visualize Wallerian degeneration using the silver impregnation procedures has provided information on the architecture of neuronal connections. Procedures have been devised that suppress normal fiber staining but enhance the staining of degenerating elements particularly axon terminals (Fink and Heimer, 1967; Beltramino *et al.*, 1993). Advantages and disadvantages of the silver degeneration procedures exist. For instance, irregular particulate deposits may become fused as evidence of terminal degeneration. In addition, incomplete staining of normal fibers or particulate deposition around myelin debris may be confused for axon degeneration. Moreover, absence of staining cannot indicate absence of neurotoxic damage. More positively however, quantitative estimates of regional degeneration may be obtained using video techniques and assessing areal involvement, and reacting axons may identify subpopulations of neurons

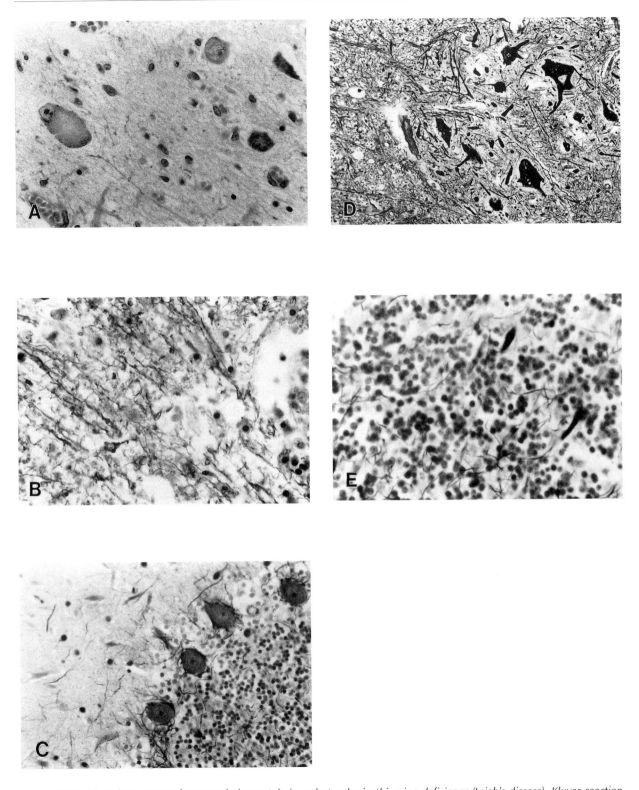

Figure 18.1 *(A) Various stages of neuronal chromatolysis and atrophy in thiamine deficiency (Leigh's disease). Kluver reaction. (B) Necrotizing leukoencephalopathy following intraventricular methotrexate. Widespread demyelination with axonal damage, status spongiosus, and modest perivascular lympho-histiocytosis is evident. Weil stain. (C) Normal cerebellar cortex showing basket fibers around Purkinje cell perikarya and molecular layer containing segments of parallel fibers. Bielschowsky silver impregnation method. (D) Abnormal neurofilamentous accumulations within swollen neurons of the gracile nucleus following intrathecal vincristine. Bielschowsky silver impregnation. (E) Axonal swellings ('torpedos') in Purkinje cell axons following intrathecal vincristine. Such swellings consist of accumulated masses of neurofilaments and degenerated organelles and maybe found in proximal axonal segments of spinal anterior horn cells following colchicine or iminodiproprionitrile. Bielschowsky silver impregnation.*

particularly vulnerable to selective toxins. The silver degeneration technique has been used to investigate neurotoxic injury due to 3-acetylpyridine (Desclin and Escubi, 1974); trimethyltin (Balaban *et al.*, 1988); organophosphate compounds (Tanaka and Bursian, 1989); and amphetamine analogues (Scallet, 1995).

Semi-thin sections

The preparation of semi-thin (1 μm thick) sections is commonly performed prior to ultra-thin sectioning for electronmicroscopy. However, such semi-thin sections following adequate fixation are valuable in the light microscopic assessment of neuronal injury. Such sections prepared following plastic embedment are usually stained with 1% toluidine blue providing a dark blue coloration to myelin and blue-purple color to cell membranes, organelles, nuclei, and neurons (Figure 18.2).

Golgi technique

The recent enthusiasm in use of the rapid Golgi technique stems from a need to interpret ultrastructural and microelectrophysiological data in terms of a more defined structural substrate. The Golgi procedure optimally reveals the dendritic processes of neurons, normally unstained in routine light microscope procedures. While the procedure is considered capricious in its ability of selective staining of individual neurons, such selectivity allows for unique examination of single neuron dendritic fields uncomplicated by excess silver reactivity. The procedure allows for the demonstration and organization of dendritic processes within defined neuropil fields, specific morphology of synapses, the pattern and type of axons and their collaterals, and in some instances may provide a morphometric analysis of spiny dendrite density. The rapid Golgi procedure is a method of choice in defining fine axonal, as well as, soma-dendrite interactions. In this respect the method may prove of value in microelectrode investigations. While application to classical neurotoxicology is somewhat meager, neuropathological and neurodevelopmental studies have been completed. For example, Brown *et al.* (1976) studied the inhibition of cerebellar dendrite development in neonatal thyroid deficiency and revealed distortion in the development of the Purkinje cell dendritic tree and patchy loss of branchelet spines in the deficient animals.

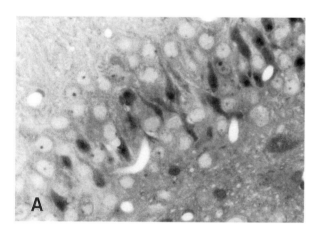

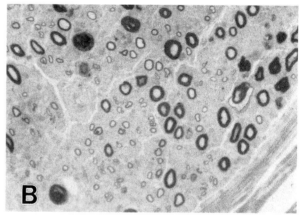

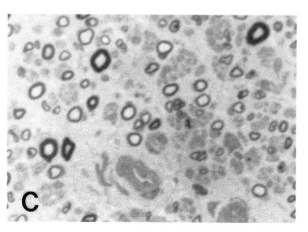

Figure 18.2 *Semi-thin (1 μm) plastic embedded sections stained with toluidine blue. (A) Trimethyltin intoxication in adult rat reveals loss of neurons throughout the pyramidal and dentate neurons of the hippocampus. Affected region shows neuron condensation, clumping of chromatin, dissolution of Nissl substance and ultimate phagocytosis. (B) Human arsenic neuropathy revealing preferential large myelinated fiber loss and ongoing degeneration eight weeks following intoxication. (C) Recovery phase of human arsenic neuropathy approximately three years postintoxication. Large myelinated fiber decrease is still present but small myelinated regenerating axon clusters and numerous hypomyelinated fibers are now evident.*

SPECIAL METHODS

Ultrastructural methods in neurotoxicology

Light microscopy provides the base for neurotoxicity studies. The recognition of early or subtle structural manifestations of cellular injury may necessitate a more detailed examination using electron microscopic techniques. Moreover, the recognition of early cellular change may provide a clue to the proximate mechanistic steps underlying the pathogenesis of the injury pathway. Transmission electron microscopy (TEM) and scanning electron microscopy (SEM) have been used successfully. Combined with autoradiography, freeze-fracture techniques or immunocytochemistry, these ultrastructural methods have proved valuable in elucidation of toxicant-induced injury.

The value of transmission electron microscopy (Figure 18.3) is dependent upon the success of obtaining technically satisfactory images following optimum tissue preparation. Such preparation includes the steps of tissue fixation, embedding, microtomy, staining, and image analysis. Details and discussion of these procedures are provided by Hayat (1981) and Bagnell *et al.* (1995). Optimum tissue fixation depends upon choice of fixative and method of fixation. Perfusion fixation has proved optimum over immersion fixation due to several advantages, including uniformity of rapid penetration via the vascular bed, minimum handling artifacts, immediate onset following circulation perfusion, and lower fixative concentration, thereby providing partial enzyme preservation. However, cell suspensions, fractions and tissue cultures may be fixed *in situ* with optimum results.

Scanning electron microscopy examines surface cellular features giving a three-dimensional appearance (Figure 18.4). Tissue preparation and methodology is well discussed by Goldstein *et al.* (1981) and summarized by Bagnell *et al.* (1995).

The combination of transmission electron microscopy with other specialized methods has proved valuable. Polak and Priestley (1992) surveyed the use of immunocytochemistry in electron microscopy. Enzyme cytochemistry and autoradiography have also been used with success (Hayat, 1993). Electronmicroscopy combined with the Golgi technique has provided data on neuronal structure in pathological conditions (Braak and Braak, 1985).

ENZYME HISTOCHEMISTRY

Enzyme histochemistry provides a means for understanding the biochemical basis of neurotoxicant-induced injury. Some advantages of the technique are summarized in Table 18.2. Enzyme histochemistry/cytochemistry is based upon the *in situ* localization of specific enzyme activity allowing for cytological localization. In this respect neurotoxicity may be reflected in a change of localization and/or activity of specific enzymes and their catalyzed activities. In contrast to biochemical studies, small tissue samples may be used and differences between neighboring neuron activities easily displayed.

Numerous examples highlight the use of enzyme histochemistry in elucidating neurotoxicant action (Figure 18.5). Organophosphate insecticides inhibit brain acetylcholine esterase. A selective loss of cholinergic neurons (identified by their acetylcholine esterase activity) has been reported following quisqualic acid exposure (Unger and Schmidt, 1993). This study reveals a principle of neuron selectivity. Similarly, NADPH-diaphorase activity reveals a select population of striatal neurons (Kowall, *et al.* 1987) preferentially involved in Huntington's disease. More sophisticated studies have utilized the principles of quantitative histochemistry in which a quantitative assessment of chromophore deposition is used for the evaluation of enzyme reaction rates. These studies rely upon complex equipment including microdensitometers but have been used in the assessment of cytochrome oxidase activity (Kugler *et al.*, 1988) and enzymes of glycolysis (Chieco *et al.*, 1988).

IMMUNOHISTOCHEMISTRY

The application of immunohistochemical procedures should be made in conjunction with correlative biochemical data and classical light microscopic or ultrastructural studies. The production of polyclonal or monoclonal antisera against specific molecules provides the basis for specificity combined with appropriate preservation of antigenic sites in the tissue following fixation and histological processing (Sternberger, 1986; Hockfield *et al.*, 1993). Immunohistochemistry provides for the recognition of specific cellular proteins. Their amount and localization demonstrate the organization and terminal arborizations of specific neuronal pathways, characterized by selective neurotransmitter molecules and their biosynthetic enzymes; provides an analysis of pharmacological alterations in neuronal

Table 18.2 *Value of enzyme histochemical methods in neurotoxicology*

1 Demonstrate cellular enzyme localization
2 Provide a semiquantitative measure of enzyme activity
3 Use in small tissue samples unsuitable for biochemical analysis
4 Allow for study of 'near neighbor' neuronal enzyme function
5 Provide for analysis of early dysfunction due to neurotoxicant interaction

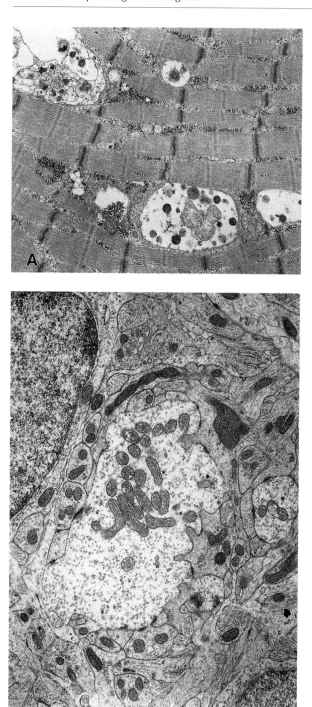

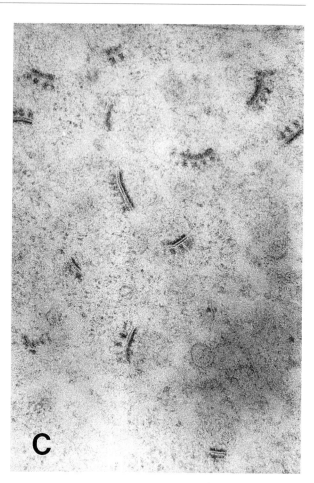

Figure 18.3 *(A) Transmission electron microscopy of colchicine neuromyopathy characterized by a lysosomal vacuolar myopathy. Vacuoles are filled with membrane aggregation and small dense bodies. There is minimal associated necrosis of adjacent sarcomeres. (B) The electron microscopy of cerebellar mossy fiber terminal (glomerulus) in 21-day hypothyroid rat. Technique used for morphometric analysis of terminal volume, organelle content, and number synaptic complexes under the influence of hypothyroid induced cerebellar development. (C) Ultrastructural study of developing cerebellar molecular layer in hypothyroid rat stained with ethanolic phosphotungstic acid which selectively reveals the detailed morphology of the synaptic complex. The presynaptic membrane containing dense projections is separated from the dense line representing the postsynaptic density. The synaptic cleft contains a fine line. Detailed morphometric analysis allows for the description of development of components of the synapse.*

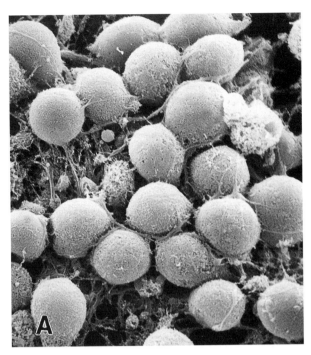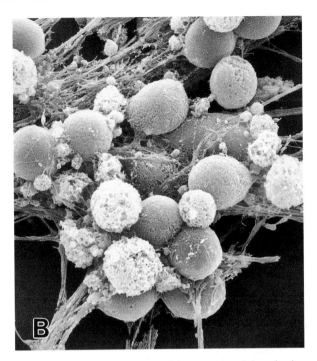

Figure 18.4 *Scanning electronmicroscopy of cerebellar granule cell neurons in culture. (A) Control. (B) Twenty-four h intoxication with 5 μM methyl mercury. Note the increased membrane vesiculation, blister formation, and multiple lytic lesions within the plasma membrane. ×3000.*

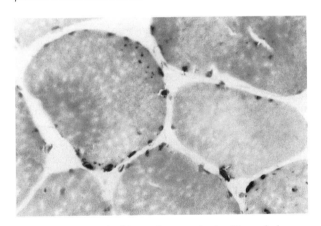

Figure 18.5 *Muscle biopsy from patient with amiodarone-induced myopathy. Sub-sarcolemmal acid phosphatase positive deposits representing lysosomes and autophagic vacuoles are present. Similar changes maybe observed with chloroquine and colchicine. Gomori acid phosphatase reaction on cryostat sections. ×800.*

systems or pathways combined with degenerative structural changes; and reveals the possibility of post-translational change, for example phosphorylation of target proteins linked to the onset of neurotoxicant injury.

While numerous examples exist, we will discuss selective examples supporting the defined principles and advantages of immunohistochemistry in elucidation of neurotoxicant injury. Immunohistochemical staining for astrocytic glial fibrillary acid protein (GFAP) is a recognized measure of neuro-injury

(Norton *et al.*, 1993). Astrocyte hypertrophy varies as a function of induced injury, likely representing increased transcription of newly synthesized GFAP and its spatial translocation throughout glial processes (Figure 18.6 and Figure 18.11C (color plate section)). GFAP reactivity and process complexity is related to the magnitude of injury (O'Callaghan and Jensen, 1993) confirmed using enzyme-linked immunosorbent assay (ELISA) immunoassay.

Immunohistochemical staining for specific neuro-transmitters and their enzymes provides a cytoarchitectonic image of specific neuropathways. Because tyrosine hydroxylase is the rate-limiting enzyme for dopamine synthesis, immunohistochemical studies delineate the nigrostriatal projection. Following 1-methyl-4-phenyl-1,2,3,6-tetrahydropyridine (MPTP), an apparent reduction in the staining intensity of the striatum is revealed suggesting that early neurotoxicity occurs in the axon terminals within the striatum with later retrograde damage within the neurons of the substantia nigra (Jensen, 1995).

Apart from evaluating neurotransmitter localization and associated biosynthetic enzyme function, immunohistochemical procedures may be used in the identification of toxicant-induced alterations in cytoplasmic organelles. Cytoskeletal pathology affecting the neurofilament system occurs in the presence of aluminum intoxication (Yokel *et al.*, 1988), dialysis encephalopathy, and Alzheimer's disease (Tomlinson, 1992). Hyperphosphorylation of tau, τ (Figure 18.6) can be detected immunohistochemically in the neurofibrillary tangles characteristic of these toxicant and

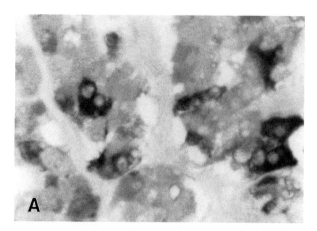

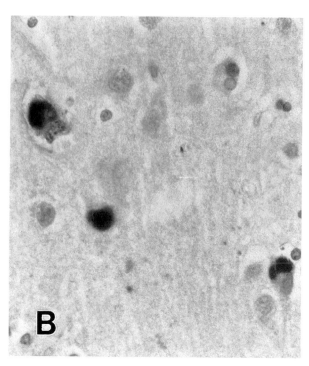

Figure 18.6 *(A) Immunohistochemistry for thyroid stimulating hormone (TSH) within individual cells of human anterior pituitary gland. The finely granular deposit fills the cytoplasm but unstained nuclei are easily visible. ×800. (B) Tau-positive neurofibrillary tangle bearing neurons in Alzheimer's disease. Similar changes have been found following aluminum intoxication. ×460.*

disease states (Saitoh *et al.*, 1991). While these studies reveal the pathologic effects of hyperphosphorylation on cytoskeletal proteins, they also suggest that the activities of selective kinases and phosphatases may be altered providing the mechanism leading to the hyperphosphorylated state, and resultant structural and functional abnormality. Ohmstede *et al.* (1989) and O'Callaghan (1994) have examined the activity of calmodulin-linked kinase activity using ultrastructural immunohistochemistry. These studies have also received support from the observations of Abou-Donia *et al.* (1988) who observed increased phospho-kinase activity in the cytoskeletal proteins of peripheral nerves following organophosphate exposure. Subsequent immunohistochemical studies demonstrated axonal degeneration associated with phosphorylated neurofilament aggregation.

Tubulin immunohistochemistry has provided valuable data on toxicant-induced alterations of microtubule function. The recognition of colchicine-induced depolymerization of microtubules, studies with β,β-iminodipropionitrile (Griffin and Price, 1981), and taxol (Schiff and Horwitz, 1981) have used *in situ* local injection or organotypic tissue cultures. Studies with methyl mercury *in vivo* and *in vitro* have suggested selective vulnerability of microtubules (Figure 18.11 (color plate section)) to the toxicant leading to defective neuroblast migration and differentiation in the developmental model of intoxication and revealing disrupted microtubule organization following *in vitro* exposure (Reuhl *et al.*, 1994; Verity, 1996).

A useful example of immunohistochemical studies has been the application of the technique to the identification of neuronal populations expressing the immediate-early gene activated proteins, c-fos and c-jun, following systemic pyrethroid insecticide administration. The immunocytochemical detection of these proteins enables their visualization in activated neurons reacting to pathophysiological stimulation with alteration in gene expression. Hassouna *et al.* (1996) demonstrated that the neurotoxicity of the insecticides involved selective changes in thalamic and hypothalamic neurons with differences in neuronal selectivity, pyrethroid type, and regional specificity throughout the brain. Such studies are valuable in identifying vulnerable neuron populations and their involvement in proto-oncogene expression, which may contribute to the neurodegenerative process and provide a molecular basis for risk assessment and mechanistic study.

IN SITU HYBRIDIZATION: NUCLEIC ACID NEUROTOXICITY ASSESSMENT

Nucleic acid hybridization allows for the specific detection, purification, and quantization of RNA and deoxyribonucleic acid (DNA). The basic principle reflects the formation and hybridization of single stranded DNA and/or RNA molecules in solution or *in situ*. While both methods have provided valuable neurotoxicology data, the latter is of interest to this discussion. In particular, the localization of specific messenger RNA (mRNA) to neuronal or glial populations has proven valuable in assessing subacute or chronic toxicant-induced change. The mRNA is fixed *in situ* following perfusion or immersion with paraformaldehyde. A variety of probes including antisense riboprobes, cyclic DNA (cDNA) or oligonucleotides are then added and detected following radioisotopic labeling or colorimetric methods. Such *in situ* hybrid-

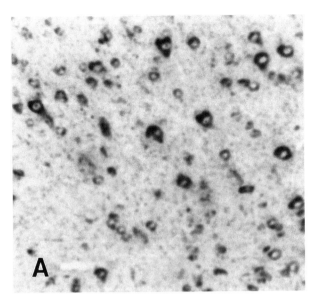
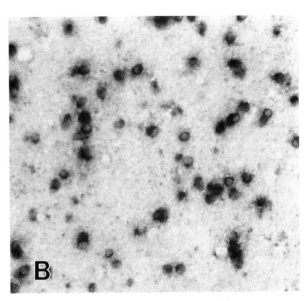

Figure 18.7 *In situ hybridization histochemistry. Riboprobes were prepared by in vitro transcription using digoxigenin-labeled UTP. Following hybridization slides were incubated with anti-DIG antibody conjugated to alkaline phosphatase and processed for color development overnight in alkaline phosphate substrate. (A) In-situ hybridization for neuronal neurofilament-68 within cerebral cortex. Note the regular staining of cytoplasm in neurons with sparing of nuclei. (B) Myelin basic protein (MBP) mRNA expressed in oligodendroglia within white matter.*

ization provides data on changes in gene expression, and especially reveals cellular subsets which may be sensitive to the toxicant. *In situ* hybridization of mRNA expression following neurotoxicant exposure may identify the mRNA as a primary target of the toxicant, be a secondary compensation for loss of neuron integrity, or represent a non-specific 'stress' response. Neuron-specific gene products would include mRNA (Figure 18.7) for neurofilaments or synaptophysin, while injury-reactive expression may involve GFAP or the immediate-early response genes, c-fos, or c-jun. c-Fos induction has been demonstrated in PC12 cells after veratridine and c-fos gene expression represents an early marker of neurotoxicity following the organochlorine pesticide, lindane (Morgan and Curran, 1986;

Vendrell *et al.*, 1991). Studies on myelin associated genes have provided data on the differential activation of specific myelin proteins in the developing mouse brain (Verity and Campagnoni, 1988) and revealed abnormalities in oligodendrocyte expression and translocation of myelin basic protein mRNA in certain mouse mutants revealing dysmyelination (Verity *et al.* 1990).

NEUROANATOMICAL STUDIES IN ISOLATED *IN VITRO* NEURAL SYSTEMS

Nerve fiber teasing of peripheral nerve

Peripheral nerve disease is a common manifestation of many neurotoxicants. Neuropathies due to environmental agents include acrylamide, carbon disulfide, *n*-hexane, metals, and organophosphate esters. Investigation of such neuropathies include routine light microscopy, one micron plastic embedded section microscopy, morphometry, electron microscopy, and single nerve fiber teasing preparations. This latter technique provides segments of peripheral nerves stained with osmium tetroxide, held in glycerin, and single nerve fibers teased with fine forceps then mounted on glass slides for microscopic examination (Figure 18.8). Individual changes in nerve fibers may be identified allowing classification as Wallerian degeneration, segmental demyelination, axonal regeneration, remyelination, and recognition of inclusion bodies, for example amiodarone (Costa-Jussa and Jacobs, 1985).

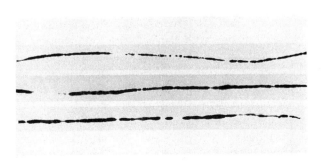

Figure 18.8 *Nerve fiber teasing from sural nerve biopsy in human case of acute and chronic alcohol abuse. Segment of nerve biopsy was incubated in osmium tetroxide overnight, softened in glycerin and single fiber teasing performed. A*

Brain slice techniques

While the hippocampus is the most commonly used brain slice preparation, use of neocortical slices, spinal cord slices, cerebellar slice, and other tissue regions have been used for electrophysiological and neuroanatomical studies. The hippocampal slice provides an intact trisynaptic circuit with defined dendritic fields and fiber systems providing the investigator with a well-defined slice preparation and control of the chemical environment. While the hippocampal slice has been used extensively for electrophysiological studies including intracellular and patch clamp methods, neuroanatomical studies have provided useful data, for example, the effect of lead on hippocampal morphology (Brinck and Wechsler, 1989).

A major neuroanatomical contribution to an understanding of the neuronal damage induced by excitatory amino acids has been presented by Hajos and Garthwaites (Hajos et al., 1986; Garthwaite et al., 1986a,b). These authors used immature rat cerebellar slice preparations in vitro examined after exposure to excitotoxic agonists. The slices were fixed in paraformaldehyde–glutaraldehyde and prepared as one micron resin embedded sections stained with toluidine blue for light microscopy (see earlier sections) or ultrathin sections for electron microscopy. The preparations allowed for the evaluation and progression of neuropathological events, reversibility, differential effects between N-methyl-D-aspartate (NMDA), kainate and quisqualate, and apparent receptor sensitivity between different cerebellar neuron populations.

Organotypic explants

Organotypic cultures are usually derived from undifferentiated embryonic tissue and develop into an integrated mature system. They provide an in vitro paradigm for chronic neurotoxicity studies, a technique introduced by Peterson and Murray, (1955) and extended by Bornstein as fragments of myelinating kitten or rodent cerebellum in the Maximow slide assembly (Figure 18.10) (Bornstein and Murray, 1958). Yonezawa et al. (1980) have described neurotoxicological studies using organotypic cultures. Whetsell and Schwarcz have used the organotypic tissue culture model to investigate mechanisms of excitotoxin action and recently demonstrated that prolonged exposure to sub-micromolar concentrations of quinolinic acid causes excitotoxic damage in organotypic cultures of rat corticostriatal systems (Whetsell and Schwarcz, 1989; Figure 18.9). Veronesi et al. (1983) examined hexacarbon neuropathy in nerve fibers undergoing giant axonal degeneration in spinal cord co-cultured with muscle.

Brain-derived reaggregating culture

Reaggregating cultures are derived from enzymatically or mechanically dissociated suspensions of individual cells. Moscona (1961) showed that dissociated undifferentiated cells could reassemble in vitro to form three-dimensional assemblies. During maturation a typical histotypic pattern emerged capable of synaptogenesis and myelination (Trapp et al., 1979; Lu et al., 1980). Advantages of reaggregating brain-derived cell suspensions include histotypic cytoarchitecture; an in vitro association between different cell species closely mirroring the in vivo state; longevity of culture allowing for maturation; direct accessibility of neurotoxicants, withdrawal and ease of concentration control. Disadvantages include large diffusional gradients between periphery and center for toxicant and metabolites; difference between individual aggregates; heterogeneity of cell types complicating electrophysiological or neurochemical studies (but valuable for in situ neuroanatomical/immunohistochemical observations); and variable aggregate representation of cellular species from small brain regions, for example substantia nigra. Such systems have been used in neurotoxicology (Honneger and Werffeli, 1988), especially to examine the neurotoxicity of organophosphate and carbamate pesticides (Segal and Federoff, 1989); morphology and synaptogenesis following low dose radiation (Dimberg et al., 1992); aluminum (Atterwill and Collins, 1988); and methyl mercury (Jacobs et al., 1986).

Cell suspensions

A variety of cell suspension techniques have been used in neurotoxicology (Verity, 1995). Cell suspensions have been obtained as primary cell dissociates from cerebrum, cerebellum and dorsal root ganglia, and have certain advantages over culture in biochemical studies but provide equivalent excellence in morphology, ultrastructure, and immunocytochemistry as culture systems. In both cases the rapidity and ease of fixation contrasts sharply with the necessity for perfusion in vivo. Cerebellar granule cell suspensions have been used in investigations of methyl mercury neurotoxicity (Sarafian et al., 1984; Sarafian and Verity, 1986). Transmission electron micrographs of seven-day-old cerebellar granule neurons demonstrated methyl mercury induced organelle and cytoplasmic changes (Verity, 1995). Other cell systems have been used rarely for morphological studies. However, Ransom et al. (1991) examined PC12 cell suspensions using flow cytometry and demonstrated different patterns of Ca^{2+} mobilization following receptor stimulation.

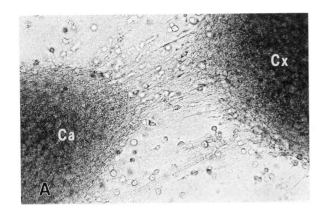

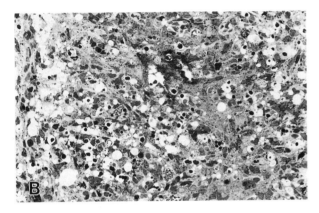

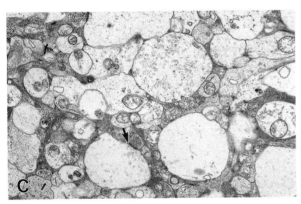

Figure 18.9 *Combination organotypic culture of rat frontal cortex and caudate nucleus prepared on collagen-coated coverslips using the Maximow double-coverslip assembly technique. (A) Twenty-one day old cortical striatal culture (Cx = cortex; Ca = striatum) demonstrating interconnecting fibers projecting from cortex towards striatum which allow for innervation of the striatum. (B) One micron, toluidine blue stained section of the striatum part of organotypic culture (21 DIV) following exposure to 1 mM quinolinic acid for 20 h. Note the granular appearance and numerous variably sized vacuoles throughout the striatum. (C) Electronmicrograph of striatal portion of organotypic culture following exposure to quinolinic acid for 20 h. Note swollen processes, especially postsynaptic swellings (arrows) characteristic of excitotoxic neurodegeneration (×8200). Striatum grown in isolation does not show a toxic response to quin or kainate. Only when the cortical portion innervates the striatum does the excitotoxic response occur. (preparations courtesy of W. Whetsell).*

Primary cell and cell line culture

Cell culture techniques provide a basic neurobiological method for the evaluation of neurotoxicant-induced injury. Methodologies utilizing fetal or neonatal brain tissue from a variety of regions have been well described. Systems include astrocytes, oligodendroglia, Schwann cells, dorsal root ganglia, retinal neurons, and a variety of neurons from different regions, for example cerebellum, mesencephalon, cortex (Figure 18.11D, E, F (color plate section)). The reader is referred to primary sources (Shahar *et al.*, 1989). Cell lines allow for continuous propagation and may be cloned providing defined cell strains. Such cultures undergo many cell divisions, reveal absence of contact inhibition, and may be propagated as monolayers. Morphological studies using tissue culture systems have been devoted principally to analyzing the onset of cytotoxicity and provide a first-tiered approach to neurotoxicity testing *in vitro*. Cytotoxicity may be measured using mitochondrial histochemistry (Atterwill *et al.*, 1991) or, more commonly, dye exclusion techniques. Cultures lend themselves to time-lapse cinemicrophotography allowing for structural observations on neurite outgrowth, differentiation, cellular aggregation, and orientation. Observations have revealed the unique characteristics of astrocyte migration and changes in morphology under the influence of neuronal co-culture (Hatten, 1987). Light and phase contrast microscopy, ultrastructure, and immunohistochemistry have all been used in tissue culture preparations to elucidate mechanistic and risk assessment aspects of neurotoxicant injury.

Pheochromocytoma clones, PC12, have become well established in investigations of catecholamine metabolism and neuronal differentiation (Hamprecht, 1977). In the presence of nerve growth factor such cultures undergo neuronal differentiation with prominent neuritic outgrowth and dense-core granule formation. For example, Burstein *et al.* (1985) demonstrated inhibition of nerve growth factor induced neurite outgrowth by lithium associated with hyperphosphorylation of microtubule associated proteins. Similar morphological observations were made by Hashimoto (1988) using K-252a, a potent protein kinase inhibitor.

Neuroblastoma cell lines have been extensively used for neurotoxicity studies. Many lines are commercially available from the American Type Culture Collection. An advantage of such lines is their ability to undergo differentiation. For example, retinoic acid induces growth inhibition and morphologic differentiation of LA-N-1 human neuroblastoma culture (Sidell, 1982). Similarly, LA-N-5 neuroblastoma cells grown in the presence of menthol exhibited increased neurite outgrowth and cellular clustering but a reduction in growth rate reflected by reduced thymidine incorporation (Sidell *et al.*, 1990), supporting the hypothesis

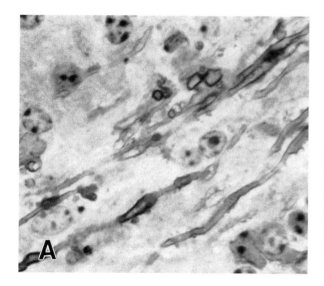

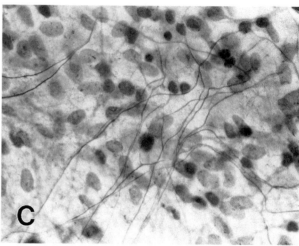

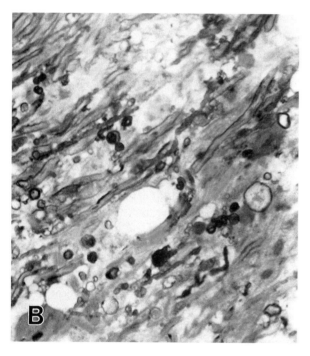

Figure 18.10 *Mouse cerebellar explant culture, 22 DIV, prepared using the Maximow technique. (A) Normal control myelination at the junction of Purkinje and internal granule neuron layer. Toluidine blue stain. (B) Neonatal cerebellar explant 48 h postinoculation with Theiler's virus. Note the extensive myelin fragmentation and vesiculation. Elsewhere, Purkinje cells appeared normal. Toluidine blue (×1000). (C) Ramifying axons in neonatal mouse explant culture, 18 DIV. Holme's silver impregnation (×600).*

that voltage-gated Ca^{2+} channels may influence morphological development of nerve cells. Hence toxicant-induced aberrations in such channels, for example methyl mercury (Atchison and Hare, 1994; Verity, 1996), would be expected to influence neuritogenesis, a well-recognized event in developmental mercury intoxication. Other morphological studies have included the effects of *n*-hexane and derivatives (Selkoe *et al.*, 1978), and co-cultures with muscle cells allow for the examination of complex cellular interactions amenable to morphological, histochemical, and electrophysiological observations (Schubert *et al.*, 1977). In this respect important observations concerning neuronal interaction with astroglial morphology and proliferation have been made (Hatten, 1987). These studies indicate that neurite outgrowth provides an *in vitro* model for the assessment of neurotoxicity. Neurite

outgrowth is a complex but increasingly well-understood process involving microtubule, neurofilament, actin, and microtubule-associated protein interactions coupled to a variety of extracellular and membrane-linked signal transduction events. Moreover, the morphological observations may be confirmed through the immunochemical assessment of neurofilament protein change (Abdulla and Campbell, 1993).

CONCLUSION

The procedures described in this chapter have been utilized in clinical and experimental neurotoxicology. Their value rests in their appropriate use and interpretation with full recognition of their limitations.

Hence, a battery of procedures is often used and may provide overlapping data. The sophisticated procedures, for example Golgi electronmicroscopy, are valuable in the hands of proficient users but need skill, repetition, and patience for optimum preparations.

By their very nature all procedures provide a visual demonstration of neuroinjury. Coupled with appropriate functional studies, varying from electrophysiology through to molecular neurobiology, their value is time honored and tested. Space has only allowed for arbitrary selection of the most often used procedures. However, more exciting neuroanatomic techniques are being utilized, including autoradiography, electronhistochemistry, and a variety of *in vitro* imaging techniques. The latter are capable of revealing rapid oscillation in Ca^{2+} movement, or pH change through the use of fluorescent indicators. A variety of *in vivo* imaging techniques have now been developed and are applicable for neurotoxic assessment. Aspects of brain metabolism, morphology, and vascular dynamics can be obtained through brain-computed tomography, magnetic resonance imaging (MRI) and positron emission tomography.

REFERENCES

Abdulla, E.M. and Campbell, I.C. 1993: Use of neurite outgrowth as an *in vitro* method of assessing neurotoxicity. *Annals of the New York Academy of Science*, **679**, 275–9.

Abou-Donia, M.B. and Gupta, R.P. 1994: Involvement of cytoskeletal proteins in chemically induced neuropathies. In *Principles of Neurotoxicology*, Chang, L.W. (ed.), pp 153–210. New York: Dekker.

Abou-Donia, M.B., Lapadula, D.M. and Suwita, E. 1988: Cytoskeletal proteins as targets for organophosphorus compound and aliphatic hexacarbon-induced neurotoxicity. *Toxicology*, **49**, 469–77.

Atchison, W.D. and Hare, M.F. 1994: Mechanisms of methyl mercury neurotoxicity. *FASEB Journal*, **8**, 622–9.

Atterwill, C.K. and Collins, P. 1988: Investigation of aluminum neurotoxicity using rat brain re-aggregate cultures. *British Journal of Pharmacology*, **94**, 441–52.

Atterwill, C.K., Johnston, H. and Thomas, S.M. 1991: Models for the *in vitro* assessment of neurotoxicity in the nervous system in relation to xenobiotic and neurotrophic factor-mediated events. In *Current Issues in Neurotoxicology*, Mutti, A., Costa, L.G., Manzo, L. and Cranmer, J.M. (eds), pp 40–53. Little Rock, AR: Intox Press.

Bagnell, R., Madden, V., Langaman, C. and Suzuki, K. 1995: Ultrastructural methods for neurotoxicology and neuropathology. In *Neurotoxicology: Approaches and Methods*, Chang, L.W. and Slikker, W. Jr (eds), pp 81–98. New York: Academic Press.

Balaban, C.D., O'Callaghan, J.P. and Billingsley, M.L. 1988: Trimethyltin-induced neuronal damage in the rat brain: comparative studies using silver degeneration stains, immunocytochemistry and immunoassay for neuronotypic and gliotypic proteins. *Neuroscience*, **26**, 337–61.

Beltramino, C.A., de Olmos, J.S., Gallyas, F., Heimer, L. and Zaborszky, L. 1993: Silver staining as a tool for neurotoxic assessment. *NIDA Research Monograph*, **136**, 101–32.

Bielschowsky, M. 1935: Allgemeine histologie und histopatologie des nervensystems. In *Handbuch Der Neurologie*, Bumke, O. and Foster, O. (eds), Vol. 1, pp 35–226. Berlin: Springer-Verlag.

Bodian, D. 1936: A new method of staining nerve fibers and nerve endings mounted in paraffin sections. *Anatomical Record*, **65**, 89–97.

Bornstein, M.B. and Murray, M.R. 1958: Serial observation on patterns of growth, myelin formation, maintenance and degeneration in cultures of new-born rat and kitten cerebellum. *Journal of Biophysics, Biochemistry and Cytology*, **4**, 499–504.

Braak, H. and Braak, E. 1985: Golgi preparations as a tool in neuropathology with particular reference to investigations of the human telencephalic cortex. *Progress in Neurobiology*, **25**, 93–139.

Brinck, U. and Wechsler, W. 1989: Microscopic examination of hippocampal slices after short-term lead exposure *in vitro*. *Neurotoxicology and Teratology*, **11**, 539–43.

Brown, W.J., Verity, M.A. and Smith, R.L. 1976: Inhibition of cerebellar dendrite development in neonatal thyroid deficiency. *Neuropathology and Applied Neurobiology*, **2**, 191–207.

Burstein, D.E., Seeley, P.J. and Greene, L.A. 1985: Lithium ion inhibits nerve growth factor-induced neurite outgrowth and phosphorylation of nerve growth factor-modulated microtubule-associated proteins. *Journal of Cell Biology*, **101**, 862–70.

Chieco, P., Hrellia, P., Lisignoli, G. and Cantelli-Forti, G. 1988: Quantitative enzyme histochemistry of rat fetal brain and trigeminal ganglion. *Histochemical Journal*, **20**, 455–63.

Costa-Jussa, F.R. and Jacobs, J.M. 1985: The pathology of amiodarone neurotoxicity. Experimental studies with reference to changes to other tissues. *Brain*, **108**, 735–52.

Desclin, J.C. and Escubi, J. 1974: The effects of 3-acetylpyridine on the central nervous system of the rat, as demonstrated by silver methods. *Brain Research*, **77**, 349–64.

Dimberg, Y., Totmar, O., Aspberg, A., Ebendal, T., Johansson, K.-J. and Walinder, G. 1992: Effects of low-dose X radiation on mouse-brain aggregation cultures. *International Journal of Radiation Biology*, **61**, 355–63.

Duchen, L.W. 1992: General pathology of neurons and neuroglia. In *Greenfield's Neuropathology*, Adams, J.H. and Duchen, L.W. (eds), 5th edn, pp 1–68. New York: Oxford University Press.

Fink, R.P. and Heimer, L. 1967: Two methods for selected silver impregnation of degenerating axons and their synaptic endings in the central nervous system. *Brain Research*, **4**, 369–74.

Gallyas, F. and Zoltay, G. 1992: An immediate light microscopic response of neuronal somata, dendrites and axons to non-contusing concussive injury in the rat. *Acta Neuropathologica (Berlin)*, **83**, 386–93.

Garthwaite, G., Hajos, F. and Garthwaite, J. 1986a: Ionic requirements for neurotoxic effects of excitatory amino acids analogues in rat cerebellar slices. *Neuroscience*, **18**, 437–47.

Garthwaite, J., Garthwaite, G. and Hajos, F. 1986b: Amino acid neurotoxicity: relationship to neuronal depolarization in rat cerebellar slices. *Neuroscience*, **18**, 449–60.

Goldstein, J.I., Newbury, E.I., Echlin, P., Joy, D.C., Fiori, C. and Lifshin, P. 1981: *Scanning Electronmicroscopy and X-ray Microanalysis*. New York : Plenum Press.

Griffin, J.W. and Price, D.L. 1991: Demyelination in experimental β,β-iminodipropionitrile and hexacarbon neuropathies. Evidence of an axonal influence. *Laboratory Investigation*, **45**, 130–41.

Hajos, F., Garthwaite, G. and Garthwaite, J. 1986: Reversible and irreversible neuronal damage caused by excitatory amino acid analogues in rat cerebellar slices. *Neuroscience*, **18**, 417–36.

Hamprecht, B. 1977: Structural, electrophysiological, biochemical and pharmacological properties of neuroblastoma – glioma cell hybrids in culture. *International Review of Psychology*, **49**, 99–170.

Hashimoto, S. 1988: K-252a, a potent protein kinase inhibitor, blocks nerve growth factor-induced neurite outgrowth and changes in the phosphorylation of proteins in PC12h cells. *Journal of Cell Biology*, **107**, 1531–9.

Hassouna, I., Wickert, H., El-Elaimy, I., Zimmerman, M. and Herbegen, T. 1996: Systemic application of pyrethroid insecticides evokes differential expression of c-Fos and c-Jun proteins in rat brain. *Neurotoxicology*, **17**, 415–41.

Hatten, M.E. 1987: Neuronal inhibition of astroglial cell proliferation is membrane mediated. *Journal of Cell Biology*, **104**, 1353–60.

Hayat, M.A. 1981: *Fixation for Electronmicroscopy*. New York: Academic Press.

Hayat, M.A. 1993: *Stains and Cytochemical Methods*. New York: Plenum Press.

Hockfield, S., Carlson, S., Evans, C., Levitt, B., Pintar, J. and Silverstein, L. 1993: *Molecular Probes of the Nervous System*. Cold Spring Harbor, NY: Cold Spring Harbor Laboratory Press.

Honegger, P. and Werffeli, P. 1988: Use of aggregating cell cultures for toxicological studies. *Experientia*, **44**, 817–23.

Jacobs, A.L., Maniscalco, W.M. and Finkelstein, J.N. 1986: Effects of methyl mercury chloride, cycloheximide and colchicine on the re-aggregation of a dissociated mouse cerebellar cells. *Toxicology and Applied Pharmacology*, **86**, 362–71.

Jensen, K.F. 1995: Neuroanatomical techniques for labeling neurons and their utility in neurotoxicology. In *Neurotoxicology: Approaches and Methods*, Chang, L.W. and Slikker, W. Jr (eds), pp 27–66. New York: Academic Press.

Kowall, N.W., Ferrante, R.J., Beal, M.F. *et al.* 1987: Neuropeptide Y, somatostatin, and reduced nicotinamide adenine dinucleotide phosphate diaphorase in the human striatum. A combined immunocytochemical and enzyme histochemical study. *Neuroscience*, **20**, 817–28.

Kugler, P., Vogel, S., Volk, H. and Schiebler, T.H. 1988: Cytochrome oxidase histochemistry in the rat hippocampus. A quantitative methodological study. *Histochemistry*, **89**, 269–75.

Lillie, R.D. 1965: *Histopathologic Technique and Practical Histochemistry*, 3rd edn. New York: McGraw-Hill.

Lu, E.J., Brown, W.J., Cole, R. and de Vellis, J. 1980: Ultrastructural differentiation and synaptogenesis in aggregating rotation cultures of rat cerebral cells. *Journal of Neuroscience Research*, **5**, 447–63.

Morgan, J.I. and Curran, T. 1986: Role of ion flux in the control of c-fos expression. *Nature*, **322**, 552–5.

Moscona, A.A. 1961: Rotation-mediated histogenetic aggregation of disassociated cells. *Experimental Cell Research*, **22**, 455–75.

Norton, W.T., Aquino, D.A., Hozumi, I., Chiu, F.-C. and Brosnan, C.F. 1993: Quantitative aspects of reactive gliosis: a review. *Neurochemical Research*, **17**, 877–85.

O'Callaghan, J.P. 1994: A potential role for altered protein phosphorylation in the mediation of developmental neurotoxicity. *Neurotoxicology*, **15**, 29–40.

O'Callaghan, J.P. and Jensen, K.F. 1993: Enhanced expression of glial fibrillary acidic protein and the cupric silver degeneration reaction can be used as sensitive and early indicators of neurotoxicity. *Neurotoxicology*, **13**, 113–22.

Ohmstede, C.A., Jensen, K.F. and Sahyoun, N.E. 1989: Ca^{2+}/calmodulin-dependent protein kinases enriched in cerebellar granule cells. Identification of a novel neuronal calmodulin-dependent protein kinase. *Journal of Biological Chemistry*, **264**, 5866–75.

Peters, A., Pallay, S.L. and Webster, H.D. 1991: *The Fine Structure of the Nervous System*, 3rd edn. New York: Oxford University Press.

Peterson, E.R. and Murray, M.R. 1955: Myelin sheaf formation in cultures of avian spinal ganglia. *American Journal of Anatomy*, **96**, 319–56.

Polak, J.M. and Priestley, J.V. 1992: *Electronmicroscopic Immunocytochemistry, Principles and Practice*. New York: Oxford University Press.

Ramon y Cajal, 1928: *Degeneration and Regeneration of the Nervous System*. New York: Oxford University Press.

Ransom, J.T., Cherwinski, H.M., Dunne, J.F. and Sharif, N.A. 1991: Flow cytometric analysis of internal Ca^{2+} mobilization via a B_2-bradykinin receptor on a subclone of PC12 cells. *Journal of Neurochemistry*, **56**, 983–89.

Reuhl, K.R., Lagunowich, L.A. and Brown, D.L. 1994: Cytoskeleton and cell adhesion molecules: critical targets of toxic agents. *Neurotoxicology*, **15**, 133–46.

Saitoh, T., Masliah, E., Jin, L., Cole, G.M., Wieloch, T. and Shapiro, I.P. 1991: Biology of disease. Protein kinases and phosphorylation in neurological disorders and cell death. *Laboratory Investigation*, **64**, 596–616.

Sarafian, T., Cheung, M.K. and Verity, M.A. 1984: *In vitro* methyl mercury inhibition of proteins synthesis in neonatal cerebellar perikarya. *Neuropathology and Applied Neurobiology*, **10**, 85–100.

Sarafian, T. and Verity, M.A. 1986: Mechanism of apparent transcription inhibition by methyl mercury in cerebellar neurons. *Journal of Neurochemistry*, **47**, 625–31.

Scallet, A.C. 1995: Quantitative morphometry for neurotoxicity assessment. In *Neurotoxicology: Approaches and Methods*, Chang, L.W. and Slikker, W. Jr (eds), pp 99–129. New York: Academic Press.

Schiff, P.B. and Horwitz, S.B. 1981: Taxol assembles tubulin in the absence of exogenous guanosine 5triphosphate or microtubule associated proteins. *Biochemistry*, **20**, 3242–52.

Schubert, D., Heinemann, S. and Kidokoro, Y. 1977: Cholinergic metabolism and synapse formation by a rat nerve cell line. *Proceedings of the National Academy of Sciences of the United States of America*, **74**, 2579–83.

Segal, L.M. and Federoff, S. 1989: The acute and subchronic effects of organophosphorus and carbamate pesticides on cholinesterase activity in aggregate cultures of neural cells from the fetal rat brain. *Toxicology In Vitro*, **3**, 111–22.

Selkoe, D.J., Lukenbill-Edds, L. and Shelanski, M.L. 1978: Effects of neurotoxic industrial solvents on cultured neuroblastoma cells: methyl *n*-butyl ketone, *n*-hexane and derivatives. *Journal of Neuropathology and Experimental Neurology*, **37**, 768–89.

Shahar, A., de Vellis, J., Vernadakis, A. and Haber, B. 1989: *A Dissection and Tissue Culture Manual of the Nervous System*. New York: A.R. Liss.

Sidell, N. 1982: Retinoic acid-induced growth inhibition and morphologic differentiation of human neuroblastoma cells *in vitro*. *Journal of National Cancer Institute*, **68**, 589–96.

Sidell, N., Verity, M.A. and Nord, E.P. 1990: Menthol blocks dihydropyridine-insensitive Ca^{2+} channels and induces neurite outgrowth in human neuroblastoma cells. *Journal of Cellular Physiology*, **142**, 410–19.

Sternberger, L.A., 1986: *Immunocytochemistry*, 3rd edn. New York: Wiley.

Tanaka, D. Jr and Bursian, S.J. 1989: Degeneration patterns in the chicken's central nervous system induced by ingestion of the organophosphorus delayed neurotoxin tri-ortho-tolyl phosphate. A silver impregnation study. *Brain Research*, **484**, 240–56.

Tomlinson, D.E. 1992: Aging and the dementias. In *Greenfield's Neuropathology*, Adams, J.H. and Duchen, L.W. (eds), 5th edn, pp 1284–410. New York: Oxford University Press.

Trapp, B.D., Honegger, P., Richelson, E. and Webster, H. de F. 1979: Morphological differentiation of mechanically dissociated fetal brain in aggregating cell cultures. *Brain Research*, **160**, 117–30.

Unger, J.W. and Schmidt, Y. 1993: Galanin–immunoreactivity in the nucleus basalis of Meynert in the rat: age-related changes and differential response to lesion-induced cholinergic cell loss. *Neuroscience Letters*, **153**, 140–3.

Vendrell, M., Zawia, N.H., Serratosa, J. and Bondy, S.C. 1991: C-fos and ornithine decarboxylase gene expression in brain as early markers of neurotoxicity. *Brain Research*, **544**, 291–6.

Verity, M.A. 1995: Cell suspension techniques in neurotoxicology. In *Neurotoxicology: Approaches and Methods*, Chang, L.W. and Slikker, W. Jr (eds), pp 537–48. New York: Academic Press.

Verity, M.A. 1996: Pathogenesis of methylmercury neurotoxicity. In *Mineral and Metal Neurotoxicology*, Yasui, M. (ed.), pp 159–67. Boca Raton, FL: CRC Press.

Verity, A.N. and Campagnoni, A.T. 1988: Myelin basic protein gene expression in the quaking mouse. *Brain Dysfunction*, **1**, 272–84.

Verity, A.N., Levine, M.S. and Campagnoni, A.T. 1990: Gene expression in the Gimpy Mutant: evidence for fewer oligodendrocytes expressing myelin basic protein genes and impaired translocation of myelin basic protein mRNA. *Developmental Neuroscience*, **12**, 359–72.

Veronesi, B., Peterson, E.R. and Spencer, P.S. 1983: Ultrastructural studies of the dying-back process. VI. Examination of nerve fibers undergoing giant axonal degeneration in organotypic culture. *Journal of Neuropathology and Experimental Neurology*, **42**, 153–65.

Whetsell, W.O. Jr and Schwarcz, R. 1989: Prolonged exposure to submicromolar quinolinic acid causes excitotoxic damage in organotypic cultures of rat corticostriatal system. *Neuroscience Letters*, **97**, 271–75.

Yokel, R.A., Provan, S.D., Meyer, J.J. and Campbell, S.R. 1988: Aluminum intoxication and the victim of Alzheimer's disease: similarities and differences. *Neurotoxicology*, **9**, 429–42.

Yonezawa, T., Bornstein, M.B. and Peterson, E.R. 1980: Organotypic cultures of nerve tissue as a model system for neurotoxicity investigation and screening. In *Experimental and Clinical Neurotoxicology*, Spencer, P.S. and Schaumburg, H.H. (eds), pp 788–802. Baltimore, MD: Williams & Wilkins.

19

The neurochemical investigation

FAITH M WILLIAMS

INTRODUCTION

Neurotoxicity may be defined as a permanent or reversible adverse effect on the structure or function of the central or peripheral nervous system by exposure to a biological, chemical or physical agent. Neurobiochemical investigations in humans comprise measures of chemical and biochemical function and must compliment neurophysiological and neurobehavioral investigations. Many specific clinical diseases and syndromes result from alterations in the chemical composition and metabolic activity of the brain and central and peripheral nervous system. These may result from inborn errors of metabolism or secondary effects on metabolism, for example, from exposure to a neurotoxin. This chapter is concerned with the use of neurochemical markers of toxicity.

THE CHOICE OF A NEUROCHEMICAL MARKER

Neurochemical studies of the human brain are restricted by the availability of tissue for analysis or to *in vivo* imaging. Neurochemical markers can be assessed in available peripheral tissue, such as blood, but must have been shown to predict or reflect changes in the nervous system *in vivo*. Markers must be developed and

validated in research strategies in animals *in vitro* and in pilot studies in humans before being used clinically. The markers act as adjuncts to more routine clinical and laboratory tests for the detection of severe poisoning or for evidence of low-level exposure to specific neurotoxins. Potential markers can be assessed in *in vitro* models but application in humans is more limited. Their value may be proposed following *in vitro* investigations but must be fully evaluated. Cell culture and organotypic models are currently being developed with human or animal tissue to give parallel mechanistic studies. (Atterwill *et al.*, 1994). Mechanistic neurochemical investigations in *in vitro* systems can be more extensive and may include measurements such as receptor density, transmitter levels, and biochemical function.

When investigating the pathological response of exposure to chemical toxins there is a need to distinguish acute from chronic and delayed effects. Doses can be further differentiated as high- or low-dose exposure, and either single or multiple exposures. There is a need to define whether the effects are reversible and whether recovery can be monitored. There are also differences in requirements for markers of acute effects compared to long-term or effects that develop with a delay.

It is important to determine whether the proposed marker is a primary or secondary response to exposure to the toxin. For example, is the appearance of raised concentrations of brain proteins in the plasma or cerebrospinal fluid due to a direct effect on the expression or metabolism of the protein or the result of damage to the blood–brain barrier? It is also important to define the specificity of the effect when proposing the use of a marker for a specific toxin. Circulating blood constituents have been extensively used as markers in extreme disease states, for example following inborn errors of metabolism, but it must be acknowledged that changes in the constituents of blood or cerebrospinal fluid may not parallel changes in brain structure or function.

The primary effect of neurotoxins is to alter the metabolic processes of neurones. At a low level of exposure the neurone may withstand the toxin but at a high level or following chronic exposure irreversible damage and cell death, leading to peripheral or central changes, may occur. Biochemical events precede structural changes or permanent lesions and dysfunction and should act as early markers before overt symptoms develop following exposure to a toxin. General neurochemical mechanisms of the initiation of neurotoxicity, as shown in Table 19.1, include, first, effects at receptors or enzymes, such as binding irreversibly or reversibly and competitively with natural endogenous substrates, and leading to altered levels of neurotransmitters and second, selective uptake of a neurotoxin may give high local concentrations, for example in brain and local areas within. Neurotoxins may use existing uptake pathways and compete with endogenous substrates. Once within the neural system neurotoxins may result in altered signaling and secondary messengers leading to damage such as apoptosis (altered natural programmed cell death). Apoptosis is an important physiological process by which multicellular organisms eliminate unwanted cells. Many diseases result from improper regulation of apoptosis which involves the dysfunction of mitochondrial oxidation and excessive production of free radicals leading to premature cell death. It has recently been suggested that neurodegenerative diseases may be linked to excessive apoptosis but specific surrogate markers are not yet available to test the suggestion.

Neurological dysfunctions may also be associated with genetically determined susceptibility to chemicals, such as toxins, in the environment. Differences in susceptibility between individuals may be for a variety of reasons. Differences in the metabolic profile of the toxin may be involved. Many toxins exert their effect following activation to the toxic metabolite, and termination of the toxic effect may involve a further metabolic step to a non-toxic and more easily excreted molecule. Therefore, a complete understanding of the metabolic pathways for the toxin in humans is necessary. It is known that many metabolizing enzymes, in particular the isoenzymes of cytochrome p450, are under genetic control and are polymorphically expressed. There may also be differences in expression between hepatic and extrahepatic tissues, and differences in the influences of environmental factors on metabolism. Possible examples of neurotoxins for which there may be genetic contributions to inter-individual susceptibility include organophosphates (Mutch et al., 1997), Ecstasy (Tucker et al., 1994), 1-methyl-4-phenyl-1,2,3,6,tetrahydropyridine (MPTP) (Steventon et al., 1989b) will be discussed in detail later. Humans are exposed to a wide range of potential neurotoxins during their lifetime such as occupational or environmental chemicals, therapeutic agents or recreational drugs, for example alcohol, lysergic acid diethylamide (LSD), Ecstasy, and narcotics. Specific neurotoxic agents are listed in Table 19.2. In addition, changes at the central nervous system (CNS) are often due to clinical disease. However, the trigger for the development of many neurodegenerative diseases, such as Alzheimer's, has not so far been identified and environmental toxins, such as toxic chemicals or natural toxins, may be involved directly or indirectly.

Neurochemical and biomarkers of exposure to neurotoxins have recently been reviewed by Silberg

Table 19.1 *Neurochemical indicators of neurotoxic effects*

Effect
Alterations in synthesis, release, uptake, degradation of transmitters
Selective uptake
Altered activity of critical enzymes (e.g. AChE)
Altered receptor function and/or second messenger systems
Neurochemical biomarkers of injury (e.g. GFAP)

Table 19.2 *Examples of neurotoxic agents*

Site	Chemical
Neuronal cell body	Methylmercury
	Domoic acid
	Acetyl ethyl tetramethyl tetralin
Schwann cell myelin	Hexachlorophene
Peripheral nerve	Acrylamide
	n-Hexane
Neuromuscular junction	Organophosphates
	Carbamates
Proximal axons	Iminodiproprionitrile
Centrals axons	Clioquinol
Nerve terminal (dopaminergic)	MPTP
Nerve terminal (serotonergic)	MDMA
Astrocytes	6-Aminonicotinimide

(1993), Costa and Manzo (1995), Tilson *et al.* (l995), Costa (1996), and Manzo *et al.* (1995, 1996).

BIOCHEMICAL STUDIES OF SURROGATE MARKERS: SELECTION OF TISSUES

Samples of human neural tissue are not generally available for investigations of neurotoxicity. Biochemical investigations must be conducted on available material such as blood, plasma or blood cells (red blood cells, lymphocytes), urine or cerebrospinal fluid. Measurements of neurotransmitters and their metabolites in peripheral fluids or receptors, or enzyme activities in peripheral cells, may indicate central activity, but such measurements in accessible body fluids must be considered with caution.

Cerebrospinal fluid

The cerebrospinal fluid acts as a buffer protecting the brain and spinal cord from both direct and chemical injury. The cerebrospinal fluid (pH 7.31) is in equilibrium with the nervous system and protected by the blood–brain barrier. Biologically active molecules such as hormones are distributed in the cerebrospinal fluid throughout the central nervous system. The normal composition includes little protein (15–45 μg/100 ml), mostly as albumin. Samples of cerebrospinal fluid can be obtained only in cases where a lumbar puncture is regarded as appropriate, for example meningitis, and therefore there is difficulty in obtaining human cerebrospinal fluid from normal subjects. Increase in total protein greater than 100 μg/100 ml can be associated with inflammation and there is a selective rise in globulin. Electrophoretic separation of cerebrospinal fluid proteins has also indicated an increase in IgG in conditions such as multiple sclerosis.

Levels of metabolites of neurotransmitters such as serotonin (5HT), dopamine (DA) and noradrenaline (NE) can be monitored by sensitive techniques in the cerebrospinal fluid. The acid metabolites, homovanillic acid (HVA) and hydroxyindoleacetic acid (HIAA), reflect the central metabolism of DA and 5HT; the alcohol metabolite, methoxyhydroxyphenyl glycol (MHPG), reflects the central metabolism of NE. It is important to know that metabolite levels represent metabolic activity in the central nervous system and not other peripheral organs. Lumbar cerebrospinal fluid is most easily obtained and this must be shown to represent ventricular cerebrospinal fluid and not local spinal cord changes. Under normal conditions 5HIAA crosses the blood/cerebrospinal fluid or blood–brain barrier by an active process. Decreased HVA directly reflects the low brain dopamine associated with parkinsonism and is altered by levodopa. Phenelzine, reserpine, probenicid, and hydrocephalus may alter cerebrospinal fluid metabolites secondarily by inhibition of the organic acid efflux system, as well as by direct cerebral effects.

There is preferential transport into the brain across the blood–brain barrier for neutral, acidic or basic amino acids, but many, such as the neurotransmitters gamma-aminobutyric acid (GABA), glutamine, aspartate, glutamate, 5HT and dopamine, are synthesized centrally. Excretion of abnormal amounts of various nervous system-derived amino acids in the urine is associated with disorders, often severe, of autosomal recessive inherited inborn errors, manifested in the new born and young. Drug or toxin levels in the cerebrospinal fluid may be closer to levels at the target site in the brain than levels in the blood, but cerebrospinal fluid samples are not often readily available for these measurements. Total concentrations of drug in the cerebrospinal fluid are generally lower than in the blood reflecting binding to plasma proteins. Further details of the analysis of cerebrospinal fluid are beyond the scope of this chapter and can be found in McConnell and Bianchine (1994) and Walton (1987a).

Metabolic markers in blood

Metabolic disorders, often severe and of hereditary origin, as seen in the new born, lead to changes in blood marker enzymes (Walton, 1987b). For example, raised blood pyruvate and metabolic acidosis due to low levels of pyruvate carboxylase are characteristic of sub-acute necrotizing encephalopathy (Leigh's disease). Mild hypoglycemia is associated with enzyme defects leading to glycogen storage disease. Elevated uric acid in serum and urine may be indicative of X-linked low hypoxanthine guanine phosphoribosyl transferase (Lesch–Nyhan syndrome).

In Wilson's disease and Menke's disease, which is autosomal recessive, copper is deposited in the brain. The deposition is associated with low copper oxidase activity, excessive urinary excretion of copper, decreased serum copper and low ceruloplasmin levels.

A low serum folate (<2 μg/ml) can be associated with polyneuropathy, myelopathy, and dementia but may not have a role in the etiology. Abnormal levels of specific excitatory amino acids in the urine are associated with disorders of cerebral metabolism, for example, impaired blood–brain barrier properties and transport systems. Catecholamine phenotyping is currently being used in diagnosis, treatment, and pathophysiology of neurogenetic disorders (Goldstein *et al.*, 1996). The application has developed following establishment of simultaneous sensitive and specific assays for catecholamines.

Brain studies

It is very rare to obtain biopsy material from the human brain although material may occasionally be available at neurosurgery following the removal of a tumor. A useful study was conducted comparing acetylcholine synthesis in biopsies of normal brain and brain from a patient with Alzheimer's disease (Bowen, 1983).

Measurement of neurone number, neurotransmitters, metabolites, receptors, enzymes, etc. in post-mortem samples of brain can potentially give an indication of events prior to death and are very useful. However, this information must be considered critically as variation may occur due to post-mortem delay, differences between brain regions, stability of neurotransmitters, storage conditions, etc. There are also differences in transmitter profile following sudden death compared to a long terminal phase.

There has been limited application of studies of drug levels and localization using post-mortem tissues. For example, amantidine (1-amino adamantane), which is clinically used in parkinsonism and in drug-induced extrapyramidal symptoms, has been shown to be a low-affinity uncompetititve antagonist of N-methyl-D-aspa-rate (NMDA) receptors. Studies in post-mortem brain, cerebrospinal fluid, and serum have indicated that brain concentrations are close to the K_i (inhibition constant) for the phonocyidine (PCP) binding site (Kornhuber et al., 1995).

SPECIFIC BRAIN MARKERS IN CEREBROSPINAL FLUID AND PLASMA

Sensitive and specific techniques have been developed to monitor cell-specific proteins using serum immunoglobulins raised against brain-derived antigens. Protein markers of neurofunction include glial fibrillary acidic protein (GFAP) – a gliotypic protein – and myelin basic protein (MBP) – a neurotypic protein. Breakdown of the blood–brain barrier associated with neurotoxicity results in the release of neural-derived molecules into the extraneural fluids.

Protein markers

Anti-MBP antibodies were detected in the serum and cerebrospinal fluid of patients, and appear to be markers of demyelinating lesions (O'Callaghan, 1991). They may act as early biomarkers at a sub-clinical level before clinical manifestation of disease. This has been tested in rats exposed to lysolecithin, which produces primary demyelination, and to tetraethyltin, which produces secondary demyelination. MBP was detected in the cerebrospinal fluid following the process of chemical demyelination by lysolecithin exposure but not following tetraethyltin (Manzo et al., 1996).

Lead and other metals produced enhanced immunogenicity to MBP and GFAP in workers exposed to the metals (Moneim et al., 1994). GFAP acts as a peripheral indicator of axonal damage (O'Callaghan, 1991). Autoantibodies to MBP have been detected in the cerebrospinal fluid of patients with demyelinating lesions from acquire immune deficiency syndrome (AIDS) and autism (Mastroianni et al., 1991; Singh et al., 1993)

A recent study has suggested that levels of iron-binding protein (P97) and AD melanotransferrin P97 in the cerebrospinal fluid may be a marker of the progression of Alzheimer's disease. These proteins are involved in uptake of iron into the CNS. Previously investigated β-amyloid protein in cerebrospinal fluid does not correlate with the progression of disease. Other possible diagnostic markers include α-1 chymotrypsin, ubiquitin CSF tau, Ab_{1-42}, apolipoprotein E (Kennard et al., 1996).

Degradation of the blood–brain barrier may occur following neurotoxic insult or after ischemic or hemorrhagic injury when the endogenous production of gelatinase D and serine proteinase promotes the opening of the blood–brain barrier. Delaying damage by proteolytic cascade enzymes, by interfering with the genes that produce MMP (metalloproteinases), or inhibiting action of the products might be protective (Rosenberg, 1995). Release of protein-like gelatinase B has been used as a marker of the integrity of the blood–brain barrier.

Neuroendocrine markers

Neuroendocrine probes allow peripheral monitoring of responses to neurotoxins that originate in the brain (Smargiassi et al., 1997).

SERUM PROLACTIN (PRL)

Prolactin measurements have been widely used to study the effects of drugs and chemicals on dopaminergic pathways. Increased serum prolactin is generally considered to indicate reduced tubero-infundibular activity since PRL is controlled by dopamine, released by TIDA (tubero-infundibular activity) in a feedback control. Impaired control of pituitary PRL secretion is common among subjects exposed to low levels of toxic chemicals known to effect the dopaminergic pathways. Therefore, prolactin levels may be used as a secondary biomarker of dopaminergic effects. The disadvantage is that there may be many confounding factors such as stress and nutritional states (Manzo et al., 1996).

Serum PRL was elevated in workers exposed to lead, styrene, and manganese compared to controls, but in the workers exposed to styrene, elevated serum PRL did not correlate with MAO-B (monoamine oxidase) and DBH, which were also affected (Mutti, 1993, 1997).

Specific receptors in peripheral blood lymphocytes (PBL)

The similarity between transmitter receptors found in the brain and those found on lymphocytes in peripheral blood (Costa, 1987) has led to the use of peripheral lymphocytes as markers of changes in the CNS.

Muscarinic receptors in lymphocytes, for example, are similar to those in the CNS and studies with ^{3}H quincyclidine beazilate have indicated that the effects of oxotremorine on muscarinic receptor function in the CNS are reflected peripherally. The organophosphate disulfoton also affected peripheral and central muscarinic receptors in parallel.

SEROTONIN (5HT) RECEPTORS

The platelet has been proposed as the peripheral model for the central serotogenic neurone. 5HT receptors on platelets act as good markers of 5HT receptor function in the CNS. Levels of serotonin in platelets and plasma were significantly reduced in Alzheimer's patients compared to controls in a similar manner in the brain (Kumar et al., 1995a, b). There were also abnormalities in the uptake of 5HT (Freo, 1996).

BLOOD ENZYMES AS MARKERS OF THE CNS

Effects on blood enzymes have been employed as biomarkers of exposure to a number of drugs and chemicals. For example, exposure to lead can be monitored by serum dopa β-hydroxylase and monoamine oxidase (MAO-B) in platelets, inhibition of aminolevulinic acid (ALA) and elevation of both zinc protoporhyrin (ZPP) and free erythrocyte porphyrin (FEP). Similarly the level of inhibition of plasma cholinesterase and red blood cell acetylcholinesterase can be used to monitor exposure to anticholinesterases. Neuropathic chemicals can be monitored by measuring inhibition of lymphocyte neuropathy target esterase (NTE).

In the diagnosis of Fabry's disease a galactosidase can be monitored in leukocytes and in cultured skin fibroblasts. Mucolipidoses are associated with enzyme deficiencies in fibroblasts.

Increases in the concentration of neural proteins in the blood may be indicative of impairment of the integrity of the blood–brain barrier. Contrast-enhanced magnetic resonance imaging (MRI) (using gaudolinium) was used to assess the permeability of the blood–brain barrier and the data were compared with blood levels of matrix mettaloproteinase (MMP), urokinase-type plasminogen activator (UPA), and tissue inhibitors of MMPs (TIMPS) in patients with multiple sclerosis. Patients with gaudolinium enhancement had elevated gelatinase B and UPA and an increased complex of gelatinase B and TIMPs. This suggests that elevation of gelatinase B is associated with opening of the blood–brain barrier and may be a marker of changes in barrier integrity (Rosenberg et al., 1995). Creatine kinase BB and myelin-based protein in the cerebrospinal fluid are elevated following damage to the blood–brain barrier associated with trauma.

Cholinesterase

Cholinesterase (EC 3.1.1.8. ChE) is found in most systems in the body including the blood plasma. Despite its widespread distribution, its physiological role is not defined although it may have some role in lipid metabolism. Cholinesterase hydrolyses a number of drugs, such as suxamethonium, aspirin, diacetylmorphine, procaine, steroid esters, and chemicals such as herbicide esters. It is inhibited by anticholinesterases, such as organophosphates and carbamates, and inhibition acts as a marker of exposure (see later).

Serum cholinesterase is controlled by at least four allelomorphic genes (ChEu, ChEa, ChEf, ChEs) at the same locus which are autosomal and codominant. Ninety-five percent of the population are homozygous for the main genotype ChEu.ChEu, whereas a proportion of the population are heterozygous for the atypical enzyme (ChEu.ChEa) or the silent enzyme (ChEu.ChEs) and display reduced enzyme activity. Heterozygous individuals are distinguished by the inhibition of enzyme activity by fluoride and dibucaine. Depression of serum ChE activity has been reported in patients with liver disease, infections, etc. Serum ChE forms a close association with LDL (low-density lipoprotein) and is depressed in starvation. Therefore when a depressed serum ChE level is detected it is necessary to consider genetic predisposition, metabolic disease or inhibition by organophosphates or carbamates.

Acetylcholinesterase

Acetylcholinesterase (EC 3.1.1.7.AChE) is found in the red blood cells attached to the plasma membrane as well as in neural tissue. A number of studies have indicated that red blood cell enzyme reasonably reflects that in the neural tissue and can therefore act as a peripheral marker of neurotoxic effects (see Organophosphates).

Neuropathy target esterase

Neuropathy target esterase is a membrane-bound protein, inhibition of which in the axon is thought to be associated with the development of delayed peripheral neuropathy following exposure to neuropathic organophosphates which can phosphorylate and age at the active site (Johnson, 1990). Neuropathy target esterase (NTE) is also present in many peripheral tissues including blood lymphocytes and platelets. Inhibition of the enzyme in lymphocytes has been used as a marker of exposure to neuropathic organophosphates (Mutch et al., 1992) and recovery of the enzyme inhibition paralleled clinical recovery from an overdose of chlorpyrifos (Lotti et al., 1986).

MONITORING EXPOSURE TO NEUROTOXINS (BIOMARKERS AND BIOLOGICAL EFFECT MARKERS)

When considering the role of a neurotoxin in the etiology of disease it is important to obtain reliable data on the nature and degree of exposure. Estimation of systemic levels of a chemical often follows biological monitoring of the level of the chemical or its metabolite in a readily accessible body fluid such as blood or urine. This may parallel the monitoring of a biological effect. However, there has generally been more development in the field of biomarkers of exposure than biomarkers of effect. When considering neurotoxins a measurement of chemical in blood or urine may not give a valid estimate of the chemical that has crossed the blood–brain barrier to produce effects in the nervous system.

The emphasis of the following discussion is on the use or potential use of neurochemical/biochemical biological effect markers for indicating exposure to specific groups of chemicals.

Adducts of hemoglobin and proteins as markers of CNS exposure and effects

Monitoring the levels of adducts of chemicals or their activated metabolites with hemoglobin and the polyamines, α and β spectrin, in red blood cells is accepted as a biomarker of exposure to chemicals. Hemoglobin and spectrin adducts of the neurotoxins hexane, carbon disulfide, acrylonitrile and acrylamide have been measured in red blood cells as markers of exposure in workers. (Farmer et al., 1987). A good correlation has been shown between neurotoxicity and hemoglobin adducts of acrylonitrile.

Neurochemistry of specific neurotoxins

Examples of specific neurotoxins are shown in Table 19.3. Several are discussed in detail below.

ORGANOPHOSPHATE AND CARBAMATE PESTICIDES

Because organophosphates and carbamates are rapidly hydrolyzed, the unchanged active chemical is not detectable in the blood except immediately following exposure or following a very high dose. The metabolites of organophosphates (alkyl phosphates) or of carbamates are detectable in the urine for up to 48 h after exposure. Methods are sensitive, involving gas/liquid chromatography with phosphorus detection or high performance liquid chromatography, and metabolites can be detected at lower doses than by monitoring the inhibition of cholinesterases (Nuttley and Cocker, 1993). However, metabolite measurements are not widely available and are not a desirable alternative to the measurement of enzyme activity.

Determination of plasma or serum cholinesterase or red blood cell acetylcholinesterase is used routinely to monitor for exposure to organophosphates and carbamates (Coye et al., 1987). Inhibition of cholinesterase is maximal within 2–3 h of exposure. Preferably both cholinesterase and acetylcholinesterase should be determined in parallel as the profile of inhibition differs; often only cholinesterase activity is offered.

Plasma cholinesterase is more labile than red blood cell acetylcholinesterase (which more closely reflects the similar enzyme at the neuromuscular junction). No physiological role has as yet been described for plasma cholinesterase or for red blood cell acetylcholinesterase. Studies in animals have shown that inhibition of both enzymes reasonably reflects the brain enzyme as determined on total homogenate (Mutch et al., 1996; Williams et al., 1997). Acetylcholinesterase exists as multiple molecular forms in equilibrium and there are

Table 19.3 Examples of biomarkers of neurotoxicity of specific neurotoxins

Biomarkers	Neurotoxicant	Neurotoxic effect
Inhibition of aminolevulinic acid dehydrogenase	Lead	Cognitive dysfunction (children)
Neuropathy target enzyme	Mipafox	Organophosphate-induced delayed neuropathy
Formation of hemoglobin adducts	Styrene	Axonopathy
Spectrin cross-linking	2,5-Hexanedione	Axonopathy
Paraoxonase polymorphism	Paroxon	Enhanced sensitivity to cholinesterase inhibitors

differences between peripheral AChE, central AChE, and red blood cell AChE (Younkin et al., 1982). Plasma cholinesterase is influenced by other factors such as liver disease, age, pregnancy, and alcohol. It is also polymorphic and a small proportion of the population is homozygous for an inactive atypical enzyme; a percentage is heterozygous with intermediate levels of enzyme activity.

Inhibition of acetylcholinesterase by organophosphates is relatively irreversible and enzyme recovery following exposure is generally due to synthesis of new enzyme. Inhibition by carbamate is more rapidly reversible; reversibility is associated with less severe toxicity. Red blood cell acetylcholinesterase activity is slightly affected by rare conditions that damage the cell membrane such as hemolytic anemia.

It is difficult to interpret low levels of inhibition of an individual's cholinesterase or acetylcholinesterase unless an appropriate baseline measurement has been made. For routine monitoring of occupational exposure to organophosphates this is very important and each laboratory must establish its own normal range (Mutch et al., 1992). Up to 70% inhibition can occur before clinical symptoms are detectable. Monitoring urine alkylphosphate levels results in the detection of exposure at levels that produce no inhibition of peripheral cholinesterase. Some organophosphates produce central–peripheral delayed neuropathy (OPIDN) associated with inhibition of another target enzyme, neuropathy target esterase (NTE), in the nervous system.

OPIDN is independent of effects on acetylcholinesterase. For example, it follows exposure to triorthocresylphosphate (TOCP), which does not inhibit acetylcholinesterase. The NTE enzyme is phosphorylated and then ages. The threshold inhibition for the expression of pathology is 50–70%. Inhibition of NTE in the nervous system is paralleled by inhibition of NTE in peripheral tissues. NTE in lymphocytes, platelets, and red blood cells has been recommended as a surrogate marker (Mutch et al., 1992). The most widely used has been lymphocyte NTE although application has been limited because of difficulties in the assay, instability of the enzyme and of the blood cells, and difficulty in interpreting the result. Best documentation of the use of lymphocyte NTE as a peripheral marker was during the recovery of a patient from a chlorpyrifos overdose (Lotti et al., 1986). Most organophosphates in use today are not neuropathic and do not inhibit NTE.

Recent reports of long-term neuropsychological and neurological problems in sheep dippers following long-term exposure to organophosphates have prompted a need for more sensitive markers of the toxic effects of organophosphates. Appropriate biomarkers will not be available until the mechanism of the toxicity is elucidated in animal models or in in vitro systems (Kelly et al., 1997; Williams et al., 1997).

Organophosphate compounds are potent anticholinesterase inhibitors either directly or following activation to the oxon by cytochrome p450 isozymes. Activation occurs mainly in the liver but, possibly more importantly, locally at the site of action, for example the brain. Interindividual differences in the major enzymes involved in activation (CYP3A) may be important in determining susceptibility to toxicity in humans. Phenotyping and genotyping of individuals may be useful in predicting effect (Mutch et al., 1997). The plasma high-density lipoprotein associated enzyme paraoxonase can hydrolyse paraoxon and a number of other organophosphates. Human serum PON1 is polymorphic occurring as two forms, differing only in the amino acid at position 191. The variant PON1 (R), which has arginine at position 191, has eight times the activity of type Q, which has glutamine at position 191. Fifty percent of Caucasians are homozygous for the Q allozyme, 40% are QR heterozygotes and the rest are RR homozygotes (La Du, 1996). The polymorphism can easily be determine in vitro from a blood sample (Primo-Parmo et al., 1996). For organophosphates commonly used these days the distribution has still to be determined. It appears that each substrate differs in its relative affinity for the isoforms and some organophosphates respond similarly to the polymorphic forms (Humbert et al., 1993). Both isoforms, for example, hydrolyze chlorpyrifos oxon at the same rate and the effects of the polymorphism are reversed for diazinon, sarin, and soman (Davies et al., 1996). Even for paraoxon, paraoxonaze may be of little importance at the low concentrations formed following occupational exposure to parathion because of the high K_m affinity constant of the enzyme. Detoxification of unbound paraoxon may be by alternative routes including spontaneous breakdown and binding to carboxylesterases (Mutch et al., 1997). However, monitoring of detoxification enzymes may be predictive markers of susceptibility. A balance exists between activation and the detoxifying hydrolytic pathways, and this may differ between brain and liver.

ECSTASY

Methylenedioxymethamphetamine (MDMA) is a popular mood-altering recreational drug. Acute effects are mediated by increases in extracellular dopamine and 5HT. Repeated high dosage has been shown to be neurotoxic to a sub-population of 5HT-containing axons. Both dopamine release and an intermediary step of MDMA-induced serotonin release are necessary for the inhibitory effects or neuronal excitability in the nucleus accumbens, affecting glutamate-evoked firing (Obradovic et al., 1996; White et al., 1996).

MDMA is converted to the catecholamine dihydroxymethylamphetamine (DHMA) by CYP2D6 which is polymorphically distributed in humans (Daly et al.,

1993; Tucker *et al.*, 1994) This may give rise to a genetically determined difference in neurotoxicity.

ALCOHOL

Chronic alcoholism can induce thiamine deficiencies leading to Wernicke–Korsakoff syndrome, associated with progressive cerebellar degeneration, in susceptible patients. There is an inborn predisposition to this syndrome due to transketolase deficiency, which results in reduced thiamine binding.

Alcohol exposure can be determined easily by monitoring blood alcohol levels by gas chromatography. Alcohol is metabolized and detoxified by oxidation by alcohol and aldehyde dehydrogenase. Polymorphisms have been identified; ADH2 and ADH3 for alcohol dehydrogenase which exists in six forms (ADH1–6). Aldehyde dehydrogenase is found in at least five forms with polymorphisms in ALDH1 and ALDH2, which may contribute to interindividual differences in CNS toxicity (Daly *et al.*, 1993). Polymorphisms of alcohol dehydrogenase may be associated with interethnic variation due to different expressions of the genetic variants. Increased frequency of ADH3*1 has been associated with alcoholic liver disease.

LEAD

Lead exposure, particularly the dust, is still seen in a number of occupations including painters and battery makers. Lead has been removed from most previous sources including lead pipes, pencils and paint, and the tetraethyl lead content of petrol has been reduced so that environmental levels of lead are reducing. The nervous system is very susceptible to the neurotoxic effects of lead. Lead produces encephalopathy particularly in children in whom the blood–brain barrier is less effective. It also produces cerebral edema, peripheral axonal degeneration, and demyelination. Absorbed lead is stored in the body in the red blood cells, bone, and soft tissue (liver, brain, etc.).

Blood lead levels

Whole blood lead levels reflect lead that is in dynamic equilibrium and is available for transport to the brain. In a child under six years with developmental delay, behavioral disorder or speech impairment, a high blood lead level should be considered particularly in countries where control on lead in the environment is not good. It is a requirement to monitor the blood levels of workers exposed to lead in the UK, Europe, and USA.

Blood and tissue lead are generally measured by atomic absorption spectrophotometry Normal blood lead in the UK and USA is now less than $10 \mu g/100$ ml. This has reduced since removal of lead from petrol. Even levels below $15 \mu g/100$ ml in children with symptoms of lead poisoning need to be reduced. In asymptomatic children levels of $25 \mu g/100$ ml indicate a need to remove the source of the lead but chelation therapy is generally not required. At higher levels in children chelation may be considered to reduce the body stores of lead. Occupational control levels in workers exposed to lead are currently $50 \mu g/100$ ml in males and $25 \mu g/100$ ml in females. Removal from the source of exposure is required to see a reduction in blood level.

BIOCHEMICAL INVESTIGATIONS

Blood erythrocyte zinc protoporphyrin levels (ZPP) and ALA dehydrogenase are routinely monitored as biological effect markers of lead exposure. Lead binds to SH groups in enzymes involved in porphyrin synthesis leading to reduced hemoglobin synthesis and anemia. Accumulation of ZPP is secondary to the inhibition of enzymes involved in hemoglobin synthesis in the red blood cell. With continuous lead exposure the effects on the enzymes lag behind the blood lead level reaching a steady state only when all the erythrocytes have turned over (120 days). The ZPP level is not sensitive to low levels of exposure; for example, with lead levels of $30 \mu g/100$ ml the ZPP level was normal ($35 \mu g/100$ ml).

Markers of specific neurological toxic effects of lead are limited and often not validated in humans or in clinical situations. Lead may cause neurotoxicity by amplification of glutamate-induced stress by protein kinase C activation (Naarala *et al.*, 1995). Lead exposure has also been shown to be associated with increased MBP in the cerebrospinal fluid, GFAP enhanced immunogenicity in blood, and elevated serum PRL (Moneim *et al.*, 1994). The elevated blood GFAP in lead workers may be a primary marker or secondary to blood–brain barrier damage.

OTHER METALS

Arsenic, manganese, mercury, and other heavy metals produce polyneuropathies under certain conditions. Similar increased levels of neuroproteins in peripheral fluids would be expected.

N-HEXANE

Symptoms of neurotoxicity, which were first investigated in shoe manufacturers exposed to hexane, included numbness of the extremities and weakness of the hands and feet. With continuous exposure there was progressive loss of sensory and motor function. This is a distal sensorimotor neuropathy. The mechanism has been shown to involve the metabolite of hexane, 2,5-hexanedione, which forms a pyrrole with lysine in neurofilaments cross-linking them. Other solvents that form γ-diketones produce the same effect (Anthony *et al.*, 1983). Activation of hexane to hexanedione involves successive metabolic steps by cytochrome p450 and alcohol dehydrogenase, and these metabolic steps can occur locally in muscle and neural tissue (Crosbie *et al.*, 1997a). P450s involved include cyp2B and 3A, depending on concentrations, and metabolism may contribute to differences in susceptibility (Crosbie *et al.*, 1997b).

Exposure has been assessed by monitoring 2,5-hexanedione in urine but this reflects only recent exposure. Measurements of pyrrole adducts peripherally should closely reflect the neural filaments. Hemoglobin and spectrin pyrrole adducts (Graham *et al.*, 1995) have been shown to be surrogate markers in rats but have not been evaluated as yet in humans.

CARBON DISULFIDE

Exposure to carbon disulfide produces a distal sensorimotor neuropathy characterized by a neurofilamentous axonopathy, similar to that produced by hexane. Carbon disulfide interacts with amino groups on proteins forming neurofilament cross-linkages leading to toxicity. Carbon disulfide combines with primary and secondary amino acids to form dithiocarbamate esters or thiourea bridges. Erythrocyte spectrin is cross linked by carbon disulfide and accumulation of spectrin dimers in rats is dose dependent. The dimers have been detected at earlier time points than classical neurotoxicity markers, although this has not been assessed in humans. Occupationally exposed workers are monitored by measuring breath carbon disulfide or urine levels of 2-thiothiazolidine-4-carboxylic acid (Cox *et al.*, 1992; Riihimaki *et al.*, 1992; Kitamura *et al.*, 1993). Carbon disulfide may also exert its neurotoxic effects by alterations in dopamine metabolism.

ACRYLAMIDE

Acrylamide exposure produces a distal axonopathy in humans (Tilson, 1981; He *et al.*, 1989). Acrylamide is covalently bound to cysteine and adducts of both brain proteins and hemoglobin have been detected. Methods for monitoring exposure to acrylamide have been developed, based on measurement of the adduct *S*-(2-carboxyethyl) cysteine using gas chromatography mass spectrometry (GCMS). Glycidamide, a metabolite of acrylamide, is thought to be involved in the toxicity. Acrylamide and glycidamide adducts of *N*-terminal valine in hemoglobin have been used as markers of exposure in workers. A neurotoxicity index for acrylamide-induced neuropathy correlated well with hemoglobin adducts of acrylamide and with the accumulated dose (inhalation plus dermal absorption) (Calleman *et al.*, 1994).

STYRENE

Styrene exposure has been reported to cause neurotoxicity and workers have reported central nervous system effects (Edling *et al.*, 1993; Pahwa and Klara,

1993). Styrene is activated by cytochrome p450 styrene 7,8-oxide which can form *N*-terminal valine adducts with hemoglobin and this has been used as a biomarker of exposure (Christakopoulos *et al.*, 1993; Korn *et al.*, 1994; Severi *et al.*, 1994). Recent exposure can also be monitored by measuring blood or breath styrene and urinary mandelic or phenylglyoxylic acid (Guillemin and Berode, 1988; Ong *et al.*, 1994). The mechanism of styrene neurotoxicity is unknown. Studies in animals and in *in vitro* systems have shown that styrene depleted brain glutathione and ATP, followed by elevation in intracellular calcium levels (Trenga *et al.*, 1991).

Styrene may also affect dopamine metabolism. Workers exposed to styrene had elevated plasma prolactin levels. Prolactin release from the anterior pituitary gland is chronically inhibited by dopamine. In addition, a decrease in brain MAO-B was seen in rats exposed to styrene and in the platelets from styrene-exposed workers who also had decreased serum dopamine β hydroxylase activity. Some of these effects appear specific for styrene and others are also produced by other solvents. Further elucidation of the mechanism of styrene interaction with the dopamine pathway may yield effect-related markers of styrene exposure.

NATURAL NEUROTOXINS

Neuroexcitatory plant amino acids, for example from *Lathyrus*, *Cycas* or *Mannihot*, cross the blood–brain barrier using uptake mechanisms for endogenous amino acids (Huxtable, 1992).

Neurolathyrism and neurocassavism (konzo) are examples of neurotoxic disorders mediated by plant amino acids that predominately target the large betz cell and produce spastic paraparesis. They are caused by the continuous intake of the neurotoxic plant products such as *Lathyrus sativus* or *Manihot esculenta*. Neurotoxic excitatory amino acids, such as β-*N*-oxalylaminoanaline or β-*N*-methylaminoaniline (cycad), which are agonists at glutamate receptors, are involved (Ludolph and Spencer, 1996). Levels of glutamate, aspartate, glycine, and taurine were elevated compared to controls indicating disturbances in amino acid metabolism (Khan *et al.*, 1995).

Cassava (manioc tuber) can produce tropical ataxic neuropathy due to excessive dietary cyanide. Similarly, West Indian or South Indian spastic paraplegia results from excessive cyanide.

Excitotoxin-induced neuronal degeneration mimics diseases such as Alzheimer's or Parkinson's disease in many of its features.

Table 19.4 *End points used in in vitro neurotoxicity testing*

Effect	Assay
General end points	
Cell necrosis	Neutral red uptake
	MTT reduction
	Fluorescein diacetate hydrolysis
	Lactate dehydrogenase leakage
	Ethidium bromide
Apoptosis	ELISA[a] for determination of nucleosomes,
DNA fragments, and nick and labeled DNA	
Proliferation	Cell counting
	[^{3}H]-Thymidine incorporation
	Flow cytometry
Differentiation	
Glia	Glial fibrillary acidic protein
	Monoamine oxidase B
	Myelin basic protein
Neurons	Transmitter metabolism, uptake and content
Cell homeostasis	Voltage-selective and ion-selective fluorescent dyes
Specific end points	
Receptors	Radioligand binding
Ionotropic	Electrophysiology
	Dye measurement (Fluo-3, Fura-2)
Metabotropic	Cyclic nucleotides (RIA[b])
	Inositol phosphates (radio-labeled or mass measurement)
	Intracellular pH (cytosensor)
Ion channels	Electrophysiology
	Ion fluxes (^{86}Rb, ^{22}Na, ^{45}Ca, ^{36}Cl)
	Dye measurements
Signal transduction	Protein phosphorylation ([^{32}P]ATP incorporation blotting)
Enzymes	Acetylcholinesterase
	Choline acetyltransferase
	Monoamine oxidase
	Neurotoxic esterase
Uptake systems	Radio-labeled ligand uptake
Release	Radio-labeled tracers
	Endogenous release (HPLC-ECDc, RIAb, bioassays for cytokines)
	Electrocapacitance
Energy metabolism	ATP levels (luciferin/luciferase assay; HPLC)

[a]Enzyme-linked immunoabsorbent assay; [b]radioimmunoassay; [c]high performance liquid chromatography – electrochemical detection.

NEUROTOXINS AND PARKINSON'S DISEASE

There is a polymorphism for thiomethyltransferase (TMT) in the population. TMT activity in circulating lymphocytes is lower in Parkinson and Alzheimer's patients compared to controls. Patients with amylotropic lateral sclerosis have high activity of TNT. MPTP (1-methyl-4-phenyl-1,2,3,6-tetrahydropyridine) was discovered as a contaminant of designer drugs that produced Parkinson-like symptoms. MPTP crosses the blood–brain barrier where it is converted to MPP$^+$ locally by the action of MAO-B and then mimics NAD$^+$. N-methylated pyridines with a quaternary nitrogen atom are more neurotoxic than the parent molecule. Methylation by TMT centrally may therefore promote toxicity but peripherally may protect (Waring et al., 1989). MAO-B is also found in the platelets where activity parallels the neural enzyme. Parkinson patients had reduced peripheral activity (Steventon et al., 1989a; Kurth et al., 1993) Peripheral MAO-B may act as a protectant by peripherally metabolizing MPTP to MPP$^+$, which cannot cross the blood–brain barrier. Therefore, low activity may increase susceptibility to the toxic effects. There may also be differences in the relative levels of isoforms of

MAO-B in Parkinson's disease, reducing metabolism of dopamine or producing metabolites of dopamine with neuroexcitatory properties, for example, hydroxylated metabolites. Neuronal and extraneuronal action of the MAO inhibitors deprenyl and debrisoquine indicated differential metabolic profiles (Eisenhofer *et al.*, 1996).

Several studies have been conducted to search for a polymorphism in the expression of MAO-B (Hsu *et al.*, 1989; Ho *et al.*, 1995). 1-Deprenyl and debrisoquine differentially inhibit neuronal and extraneuronal MAO-B and can be used as indicators of effects on catecholamine metabolism. Intraneuronal deamination of noradrenaline to DHPG was compared to extraneuronal demethylation of noradrenaline. Deprenyl and debrisoquine both had neuronal effects but deprenyl alone had extraneuronal effects (Eisenhofer *et al.*, 1996).

An earlier study linked poor metabolizers by CYP 2D6 with susceptibility to Parkinson's disease but later studies have not confirmed this (Steventon *et al.*, 1989b; Blain, 1996).

B-carbolines may be a potential natural source of inducers of Parkinson's disease. 1-Trichloromethyl, 1,2,3,4-tetrahydro-β-carboline (TaClo) causes neurodegeneration of the dopaminergic system. There is a potential for formation of this compound in humans following exposure to chloral hydrate (Bringmann *et al.*, 1996).

The mechanism of development of neurotoxicity following exposure to excitatory amino acids and free radicals has been extensively investigated and appears to involve accelerated apoptosis. The proto oncogene BCL-2 has a key role in preventing programmed cell death or apoptosis. BCL-2 protein and its analogues protect different classes of neurones from cell death, although over expression of BCL-2 in a model system has not prevented initiated degeneration experimentally. The mode of neuronal cell death initiated by excitotoxic levels of glutamate involves altered mitochondrial function. High glutamate and overstimulation of postsynaptic glutamate receptors stimulates calcineurin (Ca^{2+}/camodulin-regulated protein phosphatase) and Ca^{2+}-dependent processes. The resultant intracellular Ca^{2+} overload leads to cell death.

Interleukin-1β-converting enzyme (ICE)-like protease, is also critically involved in early stage apoptosis. The Ca^{2+}-regulated serine protease contributes to the proteolytic cascade leading to cleavage of key cytoskeletal elements, for example lamin cleavage, disolution of the microtubule network. ICE-like proteases are synthesized as pro-enzymes and are activated by limited proteolysis (Orreniius *et al.*, 1996; Sadow *et al.*, 1996). It may be possible to use neurobiochemistry and immunology to identify neurochemical markers that can be monitored *in vivo* to study the development of the disease in humans and the variables that contribute to susceptibility.

MARKERS OF INTERINDIVIDUAL DIFFERENCES IN SUSCEPTIBILITY

Genetic polymorphisms in bioactivation and detoxification enzymes, such as cytochrome p450 or glutathione transferases, may lead to particular susceptibility to neurotoxins. Metabolic polymorphisms have been reviewed by Daly *et al.* (1993). Genetic susceptibility can be determined from a blood sample by genotyping the lymphocytic DNA but this may present ethical problems, particularly for workers exposed to neurotoxic chemicals. The genetic polymorphism in 2D6 has implications for metabolism of MPTP and of Ecstasy. Polymorphisms in *N*-methyltransferase and *O*-methyltransferases found in neural tissues may have implications for neurotoxcity.

IN VIVO TECHNIQUES

Generally accepted *in vivo* monitoring in humans involves observation of clinical signs and behavioral effects. However, tracer methodology allows biochemical detection *in vivo*. Nuclear physicians can use radionuclides as tracers to measure biochemical processes or determine receptor status. For example ^{18}F-2 fluorodezoxyglucose behaves in a manner similar to glucose and has been used for imaging brain tumors; indium 111-pentetreodide localizes in somatostatin receptors. (Coleman, 1995).

Using tracer imaging with, for example, $H_2^{15}O$, it is possible to monitor regional brain activity, blood flow, etc. in disease states. Serotonin neuromodulation can be studied with positron emission tomography (PET), and $H_2^{15}O$ by measuring cerebral blood flow during challenge with a 5HT agonist buspirone (Freo, 1996). Mapping of neuroreceptor distribution in the living human brain permits direct investigation of neurochemical disorders and opens possibilities for the development of targeted pharmacological treatments and elucidation of the mechanisms of neurotoxicity (Busatto and Pilowsky, 1995). PET can be used to assess the functional consequences of changes in brain dopaminergic activity. Functional and neurochemical parameters can be studied in the same patient. Future developments in radiotracers, kinetic models, and detection methods will extend the applications (Volkow *et al.*, 1996).

In the future functional brain imaging should be able to produce information on the living human brain with simultaneous measurements of regional blood flow and cerebral activity, metabolism and neurotransmission for diagnosis of disease states and their treatment (Kuiikka *et al.*, 1996). Application of these techniques to studies of patients acutely or chronically exposed to neurotoxins has been limited but the possibilities are enormous.

IN VITRO TECHNIQUES

Other markers of the mechanism of neurotoxins can really only be defined and studied in animal models and *in vitro*, for example measures of acetylcholine release, receptor density, synthesis, and breakdown. Neurochemical mapping of the brain can be conducted in animals and using human post-mortem tissue or tissue removed at surgery. For example, there have been extensive studies in post-mortem brain tissue obtained from patients with parkinsonism.

Techniques for *in vitro* testing have been considered at a European Centre for the Validation of Alternate Methods (ECVAM) Workshop (Atterwill *et al.*, 1994). It was concluded that it was necessary to devise a three-tiered system for relevant neurotoxicity testing encompassing basic cytoxic, cell physiology, and neural cell-specific end points for predicting and studying CNS and PNS neurotoxic insults. Techniques would include use of neural cell culture of animal and human cell origins and organotopic whole-brain cultures. The important point is the need for validation in parallel with *in vivo* studies and the need for toxicokinetic data to relate the *in vitro* predictions at the concentrations of neurotoxin used to the critical concentrations achieved *in vivo* in humans in the central and peripheral nervous systems.

With the development of sensitive-specific antibodies to proteins that have been shown to be markers of toxicity *in vitro* the low levels of proteins lost from the brain to peripheral fluids will become more detectable and find a greater role as early markers of neurotoxicity.

CONCLUSION

This chapter has aimed to summarize the rather limited role played by specific neurochemical investigations *in vivo* in the management of neurotoxic exposure and the clinical manifestation of effects and in elucidating the mechanism of action of neurotoxins.

REFERENCES

Anthony, D.C., Boekelheide, K., Anderson, C.W. and Graham, D.G. 1983: The effect of 3,4-dimethyl substitution on the neurotoxicity of 2,5-hexanedione. II. Dimethyl substitution accelerates pyrrole formation and protein cross-linking. *Toxicology and Applied Pharmacology*, **71**, 372–82.

Atterwill, C.K., Bruinink, A., Drejer, J. *et al.* 1994: *In vitro* neurotoxicity testing: the report and recommendations of ECVAM Workshop. *Alternatives to Laboratory Animals*, **22**, 350–62.

Blain, P.G. 1996: Variability in susceptibility of the nervous system to toxic insult. *Environmental Toxicology and Pharmacology*, **2**, 131–3.

Bowen, D.M., Allen, S.J., Benton, J.S. *et al.* 1983: Biochemical assessment of serotinergic and cholinergic dysfunction and cerebral atrophy in Alzheimer's disease. *Journal of Neurochemistry*, **41**, 266–72.

Bringmann, G., Feineis, D., God, R. *et al.* 1996: Neurotoxic effects on the dopaminergic system induced by TaClo (1-trichlormethyl-1, 2, 3, 4-tetrahydro-beta-carboline), a potential mammalian alkaloid – *in vivo* and *in vitro* studies. *Biogenic Amines* **12**, 83–102.

Busatto, G.F. and Pilowsky, L.S. 1995: Neuroreceptor mapping with *in vivo* imaging techniques – principles and applications. *British Journal of Hospital Medicine*, **53**, 309–13.

Calleman, C.J., Wu, Y., He, F. *et al.* 1994: Relationship between biomarkers of exposure and neurological effects in a group of workers exposed to acrylamide. *Toxicology and Applied Pharmacology*, **126**, 361–71.

Christakopoulos, A., Bergmark, E., Zorcec, V., Norppa, H., Maki-Paakkanen, J. and Osterman-Golkar, S. 1993: Monitoring occupational exposure to styrene from hemoglobin adducts and metabolites in blood. *Scandinavian Journal of Work and Environmental Health*, **19**, 255–63.

Coleman, R.E. 1995: Revealing biochemistry in a single image. *Journal of Nuclear Medicine*, **36**, 32–3.

Costa, L.G. 1987: Peripheral models for the study of neurotransmitter receptors: their potential application to occupational health. In *Occupational and Environmental Chemical Hazards*, Foa, V., Emmett, E.A., Maroni, M. and Colombi, A. (eds), pp 542–8. Chichester: Ellis Horwood.

Costa, L.G. 1996: Biomarker research in neurotoxicology: the role of mechanistic studies to bridge the gap between the laboratory and epidemiological investigations. *Environmental Health Perspectives*, **104**, 55–67.

Costa, L.G. and Manzo, L. 1995: Biochemical markers of neurotoxicity; research strategies and epidemiological applications. *Toxicology Letters*, **77**, 137–44.

Cox, C., Lowry, L.K. and Que Hee, S.S. 1992: Urinary 2-thiothiazolidine-4-carboxylic acid as a biological indicator of exposure. *Applied Occupational and Environmental Hygiene*, **7**, 672–6.

Coye, M.J., Barnett, P.G., Midtling, J.E. *et al.* 1987: Clinical confirmation of organophosphate poisoning by serial cholinesterase analyses. *Archives of International Medicine*, **147**, 438–42.

Crosbie, S.J., Blain, P.G. and Williams, F.M. 1997a: An investigation into the role of rat skeletal muscle as a site for xenobiotic metabolism using microsomes and isolated cells. *Human and Experimental Toxicology*, **16**, 138–45.

Crosbie, S.J., Blain, P.G. and Williams, F.M. 1997b: Metabolism of *n*-hexane by rat liver and extrahepatic tissues and the effect of cytochrome p450 inducers. *Human and Experimental Toxicology*, **16**, 131–7.

Daly, A.K., Cholerton, S., Gregory, W. and Idle, J.R. 1993: Metabolic Polymorphisms. *Pharmacology and Therapeutics*, **57**, 129–60.

Davies, H.G., Richter, M.F., Keifer, M., Broomfield, C.A., Sowalla, J. and Furlong, C.E. 1996: The effect of the human serum paraoxonase polymorphism is reversed with diazoxon, soman and serin. *Nature Genetics*, **14**, 334–6.

Edling, C., Anundi, H., Johanson, G. and Nilsson, K. 1993: Increase in neuropsychiatric symptoms after occupational exposure to low levels of styrene. *British Journal of Industrial Medicine*, **50**, 843–50.

Eisenhofer, G., Lenders, J.W.M., Harveywhite, J. *et al.* 1996: Differential inhibition of neuronal and extraneuronal monoamine-oxidase. *Neuropsychopharmacology*, **15**, 296–301

Farmer, P.B., Neumann, H.G. and Henschler, D. 1987: Estimation of exposure of man to substances reacting covalently with macromolecules. *Archives of Toxicology*, **60**, 251–60.

Freo, U. 1996: Cerebral metabolic effects of serotonin drugs and neurotoxins. *Life Sciences*, **59**, 877–91.

Goldstein, D.S., Lenders, J.W.M., Kaler, S.G. and Eisenhofer, G. 1996: Catecholamine phenotyping – clues to the diagnosis, treatment and pathophysiology of neurogenetic disorders. *Journal of Neurochemistry*, **67**, 1781–90.

Graham, D.G., Amarnath, V., Valentine, W.M., Pyle, S.J. and Anthony, D.C. 1995: Pathogenic studies of hexane and carbon disulfide neurotoxicity. *Critical Review of Toxicology*, **25**, 91–112.

Guillemin, M.P. and Berode, M. 1988: Biological monitoring of styrene: a review. *American Industrial Hygiene Association Journal*, **49**, 497–505.

He, F., Zhang, S., Wang, H. *et al.* 1989: Neurological and electroneuromyographic assessment of the adverse effects of acrylamide on occupationally exposed workers. *Scandinavian Journal of Work and Environmental Health*, **15**, 125–9.

Ho, S.L., Kapadi, A.L., Ramsden, D.B. and Williams, A.C. 1995: An allelic association study of monoamine oxidase B in Parkinson's disease. *Annals of Neurology*, **37**, 403–5.

Hsu, Y-P.P., Powell, J.F., Sims, K.B. and Breakefield, X.O. 1989: Molecular genetics of monoamine oxidases. *Journal of Neurochemistry*, **53**, 12–18.

Humbert, R., Adler, D.A., Distecha, C.M., Hassett, C., Omiecinski, C.J. and Furlong, C.E. 1993: The molecular basis of the human serum paraoxonase activity polymorphism. *Nature Genetics*, **3**, 73–6.

Huxtable, R.J. 1992: Neurotoxins in herbs and food plants. In *The Vulnerable Brain and Environmental Risks 1*, Isaacson, R.L. and Jensen, K.F. (eds), pp 77–108. New York: Plenum Press.

Johnson, M.K. 1990: Organophosphate and delayed neuropathy – is NTE alive and well? *Toxicology and Applied Pharmacology*, **102**, 385–99.

Kelly, S.S., De Blaquiére, G.E., Williams, F.M. and Blain, P.G. 1997: Effects of multiple doses of organophosphates on evoked potentials in mouse diaphragm. *Human and Experimental Toxicology*, **16**, 72–8.

Kennard, M.L., Feldman, H., Yamada, T. and Jefferies, W.A. 1996: Serum levels of the iron binding protein p97 are elevated in Alzheimer's disease. *Nature Medicine*, **2**, 1230–5.

Khan, J.K., Kuo, Y.H., Haque, A. and Lambein, F. 1995: Inhibitory and excitatory amino acids in cerebrospinal fluid of neurolathyrism patients, a highly prevalent motorneurone disease. *Acta Neurologica Scandinavica*, **91**, 506–10.

Kitamura, S., Ferrari, F., Vides, G. and Filho, D.C.M. 1993: Biological monitoring of workers occupationally exposed to carbon disulfide in a rayon plant in Brazil: validity of 2-thiothiazolidine-4-carboxylic acid (TTCA) in urine samples taken at different times during and after the real exposure period. *International Archives of Occupational and Environmental Health*, **65**, S177–9.

Korn, M., Gfrorer, W., Filser, J.G. and Kessler, W. 1994: Styrene-7, 8-oxide in blood of workers exposed to styrene. *Archives of Toxicology*, **68**, 524–7.

Kornhuber, J., Quack, G., Danysz, W. *et al.* 1995: Therapeutic brain concentration of the NMDA receptor antagonist amantadine. *Neuropharmacology*, **34**, 713–21.

Kuikka, J.T., Belliveau, J.W. and Hari, R. 1996: The future of functional brain imaging. *European Journal of Nuclear Medicine*, **23**, 737–40.

Kumar, A.M., Kumar, M., Sevush, S., Ruiz, J. and Eisdorfer, C. 1995a: Serotonin uptake and its kinetics in platelets of women with Alzheimer's disease. *Psychiatry Research*, **59**, 145–150.

Kumar, A.M., Sevush, S., Kumar, M., Ruiz, J. and Eisdorfer, C. 1995b: Peripheral serotonin in Alzheimer's disease. *Neuropharmacology*, **32**, 9–12.

Kurth, J.H., Kirth, M.C., Poduslo, S.E. and Schwankhaus, J.D. 1993: Association of a monoamine oxidase B allele with Parkinson's disease. *Annals of Neurology*, **33**, 368–72.

La Du, B.N. 1996: Structural and functional diversity of paraoxonases. *Nature Medicine*, **2**, 1186–7.

Lotti, M., Moretto, A., Zoppellari, R., Dianese, R., Rizzutto, N. and Barusco, G. 1986: The inhibition of lymphocyte NTE predicts the development of OPIDN. *Archives of Toxicology*, **59**, 176–80.

Ludolph, C.A. and Spencer, P.S. 1996: Toxic models of upper motor-neuron disease. *Journal of Neurological Sciences*, **139**, 53–9.

Manzo, L., Artigas, F. and Martinez, E. 1996: Biochemical markers of neurotoxicity, a review of mechanistic studies and applications. *Human and Experimental Toxicology*, **15**, 20–35.

Manzo, L., Castoldi, A.F., Nicolera, P., Cocciui, T., Rossi, A.D. and Costa, L.G. 1995: Mechanisms of neurotoxicity applications to human biomonitoring. *Toxicology Letters*, **77**, 63–72.

Mastroianni, C.A., Liuzzi, G.M., Vullo, C.V., Jirillo, E., Delia, S. and Riccio, P. 1991: Detection of cerebrospinal fluid antibodies against myelin basic protein in patients with AIDS dementia complex. *Molecular and Chemical Neuropathology*, **14**, 227–35.

McConnell, H. and Bianchine, J. (eds) 1994: *Cerebrospinal Fluid in Neurology and Psychiatry*. London: Chapman & Hall.

Moneim, A.I., Shamy, M.Y., El-Gazzer, R.M. and El-Fawal, H.A.N. 1994: Autoantibodies to neurofilaments (NF), glial fibrillary acid protein (GFAP) and myelin basic proteins (MBP) in workers exposed to lead. *Toxicologist*, **14**, 291.

Mutch, E., Blain, P.G. and Williams, F.M. 1992: Interindividual variation in susceptibility to organophosphates. *Human and Experimental Toxicology*, **11**, 109–16

Mutch, E., Blain, P.G. and Williams, F.M. 1997: Involvement of cytochrome p450 3a in the metabolism of parathion by human liver. *Toxicology and Applied Pharmacology (submitted)*.

Mutch, E., Kelly, S.S., Blain, P.G. and Williams, F.M. 1996: Comparative studies of two organophosphorus compounds in the mouse. *Toxicology Letters*, **81**, 45–53.

Mutti, A. 1993: Mechanisms and biomarkers of solvent-induced behavioral and neuroendocrine effects. In *Use of Biomarkers in Accessing Health and Environmental Impact of Chemicals*, Travis, C.C. (ed.), pp 183–99. Plenum Press.

Mutti, A. 1996: Serum prolactin in subjects occupationally exposed to manganese. *Annals of Clinical and Laboratory Science*, **26**, 10–17.

Naarala, J.T., Loikkanen, J.J., Ruotsalainen, M.H. and Savolainen, K.M. 1995: Lead amplifies glutamate-induced oxidative stress. *Free Radical Biology and Medicine*, **19**, 689–93.

Nuttley, B.P. and Cocker, J. 1993: Biological Monitoring of workers occupationally exposed to organophosphorus pesticides. *Pesticide Science*, **38**, 315–22.

Obradovic, T., Imel, K.M. and White, S.R. 1996: Methylenedioxy-methamphetamine-induced inhibition of neuronal firing in the nucleus accumbens is mediated by both serotonin and dopamine. *Neuroscience*, **74**, 469–81.

O'Callaghan, J.P. 1991: Assessment of neurotoxicity: use of glial fibrillary acidic protein as a biomarker. *Biomedical and Environmental Science*, **4**, 197–206.

Ong, C.N., Shi, C.Y., Chia, S.E. *et al.* 1994: Biological monitoring of exposure to low concentrations of styrene. *American Journal of Industrial Medicine*, **25**, 719–30.

Orrenius, S., Ankarcrona, M. and Nicotera, P. 1996: Mechanisms of calcium-related cell-death. *Advances in Neurology*, **71**, 137–51.

Pahwa, R. and Kalra, J. 1993: A critical review of the neurotoxicity of styrene in humans. *Veterinary and Human Toxicology*, **35**, 516–20.

Primo-Parmo, S.L., Sorenson, R.C., Teiber, J. and La Du, B.N. 1996: The human serum paraoxonase/arylesterase gene (PON1) is one member of a multigene family. *Genomics*, **33**, 498–507.

Riihimaki, V., Kivisto, H., Peltonen, K., Helpio, E. and Aitio, A. 1992: Assessment of exposure to carbon disulfide in viscose production workers from urinary 2-thiothiazolidine-4-carboxylic acid determinations. *American Journal of Industrial Medicine*, **22**, 85–97.

Rosenberg, G.A. 1995: Matrix metalloproteinases in brain injury. *Journal of Neurotrauma*, **12**, 833–42.

Sadow R., Duboisdauphin, M., Fernandez, P.A. *et al.* 1996: Mechanisms of neuronal cell-death. *Advances in Neurology*, **71**, 419–24.

Severi, M., Pauwels, W., Van Hummelen, P., Roosels, D., Kirsh-Volders, M. and Veulemans, H. 1994: Urinary mandelic acid and hemoglobin adducts in fiberglass reinforced plastics workers exposed to styrene. *Scandinavian Journal of Work and Environmental Health*, **20**, 451–8.

Silberg, E.K. 1993: Neurochemical approaches to developing biochemical markers of neurotoxicity: review of current status and evaluation of future prospects. *Environmental Research*, **63**, 274–86.

Singh, V.K., Warren, R.P., Odell, J.D., Warren, W.L. and Cole, P. 1993: Antibodies to myelin basic protein in children with autistic behavior. *Brain, Behavior and Immunology*, **7**, 97–103.

Smargiassi, A., Mutti, A., Bergamachi, E., Belanger, S., Truchon, G. and Mergler, D. 1996: A pilot study of peripheral markers of catecholaminergic systems among workers occupationally exposed to toluene. *Neurotoxicology*, **17**, 769–75.

Steventon, G.B., Heafield, M.T.E., Sturman, S.G. *et al.* 1989a: Degenerative neurological disease and debrisoquine-4-hydroxylation capacity. *Medical Science Research*, **17**, 163–4.

Steventon, G.B., Sturman, S.G., Heafield, M.T.E. *et al.* 1989b: Platelet monoamine oxidase-B activity in Parkinson's disease. *Journal of Neural Transmission*, **1**, 255–61.

Sumner, S.J. and Fennell, T.R. 1994: Review of the metabolic fate of styrene. *Critical Review of Toxicology*, **24**, S1–33.

Tilson, H.A. 1981: The neurotoxicity of acrylamide: an overview. *Neurobehavioral Toxicology and Teratology*, **3**, 445–61.

Tilson, H.A., MacPhail, R.C. and Crofton, K.M. 1995: Defining neurotoxicity in a decision-making context. *Neurotoxicology*, **16**, 363–76.

Trenga, C.A., Kunkel, D.D., Eaton, D.L. and Costa, L.G. 1991: Effect of styrene oxide on rat brain glutathione. *Neurotoxicology*, **12**, 165–78.

Tucker, G.T., Lennard, M.S., Ellis, S.W. *et al.* 1994: The demethylenation of methylenedioxy methamphetamine (Ecstasy) by debrisoquine hydroxylase (Cyp2D6). *Biochemical Pharmacology*, **47**, 1151–6.

van Helden, H.P.M., Busker, R.W., Melchers, B.P.C. and Bruijnzeel, P.L.B. 1996: Pharmacological effects of oximes; how relevant are they? *Archives of Toxicology*, **70**, 779–86.

Volkow, N.D., Fowler, J.S., Gatley, S.J. *et al.* 1996: Pet evaluation of the dopamine system of the human brain. *Journal of Nuclear Medicine*, **37**, 1242–56.

Walton, J. 1987a: The cerebrospinal fluid, raised intracranial pressure, brain oedema, craniocerebral and spinal trauma, spinal cord compression and relevant investigations – some pathophysiological principles. In *Introduction to Clinical Neuroscience*, 2nd edn, pp 238–72. London: Baillière Tindall.

Walton, J. 1987b: Cerebral metabolism and its disorders. In *Introduction to Clinical Neuroscience*, 2nd edn, pp 213–37. London: Baillière Tindall.

Waring, R.H., Sturnam, S.G., Smith, M.C.G. *et al.* 1989: *S*-methylation in Parkinson's disease and motor neurone disease. *Lancet*, **2**, 356–7.

White, S.R., Obradovic, T., Imel, K.M. and Wheaton, M.J. 1996: The effects of methylenedioxymethamphetamine (MDMA, Ecstasy) on monoaminergic neurotransmission in the central nervous system. *Progress in Neurobiology*, **49**, 455–79.

Williams, F.M., Charlton, C., De Blaquiére, G.E., Mutch, E., Kelly, S.S. and Blain, P.G. 1997: The effects of multiple low doses of organophosphates on target enzymes in brain and diaphragm in the mouse. *Human and Experimental Toxicology*, **16**, 67–71.

Younkin, S.G., Rosenstein, C., Collins, P.L. and Rosenberry, T.L. 1982: Cellular localization of the molecular forms of acetylcholinesterase in rat diaphragm. *Journal of Biological Chemistry*, **257**, 13630–7.

20

The use of epidemiological methods in the investigation of neurotoxic disease

SARAH J O'BRIEN

The purpose of this chapter is to introduce epidemiological methods and to illustrate how these may be used in the investigation of neurotoxic disease. Some of the problems facing epidemiologists are discussed, drawing on examples from the literature as appropriate. This chapter is not, nor is it intended to be, a comprehensive review of the literature in this area. Papers have been chosen to demonstrate particular points in the design, execution, and interpretation of epidemiological studies. This chapter is not intended to replace the need to consult one of the standard texts on epidemiology before embarking on a project.

INTRODUCTION

The relationship between agent, host, and environment

We do not live in a vacuum. We inhabit a world populated by other forms of life in the presence of myriad natural and man-made phenomena. Although there might be factors in our genetic make-up which influence whether or not we develop disease, it is the way in which we interact with our environment which tends to determine our fate. In short, our degree of fitness is determined by the influence of the environ-

ment on our genetic make-up. Depending upon the disease in question, the genetic or environmental components may be quite easy to define, but for most conditions their relative contributions are subtle and much more difficult to delineate. The development of disease cannot usually be attributed to any one factor. Most diseases are multi-factorial in nature and need to be considered within an ecological framework (Mausner and Kramer, 1985).

The agent of a disease is a factor which must be present for disease to occur. For example, lead poisoning only occurs in the presence of lead. However, within an ecological framework for disease, an agent should rather be considered as a necessary but not sufficient cause of disease since suitable host and environmental influences must also exist, the former affecting susceptibility and the latter largely affecting exposure. By convention, environmental influences are divided into three major components: the physical, social, and biological environments. Aspects of the physical environment include heat, sunlight, air, water, and chemical agents. The biological environment incorporates other living things including plants and animals, micro-organisms, and the vehicles and vectors of infectious diseases. The social environment encompasses cultural, economic, and lifestyle considerations (Mausner and Kramer, 1985). The contribution of these three broad environmental categories to the development of disease will vary according to the disease being studied. However, the relationship between agent, host and environment, and the way they all interact, determines whether or not an individual, or group of individuals, will develop disease.

THE SCOPE OF EPIDEMIOLOGY

The study of any disease involves contributions from a variety of clinical and non-clinical disciplines, from the laboratory to the population. Building up a picture of disease in the population is the remit of epidemiology, and there are two basic assumptions which underpin it. The first is that human disease does not occur randomly, and the second is that causal and preventive factors can be identified by adopting a systematic approach to the study of disease in the population, or subgroups within the population (Hennekens and Buring, 1987). A widely accepted definition of epidemiology is:

> the study of the distribution and determinants of health-related events in specified populations, and the application of this study to control of health problems (Last, 1995).

The objectives of epidemiological studies encompass:

- description of the burden and distribution of diseases in the population;
- identification of etiological agents in the pathogenesis of disease;
- description of the natural history of disease;
- provision of data for the management, evaluation, and planning of services to prevent, control, and/or treat disease.

Epidemiology complements clinical and laboratory sciences so that these objectives may be met, usually by measuring associations between exposures and diseases.

The key to completing a successful study is to start by developing detailed research objectives. Once specific goals have been identified, there are three basic components for epidemiological study: populations, exposures, and outcomes. Before discussing each of these in detail, however, it is helpful to introduce the concepts of bias and confounding.

Bias

Bias is defined as any systematic error in an epidemiological study which leads to an incorrect estimation of the association between exposure and the risk of developing disease. There is a formidable list of biases which may be introduced into epidemiological studies

(Sackett, 1979) but, for convenience's sake, Hennekens and Buring (1987) divide bias into two broad classes. The first is selection bias and refers to any systematic errors which occur in selecting the study population. The second broad class is observation (or information) bias and refers to systematic errors in the measurement of information on exposure and/or outcome. If either of these categories of bias is found to be operating it means that any association found between exposure and disease may be spurious. Biases should be minimized by paying attention to the design and conduct of a study.

Confounding

By contrast, confounding is a function of the multi-factorial nature of disease. A confounding factor is a variable which is associated with exposure and, independent of that exposure, is a risk factor for the disease being studied. It may be misleading, producing estimates of risk which are not true. In the worst case scenario confounding may even completely overturn the direction of an association, leading to the belief believe that an exposure thought to be protective is in fact detrimental. Variables commonly regarded as potential confounders are characteristics of the people being studied, such as age, sex, social class, and ethnicity. Confounding may be managed during the design phase of a study but also during analysis.

Consideration of bias and confounding is essential in the design, implementation, and analysis of any epidemiological study as will now be demonstrated.

POPULATIONS

One of the secrets of a good study lies in the choice of study subjects, so that the findings may reasonably be related back to the population from which they were drawn. The term 'target population' refers to the entire set of individuals to which the findings of a study are to be extrapolated (Levy and Lemeshow, 1991). The accessible population is simply the group of individuals available for study (Hulley et al., 1988). Identifying the target population depends on the research hypothesis being clearly stated. Only when this has been established can inclusion and exclusion criteria be defined. The purpose of inclusion criteria is to define the main characteristics of the target and accessible populations.

Inclusion criteria

In terms of the target population, inclusion criteria are based on demographic and clinical characteristics. The accessible population may then be selected on geographical and temporal grounds, that is the number of people for study that can reasonably be identified in a defined area over a specified period of time.

Exclusion criteria

Exclusion criteria are then derived in order to separate out those individuals who might meet the criteria for inclusion, but whose inclusion would compromise interpretation of the study findings. A point worth noting is that as few exclusion criteria as possible should be used since they affect the ability to generalize from the study findings back to the target population.

In an ideal world it would be possible to conduct the study on the entire accessible population. In practice this is rarely possible and the investigator is faced with having to study a subset of this group. The study population is, therefore, the group of people chosen for the study. This group is selected by means of sampling. The first step is to decide upon the sampling frame. This is composed of a set of sampling units which will vary according to the study in question. For example, in a study of parkinsonism the sampling units may comprise individuals with parkinsonism, their general practitioners, or neurologists. A survey of patients recruited via general practitioners or neurologists would certainly yield information about the patients who consult them. However, consider the effect on generalizability; a survey using neurologists as the sampling frame might allow us to generalize our results to patients who are referred to secondary care, but it would not be legitimate to generalize beyond this to all patients with parkinsonism.

Sampling

Once the sampling frame has been determined there are basically two approaches to sampling: probability and non-probability sampling. For detailed discussion of the issues surrounding, and the mathematical basis for, sampling you may wish to refer to authors such as Barnett (1991), Levy and Lemeshow (1991), or Thompson (1992). The basic principles behind these two methods are discussed below.

PROBABILITY SAMPLING

Probability sampling comprises a number of different methods but, whichever method is chosen, the aim is draw a sample at random from the accessible population that may be regarded as representative of the whole group.

Simple random sampling involves listing all individuals in the accessible population, assigning a number to them, and then using a set of random number tables or a computerized random number generator to select those for inclusion in the study.

Systematic sampling similarly involves listing all individuals but in this case the sample is drawn by means of a systematic approach, having chosen the starting point at random, for example, choosing every 10th entry on the list for inclusion in the study.

Stratified random sampling involves separating the accessible population into more homogeneous subgroups and then selecting a random sample from each subgroup or stratum. There are many instances, for example, in which age might have an effect upon the likelihood of developing a disease. One way of overcoming this is to divide the target population by age, say 10-year age bands, and to select equal numbers of people from each stratum at random. The variables of interest for each age group in turn can then be examined. This is one means of controlling for confounding.

Cluster sampling is employed when individuals within an accessible population cannot be identified but groupings can be; for example households could be a grouping. A household may contain only one individual, a number of unrelated individuals or alternatively a family. The sampling frame in this case is an address list.

One-stage cluster sampling refers to the situation where it is possible to include for study all the population members in each selected cluster (Barnett, 1991). Using the household example, this means that the study would include every household member, regardless of family size. Epidemiological studies often employ two-stage cluster sampling. Extending the earlier example of a study of parkinsonism, neurologists might be selected at random from a sampling frame such as a professional association list. But in order to get at the individuals attending neurology clinics it would then be necessary to select them randomly from the list of patients provided by each neurologist in the initial sample.

NON-PROBABILITY SAMPLING

Non-probability sampling tends to compromise representativeness with a knock-on effect on generalizability. Accessibility sampling is carried out when the sole concern is to obtain information easily; only those people in the target population who are easiest to get at are chosen. This is also referred to as haphazard sampling for obvious reasons. Perhaps more sinister is judgemental (purposive) sampling which essentially involves manipulating the population sample to arrive at the desired answer. Individuals are hand-picked to produce the desired result.

Of the non-probability methods, consecutive sampling is the best (Hulley et al., 1988). This means enrolling every individual who meets the inclusion criteria either until a big enough sample has been recruited or over a predetermined duration. In other words, every member of the accessible population is recruited for as long as the study takes place. Depending upon the nature of the study and the research hypotheses, however, difficulties may arise if the study duration is not long enough to take account of seasonal variations or secular trends (Hulley *et al.*, 1988).

Sample size

Epidemiological studies commonly involve making comparisons between groups of people. So having decided upon the sampling technique, it is necessary to consider how big the sample needs to be. The principles on which sample size calculation is based should be properly understood because many mistakes are made at this stage even though several computer packages will calculate the most appropriate sample size. The following simple explanation will help understanding but an expert statistician or epidemiologist should be consulted at this point. Failing to do so could be both expensive and embarrassing when it is discovered that the study was not big enough to answer the research questions.

It should be stressed that the exact method of sample size determination depends upon the hypothesis being tested, the type of study to be performed, and the data which will be collected. Four essential details must be specified at the outset of any investigation:

- the size of the difference which is to be detected, for example a two-fold increase in the risk of developing disease;
- the amount of disease (or level of exposure) in the general population – this may be available from previously published data;
- the acceptable chance of finding a statistically significant difference when none really exists (type I error);
- the acceptable chance of failing to detect a significant difference when it does exist (type II error).

The level of a type I error (or alpha) is the significance level. Alpha represents the probability that a significant result has arisen by chance. The results from epidemiological studies are usually judged to be statistically significant, that is not to have arisen by chance, at significance levels of 0.05 or less ($p < 0.05$). The value of type II error (or beta) reflects the probability of failing to detect a significant difference when it really exists. Beta is usually chosen to be four times greater than the level of significance. The power of a study is its probability of rejecting the null hypothesis, that is that there is no difference between two groups, when to do so would be wrong. It is given by (1-beta) and depends upon sample size. In general the larger the sample the higher the power. It also depends on alpha. Unfortunately it is not possible to minimize both alpha and beta at the same time. As alpha decreases, beta increases and so power declines (Mausner and Kramer, 1985). In order to be able to maintain power, the sample size increases dramatically. As a general rule you should aim to achieve 80% or over for the power of your study.

Sometimes there may be a certain number of people available to study. It is then possible to work backwards from the sample size to decide whether or not the study would have sufficient power to detect a meaningful difference in risk. If not, it is better to decide not to proceed.

It is helpful to pause here to consider the difference between statistical significance and clinical significance. Statistical significance simply refers to the probability that the detection of a difference between two groups has occurred by chance. Clinical significance, however, concerns the relevance of study findings in the clinical context. The ability to demonstrate statistical significance partly depends on sample size so that, if it were too small, one might overlook a difference which was clinically important just because it did not have a 'p' value with enough zeros behind the decimal point! Conversely, many statistical differences reported in the literature are clinically unimportant. At this stage some form of informed judgement is required in interpreting study results.

Recruitment

Choosing the study population is the first point at which bias (selection bias) may be introduced into the study. The next task is to recruit the study subjects and the aims here are to recruit enough people, as determined by the sample size calculation, and to make sure that those who agree take part are truly representative. The response rate refers to the proportion of people who agree to take part in the study out of those originally selected and invited. The biggest danger here is non-response bias since people who do not take part may differ in certain characteristics from those who do. In the event of non-response, epidemiologists often go back to these people to determine how they differ from the responders. For example, there may be age, sex, racial or social class differences. Characterizing the non-responders in this way should allow one to determine how far the findings from the study can be extrapolated back to the accessible population let alone the target population. In epidemiological studies internal validity reflects the degree to which the investigator's conclusions accurately describe what happened in the study. External validity reflects the degree to which these conclusions are appropriate when applied to the target population. A good study should aim for both (Hulley *et al.*, 1988).

EXPOSURES

Assessment of human exposures to environmental agents is a developing field of ever increasing complexity and there are several reasons for this. First, there is the multi-factorial nature of disease. Second, there may be a considerable lag-time between exposure and development of disease, requiring study over a period of years. Third, the putative exposure may leave no easily measurable indicator of past exposure, and finally there is a burgeoning range of agents available for study (Armstrong *et al.*, 1995). This poses considerable challenges for the epidemiologist.

Environmental exposure has been defined as any contact between a pollutant present in an environmental medium and a surface of the human body (Sexton and Ryan, 1988). There is a need, however, to distinguish between the concentration and the dose of an agent. Concentration refers to the presence of an agent in an environmental medium, such as soil water or food, and can be expressed in quantitative terms. The dose refers to the amount that actually crosses from the environment to the human body, for example via the gut, skin or respiratory system (Brunekreef, 1996). Thus, knowledge of the nature of the agent, the dose, and the duration of exposure are all important (Armstrong *et al.*, 1995).

Validity and precision

The measurement of exposures for epidemiological studies needs to be both valid and precise. In this context validity gauges how far an exposure variable reflects the true exposure in the population being studied. Precision reflects the degree to which a measurement of exposure has the same value every time it is measured. Both are affected by the investigator, the subject, and the instrument(s) of measurement (Hulley and Cummings, 1988).

There are a variety of ways of estimating exposure and each method has its strengths and weaknesses. The most common method is simply to ask the study population themselves about their exposure. This may be done either by personal interview (face-to-face or by telephone) or by means of a self-administered questionnaire.

Subjective measures of exposure

INTERVIEWS

Conducting interviews maximizes the amount of information one is likely to get. The interviewer is able to clarify questions and prompt where necessary. Where more than one interviewer is speaking to people

there need to be clear rules about when and how to prompt the subjects. If one interviewer has a more interrogative style than others, and uses different means of prompting the subjects, the study might be subject to interview bias. Of course, interviewing people by telephone introduces an element of selection bias, i.e. the study only includes people who have a telephone. Nevertheless telephone sampling is a tool increasingly used in epidemiology and Potthoff (1994) wrote a useful commentary on the benefits and pitfalls of these methods. By whatever means they are conducted, interviews are an expensive way of collecting data.

The advantages of self-administered questionnaires include the fact that questions are presented in a standard way thereby reducing the bias which an interviewer might introduce. Anonymous questionnaires might also encourage a greater degree of honesty amongst the study population, especially if to admit bad practice might otherwise lead to action against the individual under Health and Safety legislation.

A poor response rate is one of the drawbacks of self-administered questionnaires, especially if they are very long and conducted as a mailshot. Non-responders might have a poorer recollection of their exposure than those who respond (response bias). Moreover, there is no means of ensuring that the questionnaires are completed properly so that missing values may cause problems in analysis. Although postal questionnaires are a relatively cheap way of gaining information about exposure there is evidence that, at least as far as occupational exposures are concerned, they leave considerable room for misclassification of exposures (Blatter *et al.*, 1997).

One of the perils of asking people, by whatever method, about their exposure is that they might not accurately remember what they have been exposed to, especially if those exposures were in the past (recall bias). For example, in an attempt to determine how accurate farmers' recollections of their use of pesticides actually was, Blair and Zahn (1993) compared the answers of farmers in Kansas with information from suppliers concerning the products available on the market at the time. The agreement between farmers and suppliers was approximately 60%. Further evidence of workers misrepresenting their occupational exposures has been provided by Joffe (1992).

PROXIES

Some studies rely on questioning relatives, especially if exposures have rapidly fatal consequences. There is conflicting evidence about the usefulness of information provided by proxies (Brown *et al.*, 1991; Johnson *et al.*, 1993; Grigoletto *et al.*, 1994), but it is clear that reporting either by self or by proxy may lead to misclassification bias. This refers to the fact that individuals may under- or overestimate their exposure.

DIARY-KEEPING

In order to gain a picture of exposures in the present, the study subjects may keep a diary. Diary-keeping reduces the possibility of forgetting facts but requires motivation on the part of the subject, especially if data collection is likely to go on for some time. Diaries can also prove quite complicated to analyze.

Objective methods for assessing exposure

All the methods of data collection described so far are subjective. In order to gain a more objective picture several strategies are available.

EXAMINATION OF RECORDS

The first of these is examining records. These are often medical and/or occupational records and may be used either in addition or as an alternative to collecting data from the subjects themselves. Anyone who has conducted studies using medical records, however, will be well aware of their shortcomings both in terms of completeness and accuracy.

ENVIRONMENTAL EXPOSURE MONITORING

Physical and/or chemical measurements can be made either on the environment or on the study groups, or both. Environmental monitoring poses considerable challenges for epidemiological studies because contaminants may be so widely dispersed in the environment, environmental contamination cannot necessarily be equated with human exposure, and environmental measurements relate only to current exposure. Although it is sometimes possible to estimate past exposure, for example through occupational health records, this becomes increasingly inaccurate the further back one goes (Armstrong et al., 1995).

Environmental monitoring may also be complicated by the effect of the environment itself on the substance(s) under investigation. For example, American Environmental Protection Agency research (Lewis et al., 1996) suggests that the public's greatest exposure to lawn pesticides actually occurs in the home. They studied the amount of lawn-applied pesticides tracked into homes up to one week after application and found they were present in dust and gathered in carpets, curtains, household surfaces, and upholstered furniture. Children are potentially at greatest risk because of pesticide residues lingering on floors and surfaces that they often touch and then transfer to their mouths. Outdoors, lawn pesticides persist for a few days before being broken down by the elements (sun, rain, etc.) but protected inside they can persist for years. Moreover, vacuum cleaning eliminates only about one-third of the contaminated dust.

Geochemical considerations need to be taken into account. For example, Taylor et al. (1995) demonstrated an inverse relationship between soluble aluminium and soluble silicon in a series of water samples collected during a case-control study examining the relationship between the risk of developing presenile dementia of the Alzheimer type (PDAT) and exposure to aluminum in drinking water, tea or medicines. Silicon determines the bioavailability of all sources of dietary aluminum (Edwardson et al., 1993) so that, in a study seeking to elucidate a relationship between PDAT the investigators need to know whether they are carrying out the work in a hard water area or not (hard water contains higher quantities of silicic acid).

The effect of geophysical elements on toxic substances is very important in deciding both what to measure and where to measure it. For example, after a chemical fire it is important to know not only what substances went up in flames, but also what the products of combustion were. Do they dissolve in water? Have they been dispersed by the wind? If so, what was the wind direction and wind speed? Did it rain? All these aspects need to be taken into account when trying to decide who was exposed and by how much.

The aftermath of disasters can provide valuable insights into some of the practical considerations facing the epidemiologist. Following the release of methyl isocyanate at Bhopal investigators quickly realized that environmental measurements would be of no value since the half-life of methyl isocyanate is so short. There was little mileage in trying to differentiate formally between people who had been exposed to the poisonous cloud and those who had not on a purely geographical basis. There was simply not enough evidence to be able to do so (Andersson, 1990). Instead the investigators adopted proximity to a high death cluster as a rough indicator of exposure (Andersson et al., 1988).

Environmental monitoring does not necessarily produce accurate insights into personal exposures. Epidemiological studies linking exposures to environmental agents with health outcomes, for example the effect of emissions from a factory on the health of the surrounding population, might use post code of residence as a proxy for exposure. This might not always be appropriate. For example, most of us spend at least 8 h a day out of the house, at work or at school, and this may be at some distance from our home, not necessarily reflecting what our exposures have actually been. Moreover, where airborne exposures around factory sites are investigated the effects of weather factors on plume dispersal must be considered.

Dispersion and emission modeling are sciences in themselves. Dispersion modeling is undertaken in order to derive estimates of the distribution of pollutants in the absence of data from the environment. A variety of models has been derived for pollutant dispersal, for example in air (including traffic), in water (streams and marine environments), and in the wider environment (Briggs, 1994). Briggs (1994) points out that the ability to apply dispersion models depends upon suitable knowledge both of the exposure pathway of the pollutant of interest and of the levels of emission into that pathway. Not surprisingly, perhaps, this combined information is rarely available.

Emission models have been developed to compensate for lack of data on emission levels. Their usefulness is limited by considerations such as the amount of experimental information which has gone into the model and technological changes which may rapidly render the model invalid (Briggs, 1994).

PERSONAL EXPOSURE MONITORING

In an attempt to determine personal exposure epidemiological studies increasingly involve personal monitoring including the use of biological markers (for example urinary mercury levels) and/or of personal exposure metering (for example a radiation badge). When using biological markers the following features need to be taken into consideration. First the validity of the biological marker should be established (Schulte, 1989). In the epidemiological context this means the extent to which a biological marker is a predictor of disease occurrence. Second, biological markers are subject to variability both because of variations within the same individual, for example diurnal variation, and also because of variations between individuals (Brunekreef et al., 1987; Hulka and Margolin, 1992; Brunekreef, 1996). People exposed to the same external dose of an agent cannot be assumed to have received the same internal dose. A further source of variation may be introduced by laboratory tests. The potential for such variations means possible sources of error in epidemiological studies and may lead to misclassification (Hulka and Margolin, 1992).

DOSE–EFFECT AND DOSE–RESPONSE RELATIONSHIPS

Dose–effect relationships provide a useful starting point for epidemiological studies (Beaglehole et al., 1993). It is convenient to pause at this point to consider the difference between dose–effect and dose–response relationships. Following exposure to an environmental agent its effect upon the human body might be to produce subtle physiological or biochemical changes. On the other hand it might lead to severe illness or even death. Usually, the higher the dose the greater the effect will be. The dose–effect relationship simply describes the relationship between dose and the severity of the effect it produces. It may be estimated for individuals or for groups but, since individuals do not all react in the same way, the value of a dose–effect relationship for an individual will differ from that of a group.

On the other hand, the dose–response relationship is defined, in epidemiological terms, as the proportion of an exposed group that develops a specific effect. Dose–response relationships in epidemiological studies, particularly in environmental and occupational studies, usually follow a sigmoid curve (Beaglehole et al., 1993). Features such as age may modify the dose–response relationship, as has been demonstrated for noise-induced hearing loss.

In practice, humans are exposed to environmental agents from a number of sources via a variety of routes. Simple measurements may indicate what the exposure has been, but not what the most important exposure route was (Brunekreef, 1996). In order to overcome this specialized modeling techniques have been developed (Stevens and Swackhamer, 1989), although these are really beyond the scope of this book.

There is no simple guide to what constitutes the best method(s) of investigation for any given study. In practice a number of techniques might be adopted. For example, a study involving an occupational hygiene assessment of practices and processes in sheep dipping used several methods for determining exposure (Niven et al., 1993). The dipping sessions were filmed so that the investigators could record aspects such as the preparation and replenishment of dip, use of protective clothing, eating, drinking and smoking habits, and accidental exposures occasioned by having to extract a distressed sheep manually from the dip. These were backed up by biological monitoring from blood and urine samples and assessing dermal exposure by ultraviolet fluorescence.

OUTCOMES

The final decision to be made is the outcome being sought in the population. This will, of course, be governed by the research question(s).

Death or disease?

The most florid outcome is, of course, death. Its advantage in epidemiological studies would appear to be that it is a straightforward outcome to define. However, the cause of death may be difficult to establish with accuracy and mortality data need to be approached with a degree of circumspection. Alderson et al. (1983) reviewed the errors in mortality data pointing out the potential for mistakes from the point of certification through coding and processing to misinterpretation of the final output. Alderson (1990) showed that up to 20% of the errors were minor, but 5% were major, that is involving a shift of the diagnosis from one body system to another.

A second alternative for study is the presence of disease. Indeed epidemiologists quite often attempt to divide up the population into those who have developed disease and those who have not in order to explain why one group should develop the disease and not the other, in other words to define risk factors. These are factors whose presence is associated with an increased probability of developing disease. Certain risk factors obviously cannot be avoided, such as genetic make-up, and may be major determinants of risk. Some risk factors, however, may be avoided altogether or, alternatively, individuals might be persuaded to change their behavior to reduce their risk of developing disease. This is the rationale for identifying risk factors and it forms the bedrock of preventive medicine (Mausner and Kramer, 1985).

In studying the presence of disease as an outcome it is necessary to be able to differentiate the diseased and non-diseased states. This is not as easy as it sounds. It may be done on clinical grounds or by using a series of diagnostic tests or, more often, both. No matter what the means of separating diseased and non-diseased individuals, the criteria must be clearly defined and reproducible. Where a clinical definition already exists, and has been agreed by others as valid, these should be used. For example, agreed criteria exist for Alzheimer's Disease (McKhann et al., 1984). The study may involve defining a variety of neurological deficits, for example neuropathological changes or neurobehavioural changes, either singly or in combination. The methods available are described in detail in the preceding chapters. But if the clinical criteria and/or diagnostic criteria used in an epidemiological study are not reliable problems are bound to arise.

Presymptomatic disease

There may be occasions when there is a need to study people who have not yet developed overt symptoms. Pathological changes are detectable but have not yet manifested themselves as clinical signs and symptoms. For example, there is good evidence that occupational exposure to mercury vapors leads to renal and neurological sequelae. Sensitive biochemical tests and neurological examinations may be able to detect pathological changes before the disease process is obvious clinically and, in certain circumstances, before irreversible damage has taken place. Boogaard et al. (1996) examined the effect of exposure to mercury vapor amongst gas industry workers where their primary interest was to detect subtle neurological and biochemical changes, not symptoms of disease. Clearly the ability to study certain diseases at the presymptomatic stage has profound implications for preventive medicine; the identification of risk factors leads to measures to reduce harmful exposures, thereby poten-

tially reversing or at least arresting pathological changes.

Susceptibility

In certain circumstances the major area of interest might be in defining susceptibility before any disease process has begun at all. For example, evidence is being amassed which supports, amongst other things, a genetic basis for schizophrenia (Eaton, 1991). Risk factors for disease which are genetically determined are, of course, unchangeable but identification of these factors and, importantly, other factors which might interact with these to trigger and/or hasten a disease process may nevertheless yield useful information for preventive medicine.

Case definition

Whatever outcome is chosen for study it is very important that it can be defined precisely. This means constructing a case definition. A good example of this can be seen by considering the issues involved in defining a case of new variant Creutzfeldt–Jakob disease (World Health Organization, 1996).

The precise means of constructing a case definition depends upon the research hypothesis but, in any event, the case definition will contain the personal (clinical and/or demographic), temporal, and geographical characteristics. For example, in their case-control study to determine risk factors for impact-related morbidity and mortality in the wake of the Plainfield tornado disaster in 1990, Brenner and Noji (1995) used the following characteristics to define a case: death or injury requiring admission to hospital for one or more days; injuries which were due to the direct mechanical effects of the tornado (i.e. excluding people whose injuries would have been sustained regardless of the tornado); and death or hospital admission within 48 h of the tornado strike. The study was conducted amongst residents of Will County, Illinois, who were in the path of the tornado, thus fulfilling the geographical characteristics.

Armed with an appreciation of some of the difficulties of making a detailed epidemiological study the various stages and protocols of the study can be identified.

DISEASE FREQUENCY AND DISTRIBUTION

The first step is to quantify the disease of interest. In order to do this two pieces of information are needed – the case count and the size of the population at risk, to which the case count relates. This enables one to calculate the disease rate. The calculation of rates is central to epidemiology because it allows the comparison of the disease experience of two or more populations directly (Hennekens and Buring, 1987). The most commonly quoted measures of disease frequency are prevalence and incidence.

Prevalence

The term prevalence means the proportion of people within a defined population who are suffering from a disease at a specified moment and is given by the formula:

$$\text{prevalence} = \frac{\text{no. of existing cases of disease at a specified time}}{\text{total population}}$$

Strictly speaking this is known as point prevalence since it measures disease burden in the population at a particular moment. Period prevalence allows assessment of disease burden over a period of time, for example a year, and is given by the formula:

$$\text{period prevalence} = \frac{\text{no. of existing cases of disease over a specified duration}}{\text{total population}}$$

Note that both these prevalence measures use the total population as the denominator. Prevalence is affected by several considerations. First, if the illness is severe and most people die from it, the point prevalence rate may underestimate the true burden of disease. Similarly, if the duration of illness is short its prevalence will appear lower than you might expect. Second, if the number of new cases of disease is high and/or diagnostic facilities improve so that more cases are recognized, the prevalence rate is raised. Finally, population migration has an effect. If a group of 'unhealthy' people who have a given disease move into a new neighborhood, prevalence will increase in the new neighborhood and decline in the old.

Prevalence measures are most useful when considering chronic diseases and repeated measurements are valuable for determining changes in disease patterns over time. Corrada *et al.* (1995) strike a note of caution in the interpretation of prevalence rates, however, by investigating sources of variability in prevalence rates of Alzheimer's disease. Their starting point was the wide variation in age-specific prevalence rates reported in the literature over a 10-year period – from 7% to 54% in those over the age of 85 years. Clearly differences in prevalence rates in different parts of the world might provide an important starting point for further studies designed to determine etiological agents. They demonstrated, however, that much of the variation could be accounted for by the use of different inclusion and exclusion criteria and case definitions.

Incidence

Incidence directly reflects risk by specifying the probability that individuals within the population at risk of developing disease will actually do so, and is given by the formula:

$$\text{incidence} = \frac{\text{no. of new cases of disease over a specified duration}}{\text{population at risk}}$$

Note that the denominator in this case should, strictly speaking, be the population at risk of developing disease, which may or may not be the same as the total population. The easiest way to illustrate this is using the example of vaccine-preventable disease and immunity. The population at risk comprises those who are susceptible, that is not immunized and who have not acquired natural immunity through suffering from the disease. These individuals may be a fraction of the total population. In practice it is often difficult to separate out those at risk from the total population but, in general terms, the inclusion of people not at risk in the denominator may underestimate the true incidence of disease (Hennekens and Buring, 1987).

Presentation of rates

Rates quoted in the literature are of three types: crude, specific or adjusted. Crude rates are the easiest to calculate and are summary rates based on the actual number of events, for example deaths or disease, in the population. Crude rates are often used for the purposes of international comparisons but are severely limited because they obscure the fact that different subgroups within the total population might have very different disease experiences. Specific rates are, therefore, calculated in order to reveal insights into disease experience in different subsets within the population so that comparisons can be made. The commonest specific rates quoted are age-specific rates. Adjusted rates are used in order to provide a summary figure for the whole population but take into account the limitations of crude rates. They have been manipulated to take into account differences in the population make-up and consequent disease experience. For a detailed discussion of these types of rates refer to standard texts such as Mausner and Kramer (1985) or Hennekens and Buring (1987).

In order to demonstrate the use of specific and adjusted rates consider the following example. In their paper using mortality data on Creutzfeldt–Jakob disease (CJD) in the USA, Holman *et al.* (1996) have presented age-specific and age-adjusted rates. Of the 3642 deaths from CJD recorded in the US between 1979 and 1994 they have been able to show that people in the 70–74 age group fared worst overall. The age-specific death rate for those in the 70–74 age band was 5.75 per million compared with 0.04 per million in the 30–34 year age band. They then wanted to compare death rates in the US with those elsewhere in the world and so calculated a single summary rate where the effect of population age structure was removed, i.e. the age-adjusted death rate. The age-adjusted death rate was 0.95 per million and was similar to published estimates elsewhere in the world.

DESCRIPTIVE STUDIES

Now that disease can be quantified it is possible to explore relationships between exposure and outcome and compare the diseased group with the rest of the population in order to identify risk factors. The first step in this process involves the use of descriptive studies – characterizing personal (for example sex, race, and social class), temporal (secular trends or seasonal patterns), and geographical (small areas, national or international) aspects of disease. These may use data from routinely available sources such as census data, vital statistics, employment and medical records, or might involve the collection of special data, for example a survey. Whatever method is chosen, it is important to recognize that descriptive studies make no attempt to analyze the links between exposure and outcome (Beaglehole et al., 1993). They simply describe what is there.

There are essentially three types of descriptive study: the case report or case series; the correlational (or ecological) study; and the cross-sectional survey. Descriptive studies are used to generate specific hypotheses about risk factors for disease, which may then be tested using analytical studies.

Case report/case series

Case reports commonly appear in the literature and comprise a patient or group of patients who exhibit characteristics which the clinician views as unusual and, therefore, worthy of comment. These studies may help in the discovery of a new disease or a new risk factor. For example, one of the earliest writers known to have made a connection between symptoms and lead mining was Hippocrates (Corn, 1992). Although many famous physicians, such as Paracelsus and Ramazzini (the father of Occupational Medicine) wrote about the effects of lead on health down the ages it was not really until the twentieth century that concerted action to control this environmental hazard was undertaken.

A somewhat extreme example of the contribution that this type of study can make is the report by Liddle et al. (1979) which described the accidental poisoning of five Jamaican fishermen with methomyl. Three of the men died within hours of eating a meal to which they had added methomyl instead of salt. The remaining two, one of whom was asymptomatic, were treated with atropine and both survived. Post-mortem examinations on the dead men yielded useful information about dose–effect levels and recovery.

Correlational (ecological) studies

In correlational studies, populations or groups of people are the category of interest, as opposed to individuals which form the basic units in case reports or case series. Relationships between exposure and outcome are examined by comparing populations on a geographical basis (for example international comparisons) or by looking at one population's experience in the same country at different times.

Correlational studies prove popular because they often use data which are already collected for other purposes and so are relatively cheap to carry out. Their chief disadvantage is that it is impossible to link exposure with outcome in individuals, and so this is one possible source of bias. Ecological fallacy refers to the situation where the investigator draws inappropriate conclusions on the basis of these data. Moreover, it is very difficult to relate multiple exposures with outcome and no account of potential confounding factors can be taken.

Cross-sectional studies

Cross-sectional studies are undertaken in order to determine the prevalence of disease and the risk factors associated with it. They are, therefore, sometimes referred to as prevalence studies. The cardinal feature of the cross-sectional study is that estimations of exposure and outcome are made together at the same point in time. Because the study is carried out at a specified moment, for example over the period of a year, it furnishes a single view of exposure and outcome in a well-defined population. In order to find out if the relationship between exposure and outcome changes another cross-sectional study would have to be performed, comparing the results of the first study with the results of the second, assuming the same method was used on each occasion.

The first step, having specified the research questions, is to define the population of interest and select the study sample. The next step is to devise a means of measuring the health status and exposures within the group bearing in mind the issues discussed in the

Exposure and Outcomes sections. As a general rule it is important to be very critical about the data to be collected. Is it really important? Will it tell you what you need to know? Will you be able to analyze it? If the answer to any of these is 'no' the data should not be collected. Do not waste energy and money collecting unanalyzable data. If a questionnaire is to be used, pilot it first. What the investigator may understand by the questions might not be what the non-specialist reader (patient) understands.

The denominator in a cross-sectional study is the whole population or, for example in the case of an occupational study, a subset of it. Since all cases of disease are collected, whether incident cases or not, cross-sectional studies yield prevalence estimates, calculated as shown in the earlier section.

In order to describe the relationship between exposure and disease, a reference group, comprising individuals judged never to have been exposed, may be recruited so that various exposure groups can be compared with it. For example, Stark *et al.* (1996) employed a cross-sectional study design in order to determine if methadone maintenance treatment reduced risk-taking behavior amongst injecting drug users in Berlin. They conducted their study amongst injecting drug users undergoing methadone maintenance treatment and compared the results with a group who were not being managed by this means between September 1992 and October 1993. They demonstrated that those drug users taking methadone maintenance treatment were significantly less likely to have either borrowed or passed on used syringes recently. They were concerned that these results might have been influenced by confounding factors such as age, level of educational achievement, and duration of drug injecting. In order to determine what effect these confounders might have had on their study results they adjusted for these in the analysis of the study by performing logistic regression. They then found that those on the methadone maintenance treatment were still less likely to borrow syringes but that the statistically significant reduction in lending syringes disappeared. They further determined that there was a statistically significant association between borrowing syringes and having injected drugs in prison, having used sedatives and having had sexual intercourse with another injecting drug user, all in the previous six months.

Advantages of conducting cross-sectional studies include the fact it is not necessary to wait to find out who will develop the outcome(s) of interest. This makes them relatively quick and cheap to carry out. They provide prevalence estimates. The biggest disadvantage is that, because exposure and outcome are ascertained at the same time, it is not possible to determine whether the risk factor was the cause of disease or a consequence of it. They favor the inclusion of people with chronic diseases who survive with the condition (survivor bias).

Those who develop symptoms and die rapidly might be missed, depending upon the completeness of both data sources and of ascertainment. Cross-sectional studies are an inefficient way of studying rare diseases. They are, however, an excellent means of generating hypotheses which can be formally tested with analytical methods.

ANALYTICAL EPIDEMIOLOGY

Analytical studies are employed to test etiological hypotheses. There are two main categories: the cohort study and the case-control study.

Cohort studies

The principal feature of a cohort study is the identification of a group of people free of disease who are then divided into two groups according to whether or not they have been exposed to a putative risk factor. They are then followed over time in order to ascertain whether or not they develop the outcome of interest. Cohort studies may be prospective or retrospective.

Prospective cohort studies involve selecting the study population and measuring details about exposure. This might be a group sampled from the general population or from an occupational group. Cohort studies are commonly employed in occupational settings. The cohort is then followed up over time and the presence or absence of disease is subsequently determined. Important variables can be measured accurately and completely but a major issue in prospective studies is the ability to keep in touch with the cohort, perhaps over a period of many years. This means, for example, being able to keep track of people who die and/or people who move house. Considerable thought needs to be given to how to do this.

Retrospective cohort studies involve the same steps, the difference being that the cohort, the exposure measurements, and the data on disease outcomes were all gathered in the past. The ability to undertake this type of study depends upon the completeness of documentation on exposure and subsequent outcome which was almost certainly collected for a different set of reasons by a different researcher. One of the biggest problems is that there is little control over the quality of these data exercised by the second investigator.

Since the population being studied is, by definition, disease-free at the outset, cohort studies (whether prospective or retrospective) provide direct estimates of incidence. Furthermore, in addition to determining whether or not an association exists between an exposure and an outcome, these studies provide information about the strength of that association. In cohort studies this is achieved by determining the relative risk.

The relative risk is defined as the ratio of the incidence rate for the group exposed to a risk factor to the incidence rate for those who were not exposed and is represented thus:

$$\text{relative risk} = \frac{\text{incidence rate among exposed group}}{\text{incidence rate among unexposed group}}$$

When analyzing the results of a cohort study the relationship between exposure and disease is described in a 2×2 table. By convention, outcome appears across the top of the table and exposure down the side:

	Outcome	
	Disease present	Disease absent
Present	a	b
Exposure		
Absent	c	d

The incidence rate in the exposed group is $a/(a+b)$, the incidence rate in the unexposed group is $c/(c+d)$, and the relative risk (RR) is

$$\frac{a/(a+b)}{c/(c+d)}$$

The higher the relative risk proves to be, the stronger the association between exposure and outcome. For example, a relative risk of two means that individuals are twice as likely to develop disease given exposure to the risk factor under consideration.

For example, Welp *et al.* (1996) undertook a retrospective cohort study in order to determine if exposure to styrene led to chronic disease of the central nervous system. They were able to make use of a cohort of workers, which had been gathered over the period 1945–1991, and who were working in 660 plants across Europe manufacturing reinforced plastic products. The cohort had originally been assembled to examine the risk of developing leukemia and lymphoma in workers exposed to styrene.

The original cohort comprised 41 167 employees although in this study 32 082 were included after taking account of missing data items for certain members of the cohort and exclusion of those who were not exposed to styrene or whose exposure status was unknown. Personal exposure was estimated by means of using historical personal measurements, extrapolation from Danish data which were very extensive and considered to represent exposures across the industry, and personal occupational histories. The outcomes of interest were deaths from all causes and deaths from central nervous system diseases as catalogued in the International Classification of Diseases manual.

The results of the study showed, amongst other things, that deaths from central nervous system diseases increased with average exposure, cumulative exposure, duration of exposure, and time since first exposure to styrene. Sources of error in the study, as the authors pointed out, included the accuracy of death certificates, other chemical exposure in the workplace acting as potential confounders, and bias brought about by the healthy worker effect (see section on Interpreting and reporting study results).

The advantages of conducting cohort studies include the fact that a temporal relationship can be established between exposure and outcome (i.e. outcome follows exposure). They are particularly useful where exposures are rare, and allow the investigation of several outcomes for each exposure. They are able to cope with the phenomenon of latency, the delay between exposure and development of symptoms. When conducted prospectively they allow accurate measurement of exposures. They yield incidence rates and a direct estimate of risk. The disadvantages include the need to involve a large number of people often over long periods of time. This means that prospective studies are very expensive to carry out and are prone to losing people in follow-up. Retrospective studies are limited by the adequacy of historical record keeping. They are not generally suitable for studying rare outcomes, except in special circumstances.

Case-control studies

The primary attribute of case-control studies is that they involve the selection of people with disease and a comparison (or control) group who do not have disease, and search historically for differences in exposures. Cases should be selected so that they represent all cases from the population with a specified disease and controls should be selected on the basis that, even though they have not developed disease, they have had similar opportunities for exposure. This means that they would have been included as cases in the study had they developed the outcome being explored. Furthermore, it means that controls are not necessarily representative of the non-diseased population as a whole.

Cases may be selected from a variety of sources, having first decided upon the case definition (see Outcomes section). In general it is easier to use incident cases unless the outcome is very rare, when existing cases might also be included. The problem with this is that the number of prevalent cases is influenced by survival times. Interpreting the findings from such a study is complicated by the fact that there are not only determinants of disease initiation to be considered but also duration.

The selection of controls is very important and is a key issue in case-control study design. Controls should be comparable to the target population from which the cases were drawn so that the exclusion criteria applied to the cases must also apply to the controls. There are three main sources from which controls may be drawn: hospital, general practice or neighborhood. Hospital controls have the advantage that they are easy to get hold of but some of the disadvantages include the fact that they have a disease, albeit not the outcome of the study, and are therefore very different from the general population.

One way of overcoming the biases introduced by the use of hospital controls is to select controls from the general population, often via a general practice list or electoral roll. One of the drawbacks of using general population controls, however, is that they might be less motivated to take part in the study especially if they are well.

A third source of controls is people from the same neighborhood as the case. Depending upon the research hypothesis, this can be a helpful means of taking into account potential confounders such as ethnicity and social background.

The next issue surrounds the question of how many control groups should be used. As a general rule it is desirable to have just one control group, but the decision to use more will be determined by the research hypothesis. The optimal case-control ratio is $1:1$ but when the sample size is limited the power of a study can be maintained by increasing the number of controls for every case. There is no point in going beyond four controls per case since the cost of collecting the additional data can be astronomical and is not rewarded by large increases in power.

The final decision is whether or not to employ matching. Matching provides a means of controlling for potential confounders, and involves defining these and selecting controls which are the same as the cases for this particular feature. A good example of a confounder for which matching might be employed is age. For example, increasing age has an influence on the development of dementia independently of any other risk factors which might be present. Investigators might therefore decide to remove the effect of age in a study by matching cases and controls on this criterion. Matching only works for controlling confounders which are recognized as such and should be employed with care. If too many variables are matched for there are few associations left to test. It is not possible to test for differences between cases and controls for matched variables since cases and controls are, by definition, the same for those features. Moreover, if matching has been employed in the design of the study this matching must be maintained in analyzing the results.

The association between an exposure and an outcome in a case-control study is measured by means of the odds ratio. The 2×2 table is drawn as before with outcome across the top and exposure down the side

(note: this is an example where matching has not been employed).

	Outcome	
	Disease present	Disease absent
Present	a	b
Exposure		
Absent	c	d

The odds ratio is essentially the odds in favor of developing the outcome of interest in the presence of and in the absence of the exposure. It is derived thus:

Odds of a case having been exposed is a/c, odds of a control having been exposed is b/d, and the odds ratio (OR) is

$$\frac{a/c}{b/d}$$

or

$$\frac{ad}{bc}$$

Case-control studies do not yield incidence directly unless the study is population based, nor do they usually provide a direct estimation of risk. However, the odds ratio reflects relative risk well when:

- the controls are representative of the general population;
- the cases which were studied are representative of all cases;
- the outcome being studied is rare in the population.

For further information on analyses for cohort and case-control studies, including how to cope with matching, refer to a standard text such as Rothman (1986).

Forster *et al.* (1995) used a case-control study design in order to investigate the relationship between presenile dementia of the Alzheimer type (PDAT) and family history, medical history, cigarette smoking, and exposure to aluminum. Potential cases were identified from specialist hospital services in the north of England and a diagnostic algorithm was applied in order to select the cases for study. Controls were randomly selected from general practice lists, and cases and controls were matched for age and sex. Exposure histories for both cases and controls were sought from a close relative by a single interviewer using previously validated methods, thus minimizing the potential for observer bias. Historical data on aluminum levels in drinking water were obtained where available.

Of the 211 cases of PDAT identified 109 were eventually eligible, and available, for study. This illustrates one of the problems facing investigators, namely that the number of cases which can eventually be included in the study might plummet. In examining the relationship between risk factors and development of PDAT, statistically significant odds ratios were obtained for first degree relative with dementia, any relative with dementia, and any relative under the age of 65 years with dementia. Exposure to cigarette smoking and to aluminium in drinking water, medicines, and diet were not statistically significant factors although some of the odds ratios exceeded one. One of the reasons for this was the problem of the drop in sample size. The authors revisited their sample size calculation on the basis of 109 case-control pairs, finding that a study of that size would have had approximately 80% power to detect odds ratios above 2.5 at the 5% significance level. The authors go on to discuss the potential biases including the dangers of misclassification bias and the influence of survivor bias in selecting cases and avoiding environmental bias in collecting controls.

Case-control studies are intuitively fairly easy to understand but their proneness to various types of bias must never be underestimated. Even the selection of cases poses problems in ensuring that they are representative of all cases. For example, for any given disease, some people might not seek medical attention, some might be seen outside the chosen study area, some might be misdiagnosed and some might either recover or die before their condition is diagnosed. Those left over are, therefore, the ones available for investigation. Further bias might be introduced in the selection of controls and, on top of these problems, there are the usual issues of accurately describing exposures, etc. Case-control studies are, however, useful for investigating rare outcomes and are a less expensive alternative to cohort studies. Unlike cohort studies, though, they might not always allow one to establish the sequence of events.

EXPERIMENTAL EPIDEMIOLOGY

Mentioned for the sake of completeness, experimental studies are rarely indicated on ethical grounds, the exception being clinical trials. Obviously the most convincing way to establish the relationship between an exposure and an effect would be to expose a group of people to the risk factor in question and follow what happens to them. The ethical difficulties inherent in this approach are obvious. However, there are certain situations where one might wish to study the effect of removal of a risk factor on the health of a population such as after a factory shut-down. Environmental disasters sometimes provide the opportunity to study the effects of, for example, a chemical release on the health of the surrounding population. An example of such a 'natural experiment' occurred in Bhopal. The local population is still the subject of studies designed to elucidate the long-term effects of their exposure to methyl isocyanate.

OCCUPATIONAL STUDIES

Occupational epidemiology is basically the study of the effects of exposures on the development of health outcomes, as applied to the workplace, and may use any of the methods described above. But another type of study favored in the occupational setting is the mortality study and involves calculating the proportional mortality ratio. It is possible to do this when the number and causes of deaths amongst the exposed group is known but the structure of the population from which they arose is not known (Hennekens and Buring, 1987). The proportional mortality ratio (PMR) is the proportion of deaths from a specific cause in the exposed group compared with the proportion of deaths from the same cause in a non-exposed or general population group, that is:

$$\text{proportional mortality ratio (PMR)} = \left(\frac{\begin{array}{c}\text{proportion of deaths from a specified}\\ \text{cause in exposed people}\end{array}}{\begin{array}{c}\text{proportion of deaths from the same specified}\\ \text{cause in a comparison population}\end{array}} \right)$$

and it is usually expressed as a percentage. For example, Schulte et al. (1996) sought to identify potential occupational risk factors for deaths from neurodegenerative diseases in 27 states of the USA between 1982 and 1991. They obtained death certification data from the National Occupational Mortality Surveillance System including cause of death, occupational and demographic characteristics. They abstracted these pieces of information relating to four groupings of neurodegenerative diseases, namely Alzheimer's disease, presenile dementia, Parkinson's disease, and motor neuron disease. They calculated PMRs by occupation for each of these disease groupings and found that excess mortality occurred for all these disease groupings in certain professions such as teachers, medical personnel machinists and machine operators, and scientists. Workers who were likely to have been exposed to solvents were found to have increased PMRs for various of the neurodegenerative diseases.

Mortality studies like this are limited by several considerations. These include the accuracy of death certification and, at least in this study, the appropriateness of occupational groupings which were determined by the investigators making a judgement about the commonality of tasks and exposures.

Studies of this sort are not suitable for describing associations between an occupational exposure and outcome but should rather be viewed as a means of generating hypotheses about such relationships which can then be tested in an analytical study.

Cohort studies are reasonably popular in the occupational setting and thought needs to be given to the most appropriate comparison group. This might not always be a general population group. One of the reasons for this is the fact that those in work are, on average, healthier than the general population, since the latter includes people who cannot work because of illness. This is known as the healthy worker effect. As a result any excess risk associated with occupational exposure and outcome might be underestimated by using the general population as a comparison group.

Another problem arises if the occupational group differs from the general population in ways which might affect exposure. A person's occupation might, for instance, mean that they differ from the general population in terms of smoking habits. Smoking might, therefore, become a potential confounder. One of the ways of overcoming this is to use another group similar in demographic characteristics to the group of interest but which is considered not to have been exposed. Stephens *et al.* (1995) tried to overcome this in a cross-sectional study designed to determine the long-term effects of exposure to organophosphates in sheep dip. They compared a group of farmers with another group of rural workers, namely quarrymen, although the appropriateness of that particular choice was subsequently the subject of some debate.

INTERPRETING AND REPORTING STUDY RESULTS

Having discovered an association between an exposure and an outcome the next task is to determine whether this is a true association or not. Could chance, bias or confounding have played a role which renders a positive association invalid?

Chance

The role of chance can be minimized by having a sample size which is large enough to answer the research hypothesis although recruiting a large enough sample can sometimes prove problematic.

The role of chance can be assessed by means of statistical significance testing. The precise method depends upon the research hypotheses, the study which has been undertaken, and the data gathered. However, all statistical significance tests end up with a statement of probability or 'p' value. Significance tests depend upon the null hypothesis as the starting point, that is that there is no association between an exposure and the outcome of interest. By convention, a 'p' value

of 0.05 or less is usually considered to be statistically significant in medical research. What this actually means is that there is, at most, a 5% probability that the positive association you have found could have occurred by chance alone.

Bias

Biases can seriously upset the conclusions of a study and should have been minimized by paying very careful attention to study design and implementation. It is essential that biases in population selection (including the healthy worker effect) and measurements of exposure and/or outcome have not led to the wrong conclusions being drawn from the data.

Confounding

Finally confounders must be considered. Confounding can be controlled for during the design phase of a study, usually by matching, or in the analysis phase, which is increasingly common these days especially in large studies. This may be achieved by performing stratified analyses or, more often, by employing regression techniques. These require the help of a statistician.

Determining cause

Epidemiologists usually adopt one of two approaches to the investigation of disease. They either start with the disease and determine its cause(s) or they identify a possible cause, for example exposure to a chemical, and look for the development of disease. In either event, the process of deciding whether or not epidemiological associations are causal is known as causal inference. The first step is to make sure that there are no flaws in the design or interpretation of a study which could render any observations invalid. The role of chance, bias and confounding must be assessed first. Once these have been ruled out, and only then, may the criteria for causation (Hill, 1965) be applied to the study findings. These are:

- A temporal relationship. The putative cause must be demonstrated to precede the development of disease.
- Plausibility. The study findings should be supported by other evidence such as knowledge of the mechanism of action of an agent or evidence from experiments on laboratory animals.
- Consistency. The study findings should be supported by similar results from other investigators.
- Strength. The stronger the association between the putative cause and development of disease, as measured by the relative risk, the more likely an association is to be causal.

- Dose–response relationship. Strong evidence for a causal relationship is provided when increased exposure to the putative cause leads to an increased effect in the population exposed.
- Reversibility. If removal of a possible cause leads to a reduction in disease occurrence, the possibility of the association being causal is strengthened.
- Specificity. This implies that the risk factor is associated with the disease being studied and no other. But in real life, a single risk factor might be causally related to more than one disease and one of the best examples of this is smoking tobacco.

The weight of evidence depends upon the type of study which has been undertaken. Although the best evidence comes from randomized control trials, it is relatively unusual. Most data are from observational or analytical studies. Well-designed and conducted cohort and case-control studies may provide good evidence for causation. Cross-sectional and ecological studies rarely provide enough evidence, particularly because they are unable to demonstrate a temporal relationship between an exposure and disease.

SURVEILLANCE

Surveillance involves the ongoing, systematic collection, collation and analysis of data, and dissemination of the results to those who need to know in order to be able to take appropriate action (Last, 1995). Surveillance is essential for:

- monitoring trends;
- detecting clusters/outbreaks/epidemics;
- detecting a newly emerging problem;
- identifying risk groups;
- evaluating the effectiveness of interventions;
- setting priorities when allocating resources;
- providing etiological clues which can be explored using appropriate epidemiological studies.

Two of the key issues which govern the usefulness of a surveillance system are its ongoing nature and the timeliness with which data are analyzed and disseminated.

Surveillance systems may be designed to collect information about the occurrence of specified health events in the population or in the workplace, about hazards, or about exposures. Thacker *et al.* (1996) describe these in the following way. Hazard surveillance is useful for providing information about substances present in the environment, for example toxic chemicals. Exposure surveillance, commonly employed in the occupational health arena, involves monitoring individuals for the presence of an environmental agent or its clinically inapparent effects. Outcome surveillance

involves documenting death, disease or disability. But, as they point out, these methods are rarely combined, although the complicated nature of environmental health surveillance merits such an integrated approach.

Surveillance data may be gleaned from a variety of sources, either making use of routinely published data, such as mortality statistics, or requiring the establishment of special recording systems. These might be for documenting biomarker measurements or for reporting cases of specific diseases to build up a disease-specific case register. These data should be of the highest possible quality and be easily accessible (Thacker *et al.*, 1996). Data which have been archived in a form which makes them difficult to retrieve will probably never be looked at again and this defeats the purpose of collecting them in the first place.

There are numerous examples of surveillance systems in the fields of communicable disease epidemiology and occupational health. An example of the latter is the system which has been set up in Fresno County, California for the surveillance of work-related pesticide illness (Maizlish *et al.*, 1995). This is an active system which has been designed to enhance the completeness and quality of reporting, to identify risk factors, to flag up high-risk sites, and to enable better targeting of preventive measures in the work place and in the community. It involves a combination of case reporting by physicians likely to treat occupationally acquired pesticide illnesses and interviews with some of the cases who meet the reporting guidelines. Work site surveys have been carried out in certain circumstances and the companies have been provided with a report highlighting inadequacies in working practices, for example deficiencies in training, and making specific recommendations based on those findings. They have supplemented this with advice on how to reduce pesticide usage. Despite flaws in the surveillance system design, which are readily acknowledged by the authors, the scheme appears to have been moderately successful. They were able to monitor trends, identify high-risk workplaces and high-risk working practices, and suggest remedial action. It is this latter aspect which has yet to be evaluated for evidence of its uptake and effectiveness.

Hall *et al.* (1994) describe a surveillance system which has been devised in order to glean information about the public health consequences of toxic releases. The system, initially operating in five states of the US, gathers data about events, chemicals, victims, injuries, and evacuations from a variety of sources including state environmental protection agencies, the emergency services, and hospitals. Surveillance definitions were assigned to the terms 'events' and 'victims.' Between January 1, 1990 and December 31, 1991 they detected 1249 events, 72% of which occurred at fixed sites with the remaining 28% being associated with transport. Only one chemical was released in the majority (80%)

of incidents. The chemicals most frequently released were herbicides, acids, volatile organic compounds, and ammonias. The surveillance system provided useful data for informing the emergency responses to incidents. The system could not, however, be regarded as furnishing data which were representative of the situation across the USA as a whole, since those who originally participated were not selected at random. This situation was expected to improve as more states joined the system.

CLUSTERS, OUTBREAKS AND EPIDEMICS

Clusters

A cluster is defined as the 'aggregation of relatively uncommon events or diseases in space and/or time in amounts that are believed or perceived to be greater than could be expected by chance' (Last, 1995). Clusters may come to light by a number of routes including observations made by the public, or sometimes by the media, or as a result of surveillance. The interpretation of clusters is difficult and many do not bear close scrutiny. The interpretation of disease clusters in small geographical areas is a specialized subject requiring specific mapping and statistical skills. Some of the issues involved are discussed by Elliott (1995) and include:

● the geographical area involved;
● the availability of relevant population data;
● the time period to be considered.

Altering geographical boundaries and/or duration can make clusters emerge or evaporate. The investigation of clusters might or might not bear fruit but can have considerable resource implications.

Krebs *et al.* (1995) describe the investigation of a neurological disease cluster amongst workers at a manufacturing plant. Eighteen people presented with neurological symptoms resembling multiple sclerosis over a 15-year period (1970–1985), all of whom worked or had worked at a factory producing carburetors. This cluster was deemed to be highly unusual and a case-control study was performed in order to explore relationships between exposures in the workplace and the development of the multiple sclerosis-like illness. Given the small number of cases the investigators recruited four controls per case, who were selected at random from the factory population and matched by age, sex, and ethnicity. The exposure assessments related to 10 chemicals and/or processes. Statistically significant levels of risk were associated with die-casting and exposure to organophosphates. Flaws in the study, acknowledged by the authors, included the small number of cases, lack of further clinical evaluation of

the cases, and misgivings about the exposure information. The association with die-casting was, however, judged to be plausible since the process had previously involved the use of hydraulic fluid products containing high levels of triarylphosphates. The practice was discontinued in 1982. One of the unresolved issues, however, is whether at least some of these cases were genuinely multiple sclerosis and unrelated to such exposures or not. Alternatively some of the cases could have had a delayed neuropathy, the presentation of which resembled that of multiple sclerosis and which was related to organophosphate exposure.

Outbreaks

Last (1995) defines an outbreak as 'an epidemic limited to localized increase in the incidence of disease, for example in a village, town or closed institution.' Recognizing an outbreak depends upon a knowledge of the background rate of the disease and a perception that what you have observed is in excess of what you would normally expect to see. An outbreak is, however, limited in scale. The objectives of an outbreak investigation are:

● to identify the agent;
● to determine the vehicle, that is the means by which the agent has been transferred into people;
● to introduce control measure to prevent further people from becoming affected.

Such investigations involve a variety of professionals whose various contributions help to paint the overall picture of the cause of the incident. Clinical, laboratory, public health (epidemiological) expertise is required in cooperation with professionals who have the authority to act within the appropriate legislative framework. A coordinated response involving such cooperation is essential in the management of incidents. Plans should already exist which detail the people who need to be involved so that an emergency response can be mounted immediately and comprehensively.

In 1986 49 people in Sierra Leone presented during May and June with an illness characterized by the sudden onset of weakness, dizziness, vomiting, and diarrhea (Etzel *et al.*, 1987). It began within half an hour of eating. A total of 14 people died – 10 children and four adults. A case-control study was performed to identify the risk factors associated with this dramatic illness. The study involved 21 of the cases (who met the case definition) and 22 household controls, and showed that cases were more likely to have eaten bread in the 4 h before the onset of symptoms – the odds ratio was 12.7 and was statistically significant. This finding prompted investigations at the flour mill and at local bakeries. Samples of bread, bread-making ingredients, and used flour bags were analyzed for chemical contamination by various methods. A loaf of bread, bread-making equipment, and empty flour sacks from one of the bakeries were contaminated with parathion. This lead the investigators to examine the floor of a truck which had been used to carry flour from the mill to a general store from where the bakers purchased their flour. Parathion was also found in the truck so it was assumed that the flour had become contaminated whilst being transported.

In October 1986 an occupational physician in Taiwan notified the public health authorities of illness amongst some of the workers in a printing factory who presented with diplopia, muscle weakness, and breathing difficulties (Chou *et al.*, 1988). Nine people were affected, four of whom were admitted to hospital and two died. Two people required mechanical ventilation to assist their breathing. At first occupational exposure to chemicals was suspected as the cause of the problem. It was subsequently ruled out, partly because the cafeteria cook, who was not exposed to chemicals in the factory, was the worst affected. All the ill workers had eaten in the staff canteen. The possibility of the problem being due to botulism surfaced approximately three weeks after the first cases occurred. A retrospective cohort study was conducted amongst the 40 factory employees seeking details about food exposures and subsequent development of symptoms. Laboratory investigations on the cases were unhelpful but clinical examination of two of the employees revealed electroincremental responses consistent with botulism. The results of the epidemiological investigation showed that eating breakfast in the staff canteen was strongly associated with illness, although no single food item was highlighted. Type A botulinum toxin was subsequently recovered from an unopened jar of peanuts in the staff canteen which had been processed by an improperly equipped, unlicensed cannery.

Both these problems illustrate the need for a swift response but as Palmer (1995) has pointed out, this does not rule out the necessity for a rigorous approach. Both problems required a multi-disciplinary team to unravel the cause of the outbreak and the latter example shows how, when confronted with a neurological illness of unknown aetiology, toxicological causes, whether environmental or occupational, might have an infectious diseases origin and should be borne in mind.

Epidemics

As implied above an epidemic is a very large outbreak. There is no magic number to define when an outbreak becomes an epidemic but it depends upon the scale of the problem, both numerically in terms of cases and geographically in terms of the overall population involved.

For example, in Spain in 1981 an epidemic occurred which eventually affected more than 20 000 people (Philp, 1995). The index case was admitted to hospital on May 1, 1991 with acute respiratory failure and died shortly thereafter. The epidemic peaked in June at which point 2000 cases per week were presenting. In the first 12 months there were 12 000 people admitted to hospital and more than 300 people died, but by December 1989 the death toll amongst people who had suffered from 'toxic oil syndrome' was over 800. The acute presentation consisted of respiratory symptoms and signs, skin rashes, and gastrointestinal problems but often progressed to severe muscle pain, muscular and neuronal degeneration, and sometimes paraplegia. It was noticed that cases tended to occur in low-income families, that nursing infants were never affected, and that the epidemic was largely confined to central and north-western Spain. The cause of the epidemic was eventually found to be cheap cooking oil which had been sold in markets in small towns and villages. Far from being the pure olive oil that the customers thought it was, it comprised low-grade olive oil mixed with various seed oils. One of these was an imported rape-seed oil which had been rendered unfit for human consumption by mixing it with aniline.

An epidemic which has yet to be satisfactorily explained affected more than 50 000 people in Cuba between 1991 and 1994 who developed optical and peripheral neuropathies (Ordunez-Garcia *et al.*, 1996). A variety of hypotheses have been tested and a combination of acute nutritional deficiency, the toxic effects of tobacco, and possible exposure to some other, as yet unidentified, toxic substance(s) has been suggested. An interesting observation made by the investigators, however, is that these events coincided with an acute deterioration in the economic fortunes of the Cuban people. A similar problem had occurred in 1897 and 1898 during the Cuban blockade when economic affairs were likewise dreadful.

Thus we come full circle – back to the multi-factorial nature of disease and the importance of the relationship between agent, host, and environment.

A PLACE FOR EPIDEMIOLOGICAL METHODS

One of the major strengths of the epidemiological approach is that risk factors for disease may be identified without the precise nature of the causative agent or its mechanism of action being understood. The finding of an epidemiological association does not, however, necessarily prove a cause–effect relationship. Furthermore, the interpretation of the findings from an epidemiological study is only as robust as the investigation itself.

REFERENCES

Alderson, M. 1990: *An Introduction to Epidemiology*. London: MacMillan.

Alderson, M.R., Bayliss, R.I.S., Clarke, C.A. and Whitfield, A.G.W. 1983: Death Certification. *British Medical Journal*, **287**, 444–5.

Andersson, N. 1990: Disaster epidemiology. In *Major Chemical Incidents – Medical Aspects of Management*, Murray, V. (ed.), pp 183–95. London: Royal Society of Medicine (International Congress and Symposium Series).

Andersson, N., Kerr Muir, M., Mehra, V. and Salmon, A.G. 1988: Exposure and response to methyl isocyanate: results of a community-based survey in Bhopal. *British Journal of Industrial Medicine*, **45**, 469–75.

Armstrong, B.K., White, E. and Saracci, R. 1995: *Principles of Exposure Measurement in Epidemiology (Monographs in Epidemiology and Biostatistics, V21)*. Oxford: Oxford University Press.

Barnett, V. 1991: *Sample Survey Principles and Methods*. London: Edward Arnold.

Beaglehole, R., Bonita, R. and Kjellstrom, T. 1993: *Basic Epidemiology*. Geneva: World Health Organization.

Blair, A. and Zahm, S.H. 1993: Patterns of pesticide use among farmers: implications for epidemiologic research. *Epidemiology*, **4**, 55–62.

Blatter, B.M., Roeleveld, N., Zielhuis, G.A. and Verbeek, A.L.M. 1997: Assessment of occupational exposure in a population-based case-control study: comparing postal questionnaires with personal interviews. *Occupational and Environmental Medicine*, **54**, 54–9.

Boogaard, P.J., Augus-Tinus, A.J.H., Journee, H.L. and Van Sittert, N.J. 1996: Effects of exposure to elemental mercury on the nervous system and the kidneys of workers producing natural gas. *Archives of Environmental Health*, **51**, 108–15.

Brenner, S.A. and Noji, E.K. 1995: Tornado injuries related to housing in the Plainfield tornado. *International Journal of Epidemiology*, **24**, 144–9.

Briggs, D.J. 1994: Mapping environmental exposures. In *Geographical and Environmental Epidemiology: Methods for Small-area Studies*, Elliott, P., Cuzick, J., English, D. and Stern, R. (eds), pp 158–76. Oxford: Oxford University Press.

Brown, L.M., Dosemeci, M., Blair, A. and Burmeister, L. 1991: Comparability of data obtained from farmers and surrogate respondents on the use of agricultural pesticides. *American Journal of Epidemiology*, **134**, 348–55.

Brunekreef, B. 1996: Exposure assessment in environmental epidemiology. In *Environmental Epidemiology: Exposure and Disease*, Bertollini, R., Lebowitz, M.D., Saracci, R. and Savitz, D.A. (eds), pp 207–215. London: Lewis Publishers.

Brunekreef, B., Noy, D. and Clausing, P. 1987: Variability of exposure measurements in environmental epidemiology. *American Journal of Epidemiology*, **125**, 892–8.

Chou, J.H., Hwang, P.H., Malison, M.D. 1988: An outbreak of Type A foodborne botulism in Taiwan due to commercially preserved peanuts. *International Journal of Epidemiology*, **17**, 899–902.

Corn, J.K. 1992: *Response to Occupational Health Hazards: A Historical Perspective*, pp 72–3. New York: Van Nostrand Reinhold.

Corrada, M., Brookmeyer, R. and Kawas, C. 1995: Sources in variability in prevalence rates of Alzheimer's Disease. *International Journal of Epidemiology*, **24**, 1000–5.

Eaton, W.W. 1991: Update on the epidemiology of schizophrenia. *Epidemiologic Reviews*, **13**, 320–8.

Edwardson, J.A., Moore, P.B., Ferrier, I.N. *et al.* 1993: Effect of silicon on gastro-intestinal absorption of aluminium. *Lancet*, **342**, 211–12.

Elliott, P. 1995: Investigation of disease risks in small areas. *Occupational and Environmental Medicine*, **52**, 785–9.

Etzel, R.A., Forthal, D.N., Hill, R.H. and Demby, A. 1987: Fatal parathion poisoning in Sierra Leone. *Bulletin of the World Health Organization*, **65**, 645–9.

Forster, D.P., Newens, A.J., Kay, D.W.K. and Edwardson, J.A. 1995: Risk factors in clinically diagnosed presenile dementia of the Alzheimer type: a case-control study in northern England. *Journal of Epidemiology and Community Health*, **49**, 253–8.

Grigoletto, F., Anderson, D.W., Rocca, W.A. *et al.* 1994: Attrition and use of proxy respondents and auxiliary information in the Sicilian neuroepidemiologic study. *American Journal of Epidemiology*, **139**, 219–28.

Hall, H.I., Dhara, V.R., Kaye, W.E. and Price-Green, P. 1994: Surveillance of hazardous substance releases and related health effects. *Archives of Environmental Health*, **49**, 45–8.

Hennekens, C.H. and Buring, J.E. 1987: *Epidemiology in Medicine*. Boston, MA: Little, Brown and Company.

Hill, A.B. 1965: The environment and disease: association or causation? *Proceedings of the Royal Society of Medicine*, **58**, 295–300.

Holman, R.C., Khan, A.S., Belay, E.D. *et al.* 1996: Creutzfeldt–Jakob disease in the United States, 1979–1994: using national mortality data to assess the possible occurrence of variant cases. *Emerging Infectious Diseases*, **2**, 333–7.

Hulka, B.S. and Margolin, B.H. 1992: Methodological issues in epidemiologic studies using biologic markers. *American Journal of Epidemiology*, **135**, 200–9.

Hulley, S.B. and Cummings, S.R. 1988: Planning the measurements: precision and accuracy. In *Designing Clinical Research: An Epidemiological Approach*, Hulley, S.B. and Cummings, S.R. (eds), pp 31–41. London: Williams & Wilkins.

Hulley, S.B., Gove, S., Browner, W.S. and Cummings, S.R. 1988: Choosing the study subjects. In *Designing Clinical Research: An Epidemiological Approach*, Hulley, S.B. and Cummings, S.R. (eds), pp 18–30. London: Williams & Wilkins.

Joffe, M. 1992: Validity of exposure data derived from a structured questionnaire. *American Journal of Epidemiology*, **135**, 564–70.

Johnson, R.A., Mandel, J.S., Gibson, R.W. *et al.* 1993: Data on prior pesticide use collected from self- and proxy respondents. *Epidemiology*, **4**, 157–64.

Krebs, J.M., Park, R.M. and Boal, W.L. 1995: A neurological disease cluster at a manufacturing plant. *Archives of Environmental Health*, **50**, 190–5.

Last, J.M. 1995: *A Dictionary of Epidemiology*, 3rd edn. Oxford: Oxford University Press.

Levy, P.S. and Lemeshow, S. 1991: *Sampling of Populations: Methods and Applications (Wiley Series in Probability and Mathematical Statistics)*. New York: Wiley Interscience.

Lewis, R., Nishioka, M. and Burkholder, H. *et al.* 1996: Measuring transport of lawn-applied herbicide acids from turf to home: correlation of dislodgeable 2,4-d turf residues with carpet dust and carpet surface residues. *Environmental Science and Technology*, **30**, 3313–20.

Liddle, J.A., Kimbrough, R.D., Needham, L.L. *et al.* 1979: A fatal episode of accidental methomyl poisoning. *Clinical Toxicology*, **15**, 159–67.

Maizlish, N., Rudolph, L. and Dervin, K. 1995: The surveillance of work-related pesticide illness: an application of the Sentinel Event Notification System for Occupational Risks (SENSOR). *American Journal of Public Health*, **85**, 806–11.

Mausner, J.S. and Kramer, S. 1985: *Epidemiology: An Introductory Text*. London: W.B. Saunders.

McKhann, G., Drachman, D., Folstein, M. *et al.* 1984: Clinical diagnosis of Alzheimer's Disease: report of the NINCDS-ADRDA work group under the auspices of the Department of Health and Human Services Task Force on Alzheimer's Disease. *Neurology*, **34**, 939–44.

Niven, K.J.M., Scott, A.J., Hagen, S. *et al.* 1993: *Occupational Hygiene Assessment of Sheep Dipping Practices and Processes. Final Report to the Health and Safety Executive on Project 1/HPD/126/269/92*. Edinburgh: Institute of Occupational Medicine (Technical Memorandum Series).

Orduñez-Garcia, P.O., Nieto, F.J., Espinosa-Brito, A.D. and Caballero, B. 1996: Cuban epidemic neuropathy, 1991 to 1994: history repeats itself a century after the 'amblyopia of the blockade'. *American Journal of Public Health*, **86**, 738–843.

Palmer, S.R. 1995: Outbreak investigation: the need for 'quick and clean' epidemiology. *International Journal of Epidemiology*, **24**, S34–8.

Philp, R.B. 1995: *Environmental Hazards and Human Health*, pp 183–4. London: Lewis Publishers.

Potthoff, R.F. 1994: Telephone sampling in epidemiologic research: to reap the benefits, avoid the pitfalls. *American Journal of Epidemiology*, **139**, 967–78.

Rothman, K.J. 1986: *Modern Epidemiology*. Boston, MA: Little, Brown and Company.

Sackett, D.L. 1979: Bias in analytic research. *Journal of Chronic Diseases*, **32**, 51–63.

Schulte, P.A. 1989: A conceptual framework for the validation and use of biologic markers. *Environmental Research*, **48**, 129–44.

Schulte, P.A., Burnett, C.A., Boeniger, M.F. and Johnson, J. 1996: Neurodegenerative diseases: occupational occurrence and potential risk factors, 1982 through 1991. *American Journal of Public Health*, **86**, 1281–8.

Sexton, K. and Ryan, P.B. 1988: Assessment of human exposure to air pollution methods, measurements and models. In *Air Pollution, the Automobile, and Public Health*, Watson, A.Y., Bates, R.R. and Kennedy, D. (eds), pp 207–38. Washington, DC: National Academy Press.

Stark, K., Muller, R., Bienzle, U. and Guggenmoos-Holzman, I. 1996: Methadone maintenance treatment and HIV risk-taking behaviour among injecting drug users in Berlin. *Journal of Epidemiology and Community Health*, **50**, 534–7.

Stephens, R., Spurgeon, A., Calvert, I.A. *et al.* 1995: Neuropsychological effects of long-term exposure to organophosphates in sheep dip. *Lancet*, **345**, 1135–9.

Stevens, J.B. and Swackhamer, D.L. 1989: Environmental pollution: a multimedia approach to modelling human exposure. *Environmental Science and Technology* **23**, 1180.

Taylor, G.A., Newens, A.J., Edwardson, J.A. *et al.* 1995: Alzheimer's disease and the relationship between silicon and aluminium in water supplies in northern England. *Journal of Epidemiology and Community Health*, **49**, 323–8.

Thacker, S.B., Stroup, D.F., Parrish, R.G. and Anderson, H.A. 1996: Surveillance in environmental public health. *American Journal of Public Health*, **86**, 633–8.

Thompson, S.K. 1992: *Sampling (Wiley Series in Probability and Mathematical Statistics)*. New York: Wiley Interscience.

Welp, E., Kogevinas, M., Andersen, A. *et al.* 1996: Exposure to styrene and mortality from nervous system diseases and mental disorders. *American Journal of Epidemiology*, **144**, 623–33.

World Health Organization 1996: Public health issues and clinical and neurological characteristics of the new variant of Creutzfeldt–Jakob disease and other human and animal transmissible spongiform encephalopathies: memorandum from two WHO meetings. *Bulletin of the World Health Organization*, **74**, 453–63.

21

Regulatory testing for neurotoxicology

SANDRA L ALLEN

INTRODUCTION

During the development of any new chemical or agent (whether drug, industrial chemical, pesticide or other) to which people may be deliberately or accidentally exposed a wide range of *in vivo* and *in vitro* studies are performed in order to show both efficacy of the chemical in its intended use and to establish margins of safety for both occupational and environmental exposures. A great majority of these studies are performed in laboratory animals and many will comply with international regulatory guidelines. Regulatory studies are designed to allow as complete an evaluation as possible of any pharmacological or toxicological effects which may impact on human health. The ultimate objective of animal toxicity studies is to provide information that will enable the safe use of chemicals through hazard identification, hazard assessment, and risk assessment.

Until very recently few countries or organizations had developed regulatory requirements for specialized neurotoxicity tests of new or existing chemicals, with the exception of the specific tests for organophosphate chemicals. Many are now developing such regulations (for example US Environmental Protection Agency, Organization for Economic Cooperation and Development (OECD)) but most regulatory authorities rely upon an extensive range of 'standard' toxicity studies in animals to indicate those chemicals which are of concern because of potential neurotoxic activity. Standard toxicity studies with rats, mice, rabbits, dogs, and possibly primates identify target organs and treatment-related effects in all organ systems including the nervous system (Steinberg, 1987; Mattsson *et al.*, 1989). Thus, a significant amount of neurotoxicity data can be obtained from standard toxicity studies.

METHODS FOR THE EVALUATION OF POTENTIAL NEUROTOXICITY

Studies designed to detect potential neurotoxicity must be able to discover a plethora of possible changes in the nervous system. Test species, age, time course, and exposure pattern are important considerations for the detection of neurotoxicity.

Although many neurotoxicological entities in humans can be readily reproduced in laboratory animals, this is not always the case. For example, the pathological manifestations associated with tri-*o*-cresyl phosphate intoxication or high doses of lovastatin in humans are not always seen in the rat (Berry *et al.*, 1988; Somkuti *et al.*, 1988). Thus, the potential neurotoxicity of a compound should be evaluated in a variety of species.

Age of the test animal also may affect detection of a neurotoxic change. For example, haemorrhagic encephalopathy is associated with administration of tunicamycins or corynetoxins in the immature rat (Berry and Vogel, 1982; Finnie and O'Shea, 1988) while organophosphorous compounds preferentially affect older rather than younger hens (Katoh *et al.*, 1990). Some neurotoxicological effects, such as those reported with amoscanate, trimethyltin, pyridoxine or tunicamycin, characteristically occur within a few days of exposure (Krinke *et al.*, 1985; Finnie and O'Shea, 1988;

Hagan *et al.*, 1988). In contrast, compounds such as acrylamide in rats (Bogo *et al.*, 1981) or high-dose lovastatin in dogs typically do not produce clinical evidence of neurotoxicity for several weeks (Berry *et al.*, 1988).

The exposure pattern for some chemicals also may be an important consideration. For example, exposure to hexane at 1000 ppm 24 h/day, five days/week for 11 weeks produced clear and long lasting neurotoxicity; however, exposure at 24 000 or 48 000 ppm for brief periods (10 min) six or 12 times per day (i.e. an equivalent or higher total exposure) produced only slight effects (Pryor *et al.*, 1982).

The design of any study should incorporate clear objectives and produce interpretable data. The World Health Organization (World Health Organization, 1986) defined the following objectives for neurotoxicity tests:

- identify whether the nervous system is altered by the toxicant (detection);
- characterize nervous system alterations associated with exposure;
- ascertain whether the nervous system is the primary target for the chemical;
- determine dose– and time–effect relationships in order to establish a no observed adverse effect level.

These objectives translate into a series of questions about the toxicity of a chemical that may be answered with standard toxicity tests and/or more specialized neurotoxicity studies.

STANDARD TOXICITY STUDIES

New and existing chemicals are evaluated routinely with standard toxicity studies that are conducted according to published guidelines (for example Organization for Economic Cooperation and Develpment, 1981; Food and Drug Administration, 1982; Environmental Protection Agency, 1983, 1984; Ministry of Agriculture, Forestry and Fisheries, 1985; European Community, 1988, 1989; Ministry of Health and Welfare, 1990; Environmental Protection Agency, 1991, 1998). The guidelines concerning toxicity/safety studies for some types of substances (for example drugs and food contact materials) contain little information on the design of studies. Rather they give guidance on the end points which must be evaluated. It is the responsibility of the manufacturer/registrant of the test substance to provide the regulatory agency with sufficient data to enable them to assess the risks of the proposed use of the substance. For other types of chemical, particularly pesticides and industrial chemicals, the regulatory guidelines are much more detailed both in terms of the type of study required (see Table

Table 21.1 *List of typical animal regulatory toxicity studies required for world-wide registration of a pesticide*

Acute oral toxicity (rat and mouse)	Subchronic (90 day) dermal toxicity
Acute dermal toxicity	Subchronic (90 day) inhalation toxicity
Acute inhalation toxicity	Chronic toxicity study (rat and dog)
Primary eye irritation	Carcinogenicity study (rat and mouse)
Primary dermal irritation	Teratogenicity/ developmental toxicity
Skin sensitization	Reproduction toxicity (one to two generations)
Subchronic (90 day) oral toxicity (rat and dog)	*In vivo* mammalian cytogenetics
Repeated dose dermal toxicity (21/28 days)	Rodent dominant lethal assay

21.1) and the detailed design of the studies. Nevertheless, information concerning potential target organs including the nervous system can be obtained from standard toxicity studies such as acute, subacute, subchronic, and chronic studies as well as reproduction studies.

Information on potential neurotoxicity from standard toxicity studies

Standard toxicity studies evaluate functional, behavioral, and morphological end points for the nervous system which may give preliminary or definite indications of the neurotoxicity of xenobiotics (Steinberg, 1987). Standard studies are important in the assessment of potential neurotoxicity of a compound because these studies are conducted at relatively high doses, with differing durations and routes of administration as well as with several species of animal (Mattsson *et al.*, 1989).

Contribution from clinical observations

Clinical observations included in standard toxicity study protocols are usually obtained by cage-side monitoring of animals as well as during handling at the time of dosing or the determination of body weight. Clinical observations may indicate changes in motor function (for example disturbances of gait, abnormal posture or muscle tone), level of arousal (for example hyperactivity, lethargy), autonomic functions (salivation, lachrymation, urination, defecation), changes in psychological status (indicated by stereotyped behavior, aggression, biting, licking, self mutilation) or may indicate pharmacological effects (sedation, anesthesia).

Clinical observation of adults or pups in standard reproduction studies may also give an indication of altered neuromotor functions. Successful mating, delivery, and rearing of pups depend on normal behavior and appropriate function of multiple organ systems including the nervous system. Also, the physical and functional landmarks of pups are sensitive parameters of development.

Contribution from morphological examinations

Standard toxicity studies generally include gross examination of most organs and tissues, measurement of the weight of organs including the brain, and histopathological evaluation of brain, spinal cord, peripheral nerve, muscle, eyes as well as many other tissues. Thus, a broad range of nervous tissues is evaluated routinely by standard toxicity studies.

Histopathology in standard toxicity studies often includes examinations of brain structures that are related to specific types of behavior. Examples include:

- the hippocampus, which is important for memory;
- components of the limbic system, which are responsible for emotion;
- the hypothalamus, which is associated with autonomic integration and control of the endocrine system.

Histopathological examination of all nervous tissue is impracticable, but representative samples of nervous tissues are considered adequate (Hirano and Llena, 1980; Thomas, 1980). Furthermore, since practically all tissues include some nervous tissue, routine microscopic sections in standard toxicity studies (for example skin, intestine, and muscle) can also contribute to the comprehensive examination of the nervous system. In addition, since the functional and structural integrity of effector organs may be altered by changes in normal control by the nervous system, histopathological examination of tissues such as muscle, exocrine glands, viscera, reproductive organs, and, in particular, sensory organs and endocrine glands may give indirect indications of neurotoxic effects.

Examples of neurotoxicity detected with standard toxicity studies

There are numerous examples of the effectiveness of standard toxicity studies in the detection of nervous system effects (see reviews by European Centre for Ecotoxicology and Toxicology of Chemicals, 1992; Eisenbrandt et al., 1994). Nevertheless there has been concern that some standard studies do not adequately assess neurotoxic potential. Therefore, many agencies,

during the periodic revision process for regulatory testing guidelines, are incorporating additional end points to enhance the ability to detect neurotoxicity. For example, the OECD guidelines for 28- and 90-day repeat dose toxicity studies (Guideline reference number 407 and 408) were revised in 1995 and 1998 to enhance the ability to detect neurotoxic substances. The guidelines now include detailed descriptions of the clinical evaluations to be performed, require functional assessments (of sensorimotor function, grip strength and locomotor activity) to be included and detail the nervous system tissues to be weighed and examined histopathologically. In 1998 most repeat dose toxicity study guidelines for the United States Environmental Protection Agency were similarly updated. It is likely that OECD will incorporate additional endpoints for neurotoxicity in most toxicity studies (e.g. 1 year studies) during its periodic review process.

REGULATORY NEUROTOXICITY STUDIES

Regulatory studies specifically designed to investigate potential neurotoxicity have been issued only for industrial chemicals and pesticides (Table 21.2). Guidelines were first introduced for organophosphorus chemicals in the early 1980s with other study types being introduced in the mid-1980s. The individual study designs are detailed below.

Delayed neurotoxicity of organophosphorus compounds

Organophosphorus compounds (OPs) have diverse effects on the peripheral and central nervous systems due to their ability to inhibit acetylcholinesterase and/

Table 21.2 Neurotoxicity testing guidelines

US EPA neurotoxicity testing guidelines
  Delayed neurotoxicity of organophosphorus substances
  following acute and 28-day exposure
  Neurotoxicity screening battery
  Developmental neurotoxicity study
  Schedule controlled operant behavior
  Peripheral nerve function
  Neurophysiology: sensory evoked potentials
OECD neurotoxicity guidelines
  418: Delayed neurotoxicity of organophosphorus
  substances following acute exposure
  419: Delayed neurotoxicity of organophosphorus
  substances: 28-day repeated dose study
  424: Neurotoxicity study in rodents
Japan MHW neurotoxicity guidelines
  Acute delayed neurotoxicity study
  Subchronic delayed neurotoxicity study

or neuropathy target esterase. Inhibition of acetylcholinesterase produces the signs seen in mammals following acute poisoning. These include excessive urination, lachrymation, diarrhea, muscular twitching, weakness, and convulsions, with death usually caused by respiratory paralysis (O'Brien, 1960, 1967). Inhibition of the membrane-bound protein neuropathy target esterase (NTE) can result, after a single dose, in a delayed polyneuropathy, and it is this effect that studies are designed to detect.

Although OP neuropathy has been demonstrated in a number of species there is considerable variation in susceptibility (Johnson, 1975). The female domestic hen (*Gallus gallus domesticus*) is classically the species of choice as the response is consistent and reproducible (Cavanagh, 1964a). Following a single dose of a neurotoxic OP there is rapid inhibition of NTE which can be detected one to two days later in the *in vitro* assay of nervous tissue from dosed hens. The percentage inhibition and, thereby the degree of phosphorylation of NTE, is highly correlated with the initiation of OP delayed neuropathy (not all OPs that inhibit NTE cause neuropathy but all those that cause neuropathy inhibit NTE). Approximately one week following a single dose, clinical signs of neuropathy first become apparent – the bird walks with an unsteady flat-footed gait. Depending on the dose the signs become more severe until the bird is unable to stand and the weakness affects the wings which may droop. The morphological pattern of OP distal axonopathy consists of symmetrical, distal axonal degeneration of ascending and descending nerve fiber tracts located in the central and peripheral nervous systems. Primarily, long, large-diameter fibers are affected (Cavanagh, 1964b; Bischoff, 1967, 1970; Prineas, 1969; Spencer and Schaumburg, 1976, 1978). In the peripheral nervous system, the longer nerve fibers to the hind limbs are affected before the shorter fibers to the forelimbs. Concurrently, the long spinal cord tracts, such as the dorsal columns (corticospinal and spinocerebellar tracts), show distal axonal degeneration. The degenerative change appears to move in a retrograde manner along the affected pathway, with neuronal damage increasing in severity from proximal to distal regions.

The regulatory studies (Table 21.3) are designed to detect the functional, biochemical, and pathological deficits of OP-induced polyneuropathy. Thus, in the acute study, hens receive a single oral dose (equivalent to the median lethal dose or an approximate lethal dose) of the test substance. Prophylaxis using atropine may be appropriate in order to prevent acute cholinergic deaths. Hens are monitored daily for a period of at least 21 days for the onset, severity, and duration of clinical signs of toxicity. Specific attention is paid to signs of gait abnormality and/or paralysis. At least twice per week animals are subjected to a period of forced locomotor activity during which a semi-quantitative assessment of locomotor deficit, for example use of rating scale of at least four points (Roberts *et al.*, 1983), should be used to grade ataxia. At predetermined time points (usually 24 and 48 h following dosing) subsets of hens are killed for the *in vitro* determination of NTE and, possibly, acetylcholinesterase. At the end of the study all survivors are given a macroscopic examination and samples of the nervous system are prepared for microscopic examination.

Table 21.3 *Generic study design for delayed neurotoxicity of organophosphorus substances*

Species, age, and sex	Hens, 8–12 (14)[a] months
Group size	≥ Six for biochemistry, ≥ six for pathology
Control groups	Vehicle control (≥ six for biochemistry, ≥ six for pathology)
Positive control	≥ Three for biochemistry, ≥ three for pathology; recent historical data acceptable
Dose levels	Acute study: one dose, single exposure
	Repeat dose study: three dose levels plus control; administered daily for 28 days
Route	Normally oral (by gavage); dermal acceptable if appropriate
Observation period	Acute: 21 days after dosing
	Repeat dose: duration of dosing plus 14/21-day posttreatment observation period
Observations and frequency	(1) signs of toxicity – daily
	(2) ataxia, paralysis on a four-point scale – daily
	(3) forced activity (e.g. ladder climbing) – twice weekly
	(4) bodyweight – weekly
NTE, AChE	Control and treated groups: three hens at 24 h, three hens at 48 h (unless otherwise indicated) for NTE (brain and spinal cord)
	Positive control: three hens at 24 h
	AChE optional for OECD
Neuropathology	Gross necropsy, *in situ* fixation, myelin and axon-specific stains
Tissues/sections	Cerebellum, medulla oblongata, spinal cord (three levels), peripheral nerves (distal region)

[a]Period of 8–12 months OECD; 8–14 months EPA and Japan.

Tissues are fixed by whole body perfusion and representative samples of both central and peripheral nervous system (see Table 21.3) prepared. Sections are stained with appropriate myelin and axon-specific stains and examined at the light microscope level.

Information on both vehicle control and positive control-treated animals is also required.

If the results of the acute study are equivocal then a repeat-dose 28-day study is required. This study is performed in essentially the same way except that repeated daily oral dosing, with at least three dose levels, is used in order to produce a dose–effect curve.

Neurotoxicity screening battery/ neurotoxicity study

A summary of the US Environmental Protection Agency guideline neurotoxicity screening battery and OECD 424 neurotoxicity study is given in Table 21.4. The design of the studies is essentially identical. The guidelines allow for single or repeat dose studies (up to two years in duration, although acute single-dose studies and 90-day repeat-dose studies are more usually performed). Studies are usually performed in the rat, although other species may be used if appropriate. The study incorporates an observation battery (functional observation battery (FOB)), assessment of locomotor activity, and detailed neuropathology. Observations are to be conducted blind, at specific times, and in a structured manner (i.e. observations in the home cage,

while the rat is moving in a standard open arena, and through manipulative tests). Specific measures to be included are:

- changes in skin, fur, eyes, mucous membranes;
- assessment of autonomic function;
- description, incidence and severity of any convulsions, tremors, or abnormal motor movements;
- reactivity to general stimuli (e.g. removal from the cage or handling);
- ranking of arousal level;
- description and incidence of any posture or gait abnormalities;
- fore limb and hind limb grip strength (quantitative assessment);
- measurement of landing foot splay;
- sensorimotor response.

Locomotor activity is assessed with an automatic device capable of detecting both increases and decreases in activity. At the end of the study a proportion of the animals are killed using *in situ* perfusion fixation and a comprehensive evaluation of the nervous system performed.

The major difference between the two guidelines is the way in which they are intended to be applied. When Environmental Protection Agency (EPA) published combined guidelines in 1991 for use under both FIFRA (Federal Insecticide, Fungicide and Rodenticides Act) and TOSCA (Toxic Substances Control Act) it was stated that they intended 'to propose requiring acute

Table 21.4 *EPA neurotoxicity screening battery/OECD neurotoxicity study in rodents*

Species and age	Young adult rat (at least 42 days old[a]/weaning to 9 weeks[b])
	Other species may be used if more appropriate
Group size	At least 10 males and 10 females per group
Control groups	Concurrent vehicle and/or untreated control required
Positive control	Historic control data acceptable. Data should demonstrate sensitivity of methods and ability of methods to detect neurotoxicity
Dose levels	At least three dose levels
Route of exposure	Most appropriate based on likely human exposure, bioavailability and practicality. Typically gavage for single dose and dietary for repeated exposures
Observations	Bodyweight
	Food consumption
	Ophthalmoscopy[b] (for studies of 90 day or longer)
	Functional observation battery (detailed clinical observations and quantitative measurement of grip strength and landing foot splay) performed blind
	Motor activity – with automated devices
Frequency of observations	Prior to exposure and:
	Acute: at estimated time of peak effect within 8 h of dosing, 7 and 14 days after dosing
	Subchronic: during 4th, 8th and 13th week
	Chronic: three monthly
Neuropathology	At least five males and five females per group. *In situ* perfusion fixation required. Special stains recommended. Representative samples of tissues to allow thorough examination of the nervous system

[a]EPA neurotoxicity screening battery; [b]OECD (424) neurotoxicity study.

and subchronic screening studies including the functional observation battery, motor activity and neuropathology for all [pesticide] active ingredients.' The OECD guideline, however, is intended for use as a 'second-tier' study to 'confirm or to further characterize the potential neurotoxicity' observed in standard studies or anticipated on the basis of structure-activity data. Additionally, the guideline has been designed so that it may be tailored to meet particular needs rather than be of a fixed design. Uniquely for OECD, the agency has an accompanying guidance document (OECD Guidance Document on Neurotoxicity Strategies and Methods, in press 1999) for use with guideline 424 giving advice on the design of the study and to facilitate the selection of additional or alternative in vivo or in vitro test methods, if appropriate. This approach will ensure that effort is applied to those test substances of concern for neurotoxicity and will avoid replicating data generated by standard procedures.

Developmental neurotoxicity study

The purpose of this study is to evaluate functional and morphological development in the offspring of females exposed during pregnancy and lactation.

This study is not required for all pesticides but is requested on a case-by-case basis. Triggers for the conduct of the study have been reported to be: agents that cause central nervous system (CNS) malfunctions; psychoactive drugs and chemicals; adult neurotoxicants; hormonally active agents; peptides and amino acids; and structurally related agents (i.e. structurally related to known developmental neurotoxicants) (Levine and Butcher, 1990). In addition, an 'exposure-based' trigger was developed in the implementation of TOSCA, under which testing may be required if the test substance is, or will be, produced in substantial quantities.

A summary of the US EPA guideline is given in Table 21.5. The study is conducted in the rat (preferably not the Fischer 344 strain as developmental timings are different to more common rat strains, for example Wistar, Sprague-Dawley) although other species may be used with adequate justification. Groups of at least 20 young adult, nulliparous, pregnant females are used. The females are dosed orally from gestation day 6 (where day of confirmed pregnancy is designated day 0) to lactation day 10 (when day of parturition is designated day 0 of lactation). The females are observed daily for changes in clinical condition. As in the adult neurotoxicity study, specific observations are detailed and it is recommended that the observations are conducted blind to minimize observer bias. Pups remain with the parent female until weaning.

On postnatal day 4 the size of each litter is adjusted, by culling extra pups, to achieve litters of four males and four females. Partial adjustment (for example three males and five females) is allowed but litters with less than seven pups cannot be used. At this point animals must be individually identified and assigned to behavioral tests, brain weight evaluation or neuropathology. One male and one female from each litter

Table 21.5 *EPA developmental neurotoxicity study*

Species and age	Young adult, pregnant female rat (not Fischer 344)
Group size	At least 20 litters ($\geq$ seven pups/litter with $\geq$ three pups/sex)
Control groups	Concurrent vehicle and/or untreated control group
Positive control	To demonstrate sensitivity of procedures
Dose levels	At least three dose levels
Route of and duration of exposure	Orally; gestation day 6 to postnatal day 10 inclusive
Observations and frequency	**Dams:** Daily clinical observations Bodyweight weekly **Pups:** Gross observations (mortality) daily Clinical observations – days 4, 11, 13, 17, 21, 22, and fortnightly until termination Developmental landmarks (vaginal opening/preputial separation) Motor activity – days 13, 17, 21, and 60 Auditory startle test – days 22 and 60 Learning and memory – days 21–24 and 60.
Neuropathology	**Postnatal day 11** One/litter for brain weights Six/sex/group for neuropathology including morphometric analysis **At termination (>day 60)** One/litter for brain weights Six/sex/group for neuropathology (*in situ* perfusion fixation) including morphometric analysis

are assigned to one of the behavioral tests (motor activity, auditory startle test, and learning and memory) and the remaining one male and one female are assigned for brain weight measurements on day 11 or at termination. In addition, six animals per sex per group (one male or one female per litter) are required for neuropathology evaluation at termination.

Detailed clinical observations and behavioral assessments of pups are performed at the time points specified in Table 21.5. Some flexibility is given in the choice of test methods and devices for behavioral assessment provided they fulfil certain criteria.

Locomotor activity must be assessed in automated activity recording devices which must be capable of recording both increases and decreases in activity. Animals should be tested individually, and activity should be collected in equal time periods of no greater than 10 minutes' duration.

Sensory function is assessed by measuring the auditory startle response which has been shown to be affected by a number of neurotoxic chemicals (Ison, 1984; Crofton, 1992). The auditory startle test requires than the mean response amplitude of the whole body startle resulting from an auditory stimulus is measured (5×10 trials per session on each day of testing). The use of prepulse inhibition is recommended, but not required.

A test of associative learning and memory should be conducted around the time of weaning and again in adulthood. The same or separate tests may be used at the two stages of development but must fulfil two criteria. First, learning must be assessed either as a change across several learning trials or sessions, or, in tests involving a single trial, with reference to a condition that controls for non-associative effects of the training experience. Second, the tests should include some measure of memory (short-term or long-term) in addition to original learning (acquisition). A difficulty in selecting tests is that many methods designed to assess learning and memory require long training periods (see Cabe and Eckerman, 1982 and Saghal, 1993 for details of methods) and, consequently, are not suitable for use in weanling animals. Similarly some methods developed to examine learning and memory in infant and weanling rats are less applicable to adults (Spear and Brake, 1983). Different tests may measure different types of learning and/or memory and may, therefore, complicate the interpretation of any treatment-related effects. As many tests of learning and memory are affected by changes in motor and sensory capacity as well as motivation and arousal, it is also important to be able to rule out such changes when interpreting the data. It is recommended, therefore, that if effects on learning and/or memory are seen then additional tests are conducted to exclude alternative interpretations.

The age of onset of sexual maturity is measured by recording the age of vaginal opening of females and cleavage of the balanopreputial gland of the males.

These two postweaning landmarks are associated with levels of sex hormones.

Neuropathology is assessed at two time points – the end of the dosing period and in adulthood. At 11 days the pups are killed by conventional means and the brain removed, weight recorded and fixed for histopathological evaluation. At the end of the study a proportion of the animals are killed using *in situ* perfusion fixation and a comprehensive evaluation of the nervous system performed. At both time points morphometric evaluation of the brain is required to allow an assessment of the rate of growth of particular brain regions as well as the evaluation of any developmental disruption.

Dose levels for the study are selected on the basis of known maternal or developmental toxicity such that the highest dose should not be expected to produce *in utero* or neonatal deaths or malformations, or a level of maternal toxicity (for example in excess of a 20% reduction in bodyweight gain) which might interfere with interpretation. Agents which produce effects in the pups at a dose that is not toxic to the maternal animal are of special concern (Environmental Protection Agency, 1995).

Interpretation of developmental neurotoxicity data may be limited but it is clear functional effects must be evaluated in the light of other toxicity data, including other forms of developmental toxicity (for example structural abnormalities, perinatal death, and growth retardation). For example, motor performance deficits may be due to a skeletal malformation rather than an effect on the nervous system.

Schedule controlled operant behavior

This guideline is designed to detect functional neurotoxic effects and is used on a case-by-case basis only for substances which have been shown to produce neurotoxic signs in other toxicity studies or are structurally related to neurotoxicants which affect performance, learning or memory.

The guideline does give information on dose levels (at least three, plus control), species (rat or mouse recommended), age (at least 14 weeks for rats, 6 weeks for mice), sex (equal numbers of males and females), and group size (6–12 per group). However, most other technical details are not constrained to allow a flexible approach. The study may be acute (single dose) or repeated dosing (subchronic or chronic, i.e. up to two years duration) and any appropriate route of exposure is acceptable. Although the guideline discusses fixed ratio and fixed interval responding as particular methods it also states that 'additional tests may be necessary to completely assess the effects of any substance on learning, memory or behavioral performance.' In reality, should this type of testing be required the regulatory agency and registrant will be involved in detailed discussions about why the study is necessary/appropriate, and also on the most appropriate study design to further investigate effects seen (see section on Specific neurotoxicity test methods). The guideline provides a forum for discussion and not a detailed protocol.

Peripheral nerve function

Nerve conduction studies can be useful in investigating possible peripheral neuropathy and is the most commonly used test of electrophysiological function in neurotoxicology (Johnson, 1980). This guideline is considered to be a 'second-tier' study for substances that have been shown to produce peripheral neuropathy (or other neuropathological change in peripheral nerves) in other neurotoxicity studies. The purpose of the study is to record amplitude and velocity of conduction in peripheral nerves *in vivo*. Protocol details are similar to those for the neurotoxicity screening battery (see Table 21.6) to allow a combination of the two components into a single study design. No specific detail is given on the timing of measurements but as surgical exposure of the nerves is allowed it is assumed that this is done at the end of the exposure and/or observation period.

Decreases in peripheral nerve conduction velocity are indicative of demyelination. For example, reduced motor nerve conduction velocity measurements in rats, guinea pigs, cats, and monkeys have been shown to be associated with segmental demyelination following acrylamide exposure (Fullerton and Barnes, 1966; Leswing and Ribelin, 1969). Decreases in response amplitude reflect a loss of nerve fibers and may occur prior to decreases in conduction velocity.

Neurophysiology: sensory evoked potentials

This guideline was published in 1998 and involves neurophysiological measurement *in vivo* in adult rats to assess sensory function. Such studies are unlikely to be required on a routine basis but may be used at any time to detect sensory dysfunction. Alternatively the study may be requested on a case-by-case basis to clarify effects seen in other studies. Similar to the guideline for peripheral nerve function, the design is such that it may be used in combination with other studies (for example neurotoxicity screening battery or standard toxicity study) and may be of any duration (acute to chronic). The guideline details a number of stimuli which may be used to assess sensory function (visual, auditory, somatosensory), and gives details of recording methods but the specific details of study design are flexible to ensure that the most appropriate test methods are used. Indeed, the guideline states that it is 'the responsibility of those submitting to justify the selection of a specific test from the categories of electrophysiological tests available.'

SPECIFIC NEUROTOXICITY TEST METHODS

Specific methods for neurotoxicological evaluation in animals are broadly similar to those applied to humans and include monitoring behavior, electrophysiology, neuropathology, neurochemistry as well as alternative *in vivo* and *in vitro* methods. Specific applications of these methods are available for developmental neurotoxicity tests. Individual test methods may be incorporated into standard toxicity studies to investigate effects seen in preliminary or previous studies. The advantage of such an approach is that it allows the evaluation of potential neurotoxicity in relation to any other toxic effects and minimizes the use of additional animals. This also helps to establish whether the neurotoxic effect is direct or secondary to toxic effects in other organs. However, the interpretation of some tests can be confounded by non-associative effects and general toxicity, and so care must be taken in the selection of tests. Certain types of test, for example complex methods for the assessment of cognitive

Table 21.6 *EPA peripheral nerve function*

Species and age	Young adult rat (at least 60 days old)
	Other species may be used if more appropriate
Group size	Twenty animals of either (or both) sex per group (e.g. 10 males and 10 females per group)
Control groups	Concurrent vehicle and/or untreated control required
Positive control	Historic control data acceptable. Data should demonstrate sensitivity of methods and ability of methods to detect neurotoxicity
Dose levels	At least three dose levels
Route of exposure	Most appropriate based on likely human exposure, bioavailability and practicality. Typically gavage for single dose and dietary for repeated exposures
Observations	Motor and sensory nerve conduction velocity and amplitude of peripheral nerve (e.g. tibial or caudal) *in vivo*. Core and nerve temperature
Frequency of observations	Not specified

function, are best conducted as stand-alone studies and, ideally, at dose levels which do not induce overt toxicity. Usually this type of study will be performed to investigate effects seen in preliminary or standard studies (or a known effect with the particular class of chemical) and can be carefully designed to avoid confounders.

Brief descriptions of approaches in broad terms (i.e. behavior, electrophysiology, neurochemistry, pathology) and their advantages and disadvantages in their incorporation into animal toxicity studies is given below. Detail of specific methodology is given in Mitchell (1982), European Centre for Ecotoxicology and Toxicology of Chemicals (1992) and World Health Organization (1986).

Behavioral tests

Behavioral changes following exposure to a neurotoxic chemical can be sensitive indicators of disturbed function of the nervous system since they may be observed earlier and/or at doses lower than demonstrable clinical symptoms or structural lesions (Alder and Zbinden, 1977, 1983; Walsh and Chrobak, 1987; Broxup et al., 1989; Schulze and Boysen, 1991). However, due to the functional reserve capacity of the nervous system there is the possibility that some structural loss may occur in the nervous system while the animal remains functionally normal (Mitchell and Tilson, 1982).

More importantly, a significant limitation of many behavioral tests is that they lack specificity. Not all behavioral changes necessarily represent the specific action of a chemical on the nervous system. Many behavioral tests are affected by changes in non-neural organs (Gerber and O'Shaughnessy, 1986; Rice, 1990) as well as by dietary restriction (Albee et al., 1987), hormonal state (Robbins, 1977), fatigue (Bogo et al., 1981), motivation (Cooper, 1981), age (Soffie and Bronchart, 1988) or housing conditions (Bouldin et al., 1981; Dyer and Howell, 1982).

The choice of behavioral test depends upon the purpose of the study; some tests may be simple to perform, but lack sensitivity, whereas others are much more sensitive, but are complex and time consuming. However, a complex test is not necessarily a sensitive one. For example, a comparison of the relative sensitivity of a functional observational battery (FOB), motor activity (MA) and schedule-controlled operant behavior (SCOB) indicated that the FOB was as sensitive or more sensitive than MA or SCOB in detecting treatment-related effects (Moser and MacPhail, 1990).

Simple observation of behavior is routinely included in all standard toxicity studies. More structured observations such as a FOB are also relatively easily included (Pryor and Rebert, 1983; Walsh and Tilson, 1984; Moser and MacPhail, 1990; Schulze and Boysen, 1991) although there are several problems related to analysis and interpretation of neurobehavioral screening data (Tilson and Moser, 1992). Most screening batteries consist of several tests that yield different types of data which are each analyzed by different statistical methods. Each measure in the battery can be viewed as a unique end point and, since there are multiple tests in the battery, some statistically significant changes might occur just by chance (Type I error). This situation is compounded by the very large amounts of data in most screening experiments.

Rodents (rat or mouse) are normally the species of choice for screening procedures. Birds and cats, however, may be a better choice for determining toxicity of the visual system (Evans, 1982; Rice, 1990). More complex and sophisticated procedures such as tests of fine motor control or some kinds of cognitive testing are usually best done in the primate (Rice, 1990).

Electrophysiological techniques

Neurophysiological techniques measure the electrical potentials of impulse transmission in the nervous system and thus reflect the function of neurons. Electrical potentials can be recorded in specific areas of the central or peripheral nervous system in vivo or from in vitro preparations. Advantages of electrophysiological methods to the neurotoxicologist include the relative ease with which the data can be quantified, analyzed, and standardized as well as the large amount of electrophysiological data that can be collected quickly. In addition, some techniques are non-invasive and allow monitoring of progression and/or recovery of functional disturbance.

Electrophysiological techniques are used extensively in human clinical neurology and are readily applied with minimal modification across species (Seppalainen, 1975; Rebert, 1983; Arezzo et al., 1985; Dyer, 1985; Mattsson et al., 1989). Most animal electrophysiology data are extrapolated easily to humans since these data are familiar to the medical community (Mattsson and Albee, 1988). In fact, the degree of comparability to humans typically is higher for electrophysiology tests than for most behavioral measures (Winneke, 1992).

The electrophysiological method for a particular experiment must be appropriate to the question being asked. If one is interested in overt changes, then macroelectrode procedures, such as electroencephalogram (EEG), may be adequate (Office of Technology Assessment,1990). More specific questions, such as whether the chemical acts on presynaptic receptors, specific ion channels, or sensory rather than motor nerves, demand more sophisticated experimental procedures (see reviews by Kerkut and Heal, 1981; Atchison, 1988). The latter techniques, perhaps in *in vitro* preparations (see Rowan, 1985), may provide specific information on the mechanism of neurotoxicity of a particular chemical. Nevertheless, a multidisciplinary approach (for example functional tests and neuropathology) will facilitate a better understanding of the effects of chemicals on the nervous system (World Health Organization, 1986; Office of Technology Assessment, 1990).

Neurochemical tests

Neurochemical methods can assess mechanisms and effects of psychopharmacological agents and are used increasingly to investigate mechanisms of neurotoxicity (Damstra and Bondy, 1980). Neurochemistry can be conducted on parts of peripheral nerves, the entire brain of animals, distinct brain structures obtained by dissecting whole brains, slices of whole brain or particular brain structures, as well as neurons or glial cells cultured *in vitro*. To increase the sensitivity of neurochemical methods, cells can be fractionated and particular cell organelles separated.

Since neuronal lesions generally are limited to specific areas of the brain and often to specific types of neurons, the sensitivity of neurochemical measurements decreases with increasing volume of nerve tissue in a single assay. In contrast, the chance of missing an effect increases with decreasing total volume of tissue.

The relationship between nervous system function and observations made in neural tissue extract in a test tube is somewhat tenuous because the concentration of many endogenous substances or the activity of enzymes may change rapidly after death. Further problems arise due to the tendency of the nervous system to compensate for neuronal loss, for example, by increasing turnover rate of transmitters or by up or down regulation of receptors (Cooper *et al.*, 1991).

Based on the above considerations, neurochemical methods are unsuitable as routine screens for neurotoxic effects (i.e. where nothing is known about the mechanism of action of the chemical). Too many different parameters need to be measured to assess comprehensively the neurotoxic potential of a given compound. In cases where the neurotoxic mechanism of a compound is known, a few critical parameters related to the neurotoxic effect can be measured in order to screen rapidly structural analogues for that specific neurotoxic mechanism.

An interesting approach which overcomes some of the problems related to neurochemical assays is the combination of neurochemical determinations and histopathology (histochemical staining techniques). Such techniques are specific, sensitive, and have the advantage of showing the topographic distribution of findings (Krinke and Hess, 1981). Immunohistochemistry and tissue radioimmunoassay also have been used to detect pathological effects in the developing and mature central nervous system (Brock and O'Callaghan, 1987; O'Callaghan, 1988; O'Callaghan and Miller, 1988). These techniques have proved valuable research tools and show potential for use in neurotoxicity screening.

Neuropathological methods

The morphological complexity of the nervous system must be taken into account in the application of pathological techniques for the assessment of the neurotoxic potential of chemicals in animals. The methods and factors that affect the ability to detect neuropathology have been reviewed (Spencer *et al.*, 1980; World Health Organization, 1986; Krinke, 1989; Mattsson *et al.*, 1989, 1990; Broxup, 1991).

Effective use of animals and resources when chemicals are tested initially for toxicity requires techniques that allow thorough examination of the nervous system, but does not disrupt pathological examination of other organs. Thus, standard pathological methods are generally incorporated when there has been no prior indication of any neurotoxic effect. Immersion fixation of nervous tissue in formalin with subsequent paraffin embedding and routine staining allows examination of large sections of nervous system. Resolution of cell detail in immersion-fixed paraffin sections is somewhat less than in plastic-embedded material, and artefactual changes may occur in these preparations (Garman, 1990); however, immersion-fixed paraffin sections are a valuable aid for the detection of neuromorphological changes.

More detailed examination of the nervous system usually requires perfusion fixation and special stains, along with other specialized procedures, to define particular effects and avoid misinterpretation of artifacts (O'Donoghue, 1989; Mattsson *et al.*, 1990). Perfusion fixation with formalin, paraformaldehyde, and/or glutaraldehyde often is used for specific investigations of neuropathological changes in the central or peripheral nervous system (Krinke, 1989; O'Donoghue, 1989; Mattsson *et al.*, 1990). Perfused tissue may be embedded in paraffin for routine light microscopy or postfixed in osmium tetroxide and processed for plastic-embedded semi-thin $(1-2\,\mu m)$ sections and stained with toluidine blue. Nervous tissue fixed by perfusion is devoid of most artefacts associated with immersion fixation (Garman, 1990). However, perfusion may be associated with other artifacts, for example those caused by inadequate control of pressure, pH or osmolarity of the fixative (Schultz and Karlsson, 1965).

Ultra-thin sections of small blocks of perfused, plastic-embedded nervous tissue can be examined with a transmission electron microscope. Although electron microscopy is a powerful tool in mechanistic studies of neurotoxicology, its application is laborious (World Health Organization, 1986). Therefore, ultrastructural studies are generally confined to those protocols where there is a specific need to characterize neuropathological changes and answer mechanistic questions.

Adequate definition of certain neuropathological changes, particularly those associated with neurodevelopmental toxicants or chemicals causing low grade peripheral neuropathy, may require quantitative morphometric methods (Rodier, 1979, 1990; Haug, 1986; Broxup et al., 1990). Other special techniques may be necessary to demonstrate subtle changes such as those found in neurites of rats exposed prenatally to lead or ethanol (Averill and Needleman, 1980; West and Hodges-Savola, 1983). Nerve fiber teasing (separation of perfusion-fixed peripheral nerve fibers embedded in epoxy resin) may provide a valuable means to characterize peripheral neuropathy (Spencer and Thomas, 1970).

Interpretation of pathological changes may be confounded by spontaneous background lesions in neurotoxicity studies (Eisenbrandt et al., 1990). For example, spinal radiculoneuropathy in the rat increases in incidence and severity with age (Burek et al., 1976; Krinke, 1983); these spontaneous lesions may complicate the interpretation of neurotoxic peripheral neuropathy in this species.

Neuropathology should be integrated with functional studies (Tilson et al., 1979; World Health Organization, 1986; O'Donoghue, 1989; Mattsson et al., 1989, 1990). While neuropathology provides clearly interpretable data and high resolution (including single neurons and axons), the methods are limited to static evaluation of discrete sections. On the other hand, functional tests evaluate dynamic system functions and populations of cells; nevertheless, functional tests are somewhat limited in resolution and interpretability and are subject to masking or compensation. Adequate definition of an encephalopathy or neuropathy may be enhanced by an understanding of the clinical or functional disturbance and the morphological effect (Spencer and Schaumburg, 1980; Dyck et al., 1986; Krinke 1989, Mattsson et al., 1989, 1990).

Developmental neurotoxicity

Examination of potential effects on the nervous system is an important aspect of the assessment of developmental toxicity (Rodier, 1990). Methods for the detection of developmental neurotoxicity have been described by Altman and Sudarshan (1975), Adams (1986), and World Health Organization (1986).

The stage of development of the nervous system at birth varies with different species. For example, the neonatal rat is at a stage of development most similar to that of humans at the beginning of the third trimester of pregnancy (Nishimura and Shiota, 1977). In addition, exposure of developing animals to a chemical may result in quantitatively and qualitatively different effects than exposure of adult animals. Examples include the developmental effects of ethanol (Meyer et al., 1990; Rees et al., 1990) and the relative resistance of the weanling rat to hexane neuropathy (Howd et al., 1983).

A number of developmental landmarks have been defined which reflect normal development (Alder and Zbinden, 1977). Some of these physical landmarks are closely connected to the development of the nervous system and their evaluation may give a first indication for an impaired nervous system development.

Parallel to physical development, evaluation of functional development of animals also may detect an impairment of neural function. Some of the functional landmarks for rats are: surface righting, negative geotaxis, disappearance of pivoting, olfactory orientation, hind limb support, auditory startle, and mid-air righting. These functional tests are easy to conduct and can be included in routine reproductive toxicity studies.

More specific measurements of behavior, sensory and cognitive functions such as odor or taste aversion, active and passive avoidance or motor activity can be conducted to characterize particular effects.

Large test batteries have been developed for comprehensive examination of developing animals. Four major test batteries have been described (Adams, 1986):

- the collaborative behavioral teratology study battery;
- the Cincinnati psychoteratogenicity screening test battery;
- the Barlow Sullivan screening battery;
- the Japanese battery for behavioral teratology screening.

Common to these test batteries is the preferential assessment of physical and functional landmarks. These landmarks seem to be more sensitive indicators than the more specific measures of behavior, sensory, and cognitive functions (Elsner et al., 1988; Elsner, 1991) and thus are valuable tools for the detection of potential developmental neurotoxicity.

Both maternal toxicity and systemic toxicity in the offspring should be taken into account in the assessment of specific effects on the developing nervous system. Test substances which induce severe maternal toxicity might generate false positive results in the pups. Developmental effects, especially altered behavior, may occur as a consequence of maternal toxicity during gestation and/or lactation rather than being a direct effect of the test substance on the offspring (Francis, 1992).

Alternative (non-mammalian) *in vivo* and *in vitro* methods

A wide range of alternative (non-mammalian) and *in vitro* methods are available and include membrane models, primary neuronal cultures, glial cell cultures, cell lines, and organotypic explants. Interest in the use of such alternatives in neurotoxicology is increasing partly because the use of such techniques in other branches of toxicology as well as their use as mechanistic tools and inexpensive prescreens. In addition cell cultures have played an extremely important role in research areas such as stroke and neuroprotection, neurodegeneration and neurotrophic factors, and developmental neurobiology. No alternative *in vivo* or *in vitro* test is widely accepted as a routine screening test for neurotoxicity. Nevertheless, various groups have put forward models and systems for prevalidation and validation, and many are being investigated (Atterwill *et al.*, 1994). A tiered testing strategy has recently been developed using *in vitro* methodology which takes into account the specific needs of screening as opposed to mechanistic studies (Atterwill, 1989) and in 1992 the US National Research Council put forward a protocol for an *in vitro* neurotoxicity screening system.

Any alternative test methods will have advantages and limitations. Some methods are more appropriate for mechanistic study, whereas others are better suited for screening. The principal advantage of *in vitro* methods is the possibility of more rigorous control of experimental conditions. Most of the variables that are relevant to the biology of the test system can be controlled in ways which are not possible in animal experiments. Other advantages include the ability to include cellular and subcellular end points (for example, cytotoxicological, morphological, biochemical, and electrophysiological). It may also be possible to include human-derived cells and tissues thereby enabling interspecies comparisons to be made. This has the potential to enhance the risk assessment process. Investigation of specific mechanisms of neurotoxicity can be very simple and, lastly, *in vitro* methods may be very cost-effective in terms of both time and amount of chemical required.

Several limitations characteristic of all alternative methods give problems in the extrapolation of *in vitro* effects to the *in vivo* situation:

1 Unless metabolic activators are incorporated in a test system neurotoxic metabolites of compounds will not be identified and metabolism of chemicals *in vitro* may be completely different from the *in vivo* situation.

2 Absence of the blood–brain barrier, although enabling direct access to the central nervous system, may impair a realistic interpretation of the results.

3 The physicochemical properties of a compound such as solubility in the test medium, changes in osmolarity, may confound interpretation of results.

4 It is necessary to discriminate between general cytotoxicity and neurotoxicity e.g. by control studies with tissues or cells of other organs.

5 The reduced complexity of most alternative test systems may be a disadvantage if the nature of the neurotoxic effect requires a complex integrative system (such as a complex behavioral response) or a long-term exposure of the whole animal to become evident.

Although regulatory authorities are aware of the large body of *in vitro* neurotoxicology work there have not as yet been any recommendations for incorporating alternative models into regulatory neurotoxicity testing. It is likely that alternative methods for neurotoxicity screening will be appropriate only in cases such as for compounds structurally related to known neurotoxicants. However, *in vitro* methods can provide important additional information on the mode of action of a neurotoxicant and should be considered complementary to whole animal tests (see Environmental Protection Agency, 1995).

LABELING FOR NEUROTOXICITY

The purpose of animal toxicology studies is to enable the safe use of chemicals and includes providing information which can be used for classification and labeling purposes. Labeling requirements are a common regulatory tool for dealing with toxic but useful substances. Pesticides, prescription and over-the-counter drugs, household products, and all commercial poisons are subject to labeling provisions incorporated in many statutes.

Labels are intended to reduce the risks of exposure to, or harm from toxic substances by alerting consumers to the dangers of a substance and providing instructions for its safe and proper use. Effective labeling relies on three tacit assumptions:

1 that consumers will read the label;
2 that they will understand and believe it;
3 that they will obey its instructions.

It has been reported (see Office of Technology Assessment, 1990) that few people read an entire label and that many people do not even read the parts of the label which relate specifically to their intended use of the chemical. Some labels may be too technical, the information difficult to read and, in some, information is vague or contradictory.

Appropriate labeling is important if adequate safety measures or precautions are to be taken by consumers.

For example, in Iraq in 1971 an epidemic of methyl mercury poisoning resulted from improper labeling. Farmers and their families ate bread made from seed treated with mercury. The bags in which the grain was imported were clearly labeled in English and Spanish (neither of which is a native language of Iraq). More than 400 people died from mercury poisoning and at least 6500 were hospitalized (Bakir *et al.*, 1973).

In order to make labels more understandable and readable to the general public there is a move to greater use of hazard symbols and standard phrases, although there are no international standards for labeling. Within the European Community (EC), labeling takes the form of symbols for the most severe hazard (for example 'skull and cross bones' symbol if classed as 'toxic'), standard risk phrases (for example R28 'Very toxic if swallowed'), and safety phrases which give advice on necessary precautions (for example S26 'In case of contact with eyes, rinse immediately with plenty of water and seek medical advice'). The symbols take a prescribed form, and the wording of risk and safety phrases is standardized in all languages of the EC. Classification, and hence labeling, is based not only on toxicological properties but also on physico-chemical properties, on the basis of specific effects on human health and on environmental effects. There are, however, no guidelines on how to label for many specific toxic effects, including neurotoxicity, although the US EPA are developing criteria for the labeling of neurotoxicants (Environmental Protection Agency, 1995).

ROLE OF THE POISONS CONTROL CENTER

Poisons control centers are a valuable source of information on the treatment of poisonings by drugs and other chemicals. They are available by phone and provide expert information and consultation to the public and health professionals (often directly to accident and emergency departments). Often information may be on recommended treatment for individuals exposed but also includes recommended actions in cases of potentially more extensive exposures (for example in the case of chemical spillages). They also provide information on poison prevention, counseling and management, and collect uniform data on poisonings and participate in nation-wide sharing of data regarding poisonings. Thus, poisons control centers have a vital role in ensuring consistent and appropriate treatment and good communications with emergency services and medical staff can ensure efficient and effective management of poisoning incidences.

REFERENCES

Adams, J. 1986: Methods in behavioral teratology. In *Handbook of Behavioral Teratology*, Riley, E.P. and Vorhees, C.V. (eds), pp 67–97. New York: Plenum Press.

Albee, R.R., Mattsson, J.L., Yano, B.L. and Chang, L.W. 1987: Neurobehavioural effects of dietary restriction in rats. *Neurotoxicology and Teratology*, **9**, 203–11.

Alder, S. and Zbinden, G. 1977 Methods in the evaluation of physical, neuromuscular and behavioral development of rats in early postnatal life. In *Methods in Prenatal Toxicology*, Neubert, D., Merker, H.J. and Kwasigroch, T.E. (eds), pp 175–85. Stuttgart: Georg Thieme Publisher.

Alder, S. and Zbinden, G. 1983: Neurobehavioural tests in single and repeated-dose toxicity studies in small rodents. *Archives of Toxicology*, **54**, 1–23.

Altman, J. and Sudarshan, K. 1975: Postnatal development of locomotion in the laboratory rat. *Animal Behaviour*, **23**, 896–920.

Arezzo, J.C., Simson, R. and Brennan N.E. 1985: Evoked potentials in the assessment of neurotoxicity in humans. *Neurobehavioral Toxicology and Teratology*, **7**, 299–304.

Atchison, W.D. 1988: Effects of neurotoxicants on synaptic transmission. Lessons learned from electrophysiological studies. *Neurotoxicology and Teratology*, **10**, 393–416.

Atterwill, C.K. 1989: Brain reaggregate cultures in neurotoxicological investigations: studies with cholinergic neurotoxins. *Alternatives to Laboratory Animals*, **16**, 221–30.

Atterwill, C.K., Bruinink, A., Drejer, J. *et al.* 1994: *In vitro* neurotoxicity testing. The report and recommendations of ECVAM Workshop 3. *Alternatives to Laboratory Animals*, **22**, 350–62.

Averill, D.R. and Needleman, H.L. 1980: Neonatal lead exposure retards cortical synaptogenesis in the rat. In *Low-level Lead Exposure: The Clinical Implications of Current Research*, Needleman, H.L. (ed.), pp 201–10. New York: Raven Press.

Bakir, F., Damluji, S-F., Amin-Zaki, L. 1973: Methyl mercury poisoning in Iraq: an inter-university report. *Science*, **181**, 230–41.

Berry, P.H., MacDonald, J.S., Alberts, A.W. *et al.* 1988: Brain and optic system pathology in hypocholesterolemic dogs treated with a competitive inhibitor of 3-hydroxy-3-methyl-glutaryl coenzyme A-reductase. *American Journal of Pathology*, **132**, 427–43.

Berry, P.H. and Vogel, P. 1982: Toxicity studies of the toxins isolated from annual rye grass (*Lolium rigidum*) infected by *Corynebacter rathayi*. *Australian Journal of Experimental Biology and Medical Science*, **60**, 129–32.

Bischoff, A. 1967: The ultrastructure of tri-*ortho*-cresyl phosphate poisoning; I. Studies on myelin and axonal alterations in the sciatic nerve. *Acta Neuropathologica*, **9**, 158.

Bischoff, A. 1970: The ultrastructure of tri-*ortho*-cresyl phosphate poisoning in the chicken; II. Studies on spinal cord alterations. *Acta Neuropathologica*, **15**, 142.

Bogo, V., Hill, T.A. and Young, R.W. 1981: Comparison of accelerod and rotarod sensitivity in detecting ethanol- and acrylamide-induced performance decrement in rats: review of experimental considerations of rotating rod systems. *Neurotoxicology*, **2**, 765–87.

Bouldin, T.W., Goines, N.D., Bagnell, C.R. and Krigman, M.R. 1981: Pathogenesis of trimethyltin neuronal toxicity. Ultrastructural and cytochemical observations. *American Journal of Pathology*, **104**, 237–49.

Brock, T.O. and O'Callaghan, J.P. 1987: Quantitative changes in the synaptic vesicle proteins synapsin 1 and the astrocyte-specific protein glial fibrillary acidic protein are associated with chemical-induced injury to the rat central nervous system. *Journal of Neuroscience*, **7**, 931–42.

Broxup, B. 1991: Neuropathology as a screen for neurotoxicity assessment. *Journal of the American College of Toxicology*, **10**, 689–95.

Broxup, B., Robinson, K., Losos, G. and Beyrouty, P. 1989: Correlation between behavioral and pathological changes in the evaluation of neurotoxicity. *Toxicology and Applied Pharmacology*, **101**, 510–20.

Broxup, B.R., Yipchuck, G., McMillan, I. and Losos, G. 1990: Quantitative techniques in neuropathology. *Toxicologic Pathology*, **18**, 105–14.

Burek, J.D., Van der Kogel, A.J. and Hollander, C.F. 1976: Degenerative myelopathy in three strains of ageing rats. *Veterinary Pathology*, **13**, 321–31.

Cabe, P.A. and Eckerman, D.A. 1982: Assessment of learning and memory dysfunction in agent-exposed animals. In *Nervous System Toxicology*, Mitchell C.L. (ed.), pp 133–98. New York: Raven Press.

Cavanagh, J.B. 1964a: The significance of the 'dying back' process in experimental and human neurological disease. *International Review of Experimental Pathology*, **3**, 219.

Cavanagh, J.B. 1964b: Peripheral nerve changes in *ortho* cresyl phosphate poisoning in the cat. *Journal of Pathology and Bacteriology*, **87**, 365.

Cooper, J.R., Bloom, F.E. and Roth, R.H. 1991: *The Biochemical Basis of Neuropharmacology*, 6th edn. New York: Oxford University Press.

Cooper, S.J. 1981: Prefrontal cortex, benzodiazepines and opiates: case studies in motivation and behavior analysis. In *Theory in Psychopharmacology*, Cooper, S.J. (ed.), Vol. 1, pp 277–322. New York: Academic Press.

Crofton, K.M. 1992: Reflex modification and the assessment of sensory dysfunction. In *Neurotoxicology*, Tilson, H.A. and Mitchell, C.L. (eds). New York: Raven Press.

Damstra, T. and Bondy, S.C. 1980: The current status and future of biochemical assays for neurotoxicity. In *Experimental and Clinical Neurotoxicology*, Spencer, P.S. and Schaumburg, H.H. (eds), pp 820–33. Baltimore, MD: Williams & Wilkins.

Dyck, P.J, Karnes, J. and Lais, A. 1986: Morphometric studies in human diabetic polyneuropathy. In *Recent Advances in Neuropathology*, Cavanagh, J.B. (ed.), pp 95–113. London: Churchill Livingstone.

Dyer, R.S. 1985: The use of sensory evoked potentials in toxicology. *Fundamental and Applied Toxicology*, **5**, 24–40.

Dyer, R.S. and Howell, W.E. 1982: Acute triethyltin exposure: effects on the visual evoked potential and hippocampal after discharge. *Neurobehavioral Toxicology and Teratology*, **4**, 259–66.

Eisenbrandt, D.L., Allen, S.L., Berry, P.H. *et al.* 1994: Evaluation of the neurotoxic potential of chemicals in animals. *Food and Chemical Toxicology*, **32**, 655–69.

Eisenbrandt, D.L., Mattsson, J.L., Albee, R.R., Spencer, P.J. and Johnson, K.A. 1990: Spontaneous lesions in subchronic neurotoxicity testing of rats. *Toxicologic Pathology*, **18**, 154–64.

Elsner, J. 1991: Animal models of behavioral defects during development. *Neurotoxicology*, **12**, 789.

Elsner, J., Hodel, B., Suter, K.E. *et al.* 1988: Detection limits of different approaches in behavioral teratology and correlation of effects with neurochemical parameters. *Neurotoxicology and Teratology*, **10**, 155–67.

Environmental Protection Agency 1983, 1984: *TSCA: Health Effects Test Guidelines. Office of Pesticides and Toxic Substances*. Washington, DC: US Environmental Protection Agency.

Environmental Protection Agency 1991: *FIFRA: Pesticide Assessment Guidelines. Subdivision F. Hazard Evaluation: Humans and Domestic Animals. Addendum 10 Neurotoxicity. Series 81, 82, 83 – Health Effects Division. Office of Pesticide Programs*. Washington, DC: US Environmental Protection Agency.

Environmental Protection Agency 1995: *Proposed Guidelines for Neurotoxicity Risk Assessment*. Federal Register, 60 No. 192, pp 52032–55. Washington, DC: US Environmental Protection Agency.

Environmental Protection Agency 1998: *Health Effects Test Guidelines. OPPTS 870.6200, OPPTS 070.6300, OPPTS 870.6500, OPPTS 870.6850, OPPTS 870.6855*. Washington, DC: US Environmental Protection Agency.

European Centre for Ecotoxicology and Toxicology of Chemicals 1992: *Evaluation of the Neurotoxic Potential of Chemicals. Monograph No. 18*. Brussels: European Centre for Ecotoxicology and Toxicology of Chemicals.

European Community 1988: *Annex V, EC Directive 67/548/EEC on the Approximation of Laws, Regulations and Administrative Provisions Relating to the Classification, Packaging and Labeling of Dangerous Substances (87/302/EEC). Part B. Methods for the Determination of Toxicity*. Luxembourg: Office for Official Publications of the European Communities.

European Community 1989: *OJEC L270 The Rules Governing Medicinal Products in the European Community Vol III: Guidelines on the Quality, Safety and Efficacy of Medicinal Products for Human Use*. Luxembourg: Office for Official Publications of the European Communities.

Evans, H.L. 1982: Assessment of vision in behavioral toxicology. In *Nervous System Toxicology*, Mitchell, C.L. (ed.), pp 81–107. New York: Raven Press.

Finnie, J.W. and O'Shea, J.D. 1988: Pathological and pathogenic changes in the central nervous system of guinea pigs given tunicamycin. *Acta Neuropathologica*, **75**, 411–21.

Food and Drug Administration 1982: *Toxicological Principles for the Safety Assessment of Direct Food Additives and Color Additives used in Food*. Washington, DC: US Food and Drug Administration, Bureau of Foods.

Francis, E. 1992: Regulatory developmental neurotoxicity and human risk assessment. *Neurotoxicology*, **13**, 77–84.

Fullerton, P.M. and Barnes, J.M. 1966: Peripheral neuropathy in rats produced by acrylamide. *British Journal of Industrial Medicine*, **23**, 210–21.

Garman, A.H. 1990: Artefacts in routinely immersion-fixed nervous tissue. *Toxicologic Pathology*, **18**, 149–53.

Gerber, G.J. and O'Shaughnessy, D. 1986: Comparison of the behavioral effects of neurotoxic and systemically toxic agents: how discriminatory are behavioral tests of neurotoxicity? *Neurobehavioral Toxicology and Teratology*, **8**, 703–10.

Hagan, J.J., Jansen, J.H.M. and Broekkamp, C.L.E. 1988: Selective behavioral impairment after acute intoxication with trimethyltin (TMT) in rats. *Neurotoxicology*, **9**, 53–74.

Haug, H. 1986: History of neuromorphometry. *Journal of Neurological Methods*, **18**, 1–17.

Hirano, A. and Llena, J.F. 1980: The central nervous system as a target in toxic-metabolic states. In *Experimental and Clinical Neurotoxicology*, Spencer, P.S. and Schaumburg, H.H. (eds), pp 24–34. Baltimore, MD: Williams & Wilkins.

Howd, R. A., Rebert, C. S., Dickinson, J. and Pryor, G. T. 1983: A comparison of the rates of development of functional hexane neuropathy in weanling and young adult rats. *Neurobehavioral Toxicology and Teratology*, **5**, 63–8.

Ison, J.R. 1984: Reflex modification as an objective test for sensory processing following toxicant exposure. *Neurobehavioral Toxicology and Teratology*, **6**, 437–45.

Johnson, B.L. 1980: Electrophysiological methods in neurotoxicity testing. In *Experimental and Clinical Neurotoxicology*, Spencer, P.S. and Schaumburg, H.H. (eds), pp 726–42. Baltimore, MD: Williams & Wilkins.

Johnson, M.K. 1975: The delayed neuropathy caused by some organophosphorus esters: mechanism and challenge. *CRC Critical Reviews in Toxicology*, **3**, 289–316.

Katoh, K., Konno, N., Yamauchi, T. and Fukushima, M. 1990: Effects of age on susceptibility of chickens to delayed neurotoxicity due to triphenyl phosphite. *Pharmacology and Toxicology*, **66**, 387–92.

Kerkut, G.A. and Heal, H.V. 1981: *Electrophysiology in Isolated Mammalian CNS Preparations*. London: Academic Press.

Krinke, G. 1983: Spinal radiculoneuropathy in aging rats: demyelination secondary to neuronal dwindling. *Acta neuropathologica*, **59**, 63–9.

Krinke, G. 1989: Neuropathological screening in rodent and other species. *Journal of the American College of Toxicology*, **8**, 141–6.

Krinke, G. and Hess, R. 1981: The value of the fluorescence histochemistry of biogenic amines in neurotoxicology. *Histochemical Journal*, **13**, 849–65.

Krinke, G., Naylor, D.C. and Skorpil, V. 1985: Pyridoxine megavitaminosis: An analysis of the early changes induced with massive doses of vitamin B_6 in rat primary sensory neurons. *Journal of Neuropathology and Experimental Neurology*, **44**, 117–29.

Leswing, R.J. and Ribelin, W.E. 1969: Physiologic and pathologic changes in acrylamide neuropathy. *Archives of International Environmental Health*, **18**, 22.

Levine, T.E. and Butcher, R.E. 1990: Workshop on the qualitative and quantitative comparability of human and animal developmental neurotoxicity. Work group IV report: triggers for developmental neurotoxicity testing. *Neurotoxicology and Teratology*, **12**, 281–4.

Mattsson, J.L. and Albee, R.R. 1988: Sensory evoked potentials in neurotoxicology. *Neurotoxicology and Teratology*, **10**, 435–43.

Mattsson, J.L., Albee, R.R. and Eisenbrandt, D.L. 1989: Neurological approach to neurotoxicological evaluation in laboratory animals. *Journal of the American College of Toxicology*, **8**, 271–86.

Mattsson, J.L., Eisenbrandt, D.L. and Albee, R.R. 1990: Screening for neurotoxicity: complementarity of functional and morphological techniques. *Toxicologic Pathology*, **18**, 115–27.

Meyer, L.S., Kotch, L.E. and Riley, E.P. 1990: Neonatal ethanol exposure: functional alterations associated with cerebellar growth retardation. *Neurotoxicology and Teratology*, **12**, 15–22.

Ministry of Agriculture, Forestry and Fisheries 1985: *Guidance on Toxicology Study Data for Application of Agricultural Chemical Registration*, 59 NohSan Number 4200. Japan: Ministry of Agriculture, Forestry and Fisheries.

Ministry of Health and Welfare 1990: *Guidelines for Toxicity Studies of Drugs Manual*. Tokyo: Yakuji Nippo Ltd.

Mitchell, C.L. (ed.) 1982: *Nervous System Toxicology*. New York: Raven Press.

Mitchell, C.L. and Tilson, H.A. 1982: Behavioral toxicology in risk assessment: problems and research needs. *CRC Critical Reviews in Toxicology*, **10**, 265–74.

Moser, V.C. and MacPhail, R.C. 1990: Comparative sensitivity of neurobehavioural tests for chemical screening. *Neurotoxicology*, **11**, 335–44.

Nishimura, H. and Shiota, K. 1977: Summary of comparative embryology and teratology. In *Handbook of Teratology: Comparative, Maternal and Epidemiologic Aspects*, Wilson, J.G. and Fraser, F.C. (eds), Vol. 3, pp 119–54. New York: Plenum Press.

O'Brien, R.D. 1960: *Toxic Phosphorus Esters*. New York: Academic Press.

O'Brien, R.D. 1967: *Insecticides, Action and Metabolism*. New York: Academic Press.

O'Callaghan, J.P. 1988: Neurotypic and gliotypic proteins as biochemical markers of neurotoxicity. *Neurotoxicology and Teratology*, **10**, 445–52.

O'Callaghan, J.P. and Miller, D.B. 1988: Acute exposure of the neonatal rat to triethyltin results in persistent changes in neurotypic and gliotypic proteins. *Journal of Pharmacology and Experimental Therapeutics*, **244**, 368–78.

O'Donoghue, J.L. 1989: Screening for neurotoxicity using a neurologically based examination and neuropathology. *Journal of the American College of Toxicology*, **8**, 97–115.

Office of Technology Assessment 1990: *Neurotoxicity: Identifying and Controlling Poisons of the Nervous System*, OTA-BA-436, 1–361. Washington, DC: US Government Printing Office.

Organization for Economic Cooperation and Development 1981: *OECD Guidelines for Testing of Chemicals; Section 4 – Health Effects*. Paris: Organization for Economic Cooperation and Development.

Prineas, J. 1969: The pathogenesis of dying-back polyneuropathies. Part I. An ultrastructural study of experimental triorthocresyl phosphate intoxication in the cat. *Journal of Neuropathology and Experimental Neurology*, **28**, 571.

Pryor, G.T., Bingham, R., Dickinson, J., Rebert, C.S. and Howd, R.A. 1982: Importance of schedule of exposure to hexane in causing neurotoxicity. *Neurobehavioral Toxicology and Teratology*, **4**, 71–8.

Pryor, G.T. and Rebert, C.S. 1983: Health effects of chemicals. IV. Behavioral and electrophysiologic evaluation of toxic effects on the nervous system. *Life Sciences Research Reports*, **13**, 1–6.

Rebert, C.S. 1983: Multisensory evoked potentials in experimental and applied neurotoxicology. *Neurobehavioral Toxicology and Teratology*, **5**, 659–71.

Rees, D.C., Francis, E.Z. and Kimmel, C.A. 1990: Scientific and regulatory issues relevant to assessing risk for developmental neurotoxicity: an overview. *Neurotoxicology and Teratology*, **12**, 175–81.

Rice, D.C. 1990: Principles and procedures in behavioural toxicity testing. In *Handbook of In Vivo Toxicity Testing*, Arnold, D.L., Grice, H.C. and Krewski, D.R. (eds), pp 383–408. New York: Academic Press.

Robbins, T.W. 1977: A critique of the methods available for the measurement of spontaneous motor activity. In *Handbook of Psychopharmacology*, Iversen, L.L., Iversen, S.D. and Snyder, S.H. (eds), Vol. 7, pp 37–82. New York: Plenum Press.

Roberts, N.L., Fairley, C. and Phillips, C. 1983: Screening acute delayed and subchronic neurotoxicity studies in the hen: measurements and evaluations of clinical signs following administration of TOCP. *Neurotoxicology*, **4**, 263–70.

Rodier, P.M. 1979: Neuropathology as a screening method for detecting injuries to the developing CNS. In *Proceedings of the Fifth FDA Science Symposium. The Effects of Foods and Drugs on the Development and Function of the Nervous System: Methods for Predicting Toxicity*, Gryder, R.M. and Frankos, V.H. (eds), pp 91–8. Washington, DC: Office of Health Affairs, Food and Drug Administration.

Rodier, P.M. 1990: Developmental neurotoxicology. *Toxicologic Pathology*, **18**, 89–95.

Rowan, M.J. 1985: Central nervous system toxicity evaluation *in vitro*: neurophysiological approach. In *Neurotoxicology*, Blum, K. and Manzo, L. (eds). New York: Marcel Dekker.

Saghal, A. (ed.) 1993: *Behavioural Neuroscience. A Practical Approach*, Vol. I. New York: Oxford University Press.

Schulze, G.E. and Boysen, B.G. 1991: A neurotoxicity screening battery for use in safety evaluation: effects of acrylamide and 3,3′-iminodiproprionitrile. *Fundamental and Applied Toxicology*, **16**, 602–15.

Schultz, R.L. and Karlsson, U. 1965: Fixation of the central nervous system for electron microscopy by Aldehyde Perfusion. II. Effect of osmolarity, pH of perfusate, and fixative concentration. *Journal of Ultrastructure Research*, **12**, 187–206.

Seppalainen, A.M. 1975: Applications of neurophysiological methods in occupational medicine: a review. *Scandinavian Journal Work, Environment and Health*, **1**, 1–14.

Soffie, M. and Bronchart, M. 1988: Age-related scopolamine effects on social and individual behavior in rats. *Psychopharmacology*, **95**, 344–50.

Somkuti, S.G., Tilson, H.A., Brown, H.R., Campbell, G.A., Lapadula, D.M. and Abou-Donia, M.B. 1988: Lack of delayed neurotoxic effect after tri-*o*-cresyl phosphate treatment in male Fischer 344 rats: biochemical neurobehavioral and neuropathological studies. *Fundamental and Applied Toxicology*, **10**, 199–205.

Spear, L.P. and Brake, S.C. 1983: Periadolescence: age-dependent behavior and pharmacological responsivity in rats. *Developmental Psychobiology*, **16**, 83–109.

Spencer, P.S., Bischoff, M.C. and Schaumburg, H.H. 1980: Neuropathological methods for the detection of neurotoxic disease. In *Experimental and Clinical Neurotoxicology*, Spencer, P.S. and Schaumburg, H.H. (eds), pp 743–66. Baltimore, MD: Williams & Wilkins.

Spencer, P.S. and Schaumburg, H.B. 1976: Central and peripheral distal axonopathy – the pathology of dying-back neuropathies. In *Progress in Neuropathology*, Zimmerman, H. (ed.), Vol. III, p 253. New York: Grune & Stratton.

Spencer, P.S. and Schaumburg, H.B. 1978: Pathobiology of neurotoxic axonal degeneration. In *Physiology and Pathobiology of Axons*, Waxman, S.G. (ed.), pp 265–82. New York: Raven Press.

Spencer, P.S. and Schaumburg, H.H. 1980: Classification of neurotoxic disease: a morphological approach. In *Experimental and Clinical Neurotoxicology*, Spencer, P.S. and Schaumburg, H.H. (eds), pp 92–9. Baltimore, MD: Williams & Wilkins.

Spencer, P.S. and Thomas, P.K. 1970: The examination of isolated nerve fibers by light and electron microscopy, with observations on demyelination proximal to neuromas. *Acta Neuropathologica*, **16**, 177–86.

Steinberg, M. 1987: The use of traditional toxicologic data in assessing neurobehavioral dysfunction. *Neurotoxicology and Teratology*, **9**, 403–9.

Thomas, P.K. 1980: The peripheral nervous system as a target for toxic substances. In *Experimental and Clinical Neurotoxicology*, Spencer, P.S. and Schaumburg, H.H. (eds), pp 35–47. Baltimore, MD: Williams & Wilkins.

Tilson, H.A., Cabe, P.A. and Spencer, P.S. 1979: Acrylamide neurotoxicity in rats: a correlated neurobehavioural and pathological study. *Neurotoxicology*, **1**, 89–104.

Tilson, H.A. and Moser, V.C. 1992: Comparison of screening approaches. *Neurotoxicology*, **13**, 1–14.

US National Research Council 1992: *Neurotoxicology and Models for Assessing Risk for New and Existing Chemicals. National Research Council Committee Report*. Washington, DC: National Academy Press.

Walsh, T.J. and Chrobak, J.J. 1987: The use of the radial arm maze in neurotoxicology. *Physiology and Behavior*, **40**, 799–803.

Walsh, T.J. and Tilson, H.A. 1984: Neurobehavioural toxicology of the organoleads. *Neurotoxicology*, **5**, 67.

West, J.R. and Hodges-Savola, C.A. 1983: Permanent hippocampal mossy fiber hyperdevelopment following prenatal ethanol exposure. *Neurobehavioral Toxicology and Teratology*, **5**, 139–50.

Winneke, G. 1992: Cross species extrapolation in neurotoxicology: neurophysiological and neurobehavioral aspects. *Neurotoxicology*, **13**, 15–26.

World Health Organization 1986: *Environmental Health Criteria 60. Principles and Methods for the Assessment of Neurotoxicity Associated with Exposure to Chemicals*. Geneva: World Health Organization.

Index